Autonomic Ganglia

Autonomic Ganglia

Edited by

Lars-Gösta Elfvin

Department of Anatomy, Karolinska Institutet,
S-104 01 Stockholm, Sweden

A Wiley-Interscience Publication

JOHN WILEY & SONS
Chichester · New York · Brisbane · Toronto · Singapore

Library of Congress Cataloging in Publication Data:

Main entry under title:

Autonomic ganglia.

"A Wiley-Interscience publication."
Includes index.
1. Ganglia, Autonomic.   I. Elfvin, Lars-Gösta.
QP368.A93 1983   596'.0188   82–17438
ISBN 0–471–10503–1 (U.S.)

British Library Cataloguing in Publication Data
Elfvin, Lars-Gösta
  Autonomic Ganglia.
  1. Nervous system, Autonomic
  I. Title
  612'.89   QP368
ISBN 0–471–10503–1

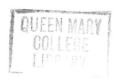
Text set in 10/12 pt Linotron 202 Times, printed and bound
in Great Britain at The Pitman Press, Bath

List of Contributors

P. Alm Department of Pathology, University of Lund, S-223 62 Lund, Sweden

L. Aloe Institute of Cell Biology, CNR, Via Romagnosi 18/A, 00196 Rome, Italy

S. Barton Department of Anatomy, School of Medicine, University of New Mexico, Albuquerque, New Mexico 87131, USA

M. Costa Centre for Neuroscience, School of Medicine, Flinders University, Bedford Park, S.A. 5042, Australia

W. G. Dail Department of Anatomy, School of Medicine, University of New Mexico, Albuquerque, New Mexico 87131, USA

C. J. Dalsgaard Department of Anatomy, Karolinska Institutet, Box 60 400, S-104 01 Stockholm, Sweden

M. Derer Laboratoire de Neurocytologie, Université Pierre et Marie Curie, 75230 Paris, France

A. Domich Laboratoire de Neurocytologie, Université Pierre et Marie Curie, 75230 Paris, France

N. J. Dun Department of Pharmacology, Loyola University, Stritch School of Medicine, Maywood, Illinois 60153, USA

B. Ehinger Department of Ophthalmology, University Hospital of Lund, University of Lund, S-221 85 Lund, Sweden

L.-G. Elfvin Department of Anatomy, Karolinksa Institutet, Box 60 400, S-104 01 Stockholm, Sweden

J. B. Furness Centre for Neuroscience, School of Medicine, Flinders University, Bedford Park, S.A. 5042, Australia

T. Hökfelt Department of Histology, Karolinska Institutet, Box 60 400, S-104 01 Stockholm, Sweden

J. Jew Department of Anatomy, University of Iowa, College of Medicine, Iowa 52242, USA

H. Kobayashi Department of Physiology, Tokyo Medical College, 1-1 Shinjuku -6- chome, Shinjuku-ku, Tokyo 160, Japan

S. C. Landis — *Department of Neurobiology, Harvard Medical School, Boston, Massachusetts 02115, USA*

N. M. Le Douarin — *Institut d'Embryologie du CNRS et du Collège de France, 49bis, Avenue de la Belle-Gabrielle, 94130 Nogent-sur-Marne, France*

R. Levi-Montalcini — *Institute of Cell Biology, CNR, Via Romagnosi 18/A, 00196 Rome, Italy*

I. J. Llewellyn-Smith — *Department of Human Morphology, School of Medicine, Flinders University, Bedford Park, S.A. 5042, Australia*

J. M. Lundberg — *Department of Pharmacology, Karolinska Institutet, Box 60 400, S-104 01 Stockholm, Sweden*

M. R. Matthews — *Department of Human Anatomy, University of Oxford, South Parks Road, Oxford OX1 3QX, UK*

L. Olson — *Department of Histology, Karolinska Institutet, Box 60 400, S-104 01 Stockholm, Sweden*

C. Owman — *Department of Histology, University of Lund, Biskopsgatan 5, S-223 62 Lund, Sweden*

M. Schultzberg — *Department of Histology, Karolinska Institutet, Box 60 400, S-104 01 Stockholm, Sweden*

Å. Seiger — *Department of Histology, Karolinska Institutet, Box 60 400, S-104 01 Stockholm, Sweden*

N.-O. Sjöberg — *Department of Obstetrics and Gynecology, University Hospital of Lund, S-221 85 Lund, Sweden*

V. I. Skok — *Bogomoletz Institute of Physiology, Bogomoltza Street, Kiev 24, USSR*

J. Smith — *Institut d'Embryologie du CNRS et du Collège de France, 49bis, Avenue de la Belle-Gabrielle, 94130 Nogent-sur-Marne, France*

F. Sundler — *Department of Histology, University of Lund, S-223 62 Lund, Sweden*

J. Taxi — *Laboratoire de Cytologie, Universitè Pierre et Marie Curie, 75230 Paris, France*

T. Tosaka — *Department of Physiology, Tokyo Medical College, 1 - 1 Shinjuku -6- chome, Shinjuku-ku. Tokyo 160, Japan*

R. Uddman — *Department of Oto-rhino-laryngology, University Hospital at Malmö, 214 01 Malmö, Sweden*

K. Unsicker — *University of Marburg, Department of Anatomy and Cell Biology, Robert-Koch-Strasse 6, D-3550 Marburg, FRG*

H. Watanabe — *Department of Anatomy, Yamagata University, School of Medicine, Yamagata, 990–23, Japan*

F. F. Weight   *Laboratory of Preclinical Studies, National Institute on Alcohol Abuse and Alcoholism, 12501 Washington Avenue, Rockville, Maryland 20852, USA*

T. Williams   *Department of Anatomy, University of Iowa, College of Medicine, Iowa 52242, USA*

A. J. Wilson   *Centre for Neuroscience, School of Medicine, Flinders University, Bedford Park, S.A. 5042, Australia*

J. D. Wood   *Department of Physiology, School of Medicine, University of Nevada, Reno, Nevada 89557, USA*

Contents

ix

Preface

The autonomic nervous system was divided by Langley, around the turn of the century, into three parts: the sympathetic, the parasympathetic and the enteric. The autonomic ganglia were thought of as being mainly relay stations passing on impulses from the central nervous system to the periphery with little or no modification. The concept of autonomic ganglia as basically relay stations has changed considerably since Langley's pioneering studies. It has become clear that the ganglia with their ability to deliver excitation and inhibition to and within the viscera possess remarkably high levels of integrative activity and in many regions function quite independently as 'little brains'.

This volume, with its nineteen contributions, reviews the rapidly growing area of neurobiological research dealing with the structure, function and development of autonomic ganglia. The contributors are all scientists actively involved in the study of these areas and they have endeavoured to review the subject assigned to them as well as report the results of their own work.

It is of course impossible to present a genuinely comprehensive account of autonomic ganglia within one volume and emphasis has thus been placed upon those areas where the recent advances in knowledge have been the most spectacular. One such area is that dealing with neuroactive peptides. The discovery that more than two dozen small peptides with powerful biological activities exist not only in the neurons of the central nervous system but some of them also in neurons of peripheral ganglia, has initiated a wealth of work dealing with the localization and action of neuropeptides in autonomic ganglia. These recent studies are reviewed in this book. The perhaps unexpected finding that neuroactive peptides may sometimes coexist in the same autonomic neurons as classical neurotransmitters such as monoamines and acetylcholine is also discussed.

It is appropriate to begin a consideration of autonomic ganglia by giving a general survey of their morphology. The chapters of the first section thus contribute much to our knowledge of the organization and structure of autonomic ganglia, with particular emphasis on fine structure where recent advances in knowledge have been very rapid. Successive chapters deal with the structure and organization of sympathetic ganglia and the ultrastructure of synapses in these ganglia, as well as with the so-called SIF cells (small intensely fluorescent cells) present in these and other autonomic ganglia; with some cranial parasympathetic ganglia, the ciliary and pterygopalatine; and with pelvic and enteric ganglia. The last chapter of this section is concerned with autonomic ganglia of amphibia.

The second section is devoted to synapses and transmitters of autonomic ganglia mainly from a functional point of view. The first two chapters deal with transmitter histochemistry of peptidergic autonomic neurons and with the fine structure of monoamine connections in sympathetic ganglia. These contributions show that anatomy is no longer a static science, but that histology can be discussed functionally. The following chapters of this section are concerned with neurophysiological and neuropharmacological aspects of synaptic transmission in mammalian sympathetic, parasympathetic and enteric ganglia as well as with synaptic mechanisms in amphibian sympathetic ganglia. The effect of peptide hormones on transmission in sympathetic ganglia is dealt with. In some instances the contributions to this section are somewhat controversial, but such points are usually made clear to the reader by the authors. For instance, some disagreement exists as to which mechanisms are responsible for the slow inhibitory postganglionic potential of sympathetic principal ganglion cells and whether it involves an interneuron such as a SIF cell or not. It is my opinion that all views on clearly controversial subjects should be presented so that the reader can then draw his own conclusions.

The final section is concerned with the development and phenotypic plasticity of autonomic ganglion cells. This is a rapidly growing field, the achievements of which are of importance not only for the understanding of the differentiation of peripheral ganglia, but also of higher nervous centres. The results of this section have been made possible by the use of modern sophisticated means for isolation of growth factors along with the refinement of organ and cell culture techniques and advanced cell and tissue transplantation methods. The contributions show clearly that ganglionic neuronal precursor cells possess a very high degree of plasticity and that the choice of transmitter substance(s) is largely influenced by environmental factors. To a certain extent this plasticity is retained also at more mature neuronal stages. A high degree of plasticity has also been demonstrated for the related SIF cells, adrenal medullary cells and the central locus coeruleus cells. No separate chapter is devoted to the issue of SIF cell plasticity. A more comprehensive account on this subject is given in the book 'Histochemistry and Cell Biology of Autonomic Neurons, SIF cells and Paraneurons'.

It is hoped that this book will be of value not only for established investigators in neurobiology but that it also will serve as an introduction to new research workers and graduate students interested in autonomic regulation. Much of the knowledge presented in the book is of importance to neuroscience in general and therefore forms part of the basis for a more complete understanding of the function of the central nervous system.

I am very grateful to the contributors to this volume for the effort and care they have put into completing their individual chapter; to many colleagues and friends in and outside the Karolinska Institutet for their suggestions about this volume; to Dr Catarína Forsman for help with reading the manuscripts; and to the secretarial staff at the Department of Anatomy for much laborious typing. I am also very much indebted to Dr S. D. Thornton and his staff at John Wiley and Sons for encouragement and counsel during the planning and preparation of this volume; and to Dr A. D. Smith at the University of Oxford, who first suggested this book to me.

LARS-G. ELFVIN

REFERENCES

Eränkö, O., Soinila, S. and Päivärinta, H. (Eds.) (1980). Histochemistry and Cell Biology of Autonomic Neurons, SIF Cells, and Paraneurons. *Advances in Biochemical Psychopharmacology*, **25,** Raven Press.

Langley, J. N. (1921) *The Autonomic Nervous System*, Cambridge, W. Heffer & Sons Ltd.

General Morphological Principles

Autonomic Ganglia
Edited by Lars-Gösta Elfvin
© 1983 John Wiley & Sons Ltd

Structure and Organization of Mammalian Sympathetic Ganglia

WILLIAM G. DAIL and SANDRA BARTON

Department of Anatomy, School of Medicine,
University of New Mexico,
Albuquerque, New Mexico 87131, USA

GENERAL CONSIDERATIONS, LOCATION OF SYMPATHETIC GANGLIA

Following development and migration of neural crest primordia, sympathetic ganglion cells come to lie in three locations throughout the body: paravertebral, prevertebral, and previsceral (Fig. 1). Sympathetic ganglia are largely found in the paravertebral position where, with their vertical interconnections, they form the bilaterally located sympathetic chain. Other ganglionated masses at the origin of the vessels of the abdominal aorta form the prevertebral or collateral sympathetic ganglia. In the third location, smaller populations of sympathetic neurons are regularly found in or near the pelvic visceral organs. Here, they are known as previsceral sympathetic ganglia, or, collectively, the short adrenergic system (Sjöstrand, 1965; Owman and Sjöberg, 1967; Owman *et al.*, 1971),

In the sympathetic chain of mammals there is usually one ganglion per segment in the thoracic, lumbar and sacral regions. The ordered segmental arrangement of the sympathetic chain is obscured in the neck where migration and fusion of primordia result in compound ganglia at each end of the cervical sympathetic chain, the superior and inferior cervical sympathetic ganglia. In the pelvis, the paired chains come together to form a single large ganglion, the ganglion impar on the front of the sacrum. Communications may occur between the two chains at lower cervical levels (Randall *et al.*, 1971) and in the lumbosacral region where fibres cross the midline.

Sympathetic ganglia are frequently found in other sites and are known as intermediate or satellite sympathetic ganglia (Fig. 1). These occur along the preganglionic connections to the chain ganglia and along the postganglionic fibre tracts from the ganglia and in the perivascular plexuses. Intermediate sympathetic ganglia occur most regularly in the cervical portion of the sympathetic chain (Foley, 1945; Boyd, 1957; Dail *et al.*, 1980), where their

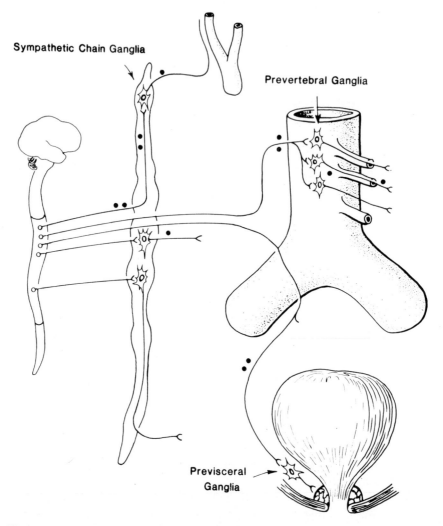

Sympathetic Chain Ganglia

Prevertebral Ganglia

Previsceral Ganglia

Figure 1 Schematic representation of the location of sympathetic ganglion cells. The small filled black circles indicate intermediate sympathetic ganglia

presence should be taken into account in determining the ratio of pregang-lionic fibres to postganglionic neurons (Brooks-Fournier and Coggeshall, 1981), and in electrophysiological studies involving stimulation of pregang-lionic input to the superior cervical ganglion. The presence of intermediate sympathetic ganglia in the perivascular plexuses distal to the major collection of neurons may well explain the variable results obtained in attempts to denervate tissues by removal of only the chain ganglia.

HISTOLOGY OF SYMPATHETIC GANGLIA: THE SUPERIOR CERVICAL SYMPATHETIC GANGLION

Our present concept of the structure and function of sympathetic ganglia is derived in large measure from studies on the superior cervical sympathetic ganglion (Fig. 2). Its large size and accessibility make it a favourite model

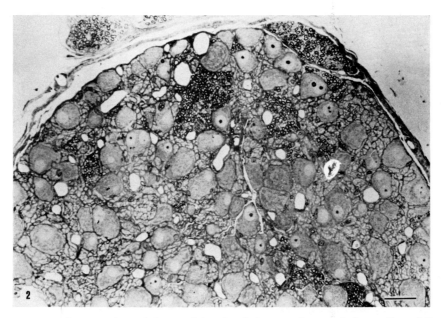

Figure 2 Cross-section of the caudal pole of the superior cervical ganglion of the rabbit, 1-μm plastic section. The ganglion is enclosed by a capsule, here artifactually separated from the ganglion. In the caudal pole myelinated fibres tend to occur in large groups concentrated on one side of the ganglion. Bar: 10 μm

and, in general, the histology of its various cell types illustrates the pattern common to chain ganglia. It is well to remember, however, that important differences exist between the sympathetic ganglia in a single species. Moreover, the compound nature of the superior cervical ganglion and the multiplicity of its target organs may impart a particular anatomy which is not found in more caudally located ganglia of the sympathetic chain. Such important differences should not be overlooked in experimental design and interpretation.

Ganglionic capsule

Sympathetic ganglion cells are isolated from their environment by a thick capsule of connective tissue which is continuous with similar layers over

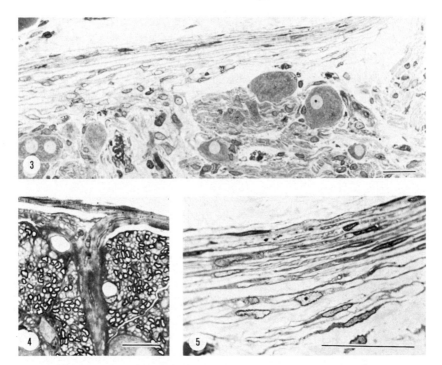

Figure 3 Transition of the ganglionic capsule into the more compact connective tissue wrapping of an efferent nerve in the rabbit superior cervical ganglion. Bar: 10 μm

Figure 4 Connective tissue septum from the capsule of rabbit superior cervical ganglion. Bar: 10 μm

Figure 5 An enlargement of part of Fig. 3 illustrating the perineurial cells of the capsule. Bar: 10 μm

afferent and efferent nerves (Fig. 3). A thin epineurium, a thick perineurium and a delicate endoneurium make up the layers of the capsule. From the capsule, connective tissue septa segregate groups of ganglion cells (Fig. 4). Septation by connective tissue imparts a lobulated appearance to the sympathetic ganglia of man (Pick, 1970). The significance of this segregation is unknown, but it is an early step in the developmental process of sympathetic ganglia (Canfield, 1978). The intermediate layer of the capsule is formed by overlapping sheets of perineurial cells which are joined by zonulae occludens and desmosomes (Arvidson, 1979a). There are two to five layers of perineurial cells surrounding the superior cervical ganglion of the rat, while as many as eight to ten layers invest the rabbit superior cervical ganglion (Fig. 5). The perineurium and connective tissue septa comprise a surprising 30% of the wet weight of the superior cervical ganglion of the rat (Matthieu, 1970). Since the concentration of various substances in the superior cervical ganglion is expressed as milligram per wet weight or per milligram of protein, the connective tissue framework of a ganglion would be a factor in determining the absolute values of the concentration of various substances.

Similar to the peripheral nerve, the perineurium of autonomic ganglia serves as a diffusion barrier (Hökfelt, 1968). Arvidson (1979a) applied horseradish peroxidase (HRP) to the surface of the superior cervical ganglion of rats and mice in a study of the diffusion barrier. After 60 minutes, the macromolecule was still excluded from the endoneurial spaces by the overlapping layers of the ganglionic perineurium. In electrophysiological studies, the capsule is often split to permit penetration of microelectrodes (Wallis and North, 1978), or in some investigations, younger animals are chosen for their thinner capsule (McLachlan, 1974).

Blood vessels

Like all nervous tissue, sympathetic ganglia are highly active metabolically and receive a rich blood supply (Fig. 2). Blood vessels arise from several sources in the neck to enter the superior cervical sympathetic ganglion over both the preganglionic and postganglionic nerve pathways. From the capsule, blood vessels accompany the septa into the ganglion and break up into a capillary plexus. The afferent vessels are small, muscular arteries (Fig. 6)

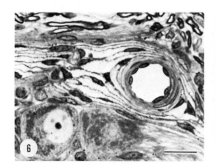
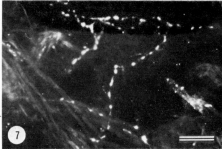

Figure 6   Small muscular vessel in the interior of the rabbit superior cervical ganglion.
Bar: 10 μm
Figure 7   Adrenergic innervation of a vessel in the interior of the superior cervical ganglion. Bar: 10 μm

which are themselves sympathetically innervated (Fig. 7). Heym and Williams (1979) have recently described vascular loops or glomeruli in the superior cervical ganglia of *Tupaia* in which chromaffin cells are clustered. From serial reconstructions it was found that the capillary beds around the principal neurons of the ganglion were downstream from the glomeruli. This arrangement suggested a means by which chromaffin cells may elaborate intraganglionic catecholamines via a portal system (Heym and Williams, 1979; see also chapter by Williams and Jew). It would be of interest to know if the glomerular arrangement is present in other species in which large clusters of chromaffin cells are known to occur. Fenestrated capillaries in sympathetic ganglia have been most often reported in association with small granule-containing cells (Siegrist *et al.*, 1968; Matthews and Raisman, 1969). Arvidson (1979b) reported that some venules as well as capillaries in the superior cervical ganglion of the mouse have fenestrations. While it has been suggested tht fenestrated capillaries might serve to distribute the secretory product of chromaffin cells within an autonomic ganglion (Benitez, *et al.*, 1974; Heym and Williams, 1979), it is also possible that this arrangement may suggest a sensory function similar to the cells of the carotid body (Kondo, 1977). Fenestrated capillaries which apparently have no relationship to small granule-containing cells also occur and, conversely, these small cells are frequently found abutted against capillaries which have a continuous lining (Jacobs, 1977). In the latter case, it has been suggested that micropinocytosis by the vascular endothelium may be the means of uptake of liberated catecholamines (Heym and Williams, 1979).

The permeability of ganglionic vessels has been investigated by Jacobs (1977) and Arvidson (1979b) using protein tracers of varying molecular size. The permeability of ganglionic vessels to HRP and ferritin led these investigators to suggest that ganglionic vessels do not offer the same protection to principal neurons as the blood–brain barrier does for neurons in the central nervous system. In a recent study, DePace (1981) found that HRP in small concentrations had not crossed the capillary endothelium of an autonomic ganglion at 15 minutes following a vascular injection. These varying results may in part be explained by the fact that larger concentrations of HRP may provoke an increase in vascular permeability (Cotran and Karnovsky, 1967). Arvidson (1979b) states, however, that HRP does not cause release of vasoactive amines and increased vascular permeability in the mouse—his animal model.

The sympathetic neuron

Early silver impregnation studies showed that sympathetic ganglion cells are multipolar neurons with a complex array of processes (Fig. 8) (Cajal, 1911; De Castro, 1932). The cell body and its processes are almost entirely enclosed by satellite cells (Fig. 9). The Schwann cell investment is deficient at sites of incoming synapses and is absent sporadically along dendrites where collections of dense core vesicles approach the plasma membrane (Fig. 11). The perfusion of multibranched processes arising from the cell soma are thought to be dendrites, since silver staining reveals a single unbranched axon. A thin axon arises from the soma or possibly from the base of a dendrite

(De Castro, 1932). In a modern study using intracellular dye injection, McLachlan (1974) determined that each neuron in the superior cervical ganglion of the guinea pig had an average of 13 dendrites. Axons were identified as single unbranched processes, an observation in agreement with classical silver studies (Cajal, 1911; De Castro, 1932).

The question of branching axons (recurrent axon collaterals) within sympathetic ganglia surfaced again with the observation by catecholamine histofluorescence of a plexus of varicose fibres in many sympathetic ganglia (Fig. 10) (Hamberger *et al.*, 1963; Norberg and Sjöqvist, 1966). Pharmacological and morphological studies of the beaded network of fibres—the autonomic ground plexus of Hillarp (1960)—in sympathetically innervated tissues had shown that this morphology represents the terminal ramifications of axons. This led some investigators to suggest that the beaded plexus in sympathetic ganglia comprised axon collaterals of ganglion cells (Norberg *et al.*, 1966; Jacobowitz and Woodward, 1968). At present, however, there is no conclusive evidence that ganglion cells have axon collaterals which ramify within sympathetic ganglia, nor is there support for the contention that some of the ganglion cells along the sympathetic trunk may contribute axon terminals to other chain ganglia (Dail *et al.*, 1980). There is a growing and persuasive body of evidence that small intensely fluorescent (SIF) cells (Jacobowitz and Green, 1974; Libet and Owman, 1974; Eränkö, 1978) and dendritic collaterals of ganglion cells (Jacobowitz, 1970; Van Orden *et al.*, 1970; Elfvin, 1971; McLachlan, 1974; Kondo *et al.*, 1980) are the major sources of the intraganglionic plexus of adrenergic terminals.

Attempts have been made to identify types of sympathetic ganglion cells based on the pattern of dendritic branching and size of the cell body. As proposed by Cajal (1911), sympathetic ganglion cells in man fall into three categories: (1) cells with long dendrites, (2) ganglion cells with short dendrities which course in the cell capsule, and (3) a class of neurons which have both long dendrites and short intracapsular dendrites. This schema is not in general use and, unfortunately, there is no modern study which has re-examined this question in detail. As cautioned by Gabella (1976), there is some evidence that age may influence the dendritic pattern (Amprino, 1938). No doubt there is some validity in Cajal's classification since modern studies using electron microscopy (Van Orden *et al.*, 1970; Elfvin, 1971), and fluorescent-dye labelling (McLachlan, 1974) have shown that a portion of sympathetic ganglion cells in small mammals have intracapsular dendrites. There is some suggestion that neurons with intracapsular dendrites can be recognized by catecholamine histofluorescence techniques [see Fig. 6 of Dail *et al.* (1975), Fig. 4 of Dail and Evan (1978a), Fig. 21 of this paper]. McLachlan (1974) was unable to separate the cells in the superior cervical ganglion of the guinea-pig on the basis of their dendritic lengths or patterns of arborization, and could not confirm early observations of dendritic glomeruli

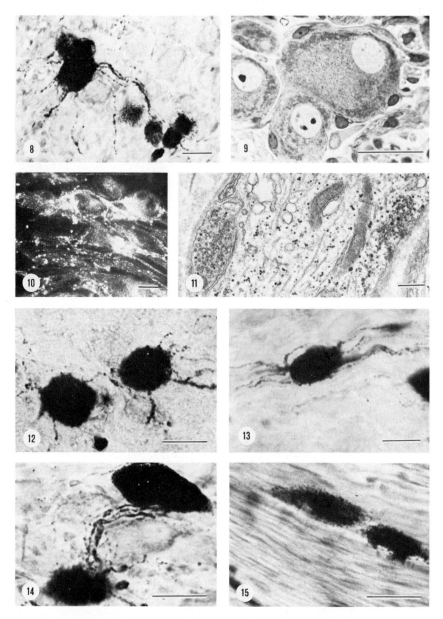

Figure 8 Multipolar neurons in the superior cervical ganglion labelled by injection of HRP into the submandibular salivary gland; 32 μm frozen section stained using the *o*-dianisidine method. Bar: 10 μm

Figure 9 One-micrometre plastic section of autonomic ganglion cells in the superior cervical ganglion of the rabbit. Note the nuclei of the satellite cells, the origin of several processes from the large neuron and the peripheral location of Nissl substance. Bar: 10 μm

or receptor plates (Cajal, 1911; De Castro, 1932). A lack of modern studies on the significance of length of dendrites and their branching patterns may in part be due to the resistance of adult mammalian sympathetic ganglia to impregnation with Golgi-like techniques. Labelling with the tracer HRP reveals a variety of dendritic patterns of sympathetic neurons (Figs. 8, 12–14). This technique may offer the opportunity to sort out the geometry of sympathetic ganglion cells since it probably shows the full extent of ganglion cell processes. In a recent electrophysiological study which used HRP, Purves and Hume (1981) elegantly demonstrated that the number of different preganglionic axons converging on the postganglionic neuron is positively correlated with the number of dendrites. For example, ganglion cells which lack dendrites receive input from only one preganglionic fibre (Purves and Hume, 1981; also see Lichtman, 1980). Whether this important principle is a determinant of neuronal geometry in sympathetic ganglia must await further study.

The wide range of cell size in sympathetic ganglia has inspired some attempts to devise a classification scheme based on the size of the cell soma. De Castro (1932) and De Castro and Herreros (1945) distinguish three size ranges in the superior cervical ganglia of rat and man and suggested that cell size was related to modality, i.e. the larger ganglion cells provided the innervation of the iridial muscles. This suggestion is indirectly supported by the observation that the superior cervical ganglion (which provides the innervation of the iris) has the largest proportion of large neurons (De Castro, 1932). A more thorough re-examination of this question is now possible since neurons can be labelled via their target organs with neuronal traces. Filling of neurons retrogradely by injecting HRP into their target organs provides a Golgi-like impregnation of ganglion cells (Figs. 8, 12). Preliminary studies in the superior cervical ganglion of the rabbit have shown that neurons destined to a target organ may show a range of sizes (injection

Figure 10   Catecholamine histofluorescence in the rabbit superior cervical ganglion. Note the abundance of varicose fibres throughout the neuropil and in relation to the cell body of ganglion cells. Glyoxylic acid-induced fluorescence in a 16 μm frozen section. Bar: 10 μm

Figure 11   In this portion of a dendrite, note the afferent synapse (left side of the photomicrograph) and the collection of small dense-cored vesicles on the opposite side. A Schwann cell process is seen in the upper left of the illustration. Bar: 0.4 μm

Figure 12   HRP-labelled neurons which project to the submandibular salivary gland. Bar: 10 μm

Figure 13   HRP-labelled neuron in which the dendrites are parallel to the surrounding nerve fibres. Bar: 10 μm

Figure 14   Dendrites from these HRP-labelled neurons enclose the unlabelled cell between them. Bar: 10 μm

Figure 15   HRP neurons which project to the submandibular salivary gland. The cells occur near the entry of the cervical sympathetic trunk into the ganglion. Bar: 12 μm

sites were in the iris, Harder's gland, parotid gland, submandibular salivary gland). In each injection site, it is presumed that vasomotor fibres in each target organ would also be labelled; therefore, two populations of cells might be revealed from each target organ injected. From these initial studies, it would appear that large neurons are as likely to innervate other targets of the superior cervical ganglion as they are to innervate the iris (Dail, personal observation).

The shape and size of ganglion cells are also being studied by this method (Dail, unpublished observations). It has earlier been suggested that some mechanical factors such as the available space for the neurons may determine shape and size (McLachlan, 1974). In our studies we have confirmed this suggestion. For example, after submandibular gland injection, HRP-labelled neurons near the centre of the superior cervical ganglion are large and round with dendrites arising radially from the soma (Figs. 12, 14). Other labelled ganglion cells near the entry point of the cervical sympathetic trunk appear compressed with their long axis parallel to incoming nerve tracks (Fig. 15). Therefore, studies on the size distribution of ganglion cells may be complicated by the position of the neuron within a sympathetic ganglion.

Small intensely fluorescent (SIF) cells

Most autonomic ganglia have a variable number of small cells which have a high content of catecholamines. The nomenclature of these cells reflects the methodology by which they may be studied: chromaffin cells, since some are positive for the chromate reaction; small intensely fluorescent (SIF) cells of catecholamine histofluorescence techniques; and small granule-containing (SGC) cells of electron microscopy. Electron-microscopic (Williams and Palay, 1969) and physiological studies indicate that some SIF cells are autonomic interneurons (for review see Libet, 1980), interposed between pre- and postganglionic neurons. Many of these terms have been used interchangeably by investigators with the understanding that there may be a variety of morphologies and functions of these small cells. (For a detailed description of the morphology of the SIF cells and their relationships to one another and to the principal neurons, see chapters by Taxi and by Williams and Jew.)

Certain synaptic relationships suggest that a very special class of SIF cells may exist that is different from the interneuronal or classical chromaffin types (see chapter by Williams and Jew). In a serial-section study of SIF cells in the rat superior cervical ganglion, Kondo (1977) reported that the predominant efferent contacts of SIF cells were to axons rather than to dendrites of ganglion cells. A single axon formed reciprocal contacts with many SIF cells. The structural resemblance of SIF cells to carotid body glomus cells and the similarity of their efferent contacts prompted Kondo (1977) to state that SIF cells are mainly in a sensory pathway, a notion contrary to the current view of SIF cells as autonomic interneurons or intraganglionic chromaffin cells. In a valuable study of the superior cervical ganglion of the rat, Grillo (1978) showed that some SIF cells indeed were presynaptic to axons. About 5% of the efferent contacts of SIF involved postsynaptic structures which resembled the sensory nerve endings in the carotid body. By sectioning the glossopharyngeal nerve, the source of sensory fibres to the carotid body, Grillo found degenerating terminals on some SIF cells in the superior cervical ganglion. These observations strongly suggest that some SIF cells mediate a chemoreceptor function within the ganglion (Grillo, 1978). Grillo (1978) and Matthews (1980) do not agree, however, that the majority of SIF cells have a chemoreceptor role as seems to be supported by Kondo (1977).

Nerve fibres connect the rat superior cervical ganglion to the glossopharyngeal nerve (ninth cranial) or to its branch, the carotid sinus nerve. Preliminary studies of HRP injection into the rat superior cervical ganglion have failed to label neurons in the petrosal ganglion along the ninth nerve (Dail, unpublished observation). However, a few ganglion cells along the ninth cranial nerve near the branching point of the carotid sinus nerve are filled with HRP following this procedure (see Fig. 23). It is significant that Hess (1981) has recently shown that cells at this site provide innervation to the carotid body. It is a reasonable hypothesis that some neurons located in the ninth nerve provided sensory fibres to SIF cells in the rat superior cervical ganglion (Fig. 23). It is further conjectured that afferent fibres from the ninth cranial nerve may be one source of substance P positive fibres present in this ganglion. This suggestion is supported by studies which show that substance P fibres in the rat superior cervical ganglion have an extraganglionic source (Hökfelt *et al.*, 1977), and that the carotid sinus nerve fibres to the carotid body are substance P positive (Hess, 1981).

CATECHOLAMINES IN SYMPATHETIC GANGLIA

Fluorescence histochemical methods have localized catecholamines in sympathetic ganglia in the cell body of ganglion cells and SIF cells. The neuropil, presumably the processes of ganglion cells and SIF cells, is also rich in catecholamines. Ganglion cells show a wide variation of fluorescence intensity with only a small percentage of cells as intensely fluorescent as those in Figs. 16 and 20. A few ganglion cells are non-fluorescent and have been presumed to be cholinergic sympathetic neurons. Fluorescence in ganglion cells is described as granular or diffuse. The basis for the granular appearance of histofluorescence images (Figs. 16, 19) of ganglion cells is the occurrence of dense-cored vesicles in clusters in the cell cytoplasm. Richards and Tranzer (1975) have shown that the clusters are made up of dense-cored vesicles of two sizes and a component of smooth endoplasmic reticulum ('tubular

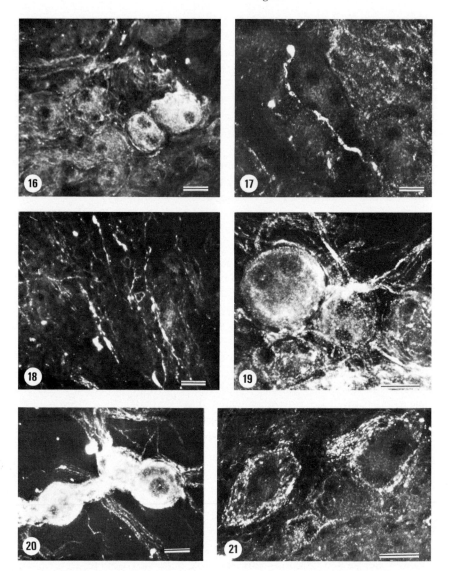

Figure 16   Glyoxylic acid-induced fluorescence in the superior cervical ganglion of the rabbit. Note the granular fluorescence in the cytoplasm of all ganglion cells and the two brightly fluorescent ganglion cells. Bar: 10 µm

Figure 17   A long fluorescent process of a SIF cell in the rabbit superior cervical ganglion. Note the irregular accumulation of catecholamine along the fibre. Bar: 10 µm

Figure 18   An area in the superior cervical ganglion containing the cell bodies of three to four SIF cells and their processes. The intensity of the fluorescence and the irregular nature of the fibres are characteristic of SIF cell processes. Bar: 10 µm

reticulum') which contains chromate-positive material. Calculations of the size of the clusters from their micrographs indicate a diameter of about 1 μm, well within the resolving power of the fluorescence microscope and approximately the size of the granular particles seen in fluorescence microscopy. The diffuse fluorescence in the cytoplasm may represent scattered granulated vesicles and the proposed soluble pool of catecholamines (Eränkö, 1972). The SIF cell is usually illustrated with very intense, even fluorescence in the cell cytoplasm. Their ultrastructure conforms to this image since granulated vesicles are not clustered in SIF cells but occur in abundance throughout the cytoplasm. The dense-cored vesicles in some SIF subtypes may be up to 3000 Å in diameter. The large size of the dense-cored vesicles may account for the granular nature of SIF cell fluorescence occasionally seen in cell processes (Fig. 17) or sections through the soma.

The neuropil of most sympathetic ganglia contains an interesting and complex array of fluorescent fibres. Descriptions of the fluorescent fibres may vary with the different applications of histofluorescence methodology. Fluorescent fibres range from delicate, granular non-varicose processes, to varicose fibres typical of an autonomic ground plexus, and to the larger irregular processes of SIF cells. The intraganglionic plexus of adrenergic fibres is a descriptive term which has been applied to this collection of fluorescent processes. The plexus of adrenergic fibres is thought to be of intraganglionic origin, contributed by SIF cells and by the principal neurons (for review, see Dail *et al.*, 1980). While it is not always possible to determine the origin of the processes by fluorescence microscopy, certain cell processes have indentifiable features. It would appear that the proximal portions of SIF cell processes can be readily identified at least in the superior cervical ganglion of the rabbit (Fig. 17). The processes are irregular and show considerable variation both in the size of the swellings along the processes and in the fluorescence intensity. It might be inaccurate to say that proximal processes of SIF cells are varicose since single granulated vesicles or small groups of them are quite large and, as such, would only reflect the irregular

Figure 19   Adrenergic ganglion cells in the rabbit superior cervical ganglion, glyoxylic acid-induced fluorescence in a 16 μm frozen section. All three ganglion cells in the photomicrograph are binucleate. Note the finely stippled fluorescent processes from the cell soma of the ganglion cell on the left. Fluorescence of a granular nature is concentrated in the peripheral part of the cell cytoplasm. Bar: 10 μm

Figure 20   Highly fluorescent ganglion cells in the superior cervical ganglion of the rabbit. Note that in the ganglion cell on the right, fluorescence is concentrated near the cell plasma membrane and around the nucleus. Bar: 10 μm

Figure 21   Glyoxylic acid-induced fluorescence surrounding two ganglion cells in the superior cervical ganglion. The section has passed through the centre of both cells. The cytoplasm of this type of cell usually has a low fluorescence. Subsequent sections show that the entire cell surface is covered by this type of delicate fluorescent structure. Bar: 10 μm

distribution of catecholamines along an otherwise smooth fibre. Areas of the ganglion in which SIF cells and their processes are plentiful can be recognized (Fig. 18). A second class of processes, the proximal portions of dendrites, also has definite histofluorescence characteristics. The initial portions of dendrites are smooth in outline and show a finely strippled fluorescence (Fig. 19). The ultrastructural counterpart of this delicate fluorescence may be the clusters of small dense cored vesicles in dendrites (Fig. 11). The background fluorescence of the neuropil is probably due in great part to fluorescence of dendrites.

A third type of fluorescence occurs less frequently around certain ganglion cells. Approximately 1–2% of the ganglion cells in the superior cervical ganglion of the rabbit appear enmeshed in a delicate web of fluorescence (Fig. 21). The individual fluorescent particles are not connected, but appear similar in size and character to fluorescence in dendrites. The arrangement is suggestive of fluorescent beads atop short processes arising from the cell body (also see Fig. 4 of Dail and Evan, 1978b). This 'halo' of fluorescence may represent the short accessory dendrites (intracapsular dendrites) shown by Van Orden *et al.* (1970) and Elfvin (1971) to contain granulated vesicles. This suggestion, however, must await further experimentation.

Finally, the system of varicose fibres in ganglia which most closely resembles an autonomic ground plexus may represent the more peripheral processes of ganglion cells or SIF cells. Varicose fibres of ganglion cells and SIF cells may indeed be indistinguishable by routine histofluorescence or ultrastructural methodology.

NEURONAL POOLS IN SYMPATHETIC GANGLIA

Any treatment of sympathetic ganglia is likely to emphasize the similarity of the organization of the different ganglia. Indeed, ganglia are encapsulated masses of neurons which reveal few clues that would suggest organizational levels. Unlike the central nervous system, subpopulations of neurons confined to a specific region are not apparent in sympathetic ganglia. The designation adrenergic neuron, which implies a common structure and function among ganglion cells, is not without justification since ganglion cell geometry is poorly understood and the great majority of ganglion cells use norepinephrine as their neurotransmitter. Several studies now clearly emphasize the rich diversity within autonomic ganglia with respect to the complexities of synaptic events and the lack of homogeneity of cell types (for reviews see Dolivo 1974; Kuba and Koketsu, 1978). In this discussion, one aspect of that heterogeneity will be reviewed, namely evidence that sympathetic ganglia may be subdivided into regions of neurons that project to specific targets.

Suggestions that there were distinct regions within sympathetic ganglia first came from catecholamine histofluorescence studies of Jacobowitz and Woodward (1968). Interruption of specific efferent nerve trunks of the superior cervical ganglion showed that only certain populations of ganglion cells responded by an accumulation of catecholamines. Ganglion cell populations nearest the sectioned nerve trunk were most affected by denervation build-up of catecholamines. Various zones of neurons could thus be identified based on their proximity to the origin of the efferent nerve bundles of the superior cervical ganglion. The existence of zones of neurons in the superior cervical ganglion, including ganglion cells which send their axons down the cervical sympathetic trunk, was considered quite important in designing electrophysiological experiments (Jacobowitz and Woodward, 1968). Similar results were obtained by Matthews and Raisman (1972) in an electron-microscopic study of chromatolysis in the superior cervical ganglion of the rat. Section of the external carotid nerve adversely affected neurons in roughly the middle and caudal third of the superior cervical ganglion. After a lesion of the internal carotid nerve nearly all of the neurons in the rostral third of the ganglion became chromatolytic.

By antidromically driving neurons of the guinea pig superior cervical ganglia, it became clear that neurons were clustered at the pole of the ganglion near the origin of the efferent nerve used to exit the ganglion (Purves, 1975). This important observation of a 'preferred' location of neurons within the superior cervical ganglion made it possible to study only one population of neurons while other nearby ganglion cells served as an intraganglionic control. Purves (1976) took advantage of this information in his study of the importance of communication between ganglion cells and their target organs in the maintenance of a normal preganglionic input. In this study, colchicine was applied to only one branch of the superior cervical ganglion. Colchicine's arrest of axoplasmic flow and the subsequent effects on preganglionic input was restricted only to those neurons whose axons travelled via the treated nerve; leaving all rostrally located neurons unaffected (Purves, 1976). In summary, these investigations were clearly suggestive of the principle that, at least in the superior cervical sympathetic ganglion, neurons tend to be clustered near the point of exit of their postganglionic branches.

In a series of elegant papers, Purves and coworkers have employed sympathetic ganglia to investigate the mechanism by which neurons establish precise connections with a specific source of innervation. Several important principles of the organization of the autonomic nervous system have emerged from these investigations and certain aspects of the experiments are relevant to the concept of subpopulations of cells within sympathetic ganglia. Each sympathetic ganglion cell in the superior cervical ganglion of the guinea-pig is innervated on the average by preganglionic fibres from four spinal cord segments. It seems a rule that one of the spinal cord segments predominates (the rule of segmental dominance) and that the segments which provide input to a single neuron are contiguous (Njå and Purves, 1977a). Stimulation of the different ventral roots produces a characteristic end-organ response, with upper spinal cord segments, (T-1 to T-3) controlling pupillary dilation and widening of the palpebral fissure, and more caudal cord segments (T-3 to T-5) controlling piloerection on the face and neck and vasoconstriction of the ear (Njå and Purves, 1977a). Neurons did not appear to be segregated in the superior cervical ganglion according to their spinal cord level of input (Njå and Purves, 1977a). That is, neurons which send their axons into either the superior carotid nerve or the inferior carotid nerve, roughly at either end of the ganglion, are just as likely to be innervated by the same spinal cord segment (Njå and Purves, 1977a). From these data it would follow, then, that ganglion cells which innervate a specific target organ, the iris for example, would be scattered throughout the superior cervical ganglion of the guinea pig. Work by Hendry *et al.* (1974) on labelling of ganglion cells by injecting a radioactive marker into the anterior eye chamber, is cited as supporting the contention that there is no clustering of neurons in the superior cervical ganglion on the basis of a common target organ (Njå and Purves, 1977a).

Njå and Purves (1977b, 1978) also investigated the reinnervation of the guinea-pig superior cervical ganglion by the cervical sympathetic trunk. Preganglionic axons largely restored their normal pattern of connections to the postganglionic cells. In addition, the rule of contiguity of innervation by spinal cord segments was again apparent. Since in one of these studies (Njå and Purves, 1978) the cervical sympathetic trunk was completely severed, it was thought unlikely that mechanical factors guided the preganglionic fibres to the appropriate postganglionic neuron. It was suggested, therefore, that the distinctiveness of the postganglionic neuron, rather than any preferred location in the superior cervical ganglion, may be the cue by which the appropriate connections are first established and re-established after denervation.

There are now several reports that show that the preferred clustering of ganglion cells near the efferent pathway used to leave the ganglion also means that there are territories within sympathetic ganglia in which neurons to a specific target organ may be found. In a systematic and quantitative study, Bowers and Zigmond (1979) applied HRP to the cut ends of postganglionic nerve trunks of the superior cervical ganglion of the rat and found that neurons were located in the rostral or caudal parts of the ganglion as a function of the postganglionic nerve trunks they utilize (the internal or external carotid nerves). It was reasoned, that, since the internal carotid nerve innervates the iris and the external carotid nerve innervates the salivary glands, experiments on defined populations of ganglion cells should be possible (that is, on neurons in the rostral or caudal part of the cervical ganglion).

Subdivision of the superior cervical ganglion into rostral and caudal regions was documented by other investigators with HRP injection of target organs.

Arvidson (1979c) injected HRP into the anterior eye chamber of rats and mice and reported that labelled neurons were distributed in the rostral part of the superior cervical ganglion, thus confirming an observation by Iversen, *et al.* (1975). In the superior cervical ganglion of the guinea pig, neurons that innervate the iris are predominantly located in the rostral part of the ganglion, while neurons to the pinna are largely found in the caudal pole (Lichtman *et al.*, 1979). Sympathetic neurons that innervate the tongue are located in the caudal region of the superior cervical ganglion of the dog (Chibuzo *et al.*, 1980).

The superior cervical ganglion of the rabbit is also composed of rostral and caudal cell groups (Dail *et al.*, 1979). The superior cervical ganglion in this animal is frequently lobulated with a rostral enlargement connected to a smaller caudal portion by a constricted segment. In some instances the rostral and caudal portions appear as independent masses, similar to that seen in the lumbar sympathetic chain ganglia at thoracic or lumbar levels (Dail, personal observation). HRP injected into the anterior chamber of the eye or into the Harderian gland in the orbit will fill cells in the rostral enlargement of the superior cervical ganglion (Fig. 22a, b), while cells in the caudal portion of the ganglion are labelled when HRP is injected into the parotid or submandibular salivary glands (Fig. 22c, d). Neurons along the cervical sympathetic trunk as

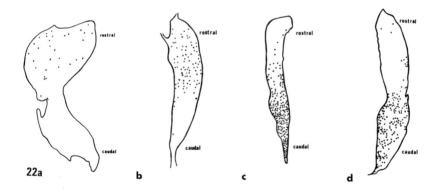

Figure 22 Drawings of histologic sections of the rabbit superior cervical ganglion showing ganglion cells labelled by HRP injection into various target organs. (a) Iris; (b) injection into Harder's gland in the orbit; (c) parotid salivary gland; and (d) the submandibular salivary gland. All sections were cut at 32 µm one day following injection of HRP

far caudal as the stellate ganglion are labelled when HRP is applied to the cut end of the external carotid nerve (Dail *et al.*, 1980). Therefore, the projection of these neurons indicates that they belong to the caudal group of neurons in the superior cervical ganglion (Fig. 23).

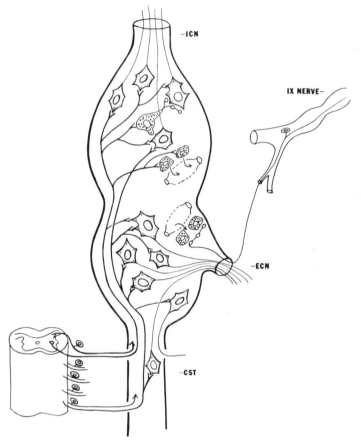

Figure 23 Schematic representation of the organization of the superior cervical sympathetic ganglion. This composite drawing summarizes data drawn from several sources and is intended to indicate only a generalized structure. Division of the superior cervical ganglion into rostral and caudal portions seems to be a feature common to many species. Whether the rostral or caudal pole receives predominant innervation from certain spinal cord segments is yet to be established for the superior cervical ganglion. Three relationships of SIF cells are shown: interneurons, chromaffin cells and sensory-type cells innervated by branches of the ninth cranial nerve. The cervical sympathetic trunk (CST) is composed of postganglionic as well as preganglionic fibres. Sensory fibres from dorsal root ganglia may also enter the superior cervical ganglion. ECN = external carotid nerve, ICN = internal carotid nerve

In a recent study of another compound ganglion, the stellate ganglion of the guinea pig, Lichtman *et al.* (1980) found that neurons were topographically related to their spinal cord preganglionic input. Neurons in the stellate receive preganglionic fibres from several spinal cord segments with ganglion cells in the upper third of the stellate innervated by more rostral segments and the lower third of the stellate by more caudal spinal cord segments. Lichtman *et al.* (1980) again emphasize that a rostrocaudal shift was not found in the superior cervical ganglion of the guinea pig (Njå and Purves, 1977a).

In summary, the superior cervical ganglion may be regarded as a fusion of at least two populations of neurons—those in the rostral pole and those in the caudal pole. The rostral part of the ganglion innervates tissues in the cranium and orbit and is probably innervated predominantly by more rostral segments of the spinal cord preganglionic outflow. The caudal pole of the superior cervical ganglion projects to tissues of the head and neck located farther caudally along the axis of the organism and is innervated by segments farther down the thoracic cord (Fig. 23). The degree of fusion of the two populations of cells probably varies among species, but in all species studied so far some segregation of neurons has been found. While it may be argued that the clustering of neurons is related only to the convenience of exiting a particular efferent nerve, the realization that the superior cervical ganglion is not a homogeneous collection of neurons is a new and important concept.

The impact of the existence of territories within an autonomic ganglion has yet to be fully assessed. Studies by Yarowsky *et al.* (1979) may foretell one future direction in research on subpopulations of sympathetic ganglion cells. In this investigation, glucose utilization was three times greater in the rostral pole of the superior cervical ganglion than in the caudal pole. Stimulation of the preganglionic nerve, which produced widening of the palpebral fissure and mydriasis, enhanced glucose utilization in the rostral pole. Biochemical studies on catecholamines, enzymes, metabolic rates and the effects of preganglionic nerve stimulation should be designed to reflect the concept of subpopulations of sympathetic ganglion cells. Similarly, there may be reason to suspect that neuronal circuitry, for example SIF cell influences, and the response to autonomic drugs may vary among the different cell populations in a sympathetic ganglion. Future studies on neuronal populations may provide new insights on the heterogeneity of sympathetic ganglion cells.

ACKNOWLEDGEMENT

Work in this manuscript was supported by the National Science Foundation, Grant BNS—791416.

REFERENCES

Amprino, R. (1938). Modifications de la structure des neurones sympathiques pendant l'accroissement et la senescence. *C. R. Assoc. Anat.*, **33**, 3–18.

Arvidson, B. (1979a). A study of the peripheral diffusion barrier of a peripheral ganglion. *Acta Neuropathol.*, **46**, 139–144.

Arvidson, B. (1979b). Distribution of intravenously injected protein traces in peripheral ganglia of adult mice. *Exp. Neurol.*, **63**, 388–410.

Arvidson, B. (1979c). Retrograde transport of horseradish peroxidase in sensory and adrenergic neurons following injection into the anterior eye chamber. *J. Neurocytol.*, **8**, 751–764.

Benitez, H. H., Masurovsky, E. B., and Murray, M. R. (1974). Interneurons of the sympathetic ganglia, in organotypic culture. A suggestion as to their function, based on three types of study. *J. Neurocytol.*, **3**, 363–384.

Bowers, C. W., and Zigmond, R. E. (1979). Localization of neurons in the rat superior cervical ganglion which project into different postganglionic trunks. *J. Comp. Neurol.*, **185**, 381–392.

Boyd, J. D. (1957). Intermediate sympathetic ganglia. *Br. Med. Bull.*, **13**, 207–212.

Brooks-Fournier, R., and Coggeshall, R. E. (1981). The ratio of preganglionic axons to postganglionic cells in the sympathetic nervous system of the rat. *J. Comp. Neurol.*, **197**, 207–216.

Cajal, S. Ramon y (1911). *Histologie du Systeme Nerveux de l'Homme et des Vertébrés*, Vol. II, Maloine, Paris.

Canfield, P. (1978). A light and electron microscopic study of developing bovine sympathetic ganglia. *Zentralbl. Veterinaermed. Reihe C*, **7**, 182–192.

Chibuzo, G. A., Cummings, J. F., and Evans, H. E. (1980). Autonomic innervation of the tongue: A horseradish peroxidase study in the dog. *J. Autonom. Nerv. Syst.*, **2**, 117–129.

Cotran, R. S., and Karnovsky, M. J. (1967). Vascular leakage induced by horseradish peroxidase in the rat. *Proc. Soc. Exp. Biol. Med.*, **126**, 557–561.

Dail, W. G., and Evan, A. P. (1978a). Ultrastructure of adrenergic terminals and SIF cells in the superior cercical ganglion of the rabbit. *Brain Res.*, **148**, 469–477.

Dail, W. G., and Evan, A. P. (1978b). Effects of chronic deafferentation on adrenergic ganglion cells and small intensely fluorescent cells. *J. Neurocytol.*, **7**, 25–37.

Dail, W. G., Evan, A. P., and Eason, H. R. (1975). The major ganglion in the pelvic plexus of the male rat: A histochemical and ultrastructural study. *Cell Tissue Res.*, **159**, 49–62.

Dail, W. G., Barraza, C., Khoudary, S., and Murray, H. M. (1979). Horseradish peroxidase studies of an autonomic ganglion. *Soc. Neurosci. Abstr.*, **5**, 332.

Dail, W. G., Khoudary, S., Barraza, C., Murray, H. M., and Bradley, C. (1980). The fate of adrenergic fibers which enter the superior cervical ganglion. In *Histochemistry and Cell Biology of Autonomic Neurons, SIF Cells and Paraneurons* (Eds. O. Eränkö, S. Soinila and H. Päivärinta), *Advances in Biochemical Psychopharmacology*, Vol. 25, pp. 287–297, Raven Press, New York.

De Castro, F. (1932). Sympathetic ganglia, normal and pathological. In *Cytology and Cellular Pathology of the Nervous System*, (Ed. W. Penfield), Vol. I, pp. 319–379, Hoeber, New York.

De Castro, F., and Herreros, M. L. (1945). Actividad funcíonal del ganglio cervical superior, en relacíon al numero y modalidad de sus fibras preganglíonicas. Models de la sinapsis. *Trab. Inst. Cajal Invest. Biol.*, **37**, 287–342.

DePace, D. (1981). A study of the permeability of the blood vessels of the rat superior cervical ganglion. *Anat. Rec.*, **199**, 66A.

Dolivo, M. (1974). Metabolism of mammalian sympathetic ganglia. *Fed. Proc.*, **33**, 1043–1048.

Elfvin, L.-G. (1971). Ultrastructural studies on the synaptology of the inferior mesenteric ganglion of the cat. I. Observations on the cell surface of the postganglionic *pericarya*. *J. Ultrastruct. Res.*, **37**, 411–425.

Eränkö, O. (1972). Light and electron microscopic histochemical evidence of granular and non-granular storage of catecholamines in the sympathetic ganglion of the rat. *Histochem. J.*, **4**, 213–224.

Eränkö, O. (1978). Small Intensely Fluorescent (SIF) cells and nervous transmission in sympathetic ganglia. *Annu. Rev. Pharmacol. Toxicol.*, **18**, 417–430.

Foley, J. O. (1945). The components of the cervical sympathetic trunk with special reference to its accessory cells and ganglia. *J. Comp. Neurol.*, **82**, 77–91.

Gabella, G. (1976). *Structure of the Autonomic Nervous System*, Chapman and Hall, London.

Grillo, M. (1978). Ultrastructural evidence for a sensory innervation of some SIF cells in rat superior cervical ganglia. *Anat. Rec.*, **190**, 407.

Hamberger, G., Norberg, K. A., and Sjöqvist, F. (1963). Evidence for adrenergic nerve terminals and synapses in sympathetic ganglia. *Int. J. Neuropharmacol.*, **2**, 279–282.

Hendry, I. A., Stockel, K., Thoenen, H., and Iversen, L. L. (1974). The retrograde axonal transport of nerve growth factor. *Brain Res.*, **68**, 103–121.

Hess, A. (1981). On the origin of substance P-positive fibres in the rat carotid body. *Anat. Rec.*, **199**, 114A.

Heym, Ch., and Williams, T. H. (1979). Evidence for autonomic paraneurons in sympathetic ganglia of a shrew (*Tupaia glis*). *J. Anat.*, **129**, 151–164.

Hillarp, N.-Å. (1960). Peripheral autonomic mechanisms. In *Handbook of Physiology* (Ed. J. Field), Section 1, Vol. II, pp. 979–1006, American Physiological Society, Washington.

Hökfelt, T. (1968). *In vitro* studies on central and peripheral monoamine neurons at the ultrastructural level. *Z. Zellforsch. Mikrosk. Anat.*, **91**, 1–74.

Hökfelt, T., Elfvin, L.-G., Schultzberg, M., Goldstein, M., and Nilsson, G. (1977). On the occurrence of substance P-containing nerve fibres in sympathetic ganglia: immunohistochemical evidence. *Brain Res.*, **132**, 29–41.

Iversen, L. L., Stöckel, K., and Thoenen, H. (1975). Autoradiographic studies of the retrograde axonal transport of nerve growth factor in mouse sympathetic neurons. *Brain Res.*, **88**, 37–43.

Jacobowitz, D. M. (1970). Catecholamine fluorescence studies of adrenergic neurons and chromaffin cells in sympathetic ganglia. *Fed. Proc.*, **29**, 1929–1944.

Jacobowitz, D., and Green, L. A. (1974). Histochemical studies on the relationship of chromaffin cells and adrenergic nerve fibres to the cardia ganglia of several species. *J. Pharmacol. Exp. Ther.*, **158**, 227–240.

Jacobowitz, D. M., and Woodward, J. K. (1968). Adrenergic neurons in the cat superior cervical ganglion and cervical sympathetic trunk. A histochemical study. *J. Pharmacol. Exp. Ther.*, **162**, 213–226.

Jacobs, J. M. (1977). Penetration of systemically injected horseradish peroxidase into ganglia and nerves of the autonomic nervous system. *J. Neurocytol.*, **6**, 607–618.

Kondo, H. (1977). Innervation of SIF cells in the superior cervical and nodose ganglia: An ultrastructural study with serial sections. *Biol. Cell.*, **30**, 253–264.

Kondo, H., Dun, N. J., and Pappas, G. D. (1980). A light and electron microscopic study of the rat superior cervical ganglion cells by intracellular HRP-labeling. *Brain Res.*, **197**, 193–199.

Kuba, K., and Koketsu, K. (1978). Synaptic events in sympathetic ganglia. In *Prog. Neurobiol.*, (Eds. G. A. Kerkut and J. W. Phillis) Vol 11, Pergamon Press, Oxford, 77–169.

Libet, B. (1980). Functional roles of SIF cells in slow synaptic actions. In *Histochemistry and Cell Biology of Autonomic Neurons, SIF Cells and Paraneurons* (Eds.

O. Eränkö, S. Soinila and H. Päivärinta), *Advances in Biochemical Psychopharmacology*, Vol. 25, pp. 111–118, Raven Press, New York.

Libet, B., and Owman, Ch. (1974). Concomitant changes in formaldehyde-induced fluorescence of dopamine interneurons and in slow inhibitory post-synaptic potentials of the rabbit superior cervical ganglion, induced by stimulation of the preganglionic nerve or by a muscarinic agent. *J. Physiol. (London)*, **237**, 635–662.

Lichtman, J. W. (1980). On the predominantly single innervation of submandibular ganglion cells in the rat. *J. Physiol. (London)*, **302**, 121–130.

Lichtman, J. W., Purves, D., and Yip, J. W. (1979). On the purpose of selective innervation of guinea-pig superior cervical ganglion cells. *J. Physiol. (London)*, **292**, 69–84.

Lichtman, J. W., Purves, D., and Yip, J. W. (1980). Innervation of sympathetic neurons in the guinea pig thoracic chain. *J. Physiol. (London)*, **298**, 285–299.

Matthews, M. R. (1980). Ultrastructural studies relevant to the possible functions of small granule-containing cells in the rat superior cervical ganglion. In *Histochemistry and Cell Biology of Autonomic Neurons, SIF Cells and Paraneurons* (Eds. O. Eränkö, S. Soinila and H. Päivärinta), *Advances in Biochemical Psychopharmacology*, Vol. 25, pp. 77–86, Raven Press, New York.

Matthews, M. R., and Raisman, G. (1969). The ultrastructure and somatic efferent synapses of small granule-containing cells in the superior cervical ganglion. *J. Anat.*, **105**, 255–282.

Matthews, M. R., and Raisman, G. (1972). A light and electron microscopic study of the cellular response to axonal injury in the superior cervical ganglion of the rat. *Proc. R. Soc. London Ser. B.*, **181**, 43–79.

Matthieu, J.-M. (1970). Effet des variations de la P_{CO_2}, du pH et de la HCO_3^- sur la production de lactate et la transmiscion synaptique du ganglion sympatique cervical insole du rat. *Brain Res.*, **18**, 1–14.

McLachlan, E. M. (1974). The formation of synapses in mammalian sympathetic ganglia reinnervated with preganglionic or somatic nerves. *J. Physiol. (London)*, **237**, 217–242.

Njå, A., and Purves, D. (1977a). Specific innervation of guinea-pig superior cervical ganglion cells by preganglionic fibres arising from different levels of the spinal cord. *J. Physiol. (London)*, **264**, 565–583.

Njå, A., and Purves, D. (1977b). Re-innervation of guinea-pig superior cervical ganglion cells by preganglionic fibres arising from different levels of the spinal cord. *J. Physiol. (London)*, **272**, 633–651.

Njå, A., and Purves, D. (1978). Specificity of initial synaptic contacts made on guinea-pig superior cervical ganglion cells during regeneration of the cervical sympathetic trunk. *J. Physiol. (London)*, **281**, 45–62.

Norberg, K.-A., and Sjöqvist, F. (1966). New possibilities for adrenergic modulation of ganglionic transmission. *Pharmacol. Rev.*, **18**, 743–751.

Norberg, K.-A., Ritzen, M., and Ungerstedt, U. (1966). Histochemical studies of a special catecholamine-containing cell type in sympathetic ganglia. *Acta Physiol. Scand.*, **67**, 260–270.

Owman, Ch., and Sjöberg, N.-O. (1967). Difference in rates of depletion and recovery of noradrenaline in 'short' and 'long' sympathetic nerves after reserpine treatment. *Life Sci.*, **6**, 2549–2556.

Owman, Ch., Sjöberg, N.-O., and Swedin, G. (1971). Histochemical and chemical studies on pre- and postnatal development of the different systems of 'short' and 'long' adrenergic neurons in peripheral organs of the rat. *Z. Zellforsch. Mikrosk. Anat.*, **116**, 319–341.

Pick, J. (1970). *The Autonomic Nervous System*, J. B. Lippincott, Philadelphia.

Purves, D. (1975). Functional and structural changes in mammalian sympathetic neurons following interruption of their axons. *J. Physiol. (London)*, **252**, 429–463.

Purves, D. (1976). Functional and structural changes in mammalian sympathetic neurones following colchicine application to post-ganglionic nerves. *J. Physiol. (London)*, **259**, 159–175.

Purves, D., and Hume, R. I. (1981). The relation of postsynaptic geometry to the number of presynaptic axons that innervate autonomic ganglion cells. *J. Neurosci.*, **5**, 441–452.

Randall, W. G., Armour, J. A., Randall, D. C., and Smith, O. A. (1971). Functional anatomy of the cardiac nerves of the baboon. *Anat. Rec.*, **170**, 183–198.

Richards, J. G., and Tranzer, J. P. (1975). Localization of amine storage sites in the adrenergic cell body. A study of the superior cervical ganglion of the rat by fine structural cytochemistry. *J. Ultrastruct. Res.*, **53**, 204–216.

Siegrist, G., Dolivo, M., Dunant, Y., Foroglou-Kerameus, G., de Ribaupierre, Fr., and Rouiller, Ch. (1968). Ultrastructure and function of the chromaffin cells in the superior cervical ganglion of the rat. *J. Ultrastruct. Res.*, **25**, 381–407.

Sjöstrand, N. O. (1965). The adrenergic innervation of the vas deferens and accessory male genital glands. *Acta Physiol. Scand., Suppl.*, **257**, 1–82.

Van Orden, L. S., Burke, J. D., Geyer, M., and Lodoen, F. V. (1970). Location of depletion-sensitive and depletion-resistant norepinephrine storage sites in autonomic ganglia. *J. Pharmacol. Exp. Ther.*, **174**, 56–71.

Wallis, D. I., and North, R. A. (1978). Synaptic input to cells of the rabbit superior cervical ganglion. *Pflügers Arch.*, **374**, 145–152.

Williams, T. H., and Palay, S. L. (1969). Ultrastructure of the small neurons in the superior cervical ganglion. *Brain Res.*, **15**, 17–34.

Yarowsky, P., Jehle, J.,7, Ingvar, D. H., and Sokoloff, L. (1979). Relationship between functional activity and glucose utilization in the rat superior cervical ganglion *in vivo*. *Soc. Neurosci. Abstr.*, **5**, 421.

Autonomic Ganglia
Edited by Lars-Gösta Elfvin
© 1983 John Wiley & Sons Ltd

The Ultrastructure of Junctions in Sympathetic Ganglia of Mammals

MARGARET R. MATTHEWS

*Department of Human Anatomy, University of Oxford,
South Parks Road, Oxford OX1 3QX, UK*

In this chapter an attempt will be made to indicate what contribution the study of ultrastructure may make, or has already made, to the elucidation of the nature and mechanisms of intraganglionic connexions, and the manner in which they are established and maintained.

That the sympathetic ganglia are sites of synaptic interaction has been evident since the work of Langley, who almost a century ago was exploring the autonomic ganglia using the block of transganglionic nervous transmission which could be produced by the local application of nicotine (Langley and Dickinson, 1889). That the mammalian sympathetic ganglion is more than a simple relay station was revealed by J. C. Eccles (1935a, b), whose pioneer studies showed more complex patterns of responses than a simple fast excitatory potential following a preganglionic volley, and demonstrated phenomena of facilitation, convergence and inhibition. The variety of functional mechanisms and the transmitter and receptor pharmacology of these ganglia have proved to be sufficiently complex to leave a number of issues still unresolved (Skok, 1973; Brooks *et al.*, 1979; see chapters in section B). The paravertebral ganglia of the sympathetic chain receive inputs primarily from the preganglionic sympathetic neurons of the spinal cord; but studies of the patterns of reflex activity associated with the alimentary tract have shown that the prevertebral ganglia receive inputs from the wall of the gut and possibly from other prevertebral ganglia as well as from the spinal cord. Their status has recently been evaluated by Szurszewski (1977). The ganglia of the pelvic (hypogastric) plexuses, from which the pelvic viscera are innervated, contain sympathetic as well as parasympathetic neurons, and their inputs and internal organization reflect this complexity (see chapter by Owman *et al.*). A knowledge at the ultrastructural level of the types and nature of the neuronal contacts, and in particular of the synapses and other specialized junctions, which are established inside the ganglia, and identification of the elements involved in such contacts, can permit correlations between structure and function, between the characteristics of presynaptic profiles and their source and transmitter content, and between their sites of termination and the particular manner in which their effects may be expressed physiologically.

Thus, it may be possible to localize sites of synaptic transmitter or modulator action to specific nerve terminals, and to exclude as well as include possible effects for known categories of endings; to establish, for example, whether adrenergic or specifically immunoreactive varicosities form true synapses and, if so, to observe on what parts of the neurons they terminate. The ultrastructural characterization, classification and counting of synapses may permit interpretation of the results of *in vitro* or *in vivo* experimental studies; the identification and study, for example, of factors determining differentiation of neurons in dissociated cell culture, or governing synaptogenesis *in vivo*.

An earlier review (Matthews, 1974) summarized the position at that stage. Since then, little that is new has been added on the situation, presynaptic organelles and general character of the pre- to postganglionic synapse, but more information has accrued on the differences between species, and between different ganglia in the same species; for example, between the prevertebral and the paravertebral ganglia, on the degree of diversity of synaptic connexions, on the plasticity of these connections and the factors governing the transmitter specification of sympathetic neurons during development, and on the level of interdependence of the elements of the various junctions. The ultrastructural investigation of ganglionic synapses has received considerable potential reinforcement and challenge lately from the immunohistochemical demonstration of systems of intraganglionic nerve networks immunoreactive for specific neuroactive peptides (see chapter by Schultzberg *et al.*), and the opportunities offered by the development of effective techniques for immunocytochemical localization (Sternberger *et al.*, 1970).

TYPES AND DISTRIBUTION OF SPECIALIZED CONTACT REGIONS

In mammals, sympathetic ganglionic neurons have numerous dendrites (Cajal, 1911; De Castro, 1932), often of considerable length, which may spread widely in the ganglion, or may form pericellular nests round other neurons, or enter into complex dendritic glomerular arborizations. In adult ganglia most of the specialized contacts involve dendrites. This is in contrast to the simple, unipolar form of amphibian sympathetic neurons, and suggests distinct possibilities of segregation of multiple inputs, or interactions between neurons. A typical dendritic field in a rat superior cervical ganglion presents a strong impression of independence of dendritic territories, coupled with scope for concurrence and the sharing of inputs. The precise arrangement and grouping of profiles could be to some extent governed by the fact that all are enclosed in satellite cell cytoplasm, which separates them from an intragang-lionic connective tissue space. Transmission electron microscopy of ganglia fixed by conventional techniques (buffered glutaraldehyde, or mixtures of glutaraldehyde with paraformaldehyde in varying proportions, followed by osmication; or osmium used as the primary fixative) shows both synaptic and non-synaptic (adhaerens-type) specialized junctions, as well as regions of simple apposition between nerve profiles. It must be remembered that any of these might represent points of transmitter or modulator action, and even that longer-range interactions might occur without close apposition, for example across connective tissue spaces, the requirement being that some type of agonist molecule reaches some receptor site in sufficient concentration to elicit a response there. This discussion concerns itself primarily with contacts of morphologically specialized nature. Detailed accounts of the fine structure of synaptic specializations may be found in the review by Elfvin (1976) and the book by Peters *et al.* (1976).

SYNAPSES

The synaptic junctions are of the chemical synapse type. No gap junctions or electrically conducting synapses have been identified between neurons, though Elfvin and Forsman (1978) have observed gap junctions and rudi-ments of tight junctions between satellite cells in sympathetic ganglia of the guinea-pig and rabbit. The elements which are postsynaptic in the ganglion are the principal ganglionic neurons, accounting for the great majority of synapses, the catecholamine-rich small granule-containing cells (the SIF cells of fluorescence microscopy) (Eränkö, 1976; Taxi, 1979; see chapter by Taxi), and occasionally, or rarely, other axon terminal profiles.

Postsynaptic elements

Principal neurons receive synapses mainly on their dendrites, less often on the soma (Fig. 1). Somatic synapses are rare in adult paravertebral ganglia of most species (the mouse is an exception: Yokota and Yamauchi, 1974), but are more frequently seen in the prevertebral ganglia and in immature ganglia. Perisomatic synapses are in any case seldom placed directly on to the soma, as in amphibia, but are more typically placed on short spurs or on spine-like processes, which may be flattened or filiform (e.g. Fig. 1c) or may be club-shaped, with expanded ends rich in organelles, often notably including a form of wide tubular network of smooth endoplasmic reticulum. This type is seen more in prevertebral than in paravertebral ganglia. Elfvin (1971) in a prevertebral ganglion of the cat noted clusters of small dense-cored vesicles in such spines, and also reconstructed the pattern of axosomatic synapses for an entire neuron soma; this neuron received 27 direct axosomatic synapses and

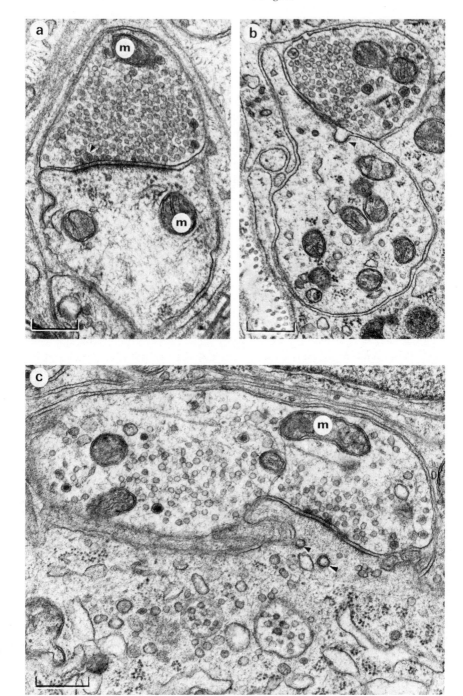

had 20 short processes, of which 17 received synapses. Other neurons almost completely reconstructed received few or no axosomatic synapses.

Dendritic synapses (Fig. 1a, b, Figs. 2, 3) are received either i) directly on to the shafts; or ii) on spine-like processes of various lengths which, like the somatic spines, may either be filiform or flattened or have expanded ends; or iii) on short blunt projections which are hardly spines but give the dendrite an irregular, knobbed contour. These blunt projections typically contain some ribosomes and/or granular endoplasmic reticulum, sacs of smooth endoplasmic reticulum and often a multivesicular body, together with a mitochondrion or two and perhaps a cytoplasmic dense body (Fig. 3a). The dendritic shaft cytoplasm beneath the base of a spine may be similarly equipped (Fig. 6). The organelle-rich cytoplasm could play a part in the response of the neuron to modulators or trophic factors which might be liberated at these synapses in addition to the transmitter which is responsible for fast synaptic action. Coated pits and coated vesicles may often be seen parasynaptically at and near the postsynaptic membrane, especially at the base of a spine (Fig. 1b, c; cf. Fig. 5b of Matthews, 1974), and might be concerned in the maintenance of the postsynaptic densities (Rees *et al.*, 1976), or in the uptake of specific macromolecules.

Slender or filiform spines have a fine web of filamentous, cytoskeletal material in their apical cytoplasm (Fig. 1b, c). Spines with expanded ends, like those of the soma, may contain tubular smooth endoplasmic reticulum or groups of small regular vesicles which are not unlike synaptic vesicles, but are not clustered toward the postsynaptic membrane at the specialized synaptic region in such way as to suggest reciprocal synaptic release (Fig. 2a). Small vesicles in such situations may often be shown after appropriate fixation

Figure 1   Three synapses of preganglionic type on to principal neurons in rat superior cervical ganglion. Scale bars represent 0.3 μm. (a) Synapse upon dendritic shaft. Among the small agranular vesicles which are crowded toward the specialized region of membrane in the presynaptic element is a single large dense-cored vesicle (arrowhead); other dense-cored vesicles lie further away, at the periphery of the mass of small vesicles. A well-defined postsynaptic 'thickening' or layer of dense filamentous material is present in the cytoplasm immediately beneath the postsynaptic membrane, and further dense material is present in the synaptic cleft. m = mitochondrion

(b) Synapse upon the base of a short spine-like process from a dendrite. The arrowhead indicates a coated pit in the postsynaptic element at the junction of the spine with the dendrite, encroaching on the margin of the synaptic zone; this association is not infrequently seen

(c) Synapse upon a short spine-like projection from the cell body of a postganglionic neuron. Arrowheads indicate coated vesicles in the base of the projection; numerous vesicles and two multivesicular bodies lie in the adjacent neuronal cytoplasm. Primary fixation in this case was by aldehydes. Reproduced from Matthews and Nelson (1975), by permission of *Journal of Physiology*.

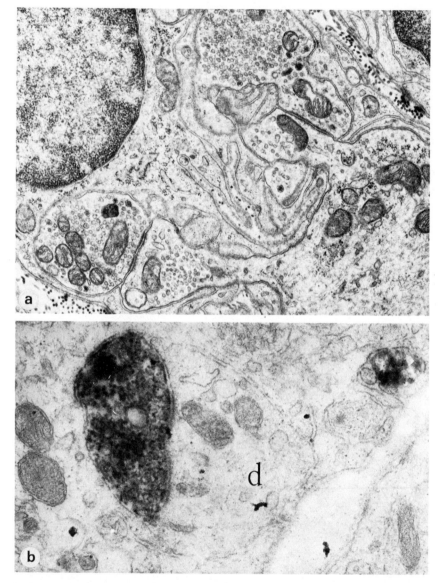

Figure 2 (a) Rat superior cervical ganglion. Problems in identification of postsynaptic profiles: this is an example of two spine-like projections from the dendrite of a principal neuron, receiving specialized contacts (synaptic on the left, symmetrical on the right) from nerve endings of preganglionic type. Both 'spines' have expanded club-like ends and contain many small vesicles in addition to a mitochondrion and sacs of smooth endoplasmic reticulum. These would be difficult to identify as dendritic projections if they were not seen in continuity with the parent dendrite. Note also the association of mitochondria in each element with the deep aspects of the junctions,

techniques, or preloading with false transmitter, to contain dense cores (see below).

Synapses received directly on to dendritic shafts or their short projections may show flanges of dendritic cytoplasm which partly surround the presynaptic terminal (Figs. 3b, 8a). It may be speculated that these flanges could assist synaptic action by restricting the free diffusion of transmitter away from the synaptic cleft or, in the case of the acetylcholine of the preganglionic nerve ending, which is rapidly hydrolysed by acetylcholinesterase, by restricting the loss of free choline by diffusion, so that it remains available to the presynaptic nerve ending for reuptake.

The ratio of spine to shaft synapses has been variously reported, in the rat superior cervical ganglion, as 4.5:1 (Raisman *et al.*, 1974) and 2.4:1 (Matthews and Nelson, 1975), the ratio probably depending on the method of sampling. (In the case of Raisman *et al.*, who counted in smaller grid squares, this specifically favoured the immediate perineuronal territory which presumably also contains more basal regions of dendrites.)

Postsynaptic specializations. Most intraganglionic synapses are asymmetric, showing a greater amount of cytoplasmic membrane-associated dense material on the postsynaptic than on the presynaptic side (Figs. 1, 3). This includes most of the synapses upon principal neurons. The major exceptions are certain synapses associated with the small granule-containing cells (see below).

Subsynaptic formations. Some dendritic shaft synapses on the larger dendrites exhibit a regular row of subjunctional cytoplasmic densities (cf. Milhaud and Pappas, 1966), with which is closely associated on its deep aspect

and the short symmetrical attachment between the right-hand presynaptic profile and its sheath of satellite cytoplasm, at the upper right border of the profile. ×22 000. Reproduced from Matthews (1976), by permission of Elsevier/North-Holland Biomedical Press.

(b) Synapse, showing two 'active zones', to a probable dendritic shaft (d, centre) from a profile immunoreactive for substance P in guinea-pig coeliac-superior mesenteric ganglion. A second immunoreactive nerve profile, which is smaller and non-synaptic, is seen at upper right. These labelled profiles represent, respectively, a varicosity and an intervaricose segment of the substance P-immunoreactive nerve networks in this ganglion. ×36 000. Immunoenzyme staining was performed using monoclonal anti-substance P antibody (NCL/34-HL; Cuello *et al.*, 1979), directly conjugated with horseradish peroxidase (Matthews and Cuello, unpublished observations). This figure illustrates also certain problems inherent in the technique of immunocytochemistry, i.e. loss of resolution in the labelled presynaptic profile, in which vesicles are partly obscured by reaction end-product, and the twin sacrifices of preservation of tissue detail and of contrast in the postsynaptic profile and in surrounding structures, the former imposed by fixation in 4% paraformaldehyde, and the latter, by minimal counterstaining with heavy metals (lead citrate and uranyl acetate) so as to avoid eclipsing the end-product.

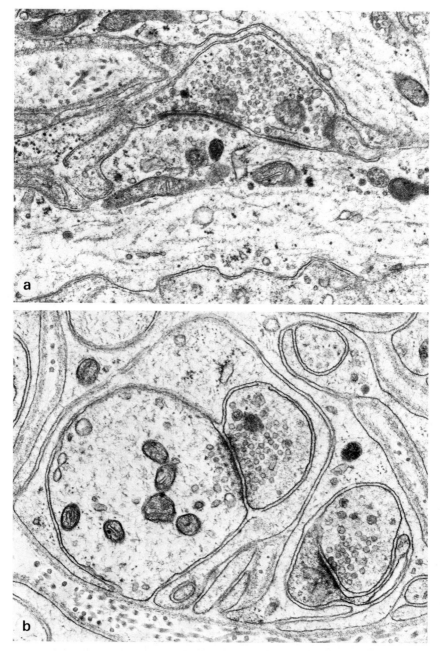

Figure 3 (a) Coupled synapse (left) and symmetrical attachment (right), from a large presynaptic profile to a large dendritic shaft, seen in longitudinal section. Rat superior cervical ganglion. The synapse has asymmetrical membrane-associated

an array of vesicles of smooth endoplamic reticulum (Fig. 3a, b; cf. Fig. 6b of Matthews, 1974). The cytoplasmic densities have a radiating, filamentous appearance and are evidently approximately spherical or stellate, arranged in a grid-like array, since they present the same aspect whether the dendrite is cut transversely or longitudinally (Fig. 3); they thus differ from the corresponding formation in the frog (the 'bandelette sous-synaptique' of Taxi, 1965), which appears to be plate-like. In both cases, however, the subsynaptic dense array is placed at a consistent depth, below and parallel to the postsynaptic surface membrane, accommodating to its contour. The array of vesicles seen in the mammalian subsynaptic formation might be concerned in some aspect of the response of the postsynaptic neuron to synaptic activation. In the frog, this position tends to be occupied by a tapering cone of cytoplasmic filaments, which sometimes contains additional, deeper dense bands. These subjunctional densities, in both frog and mammal, seem to include as at least one of their functions that of strengthening the link between the postsynaptic membrane and the cytoskeleton (see below under 'attachment plaques'). Another function in the mammal would appear to be the provision of anchorage points, temporary or permanent, for the associated vesicles.

The small granule-containing cells (SGC cells) receive synapses principally on their somata or on short spine-like projections from the soma, but may also receive them on their processes, if these are present. The presynaptic profile may lie along the surface of the SGC cell without indenting it, or may be rather deeply embedded into the SGC cell cytoplasm. In either case,

cytoplasmic densities, and there is a row of linked, subjunctional densities lying parallel to the synapse in the postsynaptic cytoplasm. An array of vesicles of smooth endoplasmic reticulum (s.e.r.) is associated with the deep aspect of this formation. The synapse is placed upon a rounded projection or spur of the dendrite which contains a variety of cytoplasmic organelles, including a multivesicular body, a cytoplasmic dense body and mitochondria, one of which is associated with the deep aspect of the adjoining symmetrical attachment. Note the mitochondrion similarly placed in the presynaptic profile, facing the symmetrical attachment, and the flattened profiles of fine tubular reticulum between each of these mitochondria and the attachment. Another multivesicular body-dense body pair is seen a little further along the dendrite, beneath a small spine-like profile, possibly from the same dendrite, which receives a synapse from the same presynaptic profile. ×30 000.
(b) Two synapses to dendritic shafts, in transverse section. Both synapses are asymmetrical. That on the left, to a large dendrite, has a distinct row of linked subjunctional densities associated on its deep aspect with vesicles of s.e.r. Deep to the junction lie several transversely sectioned mitochondria, more s.e.r. vesicles and a coated vesicle. Compare with Fig. 3a. The dendrite of the right-hand synapse is smaller but has a suggestion of a row of subjunctional densities and of associated large sacs of s.e.r. It has a projecting spur or flange which partly encircles the presynaptic profile. The two dendrites occupy different domains of satellite cell cytoplasm. Rat superior cervical ganglion, ×40 500.

cytoplasmic peripheral spines or flanges are frequently present, partly surrounding the presynaptic profile and in effect still further deepening any indentation. It is not uncommon for the foci of specialized vesicle clustering in the presynaptic profile, which are small and several in this class of synapse, to be directed toward the peripheral projections of the SGC cell, and for the central part of the contact region to be occupied by one or more attachment plaques. The small synaptic foci have little associated dense material in the post synaptic cytoplasm, i.e. they are symmetric in type. In the central nervous system also, symmetric synapses are typically multifocal (Peters *et al.*, 1976). There they are often interneuronal and intrinsic and are typically inhibitory and of local origin, either from short-axon elements or dendro-dendritic (Peters *et al.*, 1976). For the sympathetic ganglion, the reason for the symmetric–asymmetric difference is unknown: the preganglionic synapses to both principal neurons and SGC cells involve extrinsic presynaptic elements, presumably with the same cholinergic transmitter. The difference might relate to the type of receptor, i.e. whether it is nicotinic or muscarinic: the receptor for fast synaptic activation of the principal neurons is nicotinic, but that for the afferent synapse of the SGC cell has been thought to be muscarinic (Eccles and Libet, 1961), although the evidence here is indirect. Other possibilities might include the need, or absence of need, for particular mechanical stabilization of the attachment; in this respect, however, there is evidence that some of the symmetric afferent synapses upon the SGC cells require supplementary attachments (see below). Mugnaini (1970) has discussed comparable paradoxes relating to symmetrical and asymmetrical synapses in the central nervous system, chiefly in the cerebellum, concluding that it is the postsynaptic partner which determines this aspect of synaptic structure.

Identification of postsynaptic structures

It must be stressed that the nature and origin of postsynaptic elements may not always be detectable from single ultrathin sections, and that long series of consecutive sections might be needed for certain diagnosis. This point has been discussed earlier by Elfvin (1963a, b, 1971) and by Matthews (1976). In particular, the ultrastructural discrimination between axons and dendrites often rests upon the presence or absence of ribosomes or granular endoplasmic reticulum in the dendrite; but some dendrites may lack these over part of their course. The manner of fixation, or the use of specific labelling, may be of decisive importance. For such reasons it remains uncertain whether axoaxonic or dendrodendritic synapses occur in sympathetic ganglia, although examples of what may be the former are occasionally seen in prevertebral ganglia, and Kondo *et al.* (1980) have recently produced some evidence for the latter in a paravertebral ganglion.

Presynaptic elements

These may be either extraganglionic or intraganglionic in origin.

Extraganglionic sources

Preganglionic axons, from the intermediolateral and associated intercalated and intermediomedial cell columns in the thoracolumbar spinal cord, terminate in all ganglia (e.g. Chung *et al.*, 1975; Petras and Faden, 1978; Chung *et al.*, 1979; Dalsgaard and Elfvin, 1979), and their endings probably form by far the greatest proportion of the synapses in paravertebral ganglia. This last opinion is in part a generalization from observations on that most extensively studied ganglion, the superior cervical ganglion, which may simply and conveniently be decentralized by cutting the cervical sympathetic trunk (preganglionic axotomy); but the available evidence suggests that it is likely to be reasonably accurate for other paravertebral ganglia also. Preganglionic axotomy leads in the short term to loss of almost all synapses in the rat or cat superior cervical ganglion (Hámori *et al.*, 1968; Joó *et al.*, 1971; Quilliam and Tamarind, 1972; Raisman *et al.*, 1974), including in the rat synapses afferent or incoming to SGC cells (Matthews, 1971; Matthews and Ostberg, 1973). The cervical sympathetic trunk is, however, not an unmixed nerve, for it carries postganglionic adrenergic nerve fibres from the more caudal cervical and stellate ganglia, and may also include a few larger myelinated nerve fibres which could be sensory axons, in addition to some postganglionic axons running caudalward from the superior cervical ganglion itself (Bowers and Zigmond, 1979). Dail *et al.* (1980) have found in the rabbit that, after the cervical sympathetic trunk is cut, the incidence of the small proportion of synapses of adrenergic type present in the superior cervical ganglion in this species does not alter, and conclude that the adrenergic fibres ascending in the cervical sympathetic trunk pass through the ganglion without terminating there. As for sensory axons, they are unlikely to be numerous but could be diverse in character. A few profiles resembling chemosensory axons terminate in relation to SGC cells, in or near the rat superior cervical ganglion, just as they do in the adjacent carotid body (Matthews, 1976; Kondo, 1977; Matthews, 1980a). A very few substance P-immunoreactive nerve fibres are seen by immunofluorescence microscopy in the superior cervical and other paravertebral ganglia of the rat, cat and guinea-pig (Hökfelt *et al.*, 1977), but it is not known whether they form synapses there. A profuse network of enkephalin-immunoreactive nerve fibres is seen in the ganglia, and it is suggested by Schultzberg *et al.* (1979) that the enkephalin-immunoreactive material may be present in the preganglionic nerve fibres, in addition to acetylcholine (see chapter by Schultzberg *et al.*). Its release on preganglionic tetanic stimulation might account for presynaptic inhibition (Konishi *et al.*, 1980).

In the prevertebral ganglia, a substantial but unknown proportion of inputs comes from the peripheral territory which they innervate, and also from sensory nerve fibres. Inputs from the enteric nerve plexuses have been demonstrated by their reflex effects (Crowcroft *et al.*, 1971) and by intracellular recording from neurons in the prevertebral ganglia (Crowcroft and Szurszewski, 1971; Szurszewski and Weems, 1976). In these ganglia Hökfelt and his collaborators, who have pioneered the application of immuno-fluorescence microscopy to sympathetic ganglia, have by this technique shown intraganglionic networks of nerve fibres immunoreactive for neuroactive peptides of types which have been shown also to be present in neurons of the enteric plexuses (see the chapters by Llewellyn-Smith *et al.* and by Schultz-berg *et al.*). Substance P-immunoreactivity is present, both in a network of varicose fibres and in fibre bundles which traverse the ganglion; these have been shown to originate, at least in major part, centrally to the inferior mesenteric ganglion and to form synapses within it (Fig. 2b; Baker *et al.*, 1980; Matthews and Cuello, 1982; Connaughton *et al.*, 1983). Substance P is capable of mimicking a slow, nerve-mediated depolarization in sympathetic neurons of the inferior mesenteric ganglion and has been shown to be released from the ganglion on stimulation (Konishi *et al.*, 1979). Some sensory neurons of the spinal ganglia show immunoreactivity for substance P (Hökfelt *et al.*, 1975), and evidence is accumulating which indicates these as the origin of the intraganglionic substance P-immunoreactive networks, probably by way of axon collaterals (Konishi *et al.*, 1979, 1980; Baker *et al.*, 1980; Matthews and Cuello, 1982); these could subserve reflexes from gut to ganglion and back without necessitating the involvement of the central nervous system.* Other sensory axons also might give rise to nerve endings in the ganglia. All these possibilities are beginning to be explored, with the opportunity offered by immunolocalization techniques.

Other sympathetic ganglia have been suspected of providing some extra-ganglionic inputs: as noted above, Dail *et al.* (1980) in the rabbit have found evidence to the contrary in the case of the superior cervical ganglion, and the same could apply for other paravertebral ganglia; but the possibility remains, to be explored rigorously, for the prevertebral ganglia, where reflex pathways undoubtedly travel by way of interganglionic nerve connexions (Kreulen and Szurszewski 1979), and also for the pelvic ganglia, and is supported by preliminary results of tracer experiments employing horseradish peroxidase.

Intraganglionic sources

To an extent which is variable according to ganglion and to species, neurons in the same ganglion form synapses upon each other. This has long

---

* This interesting new finding implies a relationship akin to the axon reflex between substance p-containing, probably nociceptive sensory nerve fibres and peripheral autonomic ganglion cells.

been suspected as a possibility, attributable to axon collaterals, a few of which were seen by Cajal (1911), and more recently to possible dendrodendritic interactions (Elfvin, 1971). Direct proof is difficult to obtain, though Kondo *et al.* (1980) have recently adduced suggestive evidence for the existence of dendrodendritic synapses in the rat superior cervical ganglion, from serial sectioning of neurons injected with horseradish peroxidase. There is, however, no doubt that principal neurons in cultures of explanted immature (neonatal rat) sympathetic ganglia and particularly in dissociated cell culture (Mains and Patterson, 1973) may form synapses upon each other (Rees and Bunge, 1974); and the latter situation has become a powerful tool for investigating factors which control the differentiation of sympathetic neurons, since appropriate manipulation of the conditions of culture can select for the formation of either cholinergic or adrenergic synapses (see chapter by Landis).

SGC cells are presynaptic in some ganglia and in some species, such as the rat (Williams, 1967; Siegrist *et al.*, 1968; Williams and Palay 1969; Matthews and Raisman, 1969; Ivanov, 1974), rabbit (Dail and Evan, 1978; Jew, 1980), rhesus monkey (Chiba *et al.*, 1977) and the guinea-pig (Jew, 1980), though in this last species the SGC cells are found to be presynaptic only to each other (Jew, 1980). (For further details see chapter by Williams and Jew.)

Types of presynaptic profiles

The identification of the various presynaptic elements depends partly on ultrastructural criteria, partly on the results of selective nerve lesions, but also to an important extent on specific labelling techniques both of the present and of the future.

Synaptic junctions (Figs 1–3) are conventionally recognizable as specialized regions of membrane apposition between nervous profiles involving a regular intermembrane interval of about 20 nm, at which intracytoplasmic dense material is associated with each membrane and vesicles present in one profile are clustered toward the membrane in the specialized region, which typically bears triangular (pyramidal) tufts of dense fibrillar material (the presynaptic dense projections of Gray, 1963; the presynaptic grid of Akert *et al.*, 1969; Peters *et al.*, 1976). After conventional fixation for electron microscopy (aldehydes followed by osmium tetroxide, or primary fixation with osmium tetroxide), the vesicles of presynaptic profiles are seen to be of various types. These include small, regular spherical vesicles of about 20–60 nm in diameter, which may be electron-lucent ('agranular') or may contain a central or eccentric dense core (like the small granular vesicles of the catecholaminergic nerve ending), small agranular flattened or tubular vesicles (seen particularly after aldehyde fixation), and large dense-cored vesicles of various sizes and core densities, according to the type of presynaptic profile (see below).

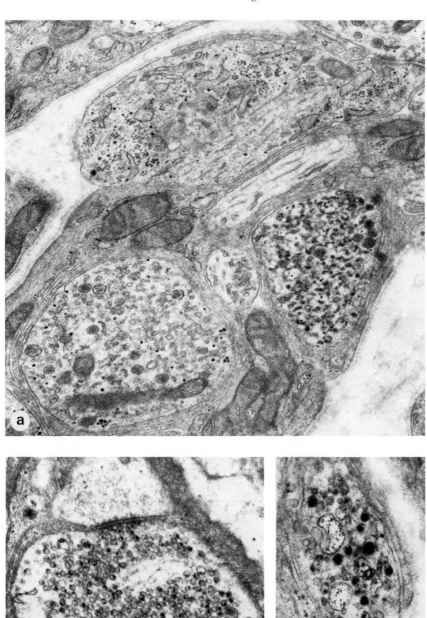

Certain combinations of vesicle types are consistently seen, and are typical for particular classes of presynaptic profiles.

Conventional fixation does not discriminate chemical differences, beyond revealing in favourable circumstances the small dense-cored or 'granular' vesicles typical of monoaminergic endings. These small dense cores are better preserved by permanganate fixation, which is also more reliably diagnostic (Richardson, 1966; Hökfelt and Jonsson, 1968; Hökfelt, 1971; Kanerva *et al.*, 1980), though that of itself may lead to ambiguities, since it does not well preserve ribosomes or pre- and postsynaptic densities, or the filamentous web of other cytoplasmic proteins, and therefore narrows the range of criteria available for discrimination. Dichromate fixation schedules (e.g. Tranzer and Richards, 1976) both preserve the cores of small dense-cored vesicles and may show cytoplasmic proteins to slightly better advantage. Permanganate and dichromate display sites of storage of endogenous catecholamines. Another way of revealing catecholamine storage capacity, which demonstrates the presence of an uptake mechanism in addition, is to load the tissue with 5-hydroxydopamine (5-OHDA) either *in vivo* (Dail and Evan, 1978) or *in vitro* (Fig. 4). This enhances the cores of small dense-cored vesicles and labels a greater proportion of vesicles per profile. A fixation schedule may

Figure 4 5-ODHA labelling of nerve profiles in a prevertebral ganglion (guinea-pig inferior mesenteric ganglion).

(a) Large, vesicle-containing nerve profile showing label in small vesicles and tubules (right), and profiles with unlabelled vesicles (left); note some labelled and some unlabelled large dense-cored vesicles with a narrow halo in the right-hand profile and contrast them with dense-cored vesicles having paler cores and a wider halo in unlabelled vesicle—containing profiles at the lower left and extreme upper right. The latter profile is forming a synapse (partly out of the frame) upon a large dendrite, to which it also has a symmetrical attachment. On its opposite face, the dendrite partly lacks satellite ensheathment and lies here directly under the basal lamina bordering the intraganglionic connective tissue space. Most of the profiles contain a few glycogen particles (see best at lower left).

(b) Synapse upon a dendritic shaft, of which the presynaptic profile contains many small dense-cored vesicles after 5-OHDA loading and some larger vesicles with core asymmetry. The eccentric localization of some cores is probably a consequence of fixation.

(c) Vesicle-containing nerve profile, in which some vesicles are heavily labelled and others show irregularly granular traces of label. The profile also contains several wide sacs of smooth endoplasmic reticulum (s.e.r.) which show irregular specks of label. It lies partly exposed to the basal lamina, and the s.e.r. sacs might represent membrane retrieved after exocytosis of granule contents, labelled by virtue of its retaining an uptake system for catecholamine. Material released from such profiles might act preferentially upon regions of dendrites exposed as in Fig. 4a. Arrangements of the type shown here appear more frequent than synapses from 5-OHDA-labelled profiles in this ganglion. Ganglion acutely labelled *in vitro* by incubation with 5-OHDA in oxygenated Krebs-Henseleit solution at 37°C; osmium fixation. Sections lightly contrasted with lead citrate.

then be used which favours the preservation of cytoplasmic proteins, in addition to retaining the 5-OHDA marker. Other combinations of preloading and fixation have also been employed; for example, Johnson *et al.* (1980b) preloaded cultured sympathetic neurons with noradrenaline and fixed with potassium permanganate; here, the system was an enclosed one and the ambiguities of permanganate fixation were subordinate to the importance of demonstrating dense cores in small synaptic vesicles. Questions of fixation and preloading of small dense-cored vesicles have also been discussed and explored by Rees and Bunge (1974).

Wider possibilities for discrimination are opened up by techniques of immunohistochemistry and immunocytochemistry, not only for neuroactive peptides, as noted earlier, but also for other transmitters such as the catecholamines or 5-hydroxytryptamine (Verhofstad *et al.*, 1981), and for specific enzymes involved in transmitter production, such as dopamine β-hydroxylase (Llewellyn-Smith *et al.*, 1981). Non-specific labelling techniques may also be of value; for example, the intracellular introduction of horseradish peroxidase (Kondo *et al.*, 1980).

Identifications that have so far been established include the following:

(1) After a lesion of preganglionic nerves, for example the cervical sympathetic trunk in the case of the superior cervical ganglion, the type of nerve ending that rapidly degenerates and disappears (Quilliam and Tamarind, 1972; Hámori *et al.*, 1968; Raisman and Matthews, 1972) is one containing small agranular synaptic vesicles which cluster toward the specialized synaptic region, and a smaller number of large dense-cored vesicles about 60–90 nm in diameter with cores of moderate electron-density (Fig. 1). Some of the large dense-cored vesicles may be included in the vesicle cluster or lie close to the presynaptic membrane, but they lie mainly at the periphery of the synaptic vesicle cluster, together with varying numbers of mitochondria, and in the preterminal axon (Figs. 1, 3, 5a, 6; Fig. 5a of Matthews, 1974). This is regarded as the preganglionic autonomic type of cholinergic nerve ending; large dense-cored vesicles are more in evidence than at the motor end-plate of skeletal muscle, where they are rarely seen. The presence of large dense-cored vesicles in a cholinergic ending has hitherto presented an enigma; recent findings, however, suggest at least one possible role for them: they may contain the enkephalin-immunoreactive material which Schultzberg *et al.* (1979) have observed in immunofluorescent intraganglionic nerve networks and have provisionally attributed to preganglionic nerve fibres. The coexistence of two transmitters, or of a transmitter and a neuromodulator, has lately been demonstrated for a number of central nervous pathways (e.g. Chan-Palay *et al.*, 1978; Hökfelt *et al.*, 1978); and in the periphery there is evidence which associates enkephalin immunoreactivity with the known cholinergic spinal innervation of the adrenal medullary chromaffin cells (Schultzberg *et al.*, 1978) and immunoreactivity for vasoactive intestinal

polypeptide with the cholinergic postganglionic innervation of the salivary glands (Lundberg *et al.*, 1980). In the latter site, bursts of stimulation delivered over a given interval have been shown to be more effective in producing non-cholinergic vasodilatation than the same number of stimuli delivered at a continuous rate over the same interval (Anderson *et al.*, 1982), and it thus seems likely that the mobilization of neuropeptide requires a minimum number of nerve impulses at a minimum frequency, which would accord well with the relative infrequency with which large dense-cored vesicles are seen actually in close apposition with the presynaptic membrane.

This type of nerve ending profile, like the preganglionic axons, shows continuous or almost continuous activity for specific acetylcholinesterase along its surface membrane. There is intense activity in the synaptic cleft. Acetylcholinesterase activity is not seen inside the actual nerve terminal, except occasionally and at a low level of activity inside coated vesicles, as if by reuptake of soluble enzyme (Jessen *et al.*, 1978). Postganglionic neurons and their dendrites show specific acetylcholinesterase activity in the cisternae of granular endoplasmic reticulum, regionally between the layers of the nuclear membranes and in some cisternae of the Golgi apparatus, but only patchily at their surface membranes (Somogyi and Chubb, 1976); studies using an irreversible inhibitor of acetylcholinesterase have suggested that the synaptic acetylcholinesterase is of preganglionic origin (Somogyi and Chubb, 1976).

(2) Nerve profiles containing small dense-cored vesicles (Fig. 8c) have not been observed to diminish following preganglionic nerve lesions (Quilliam and Tamarind, 1972; Dail *et al.*, 1980); indeed, in the longer term rather the reverse may apply (see Matthews, 1974; Ramsay and Matthews, unpublished observations). They would therefore appear to be of intrinsic origin. Most of the neurons of sympathetic ganglia are adrenergic, showing histofluorescence for endogenous catecholamines (Eränkö and Härkönen, 1965; Jacobowitz, 1970). Clusters of small vesicles, some with dense cores, are seen in normal ganglia in dendrites and in the soma, near to the surface membrane, there sometimes forming hemisynaptoid configurations. Taxi *et al.* (1969) and Elfvin (1971) noted the association of these clusters of small dense-cored vesicles with sites of dendrodendritic and dendrosomatic attachment, often adjacent to a synapse, pointing out that catecholamine might be released here and act on the membrane of the attached nervous element. In some species, and in some ganglia, a few well-defined synapses are seen in normal material in which the presynaptic element contains small dense-cored vesicles and is not obviously either the dendrite or soma of a principal neuron [guinea-pig hypogastric ganglion (Watanabe, 1971) and inferior mesenteric ganglion (Fig. 4; Baker and Matthews, unpublished observations); rabbit superior cervical ganglion (Dail and Evan, 1978; Dail *et al.*, 1980); rat coeliac-superior mesenteric ganglion (Santer *et al.*, 1980)]. In the prevertebral ganglia, such nerve profiles are also characteristically found lying immediately beneath the

basal lamina, where vesicle contents might be liberated directly into the intraganglionic connective tissue space (Fig. 4c).

While it cannot always be excluded that the presynaptic element is derived from an SGC cell (Matthews, 1976; Dail and Evan, 1978; Williams and Jew this volume), it is likely that many of these are derived instead from other principal neurons in the same ganglion, and represent either specialized regions of dendrites or axon collaterals. Without extensive serial reconstruction it will not be easy to differentiate between these possibilities, as dendritic and axonal morphology overlap: to the extent that profiles contain ribosomes or granular endoplasmic reticulum, or are traceable into continuity with such profiles, they may be identified as dendritic, with the proviso, however, that the axon of a sympathetic neuron not infrequently arises from the basal region of a large dendrite (Cajal, 1911). Cajal distinguished axons on the basis of a relatively large diameter, a smooth contour and a course toward and into nerve bundles leaving the ganglion, and saw such fibres occasionally giving rise to intraganglionic collaterals.

(3) The outgoing or efferent syanapses of SGC cells usually identifiable on morphological criteria. They are discussed in detail in the chapter by Williams and Jew. For further illustrations and discussion see Matthews, 1976.

(4) Intrinsic cholinergic synapses may arise from the small proportion of sympathetic neurons, estimated as not more than 5% in the rat superior cervical ganglion, that are cholinergic (Hill and Hendry, 1977). While there are probably minimal numbers of such synapses *in vivo*, they may increase dramatically *in vitro* among immature neurons under appropriate conditions of culture (Patterson and Chun, 1974; O'Lague *et al.*, 1974; and see chapter by Landis). The discrimination of cholinergic from adrenergic synapses at the ultrastructural level has been made by the use of permanganate fixation to display or exclude the presence of small dense cores in synaptic vesicles (Landis, 1976; Johnson *et al.*, 1976; and see Landis' chapter), and in this situation is importantly capable of being cross-checked with electrophysiological and pharmacological data.

(5) In the prevertebral ganglia, conventional electron microscopy reveals a wide variety of presynaptic profiles, characterized by a predominance of subtly varying large dense-cored vesicles, or large pale-cored vesicles, which is comparable with that seen in the ganglia of the enteric plexuses (Baker and Matthews, unpublished observations; cf. Cook and Burnstock, 1976. Llewellyn-Smith *et al.*, 1981). This is significant in the context of recent immunofluorescence findings (see chapter by Schultzberg *et al.*). Cytochemical studies over the next few years may be expected to lead to considerable clarification of the synaptic relationships of these ganglia. The nerve endings immunoreactive for substance P (Fig. 2b; Connaughton *et al.*, 1983) would seem to fall within this class.

(6) Also in the prevertebral ganglia, some of the presynaptic profiles in

which agranular vesicles predominate show particularly highly pleomorphic, flattened or tubular vesicles, rather than spherical, after aldehyde fixation and these could represent chemically distinct subclasses of synapses (Baker and Matthews, unpublished observations).

NON-SYNAPTIC JUNCTIONS: SYMMETRICAL JUNCTIONS

Specialized attachment sites, of the macula adhaerens or punctum adhaerens type (attachment plaques), involving symmetrical aggregations of intracytoplasmic dense material to a pair of apposed membranes in a region of parallel apposition with an interval of about 20 nm, are of such frequent occurrence in sympathetic ganglia that they must have considerable functional importance. Most are placed between nervous elements (Fig. 5) but a few may be found between nervous profiles and the enclosing satellite cell (e.g. Figs 2, 5; Tamarind and Quilliam, 1971); and short attachments are not uncommon along the course of a mesaxon, sometimes involving successive turns at the same point, or holding together the external or internal end of a mesaxon (Fig. 7c), or placed between a mesaxon and the Schwann or satellite cell surface. Short attachments to the basal lamina are also frequently seen along the free surfaces of satellite cells (Fig. 7c). The gap junctions between satellite cells detected after freeze-fracture by Elfvin and Forsman (1978) have seldom been observed in conventionally sectioned material, possibly because of their small extent. Symmetrical attachments between nervous profiles may be seen to involve dendrites, spines, somata and axon terminals in any combination, with the proviso that non-terminal parts of axons are probably seldom if ever involved and that the cell bodies of principal neurons are rarely in direct apposition. SGC cell somata, on the other hand, are frequently apposed to each other, and may in these regions be linked by extensive series of attachment plaques (e.g. Matthews and Raisman, 1969). The more frequent of the various possibilities have been summarized in a diagram by Elfvin (1971; reproduced in Matthews, 1974).

Some types of synapses are regularly associated with attachment plaques. One such synaptic type is the contact of an SGC cell soma with a relatively large nerve terminal profile which is presynaptic to the SGC cell. Here the two structures are frequently linked by one or more quite long attachment plaques, which together may be considerably more extensive than the specialized synaptic region or regions. As was noted earlier, the synaptic specializations, though multifocal, are short and symmetric, and it would seem that additional attachment is required here for mechanical stability. An efferent synapse from an SGC cell to a large dendrite may likewise show an accessory attachment plaque alongside the synapse. The same applies to some axodendritic synapses, similarly involving a specialized junction between large profiles. In both the latter situations, the synapse is asymmetric and thus may itself already have a greater mechanical stability than a symmetric synapse.

In the case of the afferent synapse to the SGC cell, it is usual to see one or more mitochondria aligned in the presynaptic profile parallel to and at a little distance from the attachment plaque, with a flattened sac or sacs of smooth endoplasmic reticulum, similarly parallel to the attachment plaque, lying in the intervening cytoplasm, which is more or less empty of synaptic vesicles. This arrangement appears likely to have some significance in relation to the energy metabolism required for the maintenance of adhesion at the junction, since mitochondria may be associated in this manner with both sides of a symmetrical attachment (Figs 2a, 3a), and are not infrequently associated with attachment plaques between non-synaptic profiles (Fig. 5b). Mitochondria are, however, also regularly associated with the periphery of a synaptic vesicle cluster, sometimes approaching closer to the presynaptic membrane (e.g. Figs. 1, 2, 3a) and are here presumably involved in the metabolic activity associated with synaptic transmission; and where an attachment plaque lies close to a synapse such mitochondria may gain facultative attachment there.

Another recurrent situation in which an attachment plaque appears as an adjunct to a synapse is illustrated in Fig. 3a, and in Fig. 6b of Matthews (1974); it is a special case of a large dendritic shaft of which the size indicates that it is probably near to its origin from the neuron, receiving a synapse directly on to the shaft from a large presynaptic profile. The synapse shows a row of subjunctional bodies with associated vesicles of smooth endoplasmic reticulum, and an attachment plaque of approximately equal length flanks the synapse at one side. Both this and the preceding example involve large postsynaptic structures, which are likely to have considerable inertia, and in each case a large presynaptic nerve terminal which may be close to its origin from the parent axon; and the morphological arrangements, including the subjunctional dense bodies of the dendritic shaft synapse, suggest the provision of exceptional protection against mechanical distraction. Each case thus carries the implication that the presynaptic nerve fibre has itself an appreciable inertia and is unable to follow freely movements of the post-synaptic structure, and this is interesting, since it suggests a rather direct, unbranched course from the parent axon (cf. Fig. 18 of Matthews and Raisman, 1969), and may indicate that this is an input which would therefore not be subject to much delay or attenuation in propagation through finer intraganglionic ramifications, and which might therefore have a rapid response and a high security of transmission. Proximity of a dendrite to its origin from the cell body would similarly tend to promote security of transmission. Many of the inputs to sympathetic neurons are subthreshold (Weems and Szurzewski, 1978); and the possibility of differentiating ultra-structurally terminations which are likely to have a high security of transmission is thus of some interest in terms of ganglionic physiology.

A third type of association of attachment plaques with synapses is illustrated in Fig. 6. Here, dendritic shafts bearing spine-like projections are apparently entwined by axons which form synapses upon the tips of the spines but are attached to the shafts by attachment plaques. This arrangement suggests the interpretation that the required site of synaptic action is at the apex of the spine, but that the mobility of flexibility of the spines is such that the axon needs to be secured to the dendrite for its own support. Prevention of mechanical disruption of the synapse, or of the spine itself, is less likely to be the major factor here, since the spines are likely to have relatively little inertia and to be capable of flexing and even extending a little to adapt to small movements of a large axon; but a large axon would hardly need extra support from the dendrite, and indeed this axon type (Fig. 6) appears to be a series of varicosities with slender intervaricose segments, which might well need the support of the dendritic shaft. In this case, unlike those discussed above, the immediate synaptic action is more likely to be sub- than suprathreshold, since the site of transmitter release is apparently restricted to the spine tips, away from the dendritic shaft, and the axon is a string of terminal varicosities which may well be subject to delay in impulse propagation, or even under certain conditions to failure of the impulse to invade all varicosities, by some mechanism analogous to that which has been proposed by Stjärne (1978) for adrenergic terminal arborizations.

Other intraganglionic attachment sites may be interpreted as having a mechanical function, without obvious inferences as to their deeper significance. Attachments between nerve terminal profiles (Fig. 5a) are relatively infrequent, and might facilitate transmitter-mediated interactions such as presynaptic inhibition; those between dendrites are numerous (Fig. 5b), and have been postulated by Elfvin as substrates for dendrodendritic interactions. The extensive dendrosomatic attachment of a deeply embedded dendrite (Fig. 5c) is another recurrent pattern (cf. Plate 6c of Matthews and Nelson, 1975); and here the close apposition of sacs of granular endoplasmic reticulum to the surface membrane in the neuron soma along the non-specialized part of the region of contact (Fig. 5c) may provide a clue as to its particular meaning. For example, protein or peptide material might be released here across the soma membrane from the cisternae of endoplasmic reticulum, and might influence the embedded dendrite, either through action at surface receptor sites or via uptake. As and when information becomes available on the distribution of specific receptor sites on neurons, and of release sites for effector molecules, more definite correlations may emerge. Meanwhile, it seems reasonable to infer that dendrites, particularly the long, straight radiating dendrites of some neurons, may gain support from each other and from the cell bodies of neurons across which they pass, and that to a varying extent terminal axons also are additionally fixated by attachment plaques.

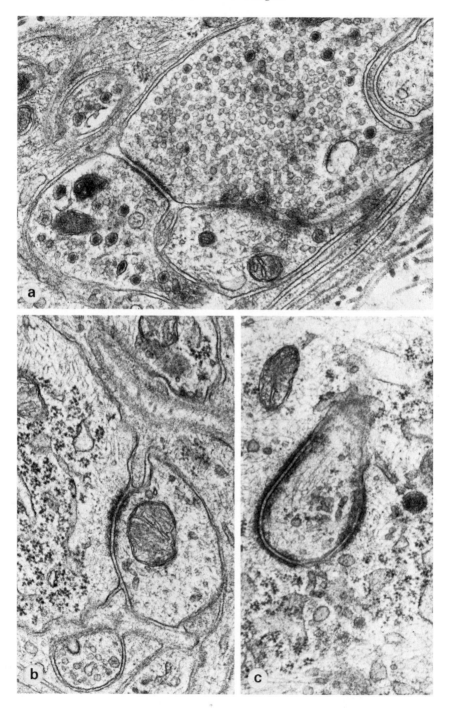

The interesting corollary of the pattern of intraganglionic symmetrical junctions is that the satellite or Schwann cell plays an enveloping but not a restraining role in supporting the neuron, maintaining its own internalized surface membrane-to-membrane relationships by its short attachments along the course of the mesaxon, and securing its attachment to the covering of basal lamina, but seldom becoming attached to neuronal elements, so that slippage and mutual movement are likely to be possible where an axon or dendrite crosses from one supporting cell to another. This is probably very necessary in a ganglion which is placed on the course of a nerve trunk (e.g. the sympathetic chain) and at a point where branches are entering or leaving it (e.g. the rami communicantes), with all the mechanical stresses which may be transmitted along these during movements of the body; in the case of the prevertebral ganglia or the cervical ganglia, transmitted arterial pulsations may also be an important source of mechanical disturbance. The satellite and Schwann cells have many intracytoplasmic filaments, a feature which indicates a highly developed cytoskeleton; and the potentiality for maintenance of shape which this implies, taken together with the internal connective tissue framework of the ganglion, to which they are linked through the basal lamina, may be their major contribution to the mechanical support of the nervous elements. The neuronal attachment plaques would in this case be left with the primary functions of resisting distraction and maintaining focal attachments. The gap junctions between satellite cells, observed by Elfvin and Forsman (1978), are likely to have a metabolically integrative function and to be

Figure 5 Symmetrical attachments between nerve profiles. Rat superior cervical ganglion.
(a) Attachment between two vesicle-containing nerve profiles, one of which is forming a synapse with a dendritic shaft (synaptic junction obliquely cut). This arrangement might mediate presynaptic inhibition, or pre-or postsynaptic facilitation. At its right margin this presynaptic profile also shows a short symmetrical attachment to the surrounding lamella of satellite cytoplasm, and this attachment is carried across to the opposite face of the narrow satellite lamella and on to an adjacent profile. Note the large dense-cored vesicle among the small agranular vesicles clustered at the presynaptic membrane. ×45 000.
(b) Attachment between a large dendrite and a smaller profile, probably a dendrite. Note the mitochondrion adjacent to the junction in the smaller profile. ×42 000. Neither in (a) nor in (b) does the attachment zone occupy the whole of the region of apposition of the two nerve profiles. Regions adjacent to the attachment zone might be sites for other interactions.
(c) A dendrite embedded into the soma of a principal sympathetic neuron and linked with it by extensive attachment zones covering more than half its circumference. A sac of granular endoplasmic reticulum in the principal neuron is closely and perhaps significantly associated with a part of the region of contact not occupied by the attachment zone (above and to right; section here slightly oblique); material might here be discharged at the surface which might influence the dendrite, for example by dendritic uptake.

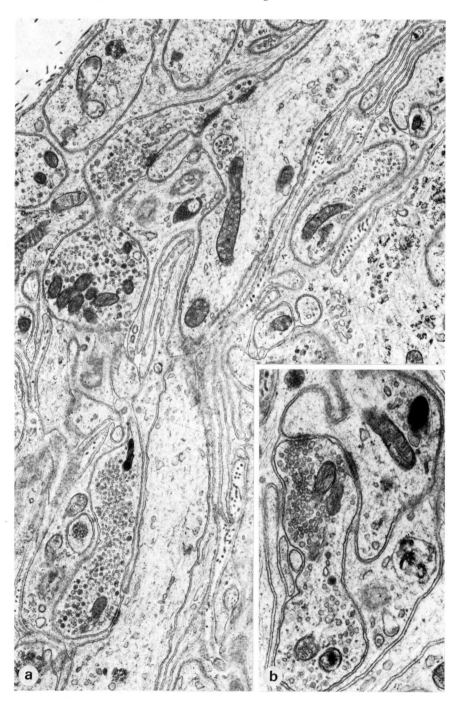

involved in maintaining the collective responsiveness of these cells to the state of the nervous tissue (e.g. Matthews and Raisman, 1972; Matthews and Nelson, 1975).

INDEPENDENCE OR INTERDEPENDENCE OF THE ELEMENTS OF THE JUNCTIONS?

As has been well established, after a preganglionic denervation the terminals of the severed axons undergo a series of characteristic degenerative changes, rapidly lose their attachment to the postsynaptic sites and are digested by the Schwann or satellite cells (Hámori *et al.*, 1968; Raisman and Matthews, 1972; Quilliam and Tamarind, 1972). As is found also in many regions of the central nervous system (Sotelo, 1973), in mature ganglia the specialized features of the postsynaptic site persist for a time, which may be considerable, recognizable and apparently unaltered (Fig. 8; Taxi, 1965; Quilliam and Tamarind, 1972; Raisman *et al.*, 1974), though the reported incidence is less than the previous incidence of synapses. If the preganglionic axons are allowed to regenerate, the incidence of synapses is restored to near its previous level (Raisman *et al.*, 1974; Purves, 1976b), and appropriate spinal levels of preganglionic inputs are re-established (Njå and Purves, 1977, 1978b). It is not clear, however, whether the original postsynaptic sites are preferentially reoccupied. In immature ganglia postsynaptic sites survive denervation less well (Smolen, 1981) or not at all (Smolen and Raisman, 1980), the differences in reported incidence possibly reflecting increased difficulty of detection; and reinnervation is also variable and may be much less complete than in the adult (Smolen and Raisman, 1980; Smolen, 1981); loss of preganglionic neurons could also be involved here.

After a lesion of postganglionic nerves the injured principal neurons become chromatolytic and unresponsive to preganglionic stimulation (Brown and Pascoe, 1954; Matthews and Nelson, 1975; Purves, 1975), losing many or all of their specialized junctions, including both synapses and symmetrical attachments (Matthews and Nelson, 1975; Purves, 1975). The loss of synapses

Figure 6 (a) Longitudinal section of a dendritic shaft and associated trail(s) of axon terminal varicosities, curving in and out of the plane of section. At three points, axon varicosities or intervaricose segments are attached to the dendritic shaft by symmetrical junctions, without distinct synaptic vesicle clustering; near the upper pair of these a well-defined synapse is formed by the same axon on the apex of a spine-like projection from the dendrite. Beneath the base of this spine lie several s.e.r. vesicles and a multivesicular body.

(b, inset) Similar arrangement upon an adjacent dendrite: a varicose axon is linked by a symmetrical attachment with the dendritic shaft (note associated mitochondria in the axon terminal cytoplasm) and forms a synapse near the apex of a spine-like projection from the dendrite. Rat superior cervical ganglion: 1, ×16 500; b, ×31 000.

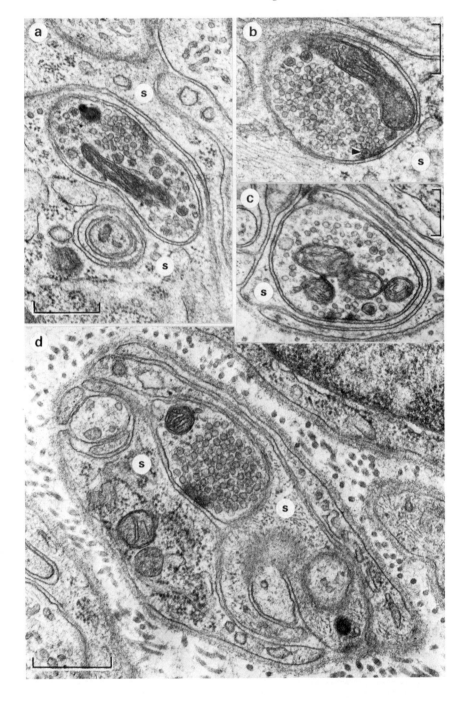

seems to occur by detachment of presynaptic endings from the injured neurons and is apparently non-selective, entailing not only a loss of pregang-lionic-to-postganglionic synapses but also a decrease in the incidence of efferent synapses from intraganglionic SGC cells to principal neurons (Case and Matthews, 1976, 1980; Matthews, 1980b). In this situation of postgang-lionic axotomy, few if any vacant postsynaptic or postattachment sites are found on the principal neurons, even in the short term, and they have evidently been resorbed or dismantled by the injured neurons, possibly even before or during the process of detachment (e.g. Plate 7 of Matthews and Nelson, 1975). Nerve terminal profiles interpreted as detached presynaptic nerve endings, (i.e. showing persistent membrane densities and typical clustering of synaptic vesicles) are, however, seen in the ganglion within the first few weeks following the injury (Fig. 7); they are rarely seen in normal ganglia. These presynaptic profiles are surprisingly normal in appearance, i.e. they do not immediately degenerate or atrophy, although they show an increased incidence of cytoplasmic dense bodies which suggests an altered turnover of components (Matthews and Nelson, 1975). Their incidence decreases postoperatively at a stage when neurons are recovering from chromatolysis and the incidence of synapses is rising again, in a manner which suggests that they may be capable of being reused in the re-establishment of synapses. Persistence of presynaptic specializations following loss of post-synaptic structures has also occasionally been observed in the central nervous system (Sotelo, 1975). The integrity of the postganglionic constitutents of the intraganglionic synapses would seem to depend upon transport in the post-

Figure 7 Detached presynaptic profiles found in rat superior cervical ganglia after injury of postganglionic axons: (a, b) two days, (c) nine days, (d) five days postoperatively. Scale bars indicate 0.5 μm in (a) and (d), 0.3 μm in (b) and (c). The presynaptic profiles show well-defined presynaptic specializations, with clustering of vesicles associated with dense material at the surface membrane [forming separate dense projections in (c)]. The profile shown in (b) has a large dense-cored vesicle in the vesicle cluster at the membrane (arrowhead). Each profile is enveloped in satellite cell cytoplasm (s), and the postsynaptic nervous element of the synapse is lacking; dense material is, however, distinctly present in the cleft between the presynaptic profile and the satellite cell membrane in the region of the membrane specialization in (b) to (d) (densest opposite the focal presynaptic dense projections). There is no definite evidence of any reciprocating membrane specialization in the underlying satellite cell cytoplasm. Satellite cells are none the less capable of forming specialized surface attachments: the upper part of (c) shows a short attachment between the two layers of the mesaxon, just before it opens out to enclose the presynaptic profile, and a short attachment of the satellite cell to the basal lamina is seen on each side of the external end of the mesaxon. Both (c) and (d) enable positive identification of the satellite cell cytoplasm as being the layer which enwraps the nervous elements and separates them across a basal lamina from the connective tissue spaces of the ganglion. Reproduced from Matthews and Nelson (1975), by permission of *Journal of Physiology*.

ganglionic axons, since application of colchicine to postganglionic nerves can mimic the effects of axotomy (Purves, 1976a); specifically, the maintenance of the synapses may depend upon the retrograde axonal transport of nerve growth factor taken up from peripheral target organs (Njå and Purves, 1978a).

The pre- and postsynaptic specializations are therefore not entirely inter-dependent, though they normally develop in specific relationship with each other. Opinions differ as to which appears first during development, whether the membrane densities or the presynaptic vesicle clustering (Westrum, 1975), and the sequence may not be uniform for all sites and for all species (e.g. Hayes and Roberts, 1973; Westrum, 1975); but, for rat sympathetic ganglionic neurons in dissociated neurone culture together with explants of embryonic spinal cord, Rees *et al.* (1976) have observed the following sequence: an initial contact between a growth cone from the spinal cord explant and a sympathetic neuron is followed by hypertrophy of the neuron's Golgi apparatus and increased formation of coated vesicles in its vicinity; the latter are also found in association with the postsynaptic membrane, at which a postsynaptic density now appears; next, a few and gradually more synaptic vesicles appear in the presynaptic profile, to be followed by the formation of a presynaptic density; maturation proceeds by way of an increase of synaptic vesicles, increasing width of the synaptic cleft and increase of the postsynaptic density. Tracer observations indicated that the coated vesicles in this synap-togenic situation were bringing material to the postsynaptic membrane from the Golgi zone, rather than taking up material from the exterior and the cell membrane via coated pit formation and endocytosis.

Most studies of the development of synapses upon mammalian neurons similarly indicate that it is the postsynaptic density which first becomes recognizable, at a stage when the presynaptic profile may have no more than one or two vesicles visible near the junctional membrane in an ultrathin section (see review by Westrum, 1975); Pick *et al* (1964) have illustrated such a stage of synaptic development as the only synapse found in sympathetic ganglia from a 15- and a 17-week human foetus.

It might thus be thought not unreasonable to survey incidences of develop-ing synapses by using a stain for synaptic densities alone, e.g. ethanolic phosphotungstic acid (E–PTA), which displays the membrane-associated dense material both of synapses and of attachment plaques (Bloom and Aghajanian, 1968), as was in fact done for the mouse superior cervical ganglion by Black *et al.* (1971). A study by Burry and Lasher (1978), however, in which the E–PTA method was compared with conventional staining techniques, has shown that counts of developing synapses (in cultures of rat cerebellum) were at all stages lower in the E–PTA-stained material, and this is probably largely attributable to the reduction in the number of criteria available for synapse identification which is inherent in the E–PTA method, though partly also to the finding that synaptic densities as visualized after E–PTA were shorter than after conventional staining. A similar disability attaches to the identification of persistent, detached or denervated, pre- or postsynaptic specializations, and is one of the considerations which must be borne in mind in evaluating numerical comparisons of their incidence with the incidence of intact synapses, after recovery or in control material (cf. Matthews and Nelson, 1975).

In the central nervous system, genetic abnormalities affecting the mouse cerebellum have permitted the observation that either the presynaptic (rarely) or the postsynaptic specialization (abundantly) may develop in the absence of the other elements (Sotelo, 1973). For the sympathetic ganglion it is possible to denervate neonatally before most of the synapses have formed, and it seems that here the postsynaptic density does not develop freely in the absence of the presynaptic element (rat superior cervical ganglion: Smolen, 1981).

LABILITY AND PLASTICITY OF SYNAPSES

As will be seen from the foregoing, in the adult principal sympathetic neuron there is some capacity for regulation of synaptic inputs, in that synapses are shed during chromatolysis and resumed during recovery, and very reasonably accurate restoration of inputs can occur by nerve regeneration following a preganglionic denervation. In the adult fully differentiated state, disturbance of the synaptic relationships of the principal neurons is followed by a strong tendency to restoration of the original state, within the limits imposed by the prevailing situation: the capacity for a change in transmitter type, found during a critical period in the young incompletely differentiated neuron, is strictly limited thereafter (Johnson *et al.*, 1980a). In respect of the interneuron-like SGC cells, however, there is much more scope for modification of synapses: in axotomized ganglia the decrease in incidence of the efferent synapses from SGC cells to the injured principal neurons is accompanied by a transient increase in the incidence of synaptic contacts between SGC cells and a more sustained increase in their synaptic inputs from preganglionic nerve fibres (Case and Matthews, 1976, 1980). A similar increase in the preganglionic inputs to SGC cells is seen also in the contralateral uninjured ganglia, after a unilateral axotomy (Case and Matthews, 1980). In this latter behaviour, the preganglionic axons seem to resemble frog somatic motor axons, which sprout bilaterally following unilateral denervation of a superficial trunk muscle (Rotshenker and McMahan, 1976), and the SGC cells are behaving like interneurons rather than like principal neurons, which do not seem to show so much flexibility in the number of inputs they will accept (Matthews, 1980b).

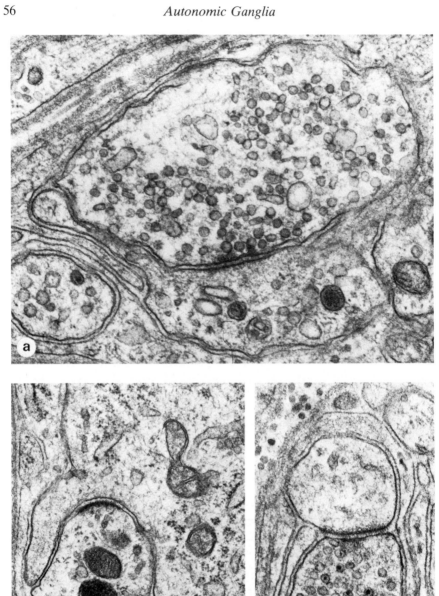

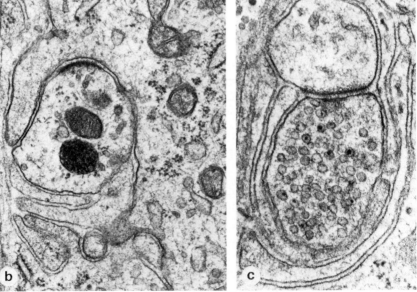

FORMATION OF HETEROTYPIC JUNCTIONS

Experiments involving ultrastructural study after anastomosis of the central end of the vagus or a somatic motor nerve (hypoglossal, or the nerve to sternohyoid) to the distal end of the divided cervical sympathetic trunk have indicated that the vagus forms fairly abundant synapses in the superior cervical ganglion (Ostberg *et al.*, 1976; Purves, 1976b), though not so many as are formed after reinnervation by the original preganglionic axons, but that the hypoglossal or the sternohyoid nerve forms relatively few synapses (McLachlan, 1974; Ostberg *et al.*, 1976). Nerve endings in the vagally innervated ganglion have not been found to differ in any major respect, either in extent of specialized synaptic region or in general appearance, from those in normal ganglia, although their synaptic action is weaker (Purves, 1976b), and this is interesting in view of the fact that the vagus is a source of cholinergic preganglionic parasympathetic nerve fibres, apart from its sensory and skeletomotor nerve fibres. Nerve endings in ganglia innervated from the hypoglossal or sternohyoid nerve, however, include some which are unlike any in normal ganglia (Fig. 8a; McLachlan, 1974; Ostberg *et al.*, 1976; Matthews, unpublished observations) and have characteristics which link them with the typical large nerve ending of the mammalian motor end-plate. These nerve endings form morphologically specialized synaptic junctions with postganglionic profiles, sometimes with a dendritic shaft but often with one or

Figure 8 (a) Synapse on to a dendritic shaft, from a ganglion six weeks after anastomosis of the central end of the hypoglossal nerve to the distal peripheral end of the severed cervical sympathetic trunk. The presynaptic profile is of a type not seen in normal ganglia, derived from a hypoglossal axon. Large axons containing similar organelles coursed through the ganglion, from the transplanted hypoglossal nerve. The presynaptic vesicles are relatively large but show a considerable range of sizes; there are also several larger expanded sacs of s.e.r. and a few microtubules and filaments. The synapse is asymmetrical, though not strongly so, and the dendrite extends a slender spur or flange part-way round the presynaptic profile. The postsynaptic cytoplasm contains irregular s.e.r. vesicles, small multivesicular bodies and a small dense body. ×58 400.
(b) Persistent postsynaptic specialization, upon a dendritic shaft, 13 months after preganglionic denervation with hypoglossal anastomosis. The dendrite has become apposed to a neuron soma, and is partly enveloped by a short process. Not only does the subsynaptic dense material persist, but also the external surface of the specialized membrane retains a fuzzy coat, which almost fills the interval between the dendrite and the neuron soma; this interval is very regular, as at the synapse, and is greater than the interval between adjacent non-specialized regions of the apposed membranes. Small vesicles are associated with the deep aspect of the postsynaptic dense material, and a mitochondrion and a mutivesicular body (dark) lie in the subjacent cytoplasm. In the neuron soma, a rather well-defined cytoplasmic web of fine filaments apposes the specialized region of the dendrite, as if it might have been induced there. ×37 000.
(c) Synapse from a profile containing small dense-cored vesicles (osmium fixation, no preloading) to a probable dendritic shaft, in a ganglion 15.5 months after preganglionic denervation with hypoglossal anastomosis; this synapse is quite unlike a hypoglossal synapse and is presumably of intrinsic origin. ×49 400.

several spine-like profiles. Apart from a few associated sensory and postgang-lionic sympathetic nerve fibres, the hypoglossal is a pure somatic motor nerve, and it is likely that these are somatic motor nerve endings. Thus, a nerve fibre whose endings normally form junctions by establishing an attachment across a basal lamina to a skeletal muscle fibre membrane is capable of forming close synaptic junctions with dendritic membranes without the intervention of any basal lamina.

These synapses are not numerous and are thus not readily formed. There may be problems of access for these somatic motor axons to suitable postganglionic sites, but they should not be greater than for the vagus nerve after a similar anastomosis. The dendritic membrane of the sympathetic neuron is, however, clearly not identical with the junctional surface membrane of the skeletal muscle fibre, and presumably differs from it more than from the parasympathetic postganglionic neurons which are the normal synaptic targets of autonomic motor fibres in the vagus nerve. For example, the nicotinic cholinergic receptor of the sympathetic ganglion is different from that of skeletal muscle: it is differentially excitable by tetramethylammonium, and more readily blockable by hexamethonium (e.g. Burgen and Mitchell, 1972), and it is not blocked by α-bungarotoxin (Brown and Fumagalli, 1977). The acetylcholine receptor is not necessarily the recognition factor utilized by the nerve fibre in the formation of the synapse, since reinnervation in muscle can occur in the presence of continuous receptor blockade with α-bungarotoxin (Jansen and van Essen, 1975), but if the receptor complex is different then other aspects of the postjunctional membrane are also likely to be different in the two sites. It is therefore of interest that the incidence per neuron of 'foreign' hypoglossal synapses after twelfth nerve anastomosis is significantly greater in ganglia in which the neurons have been injured by a postganglionic crush lesion at the time of anastomosis than in ganglia not thus injured (Matthews and Ramsay, 1980), and a discrepancy remains even after allowance has been made for neuronal loss following axotomy. The incidence of synapses of intrinsic, adrenergic type is also greater after this manoeuvre. It is possible that the chromatolytic state of the neuron which is regenerating its axon enhances some capacity for remodelling, or leads to a less differentiated state, of the postsynaptic membrane or of the somadendritic membrane in general, which allows it to be modified, albeit to a limited extent, by interactions with potential sources of synaptic input. Such a property in an adult neuron might have some adaptive significance. It might also reflect greater potentialities existing during development and the initial formation of synaptic connexions.

SUMMARY AND COMMENT

The use of the electron microscope can reveal the situation and general character of intraganglionic specialized junctions; for example, the nature of the structures involved, their features and organelle content, whether the junctions are synaptically polarized and in which direction, or whether they are symmetric attachments of the macula adhaerens type. The ultrastructural features of junctions may present clues as to their nature and possible functional importance. Markers are of particular importance in the peripheral nervous system, for this lacks both the geometrical precision of repeating patterns and the geographical advantages of highly ordered topographical organization, which exist in many parts of the central nervous system. Transmitter- or neuromodulator-specific markers visible only by light micros-copy, such as catecholamine fluorescence or specific immunofluorescence, have a limited value, in a preliminary, scanning sense, as they are not necessarily restricted in their distribution to nerve endings and cannot indicate, in the mammalian sympathetic ganglion with its highly interwoven multipolar neurons, what are the precise sites of junctions and nerve terminations. The ultrastructural counterparts of such markers are, however, particularly useful. Ultrastructural markers, and the use of experimental nerve lesions and other perturbations, in correlation with physiological and pharmacological studies, are permitting the gradual unravelling of the synaptic relationships existing in normal ganglia and revealing possibilities for modification of these relationships under experimental conditions, which throw light on factors involved in their normal maintenance or development. Quantitative studies may be of particular value here. The ultrastructural discrimination of adrenergic from cholinergic synapses has complemented physiological and biochemical studies of factors influencing the differentia-tion of sympathetic neurons as to transmitter type, in cultures of dissociated immature neurons.

There is still much that is uncertain, however, not only as between ganglia in different regions of the sympathetic system, and as between the same ganglion in different species, but also in respect of the nature of transmitters and the molecular and functional organization of junctions.

Moreover, interactions between nervous elements are almost certainly not confined to morphologically specialized junctions, and there is additional scope for the future in the localization of receptor sites, both junctional and extrajunctional, and the mapping of neuronal membranes. Recent methodo-logic developments may be expected to lead to significant advances over the next few years.

ACKNOWLEDGEMENTS

The author gratefully acknowledges research support from the Medical Research Council, the Wellcome Trust and the Royal Society. Thanks are due for certain electron micrographs: to Dr D. A. Ramsay for Fig. 3a and to Dr S. C. Baker for Fig. 4b; for technical assistance, to Mr P. J. Belk; for photographic work to Messrs B. Archer, A. C. Barclay and Miss J. Lloyd; and for secretarial assistance to Miss J. Ballinger and Miss G. Davis.

REFERENCES

Akert, K., Moor, H., Pfenninger, K., and Sandri, C. (1969). Contributions of new impregnation methods and freeze etching to the problem of synaptic fine structure. *Prog. Brain Res.*, **31**, 223–240.

Anderson, P.-O., Bloom, S. R., Edwards, A. V., and Järhult, J. (1982). Effects of stimulation of the chorda tympani in bursts on submaxillary responses in the cat. *J. Physiol. (London)*, **322**, 469–483.

Baker, S. C., Cuello, A. C., and Matthews, M. R. (1980). Substance P-containing synapses in a sympathetic ganglion, and their possible origin as collaterals from sensory nerve fibres. *J. Physiol. (London)*, **308**, 76P–77P.

Black, I. B., Hendry, I. A., and Iversen, L. L. (1971). Trans-synaptic regulation of growth and development of adrenergic neurones in a mouse sympathetic ganglion. *Brain Res.*, **34**, 229–240.

Bloom, F. E., and Aghajanian, G. K. (1968). Fine structural and cytochemical analysis of the staining of synaptic junctions with phosphotungstic acid. *J. Ultrastruct. Res.*, **22**, 361–375.

Bowers, C. W., and Zigmond, R. E. (1979). Localization of neurons in the rat superior cervical ganglion that project into different postganglionic trunks. *J. Comp. Neurol.*, **185**, 381–392.

Brooks, C. McC., Koizumi, K., and Sato, A. (Eds.) (1979). *Integrative Functions of the Autonomic Nervous System*, University of Tokyo Press and Elsevier/North-Holland, Amsterdam.

Brown, D. A., and Fumagalli, L. (1977). Dissociation of α-bungarotoxin binding and receptor block in the rat superior cervical ganglion. *Brain Res.*, **129**, 165–168.

Brown, G. L., and Pascoe, J. E. (1954). The effect of degenerative section of ganglionic axons on transmission through the ganglion. *J. Physiol. (London)*, **123**, 565–573.

Burgen, A. S. V., and Mitchell, J. F. (1972). *Gaddum's Pharmacology*, 7th edn., Oxford University Press, London.

Burry, R. W., and Lasher, R. S. (1978). A quantitative electron microscopic study of synapse formation in dispersed cell cultures of rat cerebellum stained either by Os-UL or by E-PTA. *Brain Res.*, **147**, 1–15.

Cajal, S. Ramon y (1911). *Histologie du Systeme Nerveux de L'Homme et des Vertébrés*, Vol. II, Maloine, Paris.

Case, C. P., and Matthews, M. R. (1976). Effects of postganglionic axotomy on synaptic connexions of small granule-containing (SG) cells in the rat superior cervical ganglion. *J. Anat.*, **122**, 732.

Case, C. P., and Matthews, M. R. (1980). Bilateral synaptic changes involving small granule-containing cells in the rat superior cervical ganglion after unilateral post-ganglionic axotomy. *J. Physiol. (London)*, **301**, 58P–59P.

Chan-Palay, V., Jonsson, G., and Palay, S. L. (1978). Serotonin and substance P coexist in neurons of the rat's central nervous system. *Proc. Natl. Acad. Sci. U.S.A.*, **75**, 1582–1586.

Chiba, T., Black, A. C., Jr., and Williams, T. H. (1977). Evidence for dopamine-storing interneurons and paraneurons in rhesus monkey sympathetic ganglia. *J. Neurocytol.*, **6**, 441–453.

Chung, J. M., Chung, K., and Wurster, R. D. (1975). Sympathetic preganglionic neurons of the cat spinal cord: horseradish peroxidase study. *Brain Res.*, **91**, 126–131.

Chung, K., Chung, J. M., Lavelle, F. W., and Wurster, R. D. (1979). Sympathetic neurons in the cat spinal cord projecting to the stellate ganglion. *J. Comp. Neurol.*, **185**, 23–30.

Connaughton, M., Cuello, A. C. and Matthews, M. R. (1983). Synaptic networks formed by substance P-immunoreactive sensory nerve fibres in guinea-pig prevertebral sympathetic ganglia. *J. Physiol. (London)*, **334**, 96P–97P.

Cook, R. D., and Burnstock, G. (1976). The ultrastructure of Auerbach's plexus in the guinea-pig: I. Neuronal elements. *J. Neurocytol.*, **5**, 171–194.

Crowcroft, P. J., Holman, M. E., and Szurszewski, J. H. (1971). Excitatory input from the distal colon to the inferior mesenteric ganglion in the guinea-pig. *J. Physiol. (London)*, **219**, 443–461.

Crowcroft, P. J., and Szurszewski, J. H. (1971). A study of the inferior mesenteric and pelvic ganglia of guinea-pigs with intracellular electrodes. *J. Physiol. (London)*, **219**, 421–441.

Cuello, A. C., Galfré, G., and Milstein, C. (1979). Detection of substance P in the central nervous system by a monoclonal antibody. *Proc. Natl. Acad. Sci. U.S.A.*, **76**, 3532–3536.

Dail, W. G., and Evan, A. P. (1978). Ultrastructure of adrenergic nerve terminals and SIF cells in the superior cervical ganglion of the rabbit. *Brain Res.*, **148**, 469–477.

Dail, W. G., Koudhary, S., Barraza, C., Murray, H. M., and Bradley, C. (1980). The fate of adrenergic fibres which enter the superior cervical ganglion. In *Histochemistry and Cell Biology of Autonomic Neurons, SIF Cells and Paraneurons* (Eds. O. Eränkö, S. Soinila and H. Päivärinta), *Advances in Biochemical Psychopharmacology*, Vol. 25, Raven Press, New York.

Dalsgaard, C.-J., and Elfvin, L.-G. (1979). Spinal origin of preganglionic fibres projecting onto the superior cervical ganglion and inferior mesenteric ganglion of the guinea pig, as demonstrated by the horseradish peroxidase technique. *Brain Res.*, **172**, 139–143.

De Castro, F. (1932). Sympathetic ganglia: normal and pathological. In *Cytology and Cellular Pathology of the Nervous System* (Ed. W. Penfield), pp. 319–379. Hoeber, New York.

Eccles, J. C. (1935a). The action potential of the superior cervical ganglion. *J. Physiol. (London)*, **85**, 179–206.

Eccles, J. C. (1935b). Facilitation and inhibition in the superior cervical ganglion. *J. Physiol. (London)*, **85**, 207–238.

Eccles, R. M., and Libet, B. (1961). Origin and blockade of the synaptic responses of curarized sympathetic ganglia. *J. Physiol. (London)*, **157**, 484–503.

Elfvin, L.-G. (1963a). The ultrastructure of the superior cervical sympathetic ganglion of the cat. I. The structure of the ganglion cell processes as studied by serial sections. *J. Ultrastruct. Res.*, **8**, 403–440.

Elfvin, L.-G. (1963b). The ultrastructure of the superior cervical sympathetic ganglion of the cat. II. The structure of the preganglionic end fibres and the synapses as studied by serial sections. *J. Ultrastruct. Res.*, **8**, 441–476.

Elfvin, L.-G. (1971). Ultrastructural studies on the synaptology of the inferior mesenteric ganglion of the cat. I–III. *J. Ultrastruct. Res.*, **37**, 411–448.

Elfvin, L.-G. (1976). The ultrastructure of neuronal contacts. *Prog. Neurobiol.*, **8**, 45–79.

Elfvin, L.-G., and Forsman, C. (1978). The ultrastructure of junctions between satellite cells in mammalian sympathetic ganglia as revealed by freeze-etching. *J. Ultrastruct. Res.*, **63**, 261–274.

Eränkö, O. (Ed.) (1976). *SIF Cells: Structure and Function of the Small, Intensely Fluorescent Sympathetic Cells, Fogarty International Center Proceedings*, Vol. 30, US Government Printing Office, Washington, DC.

Eränkö, O., and Härkönen, M. (1965). Monoamine-containing small cells in the superior cervical ganglion of the rat and an organ composed of them. *Acta Physiol. Scand.*, **63**, 511–512.

Gray, E. G. (1963). Electron microscopy of presynaptic organelles of the spinal cord. *J. Anat.*, **97**, 101–106.

Hámori, J., Láng, E., and Simon, L. (1968). Experimental degeneration of the preganglionic fibres in the superior cervical ganglion of the cat. *Z. Zellforsch. Mikrosk. Anat.*, **90**, 37–52.

Hayes, B. P., and Roberts, A. (1973). Synaptic junction development in the spinal cord of an amphibian embryo: an electron microscope study. *Z. Zellforsch. Mikrosk. Anat.*, **137**, 251–269.

Hill, C. E., and Hendry, I. A. (1977). Development of neurons synthesizing noradrenaline and acetylcholine in the superior cervical ganglion of the rat *in vivo* and *in vitro*. *Neuroscience*, **2**, 741–749.

Hökfelt, T. (1971). Distribution of noradrenaline storing particles in peripheral adrenergic neurons as revealed by electron microscopy. *Acta Physiol. Scand.*, **76**, 427–440.

Hökfelt, T., and Jonsson, G. (1968). Studies on reaction and binding of monoamines after fixation and processing for electron microscopy with special reference to fixation with potassium permanganate. *Histochemie*, **16**, 45–67.

Hökfelt, T., Kellerth, J.-O., Nilsson, G., and Pernow, B. (1975). Experimental immunohistochemical studies on the localization and distribution of substance P in cat primary sensory neurons. *Brain Res.*, **100**, 235–252.

Hökfelt, T., Elfvin, L.-G., Schultzberg, M., Goldstein, M., and Nilsson, G. (1977). On the occurrence of substance P-containing fibres in sympathetic ganglia: immuno-histochemical evidence. *Brain Res.*, **132**, 29–41.

Hökfelt, T., Ljungdahl, Å., Steinbusch, H., Verhofstad, A., Nilsson, G., Brodin, E., Pernow, B., and Goldstein, M. (1978). Immunohistochemical evidence of substance P-like immunoreactivity in some 5-hydroxytryptamine-containing neurons in the rat central nervous system. *Neuroscience*, **3**, 517–538.

Ivanov, D. P. (1974). Recherches ultrastructurales sur les cellules paraganglionnaires du ganglion coeliaque du rat et leurs connexions avec les neurones. *Acta Anat.*, **89**, 266–286.

Jacobowitz, D. (1970). Catecholamine fluorescence studies of adrenergic neurones and chromaffin cells in sympathetic ganglia. *Fed. Proc.*, **29**, 1929–1944.

Jansen, J. K. S., and van Essen, D. C. (1975). Reinnervation of rat skeletal muscle in the presence of α-bungarotoxin. *J. Physiol. (London)*, **250**, 651–667.

Jessen, K. R., Chubb, I. W., and Smith, A. D. (1978). Intracellular localization of acetylcholinesterase in nerve terminals and capillaries of the rat superior cervical ganglion. *J. Neurocytol.*, **7**, 145–154.

Jew, J. Y. (1980). Connections of local circuit neurons in guinea pig and rabbit superior cervical ganglia. In *Histochemistry and Cell Biology of Autonomic Neurons, SIF Cells and Paraneurons* (Eds. O. Eränkö, S. Soinila and H. Päivärinta), *Advances in Biochemical Psychopharmacology*, Vol. 25, pp. 119–126, Raven Press, New York.

Johnson, M., Ross, D., Meyers, M., Rees, R., Bunge, R., Wakshull, E., and Burton, H. (1976). Synaptic vesicle cytochemistry changes when cultured sympathetic neurones develop cholinergic interactions. *Nature*, **262**, 308–310.

Johnson, M. I., Ross, C. D., and Bunge, R. P. (1980a). Morphological and biochemical studies on the development of cholinergic properties in cultured sympathetic neurons. II. Dependence on postnatal age. *J. Cell Biol.*, **84**, 692–704.

Johnson, M. I., Ross, C. D., Meyers, M., Spitznagel, E. L., and Bunge, R. P. (1980b). Morphological and biochemical studies on the development of cholinergic properties in cultured adrenergic neurons. I. Correlative changes in choline acetyltransferase and synaptic vesicle cytochemistry. *J. Cell Biol.*, **84**, 680–691.

Joó, F., Lever, J. D., Ivens, C., Mottram, D. R., and Presley, R. (1971). A fine structural and electron histochemical study of axon terminals in the rat superior cervical ganglion after acute and chronic preganglionic denervation. *J. Anat.*, **110**, 181–189.

Kanerva, L., Hervonen, A., and Grönblad, M. (1980). Observations on the ultrastructural localization of monoamines with permanganate fixation. In *Histochemistry and Cell Biology of Autonomic Neurons, SIF cells and Paraneurons* (Eds. O. Eränkö, S. Soinila and H. Päivärinta), *Advances in Biochemical Psychopharmacology*, Vol. 25, pp. 279–285, Raven Press, New York.

Kondo, H. (1977). Innervation of SIF cells in the superior cervical and nodose ganglia: an ultrastructural study with serial sections. *Biol. Cell.*, **30**, 253–264.

Kondo, H., Dun, N. J., and Pappas, G. D. (1980). A light and electron microscopic study of the rat superior cervical ganglion cells by intracellular HRP-labelling. *Brain Res.*, **197**, 193–199.

Konishi, S., Tsunoo, A., and Otsuka, M. (1979). Substance P and noncholinergic excitatory synaptic transmission in guinea pig sympathetic ganglia. *Proc. Jpn. Acad. Ser. B.*, **55**, 525–530.

Konishi, S., Tsunoo, A., Yanaihara, N., and Otsuka, M. (1980). Peptidergic excitatory and inhibitory synapses in mammalian sympathetic ganglia: roles of substance P and enkephalin. *Biomed. Res.*, **1**, 528–536.

Kreulen, D. L., and Szurszewski, J. H. (1979). Reflex pathways in the abdominal prevertebral ganglia: evidence for a colo-colonic inhibitory reflex. *J. Physiol. (London)*, **295**, 21–32.

Landis, S. C. (1976). Rat sympathetic neurons and cardiac myocytes developing in microcultures: correlation of the fine structure of endings with neurotransmitter function in single neurons. *Proc. Natl. Acad. Sci. U.S.A.*, **73**, 4220–4224.

Langley, J. N., and Dickinson, W. L. (1889). On the local paralysis of peripheral ganglia and on the connexion of different classes of nerve fibres with them. *Proc. R. Soc. London*, **46**, 423–431.

Llewellyn-Smith, I. J., Wilson, A. J., Furness, J. B., Costa, M., and Rush, R. A. (1981) Ultrastructural identification of noradrenergic axons and their distribution within the enteric plexuses of the guinea-pig small intestine. *J. Neurocytol.*, **10**, 331–352.

Lundberg, J. M., Änggrd, A., Fährenkrug, J., Hökfelt, T., and Mutt, V. (1980). Vasoactive intestinal polypeptide in cholinergic neurones of exocrine glands: functional significance of coexisting transmitters for vasodilatation and secretion. *Proc. Natl. Acad. Sci. U.S.A.*, **77**, 1651–1655.

Mains, R. E., and Patterson, P. H. (1973). Primary cultures of dissociated sympathetic neurons. *J. Cell Biol.*, **59**, 329–366.

Matthews, M. R. (1971). Evidence from degeneration experiments for the preganglionic origin of afferent fibres to the small granule-containing cells of the rat superior cervical ganglion. *J. Physiol. (London)*, **218**, 95P–96P.

Matthews, M. R. (1974). Ultrastructure of ganglionic junctions. In *The Peripheral Nervous System* (Ed. J. I. Hubbard), pp. 111–150. Plenum, New York.

Matthews, M. R. (1976). Synaptic and other relationships of small granule-containing cells (SIF cells) in sympathetic ganglia. In *Chromaffin, Enterochromaffin and Related Cells* (Eds. R. Coupland and T. Fujita), pp. 131–146, Elsevier, Amsterdam.

Matthews, M. R. (1980a). Ultrastructural studies relevant to the possible functions of small granule-containing cells in the rat superior cervical ganglion. In *Histochemistry and Cell Biology of Autonomic Neurons, SIF Cells and Paraneurons* (Eds. O. Eränkö, S. Soinila and H. Päivärinta), *Advances in Biochemical Psychopharmacology*, Vol. 25, pp. 77–86, Raven Press, New York.

Matthews, M. R. (1980b). Dissociation and new formation of synapses in adult sympathetic ganglia. In *Ontogenesis and Functional Mechanisms of Peripheral Synapses* (Ed. J. Taxi), pp. 27–39, Elsevier, Amsterdam.

Matthews, M. R., and Cuello, A. C. (1982). Substance P-immunoreactive peripheral branches of sensory neurones innervate guinea-pig sympathetic neurones. *Proc. Natl. Acad. Sci. U.S.A.*, **79**, 1668–1672.

Matthews, M. R., and Nelson, V. H. (1975). Detachment of structurally intact nerve endings from chromatolytic neurones of rat superior cervical ganglion during the depression of synaptic transmission induced by postganglionic axotomy. *J. Physiol. (London)*, **245**, 91–135.

Matthews, M. R., and Ostberg, A.-J. C. (1973). Effects of preganglionic nerve section upon the afferent innervation of the small granule-containing cells in the rat superior cervical ganglion. *Acta Physiol. Pol.*, **24**, 215–224.

Matthews, M. R., and Raisman, G. (1969). The ultrastructure and somatic efferent synapses of small granule-containing cells in the superior cervical ganglion. *J. Anat.*, **105**, 255–282.

Matthews, M. R., and Raisman, G. (1972). A light and electron microscopic study of the cellular response to axonal injury in the superior cervical ganglion of the rat. *Proc. R. Soc. Lond. B.*, **181**, 43–79.

Matthews, M. R., and Ramsay, D. A. (1980). Evidence that chromatolysis enhances heterotypic innervation of sympathetic neurones. *J. Physiol. (London)*, **307**, 15P–16P.

McLachlan, E. M. (1974). The formation of synapses in mammalian sympathetic ganglia reinnervated with preganglionic or somatic nerves. *J. Physiol. (London)*, **237**, 217–242.

Milhaud, M., and Pappas, G. D. (1966). Post-synaptic bodies in the habenula and interpeduncular nuclei of the cat. *J. Cell Biol.*, **30**, 437–441.

Mugnaini, E. (1970). The relation between cytogenesis and the formation of different types of synaptic contact. *Brain Res.*, **17**, 169–179.

Njå, A., and Purves, D. (1977). Reinnervation of guinea-pig superior cervical ganglion cells by preganglionic fibres arising from different levels of the spinal cord. *J. Physiol. (London)*, **272**, 633–651.

Njå, A., and Purves, D. (1978a). The effects of nerve growth factor and its antiserum on synapses in the superior cervical ganglion of the guinea-pig. *J. Physiol. (London)*, **277**, 53–75.

Njå, A., and Purves, D. (1978b). Specificity of initial synaptic contacts made on guinea-pig superior cervical ganglion cells during regeneration of the cervical sympathetic trunk. *J. Physiol. (London)*, **281**, 45–62.

O'Lague, P. H., Obata, K., Claude, P., Furshpan, E. J., and Potter, D. D. (1974). Evidence for cholinergic synapses between dissociated rat sympathetic neurons in cell culture. *Proc. Natl. Acad. Sci. U.S.A.*, **71**, 3602–3606.

Ostberg, A.-J. C., Raisman, G., Field, P. M., Iversen, L. L., and Zigmond, R. E. (1976). A quantitative comparison of the formation of synapses in the rat superior cervical sympathetic ganglion by its own and by foreign nerve fibres. *Brain Res.*, **107**, 445–470.

Patterson, P. H., and Chun, L. L. Y. (1974). The influence of non-neuronal cells on catecholamine and acetylcholine synthesis and accumulation in cultures of dissociated sympathetic neurons. *Proc. Natl. Acad. Sci. U.S.A.*, **71**, 3607–3610.

Peters, A., Palay, S. L., and Webster, H. de F. (1976). *The Fine Structure of the Nervous System. The Neurons and Supporting Cells*, 2nd edn., W. B. Saunders, Philadelphia.

Petras, J. M., and Faden, A. I. (1978). The origin of sympathetic preganglionic neurons in the dog. *Brain Res.*, **144**, 353–357.

Pick, J., Gerdin, C., and De Lemos, C. (1964). An electron microscopical study of developing sympathetic neurons in man. *Z. Zellforsch Mikrosk. Anat.*, **62**, 402–415.

Purves, D. (1975). Functional and structural changes of mammalian sympathetic neurones following interruption of their axons. *J. Physiol. (London)*, **252**, 429–463.

Purves, D. (1976a). Functional and structural changes in mammalian sympathetic neurones following colchicine application to post-ganglion nerves. *J. Physiol. (London)*, **259**, 159–175.

Purves, D. (1976b). Competitive and non-competitive reinnervation of mammalian sympathetic neurones following interruption of their axons. *J. Physiol. (London)*, **261**, 453–475.

Quilliam, J. D., and Tamarind, J. P. (1972). Electron microscopy of degenerative changes in decentralized rat superior cervical ganglia. *Micron*, **3**, 454–472.

Raisman, G., and Matthews, M. R. (1972). Degeneration and regeneration of synapses. In *The Structure and Function of Nervous Tissue* (Ed. G. H. Bourne), Vol. IV, pp. 61–104, Academic Press, New York.

Raisman, G., Field, P. M., Ostberg, A. J. C., Iversen, L. L., and Zigmond, R. E. (1974). A quantitative ultrastructural and biochemical analysis of the process of reinnervation of the superior cervical ganglion in the adult rat. *Brain Res.*, **71**, 1–16.

Rees, R., and Bunge, R. P. (1974). Morphological and cytochemical studies of synapses formed in culture between isolated rat superior cervical ganglion neurones. *J. Comp. Neurol.*, **157**, 1–11.

Rees, R., Bunge, M. B., and Bunge, R. P. (1976). Morphological changes in the neuritic growth cone and target neuron during synaptic junction development in culture. *J. Cell Biol.*, **68**, 240–263.

Richardson, K. C. (1966). Electron microscopic identification of autonomic nerve endings. *Nature*, **210**, 756.

Rotshenker, S., and McMahan, U. J. (1976). Altered patterns of innervation in frog muscle after denervation. *J. Neurocytol.*, **5**, 719–730.

Santer, R. M., Lever, J. D., Lu, K. S., and Palmer, S. A. (1980). Ultrastructural studies on rat sympathetic ganglia after 5-hydroxydopamine administration. In *Histochemistry and Cell Biology of Autonomic Neurons, SIF Cells and Paraneurons* (Eds. O. Eränkö, S. Soinila and H. Päivärinta), *Advances in Biochemical Psychopharmacology*, Vol. 25, pp. 299–305, Raven Press, New York.

Schultzberg, M., Lundberg, J. M., Hökfelt, F., Terenius, L., Brandt, J., Elde, R., and Goldstein, M. (1978). Enkephalin-like immunoreactivity in gland cells and nerve terminals of the adrenal medulla. *Neuroscience*, **3**, 1169–1186.

Schultzberg, M., Hökfelt, T., Terenius, L., Elfvin, L.-G., Lundberg, J. M., Brandt, J., Elde, R. P., and Goldstein, M. (1979). Enkephalin immunoreactive nerve fibres and cell bodies in sympathetic ganglia of the guinea-pig and rat. *Neuroscience*, **4**, 249–270.

Siegrist, G., Dolivo, M., Dunant, Y., Foroglou-Kerameus, C., De Ribaupierre, F., and Rouiller, C. (1968). Ultrastructure and function of the chromaffin cells in the superior cervical ganglion of the rat. *J. Ultrastruct. Res.*, **25**, 381–407.

Skok, V. I. (1973). *Physiology of Autonomic Ganglia*, Igaku-Shoin, Tokyo.

Smolen, A. J. (1981). Postnatal development of ganglionic neurons in the absence of preganglionic input: morphological observations on synapse formation. *Devel. Brain Res.*, **1**, 49–58.

Smolen, A., and Raisman, G. (1980). Synapse formation in the rat superior cervical ganglion during normal development and after neonatal deafferentation. *Brain Res.*, **181**, 315–323.

Somogyi, P., and Chubb, I. W. (1976). The recovery of acetylcholinesterase activity in the superior cervical ganglion of the rat following its inhibition by di-isopropylphosphofluoridate: a biochemical and cytochemical study. *Neuroscience*, **1**, 413–422.

Sotelo, C. (1973). Permanence and fate of paramembranous synaptic specializations in 'mutants' and experimental animals. *Brain Res.*, **62**, 345–351.

Sternberger, L. A., Hardy, P. H., Cuculis, J. J., and Meyer, H. G. (1970). The unlabelled antibody enzyme method of immunocytochemistry. *J. Histochem. Cytochem.*, **18**, 315–333.

Stjärne, L. (1978). Facilitation and receptor-mediated regulation of noradrenaline secretion by control of recruitment of varicosities as well as by control of electro-secretory coupling. *Neuroscience*, **3**, 1147–1156.

Szurszewski, J. H. (1977). Towards a new view of prevertebral ganglion. In *Nerves and the Gut* (Eds. F. P. Brooks and P. N. Evers), pp. 244–260, Charles B. Slack, Thorofare, New Jersey.

Szurszewski, J. H., and Weems, W. A. (1976). A study of peripheral input to and its control by postganglionic neurones of the inferior mesenteric ganglion. *J. Physiol. (London)*, **256**, 541–556.

Tamarind, D. L., and Quilliam, J. P. (1971). Synaptic organization and other ultrastructural features of the superior cervical ganglion of the rat, kitten and rabbit. *Micron*, **2**, 204–234.

Taxi, J. (1965). Contribution à l'étude des connexions des neurones moteurs du système nerveux autonome. *Ann. Sci. Nat. Zool.*, **7**, 413–674.

Taxi, J. (1979). The chromaffin and chromaffin-like cells in the autonomic nervous system. *Internat. Rev. Cytol.*, **57**, 283–343.

Taxi, J., Gautron, J., and L'Hermite, P. (1969). Données ultrastructurales sur une éventuelle modulation adrénergique de l'activité du ganglion cervical supérieur du rat. *C. R. Acad. Sci.*, **269**, 1281–1284.

Tranzer, J. P., and Richards, J. G. (1976). Ultrastructural cytochemistry of biogenic amines in nervous tissue: methodologic improvements. *J. Histochem. Cytochem.*, **24**, 1178–1193.

Verhofstad, A. A. J., Steinbusch, H. W. M., Penke, B., Varga, J., and Joosten, H. W. J. (1981). Serotonin-immunoreactive cells in the superior cervical ganglion of the rat. Evidence for the existence of separate serotonin- and catecholamine-containing small ganglionic cells. *Brain Res.*, **212**, 39–49.

Watanabe, H. (1971). Adrenergic nerve elements in the hypogastric ganglion of the guinea pig. *Am. J. Anat.*, **130**, 305–330.

Weems, W. A., and Szurszewski, J. H. (1978). An intracellular analysis of some intrinsic factors controlling neural output from inferior mesenteric ganglion of guinea pigs. *J. Neurophysiol.*, **41**, 305–321.

Westrum, L. E. (1975). Electron microscopy of synaptic structures in olfactory cortex of early postnatal rats. *J. Neurocytol.*, **4**, 713–732.

Williams, T. H. (1967). Electron microscopic evidence for an autonomic interneuron. *Nature*, **214**, 309–310.

Williams, T. H., and Palay, S. L. (1969). Ultrastructure of the small neurons in the superior cervical ganglion. *Brain Res.*, **15**, 17–34.

Yokota, R., and Yamauchi, A. (1974). Ultrastructure of the mouse superior cervical ganglion, with particular reference to the pre- and postganglionic elements covering the soma of its principal neurons. *Am. J. Anat.*, **140**, 281–298.

Morphology and histophysiology of SIF cells in the autonomic ganglia

JACQUES TAXI, MICHÈLE DERER and ANNAMARIA DOMICH

*Laboratoire de Cytologie, Université P. et M. Curie (Paris VI),
and ERA-CNRS No. 884 'Organisation des Tissue Excitables', Paris, France*

INTRODUCTION: TERMINOLOGY

Although 'small intensely fluorescent' cells were first mentioned in the rat superior cervical ganglion (SCG) by Eränkö and Härkönen (1963), using the fluorescence method for catecholamines, the name 'SIF' was proposed by Norberg *et al.* (1966). Independently, they were identified as chromaffin cells by Siegrist *et al.* (1966) and Grillo (1966) using electron microscopy, but direct evidence that it was the same cells that were being observed by the two was provided much later (Grillo *et al.*, 1974). Thus, it could appear that the terms are synonymous; in fact, this is not so, for even if all chromaffin cells are SIF, not all SIF cells are chromaffin cells when stained using a classical technique for the chromaffin reaction (Eränkö and Härkönen, 1965; Norberg *et al.*, 1966; Matthews and Raisman, 1969; Jacobowitz, 1970), or even with a more sensitive modification of that reaction (Lever *et al.*, 1974). Considering that the ultrastructural features of all these cells are very similar, whether chromaffin or not, Jacobowitz (1970) concluded that they must be called chromaffin cells because of the historical priority of this denomination (Kohn, 1903). Other authors, however, considered that the term chromaffin cell cannot be properly used on the basis of the electron-microscopic appearance of these cells (Williams and Palay, 1969) or of their appearance in fluorescent preparations (Eränkö and Eränkö, 1971).

According to the feature which appeared most significant to different authors, these cells have been variously called interneurons (Williams, 1967), small granule-containing (SGC) cells (Matthews and Raisman, 1969) and granule-containing (GC) cells (Ellison and Hibbs, 1974; Chiba, 1977). They have also been included with the paraneurons (Chiba, 1977; Chiba *et al.*, 1977), which is a new concept proposed by Fujita (1977), challenging the amine precursor uptake and decarboxylation (APUD) cells of Pearse (1969), to which SIF cells also undoutedly belong. Such a string of names for one and the same type of cell is confusing, and since a large number of them were first described a long time ago as chromaffin cells, although some that are not chromaffin cells, exhibit similar fluorescence reactions or ultrastructures to chromaffin cells, it would seem that a good compromise is to call them 'chromaffin and chromaffin-like cells' (Taxi, 1979), a terminology previously used by Van Orden *et al.* (1970) and Yamauchi (1976). However, to keep in line with the terminology of this book, the term SIF cells will be used herein.

SHAPE AND SIZE OF SIF CELLS IN MAMMALS

Only the SIF cells of the autonomic ganglia will be considered here. These cells are localized within the space delimited by the connective capsule of the ganglia; they have to be distinguished from paraganglia found beside the ganglia. There are also SIF cells within the ganglionic capsule, or even clusters half outside and half inside the ganglion.

The most suitable method for studying the distribution, shape and size of SIF cells at present remains the fluorescence method or its modification using glyoxylic acid (Furness and Costa, 1975; Chiba *et al.*, 1976). In such preparations, SIF cells are very distinct from the surrounding structures because of their fluorescence; moreover, this method allows rather thick sections or whole mounts of thin material to be used (Costa and Furness, 1973). Other information can be obtained from materials prepared with the routine methods for electron microscopy, but cut and stained in semithin sections (Hökfelt, 1965; Matthews and Raisman, 1969).

SIF cells are oval, sometimes spherical or elongated when isolated, and polyhedral when tightly packed in clusters (Figs. 1–7). In all cases they are small compared to 'principal neurons', although their size varies a little according to the species. In the rat ganglia the extreme values were 5 μm (Tamarind and Quilliam, 1971) and 18 μm (Siegrist *et al.*, 1968; Jacobowitz, 1970), the mean value being around 10 μm (for references see Taxi, 1979). The mean value given for a range of species (cow, cat, rabbit, pig, monkey) was 10–15 μm (Chiba and Williams, 1975), and the same for man (Chiba, 1978). Watanabe (1971) indicated 10–20 μm in the hypogastric ganglion of the guinea-pig. In the rabbit, Elfvin (1968) found 10–25 μm in the inferior mesenteric ganglion, but Libet and Owman (1974) spoke of a mean value of 10 μm, and Dail and Evan (1978a) 6–9 μm in the superior cervical ganglion (SCG).

Certain SIF cells have one, two or even more processes (Figs. 1–7), as first mentioned by Owman and Sjöstrand (1965) and Norberg *et al.* (1966). Processes are commonly reported to be 30–40 μm in length in 10-μm-thick sections of rat ganglia, but in favourable circumstances, processes of up to

130 μm were described in the dog stellate ganglion (Jacobowitz, 1970), 170 μm in the monkey SCG (Chiba and Williams, 1975) and 120 μm in man (Chiba, 1978). Libet and Owman (1974) reported a value of several tenths of a millimeter in the rabbit SCG. A process longer than 500 μm was seen in a whole mount of guinea-pig hypogastric plexus (Furness and Costa, 1976). The mean diameter was evaluated at 1–3 μm, but locally it seems to be much greater in some cases (6 μm in the cat coeliac ganglion, according to Autillo-Touati, 1979).

These processes may ramify but it is not generally considered that the bulk of beaded fluorescent fibres in ganglia originate from SIF cells, except by Libet and Owman (1974) in the rabbit. As the number of SIF cells in this ganglion has been found to be 284 ± 110 (Domich, unpublished data), whereas principal neurons have been estimated at $67\,000 \pm 577$ (Gabella, 1976), there must be an enormous development of the ramifications of the rabbit SIF cells, yet no other example of this is available. The identification of SIF cell processes in fluorescence is straightforward when they are attached to the cell body; problems of identification may occur when they are separated from the cell body, because these processes may sometimes resemble neurites (Fig. 4), especially when they are long.

Clusters of SIF cells usually range from a few to 30 cells per section (Figs. 2, 3) or even more (Norberg and Sjoqvist, 1966). Heym and Williams (1979) counted 300 SIF cells in a cluster of an SCG and 120 in the stellate ganglion of the shrew *Tupaïa glis*. The number, size and repartition of cell clusters are specific to the ganglion and the animal species. Such clusters often lie against small blood vessels, usually capillaries, which may pass through them (Fig. 2). Clusters are either loosely or densely packed (Figs. 2, 3); the same cluster may be subdivided into several subunits (Dail *et al.*, 1975).

It soon appears from fluorescence as well as from electron-microscopic studies (Norberg *et al.*, 1966; Siegrist *et al.*, 1966), that there are two morphologically different SIF cells: those provided with processes and those which are not. In the rat they both occur within the same clusters (Fig. 3). But the rat, guinea-pig and hamster are exceptions in this respect. In several other species of Mammals of varying orders (cow, cat, rabbit, pig, monkey), Williams *et al.* (1975) and Chiba and Williams (1975) noticed that the cells displaying processes were isolated, whereas cells in clusters were devoid of them. These cells were named type I and type II, respectively. The same situation has been observed in human ganglia (Hino and Tsunekawa, 1978). Biochemical and physiological correlates suggest that type I cells are interneurons, whereas type II may be purely endocrine cells (Williams *et al.*, 1975; Chiba *et al.*, 1977). Both types were also identified in SCG and coeliac ganglia of the cat by Autillo-Touati (1979), who called Chiba and William's type II (1975) type I, and vice versa.

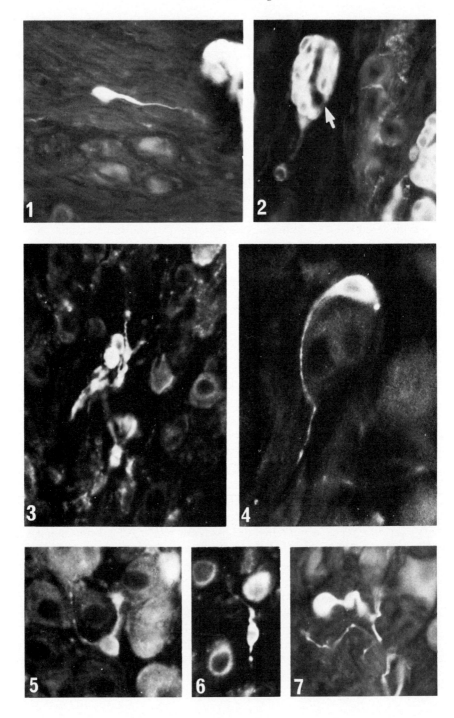

STRUCTURE AND ULTRASTRUCTURE OF SIF CELLS IN MAMMALS

Light microscopy

The fluorescence method reveals nothing of the structure of the cell except for the position of the nucleus. Semithin sections stained with basic dyes are suitable for identifying SIF cells, when this has not previously been done by fluorescence according to the method of Grillo *et al.* (1974), Chiba *et al.* (1976), or Furness *et al.* (1978). Identification relies upon size, shape, arrangement and staining affinity (Matthews and Raisman, 1969), but these characteristics vary, probably in relation to the nature of the stored catecholamines.

The nucleus is central, or more rarely eccentric, with patches of condensed chromatin forming a discontinuous ring against the nuclear envelope, that is much more prominent after aldehyde fixatives. The nucleolus is rarely conspicuous, and often absent in the rat, but this does not seem to be the case with other material such as kittens (see Figs. in Mascorro and Yates, 1980). The cytoplasmic area is small and clear, without stained organelles; Nissl bodies especially are lacking in osmium-fixed tissue. In SIF cells that have first been fixed in aldehyde, granules are visible in phase-contrast microscopy or with immersion, when they are large enough (Mascorro and Yates, 1980). Although SIF cells are rather easy to identify in semithin sections when in groups, it is more difficult to recognize them when they are isolated.

Ultrastructure

Our basic description will be from data coming mainly from the rat SCG, which is the most frequently studied material due to its uniquely high proportion of SIF cells, in particular data of Siegrist *et al.* (1966, 1968), Matthews and Raisman (1969) and Williams and Palay (1969), and personal observations (Taxi *et al.*, 1969; Taxi, 1973, 1979). The cytological features

Figures 1–7 Morphology of SIF cells as seen using the Falck–Hillarp fluorescence method.
(1) Isolated monopolar cell. Cat inferior mesenteric ganglion (×470).
(2) SIF cell cluster traversed by a capillary (arrow); it is separated from another cluster by a group of neurons. Cat inferior mesenteric ganglion (×470).
(3) A small cluster of SIF cells, one of which has a short process terminating in a varicosity. Rat, SCG (×470).
(4) A large monopolar SIF cell with a rather long process quite similar to a varicose neurite. Rabbit SCG (×600).
(5) A bopolar SIF cell, the processes of which 'encircle' a principal neuron. Hamster SCG (×600).
(6) A bipolar SIF cell. Mouse coeliac ganglion (×470).
(7) A monopolar SIF cell with a dividing process. Cat SCG (×470)

have been confirmed in many additional papers dealing with other ganglia in the rat and in various other species (for references see Taxi, 1979).

The most characteristic feature of the SIF cells is the large number of granular vesicles (GV), which will be discussed in the next section.

The nuclear profiles are usually regular (Fig. 8), although not always devoid of indentations, with fine granular contents in which chromatin clumps can be seen mainly along the nuclear envelope. However, there are SIF cells in which the nucleus is devoid of condensed chromatin, similar to that of principal neurons (Ellison and Hibbs, 1976). When present, the nucleolus is usually not conspicuous as in principal neurons (Fig. 8). A case of mitosis in the adult animal was reported by Yokota and Burnstock (1978), who also gave a list of such an occurrence in fetus and newborns (Fig. 14).

The cell membrane may form microvilli devoid of organelles, $0.1\,\mu m$ in width and $0.5\,\mu m$ in length. Coated pits are not very frequent. Pictures of exocytosis are extremely rare from normal ganglia; the only cases described are from the guinea-pig inferior mesenteric ganglion (Elfvin *et al.*, 1975). In the rat, exocytosis was observed only after stimulation (Matthews, 1978).

The cell membrane can be apposed to various other cells, for instance satellite glial cells, another SIF cell, or, exceptionally, a principal neuron (Matthews and Nash, 1970). Usually a whole cluster of SIF cells is isolated by a glial sheath, formed by one or several thin lamellae of cytoplasm; within a cluster, SIF cells can be directly apposed to each other over large surfaces (Fig. 8). In some places, the cell membrane is separated from the intraganglionic connective space only by a basement membrane. Such 'naked' surfaces are often situated just opposite the wall of a fenestrated capillary, suggesting an endocrine function. SIF cells may form several types of junctions with the other cells, including afferent and efferent synapses; these are considered in the chapters by Matthews and by Williams and Jew.

The mitochondria, apparently dispersed at random throughout the cytoplasm, appear more globular in shape than in principal neurons, and are $1–1.5\,\mu m$ in diameter. They are characterized by regularly spaced, parallel cristae. They appear rather sensitive to fixation and easily become swollen, even when the rest of the cell is quite well preserved. The endoplasmic reticulum is poorly to moderately developed, usually as ergastoplasmic cisternae scattered throughout the cell. Free ribosomes are usually very numerous. Lying in a juxtanuclear position, the Golgi apparatus is well developed. It is made up of several dictyosomes, often arranged in an arc or circle (Fig. 9), which outlines a distinct area poor in GV. The saccules are flattened or swollen and have no visible contents. Sometimes there are vesicles of variable size, with more or less dense contents in the vicinity of dictyosomes (Fig. 10), which has been considered as evidence of the Golgian origin of these vesicles (Siegrist *et al.*, 1966); in fact, as far as we know, there has been no special study made on SIF cells concerning the origin of GV, and

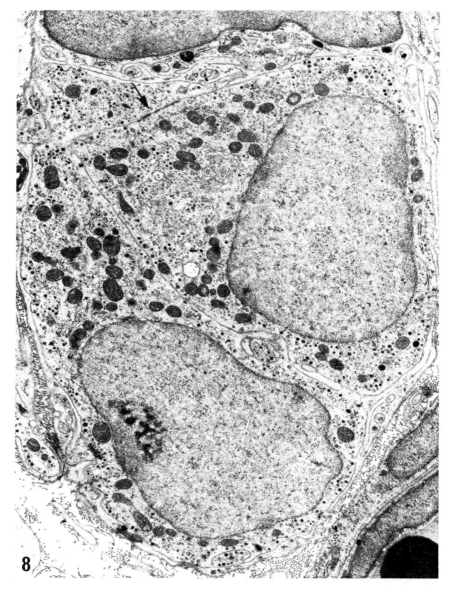

Figure 8 Small cluster of SIF cells. Osmium fixation. The cell group is surrounded by a thin glial envelope, but there are large zones of direct apposition between the SIF cells, sometimes displaying an attachment plate (arrow). The peripheral chromatin in the nuclei is poorly contrasted. A nucleolus is visible in the bottom nucleus. Rat SCG (×11 200)

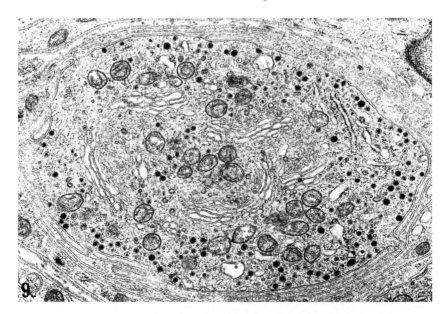

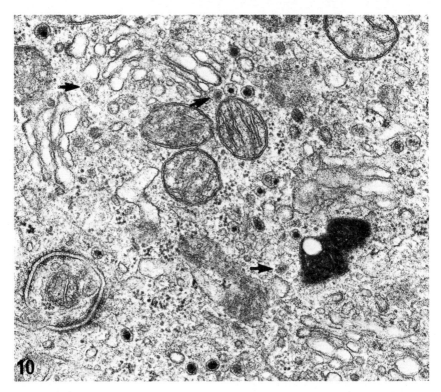

conclusions are extrapolated on the basis of studies on adrenomedullary cells (see Winkler, 1977).

Membrane-bounded dense bodies, presumably lysosomes, are few, and the same applies to the multivesicular bodies (Fig. 10). Microtubules and filaments are distributed in small amounts apparently at random throughout the cytoplasm, except in the processes where they are roughly parallel to the longitudinal axis. However, there are large discrepancies between authors concerning the amount of microfilaments. In the cat, Autillo-Touati (1979) described a special cytoplasmic differentiation in the form of microfilament bundles. Occasionally one or two centrioles are encountered, one of which may be the basal corpuscle of a cilium (Taxi, 1979). It is difficult to know if they are present in each cell. Glycogen granules, about 300 Å in diameter, are sometimes dispersed throughout the cytoplasm or grouped in rosettes. The hyaloplasm is more or less dense, as noted by Siegrist *et al.* (1968), but the significance of this fact is not established.

Two kinds of processes can be distinguished: there are large, long processes that are well seen with fluorescence methods; there are also thin, presumably short, processes, which are intercalated between SIF cells in clusters (Fig. 8), and visible only by electron microscopy. Although they do not leave the cluster, they can be finger-like and penetrate other cells (Fig. 10) to which they are bound by symmetrical 'attachment plates'. In many instances processes contain the same organelles as the cell body, but in different proportions. One of the peculiarities is that, in places, mitochondria are enveloped by a flattened saccule of smooth endoplasmic reticulum. The heterogeneity of GV is marked. In some areas there are only a few vesicles, the prominent organelles being free ribosomes which bathe in a fluffy hyaloplasmic material. Siegrist *et al.* (1968) referred to axonic and dendritic processes of SIF cells, but they admitted to being unable to distinguish them. They can behave as neurites belonging to compound unmyelinated fibres.

GRANULAR VESICLES AND SIF CELL TYPES IN MAMMALS

The characteristic organelles of the SIF cells, first mentioned by Eränkö and Härkonen (1965) and illustrated by Grillo (1966) and Siegrist *et al.* (1966), are granular (or granule-containing, or dense-cored) vesicles (GV).

Figure 9 Section through a juxtanuclear region of a SIF cell. Typical circular arrangement of dictyosomes; the bulk of the GV is located in the peripheral part of the cell beneath the membrane. Rat SCG (×16 200)

Figure 10 A more greatly enlarged Golgi zone. The Golgi zone is poor in GV; however, in the immediate vicinity of the dictyosomes, there are some GV, the contents of which are low in density (arrows), suggesting immature forms. At the bottom left, there is a finger-like invagination bound to the cell by an attachment plate. Rat SCG (×44 000)

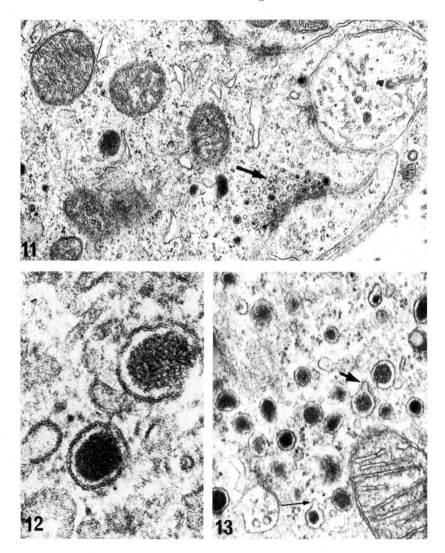

Figure 11   A part of a SIF cell process which contains a group of small (type 5) GV (arrow) along an efferent synaptic contact. Osmium tetroxide fixation. Rat SCG (×31 000)

Figures 12, 13   Some aspects of GV. Hamster coeliac ganglion. Glutaraldehyde fixation.

(12) The triple-layered membrane of the GV is visible; when the GV contents are not too dense, the heterogeneous structure is apparent (×135 000).

(13) In this field one vesicle shows a short, coated evagination which could be interpreted as a fusion with a coated vesicle or the formation of one (thick arrow). Another vesicle bears an evagination with no coating (thin arrow) (×37 500).

They are also called granules, probably because their dense contents are more conspicuous than the thin membrane; but this may lead to the part of the organelle being confused with the whole. The term membrane-bounded granule (Lu *et al.*, 1976) is also correct. The appearance of GV depends largely on the method of fixation. In osmium tetroxide-fixed cells, the granules are usually moderately to highly dense, and occupy almost all the space inside the vesicle, except a clear narrow peripheral halo. In certain vesicles the dense granule is smaller, and sometimes even reduced to a dense spot. In other cases, the dense contents are heterogeneous: there is a large area of moderate density with a small, often eccentric, granule of higher density. GV of all appearances can be found in a limited area of the same cell.

The appearance can differ somewhat after glutaraldehyde primary fixation. The triple-layered structure of the GV membrane is visible upon sufficient enlargement (Fig. 12). The dense contents can be in the form of a full, half or crescent moon lying against the membrane or even protruding through it, as in the noradrenaline-containing cells of the adrenal medulla. The GV often have a smooth contour. In certain cells the membrane of some GV forms a short evagination (Fig. 13), which might represent the ultimate fate of coated vesicles opening into the GV, according to the schema of Winkler (1977). There are also similar protrusions devoid of any coating (Fig. 13). Elongated profiles are present in certain cells. These last aspects might correspond to stages of granule synthesis or remodelling. The vesicular contents appear homogeneous when highly dense, but when they are of moderate to weak density they have a spongy structure (Fig. 12).

There is a lot of data on the size of the GV, and on the size, form, electron density and positioning of their contents. From these data, summarized in Table 1, some general conclusions may be drawn on the morphological types of SIF cells which might be directly related to their putative functions. Taking the size of GV into consideration as well as the characteristics of their contents in all species examined up to now, it seems that five kinds of GV may be found in SIF cells, of which three can be used for defining cell types in adult animals: (1) Medium-sized GV, 70–120 nm in diameter, with a core of moderate to high electron density, filling almost the entire vesicle. Such vesicles are predominant in rat adrenomedullary cells at the early developmental stages (Diner, 1965). They are numerous in the rat SCG, where it is generally accepted that SIF cells contain dopamine (Björklund *et al.*, 1970) (Figs. 8, 9, 12). (2) Large GV, from around 120 to 300 nm or more in diameter, with a dense to highly dense core; the dense core does not completely fill the vesicle, and it is eccentric in the larger GV. By analogy with what is well established in adrenomedullary cells, the GV can be considered as organelles for noradrenaline storage. (3) Large GV of the same size as type 2, but with a core of high to low density, more or less filling the

Table 1 Granular vesicles (GV) size and contents in different materials

Material	Primary fixation	GV size (nm)	Vesicular contents*	References
Rat SCG	Osmium tetroxide	65–120	Round, m.d. to h.d.	Matthews and Raisman (1969)
		70–100	Round, m.d. to h.d.	Taxi et al. (1969)
		40–140	Round, m.d. to h.d.	Tamarind and Qulliam (1971)
	Glutaraldehyde	100–150	Round, h.d.	Siegrist et al. (1968)
		200–400 (mean 140)	Eccentric, h.d.	Williams and Palay (1969)
	Potassium permanganate	150–250	h.d. or m.d.	Van Orden et al. (1970)
		80–120		Hökfelt (1969)
Rat coeliac ganglion	Osmium tetroxide	· 90–160 45–50		Ivanov (1974)
Rat, pelvic ganglion	Aldehydes (?)	160–200 Around 280	d. d.	Scott and Hung (1971)
	Glutaraldehyde	50–120 150–270	Central d. Eccentric d.	Dail et al. (1975)
Female, rat paracervical ganglion	Glutaraldehyde	80–140 200–300	Central d. Eccentric d.	Kanerva and Terävaïnen (1972)
Rat SCG and coeliac ganglion	Glutaraldehyde Paraformaldehyde	I. 50–150 II. 100–300 III. Oblong, 70 × 50	Round, m.d. Polymorphic, h.d. m. to l.	Lu et al. (1976)
Rabbit inferior mesenteric ganglion	Osmium tetroxide	70–300 most, 150–250	h.d.	Elfvin (1968)
Rabbit SCG	Glutaraldehyde + paraformaldehyde	110–210	Eccentric in large GV Central in smaller GV	Dail and Evan (1978a)
Kitten abdominal ganglion	Glutaraldehyde	100–150	h.d. m. to d.	Mascorro and Yates (1980)
Rhesus monkey SCG	Paraformaldehyde + glutaraldehyde	150–200	Variable d.	Chiba et al.
Man thoracic and lumbar ganglia	Glutaraldehyde	200–300 300–400	d.	Chiba (1978) Hervonen et al. (1979)
Cat coeliac ganglion	Glutaraldehyde + formaldehyde	120–220 60–120	h.d., polymorphous round, m. to l.	Autillo-Touati (1979)

Table 1 (*continued*)

Material	Primary fixation	GV size (nm)	Vesicular contents*	References
Guinea-pig hypogastric ganglion	Glutaraldehyde	I. 200–250 II. 100–150 III. elongated (50 × 170) VI. 200–250	l. to d. Polymorphous, h.d. l.d.	Watanabe (1971)
Guinea-pig heart ganglia	Glutaraldehyde	I. 100 II. 100	Eccentric, h.d. m.d.	Ellison and Hibbs (1974)
Guinea-pig inferior mesenteric ganglion	Glutaraldehyde	100–300 50	Homogeneous, m.d.	Elfvin *et al.* (1975)
Guinea-pig SCG	Glutaraldehyde	About 100	Eccentric, h.d.	
Mouse paracervical ganglion	Glutaraldehyde	I. 50–250 II. 50–300 up to 450	h.d. to l.d. in small GV Polymorphous, eccentric GV	Becker (1972)
Tupaïa glis SCG	Glutaraldehyde	60–80 100–120	m.d. h.d.	Heym and Williams (1979)

* Weakly (l.), moderately (m), or highly (h.), electron-dense (d.).

vesicle, yet never eccentric. They could be considered as adrenaline-storing GV (Coupland *et al.*, 1964), at least as a working hypothesis. (4) Small GV (mean diameter 45 nm) of the same size and aspect as vesicles of the sympathetic terminals (Fig. 11). It is well known that the dense granule is more or less well preserved in these small GV (Taxi *et al.*, 1969). They are restricted either to synaptic areas (see chapters by Matthews and by Williams and Jew) or to some regions in the processes, suggesting that they are related to amine release (Elfvin *et al.*, 1975). (5) Elongated vesicles of variable length, but having a minimum diameter of about 120 nm. The elongated forms are much more numerous when fixative contains formaldehyde, alone or in a glutaraldehyde mixture. For instance, they were found in rat SCG fixed by a formaldehyde–glutaraldehyde mixture, whereas such pictures are not frequent when other fixatives have been used. It may also correspond to certain stages of activity (GV genesis ?).

Since types 4 and 5 (small and elongated GV) are thought to be related to special functions, for example GV genesis or the release of a catecholamine, three types of vesicles remain, each of which can be taken as the basis of the definition of a single SIF cell type:

—type A, containing medium-sized GV (type 1);
—type B, containing large GV (type 2) with a dense to highly dense, often eccentric core;

—type C, containing large GV (type 3) with a dense core of varied density, but usually filling the entire vesicle except for a regular clear halo.

The distribution of the cell types is different according to species and ganglia.

COMPARATIVE DATA

There is little work devoted to SIF cells in non-mammalian vertebrates, except amphibia, which are treated in a special chapter by Watanabe. For classical data, which are mainly based on the chromaffin reaction, the reader should refer to Coupland's book (1965).

Birds

In the chick embryo, highly fluorescent, presumably SIF cells were observed by Enemar *et al.* (1965) as early as after six days of incubation. Using electron microscopy, Wechsler and Schmeckel (1967) noticed that by 4–5 days all primitive sympathicoblasts contained GV that were 80–160 nm in diameter, and at 6–7 days all sympathicoblasts were still similar to adult SIF cells, as confirmed by Eränkö (1972); only when embryos grew older did the principal neurons lose their GV.

The normal ganglia of adult birds have hardly been studied. SIF cells, 5–10 μm in diameter, were recorded as interneurons in the heart of domestic fowl (Bennett and Malmfors, 1970) by means of the fluorescence technique. Ultrastructural data concerning adult bird ganglia are completely lacking, as far as we know.

Reptiles

Data on SIF cells in reptile autonomic ganglia are very scarce. They were described in the heart of a turtle by Chiba and Yamauchi (1973). Their nucleus may be triangular or indented; their cytoplasm is loaded with numerous GV, 40–200 nm in diameter, the morphology of which depends on the method of fixation, as for mammals. The size, shape and density of the core vary greatly, even in the same cell; cell types are not distinct. Glycogen is abundant, as in many tissues of lower vertebrates. Other cytological features are quite similar to those of mammalian heart SIF cells, included reciprocal synapses (Yamauchi *et al.*, 1975).

Fish

The data concerning SIF cells in fish are poor and practically limited to teleosts. With the fluorescence method, they have been recognized in various ganglia of *Gadus morrhua* (Nilsson, 1976) and in the splanchnic plexus of *Salmo trutta* by Campbell and Gannon (1976). Watson (1980) studied their ultrastructure in *Myoxocephalus scorpio*. Their shape and size are very similar to those of mammalian SIF cells; GV, 300–600 nm in diameter, were found in the cell body and its processes. The value of 600 nm for GV is larger than that of mammals, but it is comparable to that of anurans. The density of the granule after glutaraldehyde fixation suggests that they contain noradrenaline. In the dipnoan *Protopterus aethiopicus*, Abrahamsson *et al.* (1979) demonstrated SIF cells adjacent to non-fluorescent peripheral neurons.

Cyclostomata

Cyclostomata raise specific problems because they represent the only class of living vertebrates in which the autonomic nervous system is not anatomically distinct. However, chromaffin cells have long been known to exist in the heart (Coupland, 1965). Nevertheless, it has only recently been established that SIF cells do not coexist with neurons (Caravita and Coscia, 1966; Lignon and Le Douarin, 1978), and they do not exhibit neuronal or intermediate features. They are 6–18 µm in diameter, many of them being endowed with processes. The main cytological features are similar to those of certain mammalian SIF cells, their GV attaining 100–300 nm in diameter in adults (Bloom *et al.*, 1961).

In the ammocoetes, in which the chromaffin reaction is negative, GV are only 120 nm in diameter (Lignon and Le Douarin, 1978). SIF cells are sensitive to reserpine, the fluorescence reaction disappearing after 3–4 days treatment (2 mg/kg/day); in electron microscopy the vesicles become degranulated, and the number of lipidic inclusions increases, as well as the endoplasmic reticulum (Caravita and Coscia, 1966). In some cells, granular contents remain, but with reduced contrast. They are the only type of aminergic cells in the heart of Cyclostomata, which suggests that this system is phylogenetically anterior to the sympathetic system.

MORPHOLOGICAL CHANGES DURING DEVELOPMENT AND AGING

The development of SIF cells in rat embryos was first studied by Champlain *et al.* (1970), who described highly fluorescent cells provided with processes, presumably SIF cells, in the three-week fetus. Soon after, Hervonen (1971) observed highly fluorescent cells in the sympathetic ganglia of man in the 14-week fetus, but mentioned that GV appear as early as eight weeks; the diameter of GV change from 110 to 260 nm between the 8th and 19th weeks and are of the very electron-dense type (Hervonen and Kanerva, 1972). Extensive studies on prenatal stages have been carried out in the rabbit by

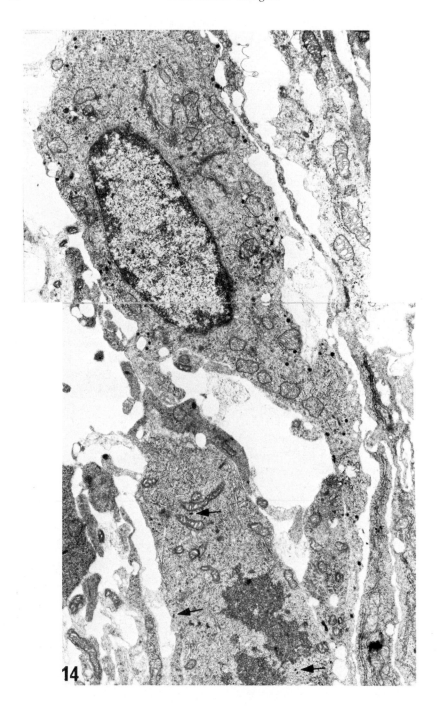

Mytilineou and Tennyson (1973) and Tennyson and Mytilineou (1976). Clusters of highly fluorescent cells were recognized in the 12-day-old embryo; although such cells were identified by their GV in electron microscopy, they were considered as SIF cells only at the end of fetal life, when the migration of 'paraganglionic' cells ended and neurons already possessed the main characteristics of maturity. Using electron microscopy in the rat, Derer (unpublished data) observed elongated cells at 15 days of gestation ($12 \times 5 \mu m$ to $20 \times 9 \mu m$ in size), endowed with processes, containing some GV that were 90–130 nm in diameter; their cytology combined adult (nuclear aspect) and embryonic features (abundance of ribosomes). Such cells were found in mitosis (Fig. 14). They are distinguishable both from principal neurons, the nucleus of which is round and clear, and from undifferentiated cells with a lobate nucleus. According to Eränkö and Eränkö (1971), SIF cells are isolated in newborns, but bunched together in adults. In electron microscopy, no GV can be found in young sympathicoblasts (Eränkö, 1972). Then come 'late sympathicoblasts', with vesicles 60–110 nm in diameter. At birth, Kanerva (1972) and Eränkö (1972) distinguished only one type of SIF cells, with GV of 80–200 nm and 90–150 nm in diameter. Recently, Partanen *et al.* (1980) distinguished two types of SIF cells in the newborn rat on the basis of GV size, respectively 50–150 nm and 50–250 nm. A third type of cell appears in grown animals, with more polymorphous GV. Kanerva (1971) and Kanerva and Hervonen (1976) suggest that maturation, of neurons as well as of SIF cells, is more advanced at birth in paracervical ganglia than in the SCG. In the first postnatal week, rearrangements occur in the SCG, as evidenced by the existence of both degenerating SIF cells and mitosis.

MORPHOLOGY OF SIF CELLS IN CULTURE

Organotypic cultures

SIF cells in cultures of sympathetic ganglia were first recognized by Lever and Presley (1971) from chick embryo ganglia; SIF cell bodies and processes were identified by fluorescence and characterized in electron microscopy by their numerous GV. Similar cultures were also obtained by Chamley *et al.* (1972), Benitez *et al.* (1974), Hervonen and Eränkö (1975) and others. Hervonen and Eränkö (1975) noted that certain cells having the nuclear and cytoplasmic features of principal neurons contain many GV; one can thus wonder whether they represent a special type of SIF cell, falling between

Figure 14   Rat SCG at 15 days of gestation. The top cell is identified as a SIF cell, due to the peripheral condensation of chromatin in its nucleus and to the presence of some typical GV in its cytoplasm. The other cell is in mitosis. It contains only a few small GV (arrows); it cannot be said whether it is a SIF cell or a sympathicoblast ($\times 10\,250$)

principal neurons and SIF cells of mammals, or only chick sympathicoblasts, which would all contain numerous GV.

SIF cells have been described in cultures of rat ganglia, by Eränkö and Eränkö (1972a), Chamley *et al.* (1972) and Benitez *et al.* (1974). In electron microscopy, Eränkö *et al.* (1972a) observed that GV were polymorphous; elongated GV (40–150 × 150–200 nm) were more numerous than in ganglia taken *in situ*, where SIF cell GV were usually round; Benitez *et al.* (1974) considered that GV were similar to those found in the adult animals.

Dissociated cell cultures

Cultures of cells from chick ganglia dissociated by trypsinization and/or dilaceration and shaking were made by Jacobowitz and Greene (1974). Highly fluorescent small cells (chromaffin in those authors' terminology) were seen in cultures from one day to a month, with or without NGF (nerve growth factor). They had long processes (up to 500 μm) with 'en passant' and terminal varicosities. In the absence of NGF, the processes grew more slowly.

Although several authors did not find SIF cells in their cultures (see Johnson *et al.*, 1980), isolated, elongated and highly fluorescent cells were seen in cultures of newborn rat ganglia by Derer (unpublished observations) (see also Landis, this volume). When cultivated in a medium supplied with NGF, these cells are endowed with a unique process, sometimes varicose or branched. In the absence of NGF, SIF cells exhibit a more varied morphology, and stellate forms are numerous. Their mean diameter was about 18 μm, the mean diameter of neurons being 46 μm in the same conditions. Although whole dissociated ganglia were put into culture, there were no SIF cells in each culture, which may explain the results of other authors. Their size is somewhat larger than *in vivo* (see above), probably due to the fact that in cultures cells spread out. The consequence is that for certain cells in fluorescence preparations it is difficult to say whether they are SIF cells or principal neurons.

The morphological differences of SIF cells grown in a medium with or without NGF, or even their absence, might be related to differences in culture media, especially in corticoids, due to the serum added (for instance, horse serum is known for its high level of hydrocortisone) and the antagonistic action of corticoids and NGF (see chapters by Landis and by Unsicker).

HISTOPHYSIOLOGY OF SIF CELLS

Uptake and storage properties

Since SIF cells were considered as interneurons of the rat SCG (Williams, 1967), it was interesting to test their properties of uptake and storage of exogenous catecholamines, in order to compare them with those of principal neurons. Libet and Owman (1974) reported by means of the fluorescence method that SIF cells of rabbit SCG, partially depleted by α-methyl-*p*-tyrosine, are capable of accumulating exogenous dopamine (about 6×10^{-5} M) in the presence of a monoamine oxidase inhibitor and ascorbic acid.

Using [³H]dihydroxyphenylalanine ([³H]DOPA), [³H]dopamine or [³H]noradrenaline injected *in vivo*, Taxi and Mikulajova (1976) obtained a moderate labelling of not previously depleted SIF cells by [³H]DOPA alone. In what way should these results be interpreted? As it has been shown that dopamine is the catecholamine of the bulk of SIF cells in the rat SCG (Björklund *et al.*, 1970), the absence of labelling of SIF cells by noradrenaline is not surprising. For dopamine, as it is generally accepted that in chromaffin cells this catecholamine is synthesized in the hyaloplasm and then stored in GV, the failure of labelling would be due to the fact that dopamine does not enter the SIF cells, because their membrane offers no high-affinity transport for this substance. However, other interpretations are possible. For instance, it could be that the turnover of amines in SIF cells is much lower than in neurons and dopamine does not enter the GV in amounts large enough to give a positive radioautographic reaction; this result could be modified if SIF cells were previously deprived of their amine, which would explain the contradiction between our results and those of Libet and Owman (1974). These discrepancies could also be due to differences in experimental conditions, especially in the concentration of dopamine, which is not actually known at the cellular level; the difference in labelling properties of SIF cells and principal neurons would be obvious only at low concentrations of dopamine, which corresponds to a high-affinity uptake, or uptake I (see Iversen, 1975).

Effect of reserpine

Norberg *et al.* (1966) reported that SIF cells of the rat were largely resistant to depletion by reserpine (5 mg/kg i.p.), as tested by the fluorescence method. In parallel observations with that method together with electron microscopy, Van Orden *et al.* (1970) were unable to obtain depletion ascertained by significant changes in ultrastructure after acrolein–osmium fixation. It seems that, contrary to principal neurons, several injections are needed to obtain even incomplete depletion as judged by fluorescence (Furness and Costa, 1976). In the turtle heart, Chiba and Yamauchi (1973) noted that SIF cells were still not depleted of their fluorescence by three injections given one daily prior to sacrifice.

Effect of synthesis inhibitors

α-*methyl*-p-*tyrosine*   This drug inhibits tyrosine hydroxylase, the first enzyme involved in catecholamine synthesis from tyrosine. At a dose of 500 mg/kg i.p., Van Orden *et al.* (1970) observed a progressive loss of electron density in GV in such a way that more than 50% of the granules were of low density 24 hours after the injection, instead of 10% in the normal rat ganglia.

α-*Methyl*-m-*tyrosine*   This drug diverts the normal synthesis of catecholamines in abnormal ways, leading to methylated derivatives and finally to depletion of normal catecholamines. Van Orden *et al.* (1970) reported that it gives the same results as reserpine.

Disulfiram   Disulfiram (tetraethylthiuram disulfide), an inhibitor of dopamine β-hydroxylase, produces variable individual responses of SIF cells. In most cases there is a decrease in the number of GV, but in some cells there is an increase in the number and size of GV, and a swelling of them (Heym, 1976). These differences might be related to different types of SIF cells.

Chlorophenylalanine   Chlorophenylalanine, an inhibitor of tryptophan hydroxylase, was found to deplete GV in SIF cells of the rat SCG by Heym *et al.* (1974) and Heym (1976). After 20 days of daily treatment, about half of the granular contents remained in the cells. This was thought to be due to interference with the tyrosine hydroxylase in the amine-containing cells.

Compound 48/80   This condensation product of *p*-methoxyphenethyl-methylamine and formaldehyde is a potent inhibitor of histamine. It was reported by Behrendt *et al.* (1976) to quickly (2 minutes) modify the ultrastructure of SIF cells in the rat SCG *in vitro*, bringing about hypertrophy of the Golgi apparatus, an increase in the number of GV and their accumulation in cell processes, all of these changes being interpreted as a stimulation of SIF cell activity.

Guanethidine   This adrenergic blocking agent brought on morphological effects that were quite similar to those of disulfiram, although its mode of action is not so well understood. It produced hyperplasia of the SIF cells in ganglia of newborn rats (Eränkö and Eränkö, 1971). This effect was not found in adults (Burnstock *et al.*, 1971), wherein, however, Heym and Grube (1975) had noted various ultrastructural changes after long-term treatment: the number of GV, the aspect of which remained unchanged, decreased in certain clusters, but in others the GV roughly doubled in diameter and their dense core became eccentric.

Effect of false transmitters:—6-hydroxydopamine (6-OHDA)

This drug is responsible for rapid degeneration of sympathetic terminals (Thoenen and Tranzer, 1968). Eränkö and Eränkö (1972b) did not find any modification of SIF cells after the administration of 6-OHDA to newborn rats, but Papka (1973) reported that in an 8-day-old rabbit a small proportion of SIF cells did degenerate. This might be related to the existence of several types of SIF cells that are more or less sensitive to the drug. After repeated injections, Kanerva *et al.* (1974) mentioned conspicuous ultrastructural changes in the three types of SIF cells of the rat paracervical ganglia, such as swelling of rough endoplasmic reticulum and formation of large vacuoles in the cytoplasm. The density of the intravesicular granule was reduced.

Corticoids

Hydrocortisone effects on the SCG of newborn rats were observed with the fluorescence method by Eränkö and Eränkö (1972a), who emphasized the increase in number (tenfold) of SIF cells devoid of processes. The number of GV is increased, but not their size (Eränkö *et al.*, 1973). These new cells are distributed throughout all parts of the ganglia, and do not represent an enlargement of pre-existing clusters. In adults, there are no detectable effects (Eränkö and Eränkö, 1972a), even as early as 12 days post partum (Ciaranello *et al.*, 1973). The action of hydrocortisone seems to be reversible *in vivo* (Eränkö and Eränkö, 1980). The action of hydrocortisone on cultures of rat ganglia was rather comparable to that obtained *in vivo*, inasmuch as it results in an increase in both number and fluorescence intensity of SIF cells (Eränkö *et al.*, 1972b, 1976). Cytologically, there is an increase in the size and number of their GV.

In the chick, effects of corticoids were tested by Hervonen and Eränkö (1975) on cultures of 12-day-old sympathetic chains, in a medium supplemented with hydrocortisone (succinate). There was a remarkable increase (tenfold) in the number of highly fluorescent cells, which were seen in electron microscopy to contain hundreds of GV per cell, measuring 80–410 nm in diameter (mean 250 nm), instead of the 105–275 nm of normal cultures. However, these cells conserved some neuronal features such as size, nuclear aspect and ergastoplasm. In short-term cultures of some aged embryos, at variance with the preceding results, Santer *et al.* (1976) noticed an increase in fluorescence intensity, but not in the number of highly fluorescent cells.

Deafferentation

In the rat SCG it was early established that SIF cells receive an afferent innervation, as do principal neurons (Williams, 1967; Siegrist *et al.*, 1968),

which disappears after preganglionic section (Taxi *et al.*, 1969). Dail and
Evan (1978b) observed that SIF cells in rat pelvic ganglia are endowed with
more processes following chronic deafferentation. According to Matthews
(1980), the morphology of the SIF cells is modified after disturbance of the
synaptic relationships, especially the size and shape of their processes.
Moreover, SIF cells of certain clusters become enlarged after a while.

SUMMARY AND CONCLUDING REMARKS

From the numerous studies on morphology and histophysiology of SIF
(small intensely fluorescent) cells located in the autonomic ganglia of
mammals, it would appear that for differing points of view different classifications of SIF cells can be proposed. From the general morphology of the cells,
two types are obvious: type I SIF cells endowed with process(es), and type II,
without them. Type I cells are isolated in many, but not all species. Type II
cells are more or less tightly packed into clusters, often traversed by small
vessels.

From the ultrastructure, several cytological types can be distinguished.
They have numerous features in common, like a nucleus with peripheral
chromatin condensations, a prominent Golgi apparatus, paucity of endoplasmic reticulum and abundance of free ribosomes. The differences mainly
involve the size and contents of granular vesicles (GV). Five types of GV are
discernible which provide a basis for the identification of at least three types
of SIF cells according to the predominant GV they contain:

—type A, with GV of medium size, having highly to moderately dense
   contents;
—type B, with large GV, having highly dense, often eccentric contents;
—type C, with large GV, having contents of varied density which fill the
   vesicle.

Another way in which cell types may be defined is by studying their
connections; this is dealt with in the chapters by Matthews and by Williams
and Jew. Three possibilities are thus to be considered: interneurons, endocrine cells and perhaps receptor cells. Endocrine functions may coexist with
the others.

There are already some correlations between cytological types and functions. For instance, rat interneurons are type A SIF cells. But in other
species, like the cat, there are claims that the interneurons are of type B.
Different authors have confirmed that in animal species where the distinction
is valid, type I are interneurons and type II endocrine cells.

Comparative data are meager in non-mammalian vertebrates. The case of
the heart is of interest: there are already SIF cells in the Cyclostomata, where
the heart is not innervated. In higher groups, when the heart becomes

innervated, SIF cells are integrated within the ganglia; SIF cell interneurons are already present in urodeles (see chapter by Watanabe), and have also been found in turtles and mammals.

The histophysiology of SIF cells has been thoroughly studied. Their high-affinity uptake properties seem to differ greatly from those of sympathetic neurons, even when they are interneurons. Their responses to certain drugs are fascinating, especially in newborns or in tissue culture. It is probable that the sensitivity to corticoids at certain stages of development plays an important role among other as yet unidentified factors, in their final differentiation into several cytological types.

REFERENCES

Abrahamsson, T., Holmgren, S., Nilsson, S., and Pettersson, K. (1979). Adrenergic and cholinergic effects on the heart, the lung and the spleen of the African lungfish *Protopterus aethiopicus*. *Acta Physiol. Scand.*, **107**, 141–147.

Autillo-Touati, A. (1979). A cytochemical and ultrastructural study of the 'SIF' cells in cat sympathetic ganglia. *Histochemistry*, **60**, 189–223.

Becker, K. (1972). Paraganglienzellen im Ganglion cervicale uteri der Maus. *Z. Zellforsch. Mikrosk. Anat.*, **130**, 249–261.

Behrendt, H., Lindl, T., and Cramer, H. (1976). *In vitro* effects of histamine liberator compound 48/80 on rat superior cervical ganglia with special regard to the small granule-containing cells. *Cell Tissue Res.*, **166**, 71–81.

Benitez, H. H., Masurovsky, E. B., and Murray, M. R. (1974). Interneurons of the sympathetic ganglia in organotypic culture. A suggestion as to their function, based on three types of study. *J. Neurocytol.*, **3**, 363–384.

Bennett, T., and Malmfors, T. (1970). The adrenergic nervous system of the domestic fowl (*Gallus domesticus* L.). *Z. Zellforsch. Mikrosk. Anat.*, **106**, 22–50.

Björklund, A., Cegrell, L., Falck, B., Ritzén, M., and Rosengren, E. (1970). Dopamine-containing cells in sympathetic ganglia. *Acta Physiol. Scand.*, **78**, 334–338.

Bloom, G., Östlund, E., von Euler, U.S., Lishajko, F., Ritzén, M., and Adams-Ray, J. (1961). Studies on catecholamines containing granules of specific cells in cyclostomes hearts. *Acta Physiol. Scand.*, **53** (Suppl. 185), 1–34.

Burnstock, G., Evans, B., Gannon, B. J., Heath, J. W., and James, V. (1971). A new method of destroying adrenergic nerves in adult animals using guanethidine. *Br. J. Pharmacol.*, **43**, 295–301.

Campbell, G., and Gannon, B. J. (1976). The splanchnic nerve supply to the stomach of the trout, *Salmo trutta* and *Salmo gairdneri*. *Comp. Biochem. Physiol.*, **55C**, 51–53.

Caravita, S. and Coscia, L. (1966). Les cellules chromaffines du coeur de la Lamproie (Lampetre Zamandreai). Etude an microscope électronique avant et aprés un traitement à la réserpine-Arch. Biol., Liège, **77**, 723–753.

Chamley, J. H., Mark, G. E., and Burnstock, G. (1972). Sympathetic ganglia in culture. I. Neurones. II. Accessory cells. *Z. Zellforsch. Mikrosk. Anat.*, **135**, 287–314, 315–327.

Champlain, J. de, Malmfors, T., Olson, L., and Sachs, C. (1970). Ontogenesis of peripheral adrenergic neurons in the rat: pre- and postnatal observations. *Acta Physiol. Scand.*, **80**, 276–288.

Chiba, T. (1977). Monoamine-containing paraneurons in the sympathetic ganglia of mammals. *Arch. Histol. Jpn.*, **40** (Suppl.), 163–176.

Chiba, T. (1978). Monoamine fluorescence and electron microscope studies on small intensely fluorescent (granule-containing) cells in human sympathetic ganglia. *J. Comp. Neurol.*, **179**, 153–168.

Chiba, T., and Williams, T. H. (1975). Histofluorescence characteristics and quantification of small intensely fluorescent (SIF) cells in sympathetic ganglia of several species. *Cell Tissue Res.*, **162**, 331–341.

Chiba, T., and Yamauchi, A. (1973). Fluorescence and electron microscopy of the monoamine-containing cells in the turtle heart. *Z. Zellforsch. Mikrosk. Anat.*, **140**, 25–37.

Chiba, T., Hwang, B. H., and Williams, T. H. (1976). A method for studying glyoxylic acid induced fluorescence and ultrastructure of monoamine neurons. *Histochemistry*, **49**, 95–106.

Chiba, T., Black, A. C., Jr., and Williams, T. H. (1977). Evidence for dopamine-storing interneurons and paraneurons in rhesus monkey sympathetic ganglia. *J. Neurocytol.*, **6**, 441–453.

Ciaranello, R. D., Jacobowitz, D., and Axelrod, J. (1973). Effect of dexamethasone on phenylethanolamine-*N*-methyl transferase in chromaffin tissue of the neonatal rat. *J. Neurochem.*, **20**, 799–805.

Costa, M., and Furness, J. B. (1973). Observations on the anatomy and amine histochemistry of the nerves and ganglia which supply the pelvic viscera and on the associated chromaffin tissue in the guinea pig. *Z. Anat. Entwicklungsgesch.*, **140**, 85–108.

Coupland, R. E. (1965). *The Natural History of the Chromaffin Cell*, Longman, London.

Coupland, R. E., Pyper, A. S., and Hopwood, D. (1964). A method for differentiating between adrenaline and noradrenaline-storing cells in the light and electron microscope. *Nature*, **201**, 1240–1242.

Dail, W. G., and Evan, A. P. (1978a). Ultrastructure of adrenergic terminals and SIF cells in the superior ganglion of the rabbit. *Brain Res.*, **148**, 469–477.

Dail, W. G., and Evan, A. P. (1978b). Effects of chronic deafferentation on adrenergic ganglion cells and small intensely fluorescent cells. *J. Neurocytol.*, **7**, 25–37.

Dail, W. G., Evan, A. P., and Eason, H. R. (1975). The major ganglion in the pelvic plexus of the male rat. A histochemical and ultrastructural study. *Cell Tissue Res.*, **159**, 49–62.

Diner, O. (1965). Observations sur le développement de la médullo-surrénale du rat: l'évolution de la partie non chromaffine. *Arch. Anat. Microsc. Morphol. Exp.*, **54**, 671–718.

Elfvin, L. G. (1968). A new granule-containing nerve cell in the inferior mesenteric ganglion of the rabbit. *J. Ultrastruct. Res.*, **22**, 37–44.

Elfvin, L. G., Hökfelt, T., and Goldstein, M. (1975). Fluorescent microscopical immunohistochemical and ultrastructural studies on sympathetic ganglia of the guinea pig, with special reference to the SIF cells and their catecholamine content. *J. Ultrastruct. Res.*, **51**, 377–396.

Ellison, J. P., and Hibbs, R. G. (1974). Catecholamine-containing cells of the guinea pig heart: an ultrastructural study. *J. Mol. Cell. Cardiol.*, **6**, 17–26.

Ellison, J. P., and Hibbs, R. G. (1976). An ultrastructural study of mammalian cardiac ganglia. *J. Mol. Cell. Cardiol.*, **8**, 89–101.

Enemar, A., Falck, B., and Håkanson, R. (1965). Observations on the appearance of norepinephrine in the sympathetic nervous system of the chick embryo. *Dev. Biol.*, **11**, 268–283.

Eränkö, L. (1972). Ultrastructure of the developing sympathetic nerve cell and the storage of catecholamines. *Brain Res.*, **46**, 159–175.

Eränkö, L., and Eränkö, O. (1972a). Effect of hydrocortisone on histochemically demonstrable catecholamines in the sympathetic ganglia and extraadrenal chromaffin tissue of the rat. *Acta Physiol. Scand.*, **84**, 125–133.

Eränkö, L., and Eränkö, O. (1972b). Effect of 6-hydroxydopamine on the ganglion cells and the small intensely fluorescent cells in the superior cervical ganglion of the rat. *Acta Physiol. Scand.*, **84**, 115–124.

Eränkö, O., and Eränkö, L. (1971). Small, intensely fluorescent granule-containing cells in the sympathetic ganglion of the rat. *Prog. Brain Res.*, **34**, 39–51.

Eränkö, O., and Eränkö, L. (1980). Induction of SIF cells by hydrocortisone or human cord serum in sympathetic ganglia and their subsequent fate *in vivo* and *in vitro*. In *Histochemistry and Cell Biology of Autonomic Neurons, SIF Cells and Paraneurons* (Eds. O. Eränkö, S. Soinila and H. Päivärinta), *Advances in Biochemical Psychopharmacology*, Vol. 25, pp. 17–26, Raven Press, New York.

Eränkö, O., and Härkönen, M. (1963). Histochemical demonstration of fluorogenic amines in the cytoplasm of sympathetic ganglion cells of the rat. *Acta Physiol. Scand.*, **58**, 285–286.

Eränkö, O., and Härkönen, M. (1965). Monoamine-containing small cells in the superior cervical ganglion of the rat and an organ composed of them. *Acta Physiol. Scand.*, **63**, 511–512.

Eränkö, O., Heath, J., and Eränkö, L. (1972a). Effect of hydrocortisone on the ultrastructure of the small, intensely fluorescent, granule-containing cells in cultures of sympathetic ganglia of newborn rats. *Z. Zellforsch. Mikrosk. Anat.*, **134**, 297–310.

Eränkö, O., Eränkö, L., Hill, C. E., and Burnstock, G. (1972b). Hydrocortisone-induced increase in the number of small intensely fluorescent cells and histochemically demonstrable catecholamines content in cultures of sympathetic ganglia of the new born rat. *Histochem. J.*, **4**, 49–58.

Eränkö, O., Heath, J. W., and Eränkö, L. (1973). Effect of hydrocortisone on the ultrastructure of the small, granule containing cells in the superior cervical ganglion of the new-born rat. *Experientia*, **29**, 457–459.

Eränkö, O., Eränkö, L., and Hervonen, H. (1976). Cultures of sympathetic ganglia and the effect of glucocorticoids on SIF cells. *Fogarty Int. Cent. Proc.*, **30**, 196–214.

Fujita, T. (1977). Concept of paraneurons. *Arch. Histol. Jpn.*, **40** (Suppl.), 1–12.

Furness, J. B., and Costa, M. (1975). The use of glyoxylic acid for the demonstration of peripheral stores of noradrenaline and 5-hydroxytryptamine in whole mounts. *Histochemistry*, **41**, 335–352.

Furness, J. B., and Costa, M. (1976). Some observations on extra-adrenal chromaffin cells in the lower abdomen and pelvis. In *Chromaffin, Enterochromaffin and related cells* (Eds. R. Coupland and T. Fujita), pp. 25–34, Elsevier, Amsterdam.

Furness, J. B., Heath, J. W., and Costa, M. (1978). Aqueous aldehyde (Faglu) methods for the fluorescence histochemical localization of catecholamine and for ultrastructural studies of central nervous tissue. *Histochemistry*, **57**, 285–295.

Gabella, G. (1976). Structure of the autonomic nervous system. Chapman and Hall. London.

Grillo, M. A. (1966). Electron microscopy of sympathetic tissues. *Pharmacol. Rev.*, **18**, 387–399.

Grillo, M. A., Jacobs, L., and Comroe, J. M., Jr. (1974). A combined fluorescence histochemical and electron microscopic method for studying special mono-amine-containing cells (SIF cells). *J. Comp. Neurol.*, **153**, 1–14.

Hervonen, A. (1971). Development of catecholamine storing cells in human foetal paraganglia and adrenal medulla. *Acta Physiol. Scand., Suppl.*, **368**, 1–94.

Hervonen, A., and Eränkö, O, (1975). Fluorescence histochemical and electron microscopical observations on sympathetic ganglia of the chick embryo cultured with and without hydrocortisone. *Cell Tissue Res.*, **156**, 145–166.

Hervonen, A., and Kanerva, L. (1972). Cell types of human foetal superior cervical ganglion. *Z. Anat. Entwicklungsgesch.*, **137**, 257–269.

Heym, Ch. (1976). Monoamine storage sites in the rat superior cervical ganglion following synthesis inhibition. *Cell Tissue Res.*, **165**, 239–248.

Heym, Ch., and Grube, D. (1975). Effects of guanethidine on paraganglionic cells in the superior cervical ganglion of the rat. *Anat. Embryol.*, **148**, 89–97.

Heym, Ch., and Williams, T. H. (1979). Evidence for autonomic paraneurons in sympathetic ganglia of a shrew (*Tupaia glis*). *J. Anat.*, **129**, 151–164.

Heym, Ch., Grube, D., and Forsmann, W. G. (1974). Ganglienzellen und para-ganglionäre Zellen des Ganglion cervicale superius der Ratte nach Parachloro-phenylalanin (PCAP). *Z. Anat. Entwicklungsgesch.*, **143**, 223–237.

Hino, O., and Tsunekawa, K. (1978). The occurrence of small intensely fluorescent (SIF) cells in human sympathetic ganglia. *Experientia*, **34**, 1359.

Hökfelt, T. (1965). A modification of the histochemical fluorescence method for the demonstration of catecholamines and 5-hydroxytryptamine, using Araldite as embedding medium. *J. Histochem. Cytochem.*, **13**, 518–519.

Hökfelt, T. (1969). Distribution of noradrenaline storing particles in peripheral adrenergic neurons as revealed by electron microscopy. *Acta Physiol. Scand.*, **76**, 427–440.

Ivanov, D. P. (1974). Recherches ultrastructurales sur les cellules paraganglionnaires du ganglion coeliaque du rat et leurs connexions avec les neurones. *Acta Anat.*, **89**, 266–286.

Iversen, L. L. (1975). Uptake of circulating catecholamines into tissues. In *Handbook of Physiology*, Section 7, *Endocrinology*, Vol. VI, pp. 713–722. Amer. Soc. Physiol. Washington D.C.

Jacobowitz, D. (1970). Catecholamine fluorescence studies of adrenergic neurons and chromaffin cells in sympathetic ganglia. *Fed. Proc.*, **29**, 1929–1944.

Jacobowitz, D. M., and Greene, L. A. (1974). Histofluorescence study of chromaffin cells in dissociated cell cultures of chick embryo sympathetic ganglia. *J. Neurobiol.*, **5**, 65–83.

Johnson, M. I., Ross, C. D., Meyers, M., Spitznagel, E. L., and Bunge, R. P. (1980). Morphological and biochemical studies on the development of cholinergic prop-erties in cultured sympathetic neurons. I. Correlative changes in ChAT and synaptic vesicle cytochemistry. *J. Cell Biol.*, **84**, 680–691.

Kanerva, L. (1971). The postnatal development of monoamines and cholinesterases in the paracervical ganglion of the rat uterus. *Prog. Brain Res.*, **34**, 433–444.

Kanerva, L. (1972). Ultrastructure of sympathetic ganglion cells and granule-contain-ing cells in the paracervical (Frankenhauser) ganglion of the newborn rat. *Z. Zellforsch. Mikrosk. Anat.*, **126**, 25–40.

Kanerva, L., and Hervonen, A. (1976). SIF cells, short adrenergic neurons and vacuolated nerve cells of the paracervical (Frankenhauser) ganglion. *Fogarty Int. Cent. Proc.*, **30**, 19–34.

Kanerva, L., and Teräväinen, H. (1972). Electron microscopy of the paracervical (Frankenhauser) ganglion of the adult rat. *Z. Zellforsch. Mikrosk. Anat.*, **129**, 161–177.

Kanerva, L., Hervonen, A., Eränkö, O., and Rietzén, R. (1974). Fine structural changes caused by 6-OH-dopamine in the small intensely fluorescent cells of the paracervical ganglion of the rat. *Cell Tissue Res.*, **152**, 437–447.

Kohn, A. (1903). Die paraganglien. *Arch. Mikrosk. Anat.*, **62**, 263–365.

Lever, J. D., and Presley, R. (1971). Studies on the sympathetic neuron *in vitro*. *Prog. Brain Res.*, **34**, 499–512.

Lever, J. D., Lu, K. J., Presley, R., and Santer, R. M. (1974). The distribution of small intensely fluorescent (SIF) and of chromaffin-positive (CH^+) cells in rat sympathetic ganglia. *J. Anat.*, **117**, 643–644.

Libet, B., and Owman, Ch. (1974). Concomitant changes in formaldehyde-induced fluorescence of dopamine interneurons and in slow inhibitory postsynaptic potentials of the rabbit superior cervical ganglion, induced by stimulation of the preganglionic nerve or by a muscarinic agent. *J. Physiol. (London)*, **237**, 635–662.

Lignon, J. and Le Douarin, G. (1978). Small intensely fluorescent (SIF) cells and myocardic cells in the ammocoete heart; a correlative histofluorescence, light and electron microscopic study with special reference to the action of reserpine. *Biol. Cell*, **31**, 169–176.

Lu, K. S., Lever, J. D., Santer, R. M., and Presley, R. (1976). Small granulated cell types in rat superior cervical and coeliac-mesenteric ganglia. *Cell Tissue Res.*, **172**, 331–343.

Mascorro, J. A., and Yates, R. D. (1980). Paraneurons and paraganglia: histological and ultrastructural comparisons between intraganglionic paraneurons and extra-adrenal paraganglion cells. In *Histochemistry and Cell Biology of Autonomic Neurons, SIF Cells and Paraneurons* (Eds. O. Eränkö, S. Soinila and H. Päivärinta), pp. 201–213, Raven Press, New York.

Matthews, M. R. (1978). Ultrastructural evidence for discharge of granules by exocytosis from small granule-containing cells of superior cervical ganglion in the rat. In *Peripheral Neuroendocrine Interactions* (Eds. R. E. Coupland and W. G. Forsmann), pp. 80–85, Springer, Berlin.

Matthews, M. R. (1980). Ultrastructural studies relevant to the possible functions of small granule-containing cells in the rat superior cervical ganglion. In *Histochemistry and Cell Biology of Autonomic Neurons, SIF Cells and Paraneurons* (Eds. O. Eränkö, S. Soinila and H. Päivärinta), *Advances in Biochemical Psychopharmacology*, Vol. 25, pp. 77–86, Raven Press, New York.

Matthews, M. R., and Nash, J. R. G. (1970). An efferent synapse from a small granule containing cell to a principal neurone in the superior cervical ganglion. *J. Physiol. (London)*, **210**, 11–14P.

Matthews, M. R., and Raisman, G. (1969). The ultrastructure and somatic efferent synapses of small granule-containing cells in the superior cervical ganglion. *J. Anat.*, **105**, 255–282.

Mytilineou, C., and Tennyson, V. M. (1973). Development of sympathetic neuroblasts in the foetal rabbit: a fluorescence and electron microscopic study. *J. Cell Biol.*, **59**, 241.

Nilsson, S. (1976). Fluorescent histochemistry and cholinesterase staining of sympathetic ganglia in a teleost, *Gadus morrhua*. *Acta Zool. (Stockholm)*, **57**, 69–77.

Norberg, K. A., and Sjöqvist, F. (1966). New possibilities for adrenergic modulation of ganglionic transmission. *Pharmacol. Rev.*, **18**, 743–751.

Norberg, K. A., Ritzén, M., and Ungerstedt, U. (1966). Histochemical studies on a special catecholamine-containing cell type in sympathetic ganglia. *Acta Physiol. Scand.*, **67**, 260–270.

Owman, C., and Sjöstrand, N. O. (1965). Short, adrenergic neurons and catecholamine-containing cells in vas deferens and accessory male genital glands of different mammals. *Z. Zellforsch. Mikrosk. Anat.*, **66**, 300–320.

Papka, R. E. (1973). The ultrastructure of adrenergic neurons in sympathetic ganglia of the neaborn rabbit after treatment with 6-hydroxydopamine. *Am. J. Anat.*, **137**, 447–466.

Partanen, M., Hervonen, A., and Santer, R. M. (1980). Effect of aging on SIF cells of the rat. In *Histochemistry and Cell Biology of Autonomic Neurons, SIF Cells and Paraneurons* (Eds. O. Eränkö, S. Soinila and H. Päivärinta), *Advances in Biochemical Psychopharmacology*, Vol. 25, pp. 143–147, Raven Press, New York.

Pearse, A. G. E. (1969). The cytochemistry and ultrastructure of polypeptide hormone-producing cells of the APUD series and the embryologic, physiologic and pathologic implications of the concept. *J. Histochem. Cytochem.*, **17**, 303–313.

Santer, R. M., Presley, R., Lever, J. D., and Lu, K. S. (1976). Quantitative fluorescence studies of the effects of catecholamines and hydrocortisone on endogenous amines levels in neurons and SIF cells of embryonic chick sympathetic ganglia *in vivo* and *in vitro*. *Cell Tissue Res.*, **175**, 333–344.

Scott, E. B., and Hung, K. S. (1971). Observations on the nerve cells and chromaffin-like cells of the sympathetic ganglion in the seminal vesicle of the rat. In *29th Annu. Meet. Electron Microsc. Soc. America Proc.*, Boston, 1971, pp. 278–279.

Siegrist, G., Ribaupierre, F. de, Dolivo, M., and Rouiller, C. (1966). Les cellules chromaffines des ganglions cervicaux supérieurs du rat. *J. Microsc.*, **5**, 791–794.

Siegrist, G., Dolivo, M., Dunant, Y., Foroglou-Kerameus, C., and Ribaupierre, F. de (1968). Ultrastructure and function of the chromaffin cells in the superior cervical ganglion of the rat. *J. Ultrastruct. Res.*, **25**, 381–407.

Tamarind, D. L., and Quilliam, J. P. (1971). Synaptic organization and other ultrastructural features of the superior cervical ganglion of the rat, kitten and rabbit. *Micron*, **2**, 204–234.

Taxi, J. (1973). Observations complémentaires sur l'ultrastructure des ganglions sympathiques de mammifères. *Trab. Inst. Cajal. Invest. Biol.*, **65**, 9–40.

Taxi, J. (1979). The chromaffin and chromaffin-like cells in the autonomic nervous system. *Int. Rev. Cytol.*, **57**, 283–343.

Taxi, J., and Mikulajova, M. (1976). Some cytochemical and cytological features of the so-called SIF cells of the superior cervical ganglion of the rat. *J. Neurocytol.*, **5**, 283–295.

Taxi, J., Gautron, J., and L'Hermite, P. (1969). Données ultrastructurales sur une éventuelle modulation adrénergique de l'activité du ganglion cervical supérieur. *C. R. Acad. Sci.*, **269**, 1281–1284.

Tennyson, V. M., and Mytilineou, C. (1976). Fluorescence and electron microscopic studies of sympathicoblasts in the fetal rabbit. *Fogarty Int. Cent. Proc.*, **30**, 35–53.

Thoenen, H., and Tranzer, J. P. (1968). Chemical sympathectomy by selective destruction of adrenergic nerve endings with 6-hydroxydopamine. *Naunyn-Schmiedebergs Arch. Pharmakol. Exp. Pathol.*, **261**, 271–288.

Van Orden, L. S., Burke, J. P., Geyer, M., and Lodoen, F. W. (1970). Localization of depletion-sensitive and depletion-resistant norepinephrine storage sites in auto-nomic ganglia. *J. Pharmacol. Exp. Ther.*, **174**, 56–71.

Watanabe, H. (1971). Adrenergic nerve elements in the hypogastric ganglion of the guinea pig. *Am. J. Anat.*, **130**, 305–330.

Watson, A. H. D. (1980). The structure of the coeliac ganglion of a teleost fish *Myoxocephalus scorpius*. *Cell Tissue Res.*, **210**, 155–165.

Wechsler, W., and Schmekel, L., 66. (1967). Elektron–mikroskopische Untersuchung der

Entwicklung der vegetativen (Grenzstrang) und spinalen Ganglien bei *Gallus domesticus. Acta Neuroveg.*, **30**, 427–444.

Williams, T. H. W. (1967). Electron microscope evidence for an autonomic interneuron. *Nature*, **214**, 309–310.

Williams, T. H., and Palay, S. L. (1969). Ultrastructure of the small neurons in the superior cervical ganglion. *Brain Res.*, **15**, 17–34.

Williams, T. H., Black, A. C., Jr., Chiba, T., and Bhalla, R. C. (1975). Morphology and biochemistry of small, intensely fluorescent cells of sympathetic ganglia. *Nature*, **256**, 315–317.

Winkler, H. (1977). The biogenesis of adrenal chromaffin granules. *Neuroscience*, **2**, 657–683.

Yamauchi, A. (1976). Ultrastructure of chromaffin-like interneurons in the autonomic ganglia. In *Chromaffin, Enterochromaffin and Related Cells* (Eds. R. E. Coupland and T. Fujita), pp. 117–130, Elsevier, Amsterdam.

Yamauchi, A., Yokota, R., and Fujimaki, Y. (1975). Reciprocal synapses between cholinergic axons and small granule-containing cells in the rat cardiac ganglion. *Anat. Rec.*, **181**, 195–209.

Yokota, R. and Burnstock, G. (1978). A dividing granule-containing cell in the pelvic ganglion of the guinea pig. *Cell Tiss. Res.* **192**, 187–192.

Autonomic Ganglia
Edited by Lars-Gösta Elfvin
© 1983 John Wiley & Sons Ltd

Functional Morphology in Two Parasympathetic Ganglia: the Ciliary and the Pterygopalatine

B. EHINGER, F. SUNDLER and R. UDDMAN

*Departments of Ophthalmology and Histology, University of Lund,
Lund, and Department of Oto-rhino-laryngology, University Hospital
at Malmö, Malmö, Sweden*

INTRODUCTION

Generally, the parasympathetic ganglia have been less thoroughly studied with modern morphological and cytochemical techniques than the sympathetic ganglia. This is probably due to the fact that most parasympathetic ganglia are less accessible and less well defined. Further, there has been no technique for demonstrating parasympathetic neurons with a specificity and sensitivity comparable with the histofluorescence method of Falck and Hillarp for sympathetic neurons. However, the recognition of the relative accessibility of the ciliary ganglion in birds has resulted in a striking accumulation of both morphological and physiological knowledge about it within the last two decades. Further, immunohistochemical techniques are now rapidly evolving for the localization of neuropeptides, which are of pertinence to the autonomic ganglia. The following is a summary of what is known of the morphology of two discrete and fairly well studied parasympathetic ganglia—the ciliary and pterygopalatine ganglia—with some special reference to work in progress on neuropeptides. Since morphology is of little interest if it has no relation to function, physiological information is also included when appropriate.

The first light-microscopic study of the ciliary and pterygopalatine ganglia dates back to Retzius (1880) who performed a systematic investigation of the different cranial ganglia. Using osmium staining he noted that the ganglia harbour both bipolar and multipolar cells. Subsequent work showed that the multipolar cells were surrounded by a meshwork of fine fibres (Müller and Dahl, 1910; Carpenter, 1912).

THE CILIARY GANGLION

Macroscopic anatomy

The ciliary ganglion is situated deep in the orbit behind the eye. Most of its preganglionic fibres stem from the oculomotor nerve and in primates (but not in cats or rabbits) fibres also reach the ganglion from the cervical sympathetic chain by way of the perivascular nerve net, from the nasociliary branch of the ophthalmic division of the trigeminal nerve and from the maxillary division of the trigeminal nerve by means of the recently described orbitociliary nerve (Ruskell, 1974). It sends varying numbers of short ciliary nerves to the eye (Lele and Wedell, 1959; Grimes and von Sallman, 1960; Prince *et al.*, 1960; Duke-Elder and Wybar, 1961; Malmfors and Nilsson, 1964; Rohen, 1964; Ruskell, 1964). Accessory ganglia are common along the short ciliary nerves (see, for example, Wolf, 1941). At least in rats and cats it is possible to perform ciliary ganglionectomy without severely disturbing the supply of sympathetic nerves to the eye (Ehinger and Falck, 1966; Ehinger *et al.*, 1969).

In chicken there are three postganglionic nerve trunks. Each branch innervates a separate and defined region in the eye (Pilar *et al.*, 1980). Lele and Grimes (1960) noted segmental contractions of the iris upon stimulation of individual short ciliary nerves in cats but otherwise there is no information on whether there might be any organization in mammals similar to that of chicken.

It has long been held that all cholinergic axons to the eye synapse in the ciliary ganglion. Westheimer and Blair (1973) questioned this when they were unable to block accommodation completely in monkeys by applying nicotine to the ganglion, and they received support from experiments with retrograde horseradish peroxidase tracing in rabbits and monkeys (Jaeger and Benevento, 1980). However, Ruskell and Griffiths (1979) were unable to find any degenerating terminals in the monkey ciliary muscle after severing the oculomotor nerve intracranially such as they should have had there been a large uninterrupted pathway from the oculomotor nucleus. Since the number of brain cells labelled by horseradish peroxidase in the rabbit and monkey was low, and aberrant ganglion cells are well known to occur in the uvea (e.g. Ashton, 1952; Kurus, 1955; Wolter, 1960; Valu, 1962), it seems possible that the results of Westheimer and Blair (1973) and Jaeger and Benevento (1980) are due to presynaptic axons reaching as far as to the uvea before forming any synapse on aberrant ganglion cells. It is not disputed that most cholinergic nerves in the iris and ciliary body muscles arise in the ciliary ganglion (Warwick, 1954, 1956; Duke-Elder and Wybar, 1961; Pilar *et al.*, 1980).

Microscopic anatomy

Mammals

A number of subtypes have been described among the nerve cells of mammalian ciliary ganglia (e.g. Pines, 1927; Kurus, 1956; Rohen, 1964; Gabella, 1976) but their correlation with function has not been established.

Generally, the cells are larger than in the sympathetic ganglia and in other parasympathetic ganglia (see Gabella, 1976). On the other hand, they are, at least in rabbits, smaller than the nerve cells in the trigeminal ganglion (Ruskell, 1964). The dendrites are usually short. In humans, the total cell number is about 3500 (Pearson and Pytel, 1978) and in cats it is about 4500 (Wolf, 1941).

Ultrastructurally, the ganglion cells have a number of features in common with other autonomic ganglia (Yoshida, 1968, 1971; Huikuri, 1969; Tobari, 1971a, b; Watanabe, 1972). They are surrounded by satellite cells containing abundant 10 nm filaments and often also a cilium (Watanabe, 1972). Mitochondria abound in the cytoplasm of the neuron perikaryon which is also rich in rough endoplasmic reticulum but comparatively poor in smooth endoplasmic reticulum. Large (about 100 nm) dense-cored vesicles are readily seen, particularly near the usually well developed Golgi complex. Small (40–50 nm) clear vesicles are less common. Different multivesiculated bodies have been observed.

The synapses are of the conventional chemical type with an accumulation of clear 40–50 nm vesicles on the presynaptic side and with increased electron density both in the synaptic cleft and at the membranes on each side. They are usually axosomatic. Dense-cored vesicles are regularly seen; they are larger than those usually associated with adrenergic neurons.

Chicken

The ganglion has been investigated in chicken in some detail (Fig. 1). It has long been known to contain cells of two sizes, and Marwitt *et al.* (1971) showed that the small cells contact only choroidal vessels in the eye whereas the large cells innervate the muscles of the iris and ciliary body. The two cell types were therefore named choroidal and ciliary cells, respectively. The ciliary cell bodies are unipolar and myelinated (Takahashi and Hama, 1965a, b). They appear to be the only known myelinated perikarya with synapses (Hess, 1965), which may relate to the type of myelin found in the chicken ciliary ganglion (Takahashi and Hama, 1965a). In contrast, the ciliary ganglia of mammals contain only unmyelinated, usually multipolar cells. The nucleus of the ciliary cell (Fig. 2) is located in one end of the ovoid cell body (the nuclear pole) whereas the opposite end (the hilar pole) receives the innervation and gives off the axon (e.g. Hámori and Dyachkova, 1964; Szentágothai, 1964; Cantino and Mugnaini, 1975). In adult birds, the usually oval ciliary cells are 30–50 μm in diameter and the choroid cells are 15–20 μm (e.g. Hess, 1965; Cantino and Mugnaini, 1975). The latter are located together in one group situated ventromedially in the chicken ganglion. The two cell types occur in equal numbers, adding up to a total of about 3000 in chicken (Martin *et al.*, 1971). Only one presynaptic cholinergic fibre is thought to impinge on

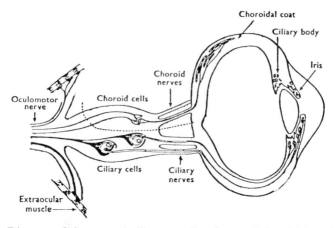

Figure 1 Diagram of the normal ciliary ganglion from a 1-day chick and postganglionic structures innervated by it. The preganglionic fibres run together in the oculomotor nerve with motor fibres to the extraocular muscles. Ciliary cells, with calyciform synapses, send axons in ciliary nerves to striated iris and ciliary muscles. Multiple-innervated choroid cells send axons in choroid nerves to innervate smooth vascular muscle in choroidal coat. Note that optic cup is drawn much reduced with respect to ganglion. From Martin and Pilar (1973); reproduced by permission of *Journal of Physiology.*

each ciliary cell, whereas each choroid cell is said to be reached by two or three axons (Johnson and Pilar, 1980). The number of neurons is higher in the ganglion of pigeons and turkeys (Marwitt *et al.*, 1971; Terzuolo, 1951).

The cell bodies giving off the axons in each of the three short ciliary nerves are scattered throughout the ganglion, although with a clear tendency for the cell bodies of a given nerve to dominate in a distinct part of the ganglion (Pilar *et al.*, 1980). No size differences were noted for the ciliary ganglion cells sending axons to different ciliary nerve branches.

Each of the two cell types in the bird ciliary ganglion is postsynaptic to a separate class of preganglionic fibres in the oculomotor nerve. The fibres to the ciliary cells conduct at a faster rate than those to the choroid cells (Landmesser and Pilar, 1972).

The synapse on the ciliary cells (Marwitt *et al.*, 1971) is peculiar and is found in birds and reptiles but not in mammals (De Lorenzo, 1960, 1966; Szentágothai, 1964; Hámori and Dyachkova, 1964; Takahashi and Hama, 1965a; Koenig, 1967; Takahashi, 1967; Cantino and Mugnaini, 1975). In the newly hatched bird the single cholinergic presynaptic terminal expands to form a calyx which engulfs a large part of the postganglionic cell body. In the growing chick, this calyx is gradually broken up into smaller but still voluminous endings forming a calyciform structure. The process begins a few days after hatching. Ultrastructurally, the presynaptic fibre is readily distinguished from postsynaptic ones. Dendrites do not occur, but short

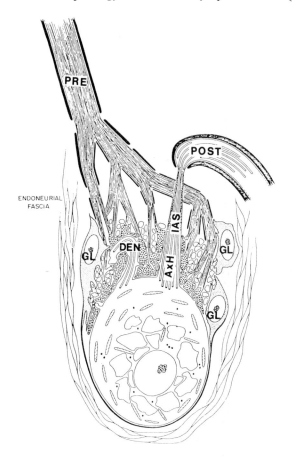

Figure 2 Schematic representation of the relationships between the preganglionic fibre (PRE) and the ciliary neuron in the adult chicken. GL indicates satellite cells; DEN, a dendrite; AxH, IAS and POST, the axon hillock, the initial axon segment and the myelinated portion of the postganglionic axon, respectively. The compact myelin sheaths are indicated by heavy lines. The distribution of various cytoplasmic organelles has been simplified. The presynaptic terminals are represented with synaptic vesicles only and the presynaptic fibre branches with neurofilaments. The synaptic and gap junctions are not shown. Note the difference in the magnitude of the extracellular compartments at the hilar region near to and more distant from the cell body. From Cantino and Mugnaini (1975); reproduced by permission of *Journal of Neurocytology*.

processes extend from the cell body into the calyx of the newly hatched bird. In adult animals they extend short distances into the cluster of end-bulbs which replace the calyx. However, transient dendrites appear during the development. Four types of specialized areas have been described on apposed plasma membranes: (1) contact areas without membrane specialization but with extensive interdigitation of the cells; (2) desmosome-like structures; (3) conventional synaptic complexes (resembling Gray's type I); and (4) gap junctions. The synaptic complexes show a 30 nm synaptic cleft, some pre- and postsynaptic electron-dense material at the membrane and clusters of pre-synaptic 40–60 nm clear vesicles. These synapses are at times seen on small spines issuing from the cell body, and the spine then has a central rod-like cytoplasmic density (Takahashi, 1967). The significance of this arrangement is unknown. The gap junctions were about 500 nm long and showed a narrow (2–8 nm) gap between the plasma membranes and some aggregation of electron-dense material at the membrane on both sides of the junction. They were found to occupy 0.17% of the extremely large ($16\,000\,\mu m^2$) total appositional area at the hilar pole (Cantino and Mugnaini, 1975). It was calculated (Cantino and Mugnaini, 1975) that the observed gap junctions were sufficient to account for the electrical behaviour of the synapse. By comparison, the conventional synapses occupied 9% of the total appositional area (Cantino and Mugnaini, 1975). In freeze fractures the gap junctions had the typical appearance with a cluster of small (9 nm) particles closely packed with centre-to-centre distances of about 10 nm. Gap junctions were not seen in embryonic or newly hatched chicken (Takahashi and Hama, 1965a).

The synapses on the ciliary cells are apparently both chemical and electrotonic with no or only little electrical rectification in chicken (Martin and Pilar, 1963a, b). The rearrangement of the single calyx to a calyciform cluster of end-bulbs does not impair the electrical transmission (Hámori and Dyachkova, 1964; Hess et al., 1969; Landmesser and Pilar, 1972).

Histochemistry of the ciliary ganglion

Acetylcholinesterases occur in the preganglionic terminals and in nerve cell bodies of the ciliary ganglion (Koelle, 1955; Koelle and Koelle, 1959; Giacobini, 1959; Taxi, 1961; Okinaka et al., 1963; Huikuri, 1966). Fukuda and Koelle (1959) showed that the enzyme is synthesized centrally and transported to the periphery of the cell body. Non-specific cholinesterases are in many animal species absent from most neurons of the ciliary ganglion but they occur in a few cells in the rat (Huikuri, 1966). They are prominent in the Schwann cells and in capillaries.

The chicken ciliary ganglion contains significant amounts of acetylcholine (Marchi et al., 1979; Johnson and Pilar, 1980), 60–70% of which is likely to be in presynaptic terminals (Pilar et al., 1973; Johnson and Pilar, 1980). The synthesizing enzymes, choline acetylase, is similarly distributed (Giacobini et al., 1979). The chicken ganglion cells synthesize acetylcholine (Johnson and Pilar, 1980), and antidromic stimulation, potassium ions (50 mM) or nicotine (1 mg/ml) will release newly synthesized acetylcholine from preganglionically denervated ganglia. The potassium-induced release is calcium-dependent

(Johnson and Pilar, 1980). Finally, the ciliary cells form cholinergic nicotinic junctions (Pilar and Vaughan, 1969) in all the muscles of the iris and ciliary body (which are of the striated type). The postsynaptic receptors of the choroid neuron terminals are muscarinic (Landmesser and Pilar, 1970). Thus, all the requirements for establishing neurons as cholinergic have been fulfilled for cells in the chicken ciliary ganglion.

The ciliary ganglion contains a variable number of so-called small intensely fluorescent cells (SIF cells) in rats, cats and Cebus monkeys (Ehinger and Falck, 1970). These cells contain substantial amounts of catecholamines and have been suggested to be a special type of interneuron (cf. Eränkö *et al.*, 1980). Their function in the ciliary ganglion remains obscure, but because of their variability it would seem they are dispensable. Another population of cells in the ciliary ganglion is characterized by only a low or no endogenous noradrenaline content, but they nevertheless have the ability to accumulate exogenous or endogenous catecholamines and to convert L-dihydroxypheny-lalanine (L-DOPA) to catecholamines (Ehinger, 1966a, b; Huikuri, 1966; Ehinger and Falck, 1970). As studied in rats, the axons of these neurons remain within the ganglion so that they form a class of intraganglionic interneurons. Their function remains undertermined.

There are in birds substantial numbers of adrenergic (perhaps sympathetic) fibres around the small (choroidal) nerve cells and a lesser but still sizable supply at the large (ciliary) nerve cells (Ehinger, 1967). The adrenergic fibres are also identifiable in the electron microscope with potassium-permanganate fixation (Cantino and Mugnaini, 1974). However, this technique is not well suited for showing synaptic contacts which therefore remain unseen at the ultrastructural level. The function of these fibres is also unknown.

Huikuri (1966) demonstrated histochemically non-specific esterases of various types, acid and alkaline phosphatases, and a number of mitochondrial respiratory enzymes in the ciliary ganglion of rats. Preganglionic denervation or sympathetic denervation had no effect on the phosphatases or the dehydrogenases. Giacobini *et al.* (1979) obtained similar results in chicken. Axotomy increased the activity of the dehydrogenases and the acid phosphatase for about two weeks. The alkaline phosphatase showed no change but the adenosine triphosphatase and cytochrome oxidase showed a decrease, with return to normal levels within two months. The presence of these enzymes and their changes are likely to reflect various aspects of the cell metabolism, but the exact significance remains uncertain. Monoamine oxidases have also been found in the ganglion (Koelle and Valk, 1954; Huikuri, 1966) but this ubiquitous mitochondrial enzyme has no specificity for any special nerve type. Axotomy was found to decrease the monoamine oxidase activity (Huikuri, 1966).

The neuropeptides, VIP (Vasoactive Intestinal Peptide) and substance P have only recently been detected in the uvea (VIP: Uddman *et al.*, 1980) (substance P: Bill *et al.*, 1979; Mandahl *et al.*, 1981). However, VIP was not detected in the cat ciliary ganglion (Uddman *et al.*, 1980), not even after colchicine treatment (Ehinger *et al.*, unpublished results). The uveal VIP nerves were found to originate in the pterygopalatine ganglion (Uddman *et al.*, 1980), presumably reaching the eye in the feline counterpart of the rami oculares described in rabbits and primates (Ruskell, 1965, 1970a, b, 1971).

Very recently, substance P and enkephalins have been observed immunohistochemically in preganglionic terminals in the avian ciliary ganglion (Karten, Erichsen, Eldred and Brecha, 1982). The terminals originate in the Edinger–Westphal nucleus. The two peptides were observed in both calyceal and boutonal terminals. Electron microscopy showed immunoreactivity in 85 nm dense-core vesicles in terminals also containing 58 nm clear vesicles. The observations suggest that the two neuropeptides may coexist with acetylcholine in preganglionic axons of the ciliary ganglion.*

Receptors in the ciliary ganglion

Cholinergic receptors

Cholinergic nicotinic receptors are present on mammalian ciliary ganglion cells (Perry and Talesnik, 1953) but have not been demonstrated morphologically. In chicken, both the ciliary and the choroid neurons have nicotinic, α-bungarotoxin- and najatoxin-sensitive receptors (Fumagalli *et al.*, 1978; Chiappinelli and Giacobini, 1978; Chiappinelli and Zigmond, 1978). The synapses on the choroid cells are more sensitive to hexamethonium and more resistant to D-tubocurarine or najatoxin than the synapses on the ciliary cells (Marwitt *et al.*, 1971; Conti-Tronconi *et al.*, 1979). In an autoradiographic analysis of the adult chicken ganglion, α-bungarotoxin-binding sites were found to be located near the plasma membranes of both cell populations. The binding sites on the choroid cells were arranged in patches at the cell circumference whereas the axon hillock was the most heavily labelled part in the ciliary cells (Fumagalli *et al.*, 1978). The total number of binding sites on ciliary cells was less than on choroid cells. The distribution of binding sites was different in developing embryos. Autoradiography of najatoxin-binding sites failed to show any differences between ciliary and choroid cells (Ciofi-Luzzatto *et al.*, 1980). However, it is not known to what extent the observed radioactivity represented neuronal uptake of the toxins rather than true receptor binding.

---

* Note added in the proofs: Kondo, Katayama and Yui have recently (1982) demonstrated terminals with *somatostatin*-like immunoreactivity in the cat ciliary ganglion and also found that somatostatin hyperpolarized many of the neurons in the ganglion.

Adrenergic receptors

Adrenergic blockers did not affect the transmission through the chicken ciliary ganglion (Marwitt *et al.*, 1971). There have been brief reports of inhibition of transmission in mammalian ciliary ganglia by adrenergic drugs (Tum Suden *et al.*, 1951, Marazzi, 1954) but, on the whole, the role of the adrenergic neurons in the ciliary ganglion remains to be demonstrated. Adrenergic receptors have not been localized microscopically.

Development in chicken

The site and cells of origin of the ciliary ganglion during ontogeny have been a matter of several opinions and were recently investigated by Narayanan and Narayanan (1978). They transplanted embryonal quail nerve tissue to chick embryos and studied the distribution of quail cells in the resulting chimaeras. Such cells end up in the chick ciliary ganglion only when they are taken from the mesencephalic neural crest which therefore should be the origin of the ciliary ganglion.

A large number of neurons in the peripheral ganglia die during the normal ontogeny, and the chick ciliary ganglion has been used for studying the factors governing this process in cholinergic neurons. The ganglion is formed at stage 25 (staging according to Hamburger and Hamilton, 1951) and both choroidal and ciliary cells seem to develop independently of the target organ until stage 30–33, with formation of functioning cholinergic synapses on all ciliary cells (Landmesser and Pilar, 1972, 1974a, b, 1976; Pilar and Landmesser, 1976). Transient dendrites appear at the time ganglion cell synapses are formed but they are later retracted when the calyces appear (Landmesser and Pilar, 1974) (Fig. 3). At stages 34–40, a number of neurons die, even though they have functioning synaptic input on their target (Landmesser and Pilar, 1974b). Eight-day chicken embryos have about 6000 cells per ganglion whereas 15-day embryos have only about 3000 (Landmesser and Pilar, 1974a; Nishi and Berg, 1977). Remarkably, in animals with an eviscerated eye, about half of the ganglion cells migrate into the remnant optic cup forming an aberrant ganglion there (Landmesser and Pilar, 1974a). Acetylcholine production (measured as choline acetyltransferase level) rises in the peripheral axons at the time of formation of peripheral synapses (Landmesser and Pilar, 1974b).

It has been shown that the cells that die are not genetically preprogrammed to do so (Narayanan and Narayanan, 1978; Pilar *et al.*, 1980). Chick ciliary ganglia are sensitive to a special cholinotrophic growth factor (e.g. Collins, 1978; Adler and Varon, 1980) which could be involved in regulating cell death and survival. However, the mechanisms governing this may be quite complex. In cells dying naturally, Pilar and Landmesser (1976) found ribosomes freed from the dilated rough endoplasmic reticulum and suggested that an accumulation of transmission-related proteins caused the cell death. On the other

Stage 25
(4½ days)   31 (7)   36 (10)   45 (20)

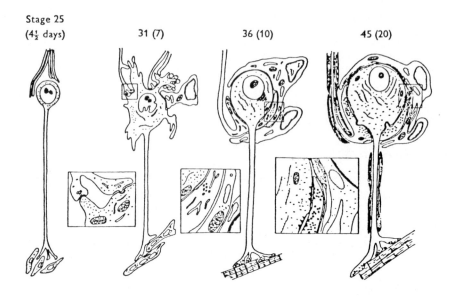

Figure 3 Ultrastructural maturation of a chicken ganglion cell of the ciliary population. At stage 25 the spheroidal unipolar cells have conducting axons. There is no
transmission through the ganglion and no ganglionic synapses are observed. By stage
31 when transmission is 100% ganglion cells have sent out processes forming a
complex neuropil. The first synapses are small boutons with few vesicles (see left
inset). By stage 36, the ganglion cell processes have been retracted and a single
preganglionic fibre now forms a calyciform ending over much of the cell surface.
Synaptic specializations with sparse vesicles occur at points along the calyx (see middle
inset). Ganglion cells have formed synapses with the iris. By stage 45 the major change
has been myelinization of axons as well as large areas of the ganglion cell soma. Gap
junctions between the calyx and ganglion cell occur and synaptic vesicles are much
more numerous (see right inset). From Landmesser and Pilar (1974a); reproduced by
permission of *Journal of Physiology*

hand, cell death induced by axotomy (peripheral ablation) very noticeably
followed a different course of morphological events with much more marked
nuclear changes and less dilatation of the rough endoplasmic reticulum.

α-Bungarotoxin was found to bind in a saturable and irreversible fashion to
membrane-associated receptors in chick ciliary ganglia (Gangitano *et al.*,
1978). The binding is selectively inhibitable with nicotinic but not muscarinic
ligands. Autoradiography showed the early labelling (incubation day 7) to be
rather diffuse, but by incubation day 19 some choroid cells had a patchy
peripheral labelling similar to the adult type. The labelling had developed
fully into the adult type at hatching. Patches of labelling also occurred on
ciliary cells on incubation day 7, but the adult type of labelling at the hilus of
the cell was not fully reached in all cells until 40 days after hatching. It

remains to be shown to what extent the reorganization of the labelling is a consequence of the formation of functioning synapses with the target organ.

Davis, Ericksen and Karten have recently (personal communication, 1981) noted that enkephalin immunoreactivity appears in nerve terminals in the ganglion just before the appearance of functioning synapses.

The ciliary ganglion in glaucoma and other diseases

The ciliary processes are supplied with cholinergic nerves which are likely to originate in the ciliary ganglion, and their production of aqueous humour is decreased with parasympathomimetics. Electrical stimulation of the ciliary ganglion affects intraocular pressure: it falls in the intact animal but rises in excised eye–ciliary ganglion preparations (Lele and Grimes, 1960; Macri and Cevario, 1975a, b). The relations between the state of the ganglion and glaucoma (a common and blinding disease with raised intraocular pressure) is therefore of interest. Tschernjawsky and Pletschkowa (1979) reported that the number of nerve cells of the human ciliary ganglion decreases with age. This could possibly affect the usefulness of indirectly acting drugs like the cholinesterase inhibitors, commonplace in ophthalmic practice. They further found that ganglion cells are entirely lacking in absolute glaucoma. However, this may well be a secondary effect and the relationship to the disease remains uncertain.

In five cases of familial dysautonomia, the size and number of cells of the ciliary ganglion were only slightly decreased, in contrast to sharp reductions in the pterygopalatine ganglion (Pearson and Pytel, 1978). Nevertheless, these patients show supersensitivity in the pupillary sphincter, but are still able to accommodate, perhaps suggesting that the neurons to the sphincter are more affected than the ones to the ciliary muscle—which constitute the great majority (Warwick, 1954). Severe degeneration of ciliary ganglion neurons has been found in Adie's syndrome in which the pupil reacts only very slowly in response to light stimulation (Harriman and Garland, 1968; Walsh and Hoyt, 1969, p. 501).

THE PTERYGOPALATINE GANGLION

Macroscopic anatomy

The pterygopalatine ganglion is situated in the pterygopalatine fossa. Preganglionic visceral motor fibres arise in the medulla oblongata and travel in the nervus intermedius and the facial nerve. They pass through the geniculate ganglion and the greater superficial petrosal nerve to form synapses in the pterygopalatine ganglion. A number of somatic sensory neurons with cell bodies located in the geniculate ganglion are also conveyed in the greater superficial petrosal nerve. These sensory neurons seem to serve areas of the soft palate and the pharynx (Ruskin, 1979). Fibres from the

cervical sympathetic chain pass through perivascular plexa and form the deep
petrosal nerve and, like fibres from the maxillary division of the trigeminal
nerve, they seem to pass uninterrupted through the ganglion (Tschallusow,
1913; Larsell and Fenton, 1928; Klepper, 1928; Christensen, 1934). The
greater superficial petrosal nerve and the deep petrosal nerve unite to form
the nerve of the pterygoid canal (the vidian nerve).

Fibres to the nose travel from the pterygopalatine ganglion in the posterior
nasal nerve. The terminals of these fibres are associated with small blood
vessels, seromucous glands and the surface epithelium. Similar structures in
the pharynx and palate are innervated via descending palatine branches.
Also, the lacrimal gland, as studied in rabbits, cats and monkeys, is
innervated by the pterygopalatine ganglion, either via direct branches or via a
retro-orbital plexus (Ruskell, 1965, 1971a; Uddman *et al.*, 1980). For details
on the neuronal connections, see Fig. 4. In cats, stimulation of the vidian

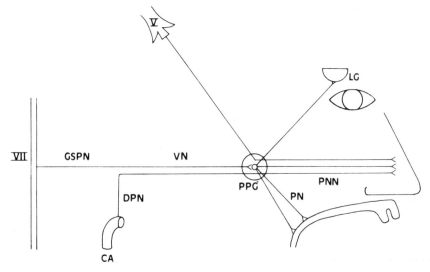

Figure 4 Neuronal connexions and projections of the pterygopalatine ganglion.
CA = carotid artery; DPN = deep petrosal nerve; GSPN = greater superficial petrosal
nerve; LG = lacrimal gland; PN = palatine nerves; PNN = posterior nasal nerve;
PPG = pterygopalatine ganglion; VN = vidian nerve

nerve evokes secretion from the lacrimal gland. This secretion is abolished by
applying nicotine to the pterygopalatine ganglion (Arenson and Wilson,
1971), indicating that they have a synapse in it. In the cat, fibres probably
arising in the pterygopalatine ganglion also reach other orbital structures such
as the Harderian glands and the tarsal glands (Uddman *et al.*, 1980). In man,
dorsal branches from the ganglion travel to the orbit. In monkeys, Ruskell
(1970a, b) demonstrated that the choroidal vessels were reached by neurons
originating in or passing through the pterygopalatine ganglion.

Microscopic anatomy

The early findings of Retzius (1880) and Müller and Dahl (1910) were later confirmed and extended in studies using various silver staining methods (Larsell and Fenton, 1928; Christensen, 1934). The ganglion was found to consist of mostly multipolar cells issuing several long branched dendrites. Both myelinated and unmyelinated fibres could be seen entering and leaving the ganglion.

Modern studies on the ganglion are few compared with work done on the ciliary ganglion. In a study of the ciliary and pterygopalatine ganglia, Pearson and Pytel (1978) found that the total number of neurons in the pterygopalatine ganglion was 56 000 in control patients. This was in sharp contrast with cases with familial dysautonomia where the number of neurons was reduced to about 1500. Koelle and Koelle (1959) demonstrated acetylcholinesterase in both preganglionic fibres and in the perikarya. Some cells showed much less enzyme activity than the others. The ultrastructure has been given some attention in two previous reports (Grillo and Palay, 1962; Yoshida, 1968). The recent immunohistochemical demonstration of the neuropeptide, VIP, in the pterygopalatine ganglion (Uddman *et al.*, 1980a, b; Lundberg *et al.*, 1980) has renewed the interest in it. We are therefore currently analysing it histochemically and ultrastructurally and the following descriptions are progress results of this work. Most of the studies have been performed on cats.

Nerve cell bodies

Light-microscopically the ganglion consists of nerve cell bodies of different sizes lying close together. Two main classes can be recognized—small cells and large cells—with some intermediates. The large ones predominate in all areas. Adrenergic cell bodies have not been observed and the ganglion has been found to contain no, or only very few, adrenergic fibres. All nerve cell bodies seem to be surrounded by satellite cells.

Ultrastructurally, nerve fibre profiles are numerous in all parts of the ganglion. Most of them are thin and unmyelinated, but myelinated ones are also regularly encountered (Fig. 5a). The former are often arranged in small bundles. Occasionally, single fibres penetrate the cytoplasm of satellite cells to form axosomatic synapses. Many fibres contain only clear 40–50 nm vesicles, whereas others contain a mixture of such vesicles and larger ones (around 100 nm) with a dense core (Fig. 5a). Previously, Grillo and Palay (1962) also described large dense-cored vesicles in presynaptic terminals in the murine pterygopalatine ganglion. Occasionally, fibre profiles containing abundant mitochondria are encountered. They presumably represent dendrites.

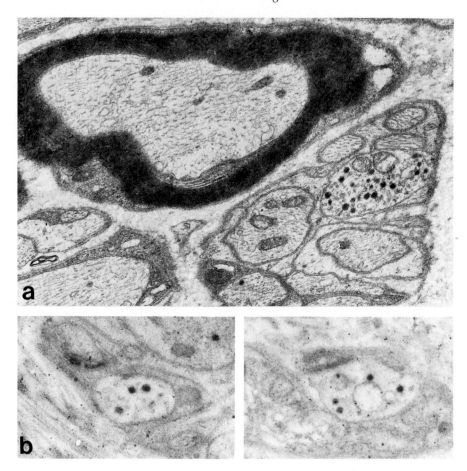

Figure 5 Feline pterygopalatine ganglion. (a) Cross-section of nerve fibres, one of which is myelinated (above). Note the occurrence of numerous small clear vesicles and larger dense-cored vesicles in one axon profile within a bundle of several others (×18 000). (b) Electron-immunocytochemical (immunoperoxidase) demonstration of VIP in axonal profiles. Immunoreactive material is confined to large dense-cored vesicles (×19)

The axosomatic synapses in the ganglion are characterized by a presynaptic cluster of 40–50 nm clear vesicles, symmetrically increased membrane densities on both the pre- and postsynaptic side, an occasional large dense-cored vesicle (100 nm), and some electron-dense material in the synaptic cleft. Fibre profiles with small dense-cored vesicles of the type commonly associated with adrenergic fibres have not been observed.

There are differences in the ultrastructure of the large and the small cells. The large ones have a well-developed endoplasmic reticulum with dilated

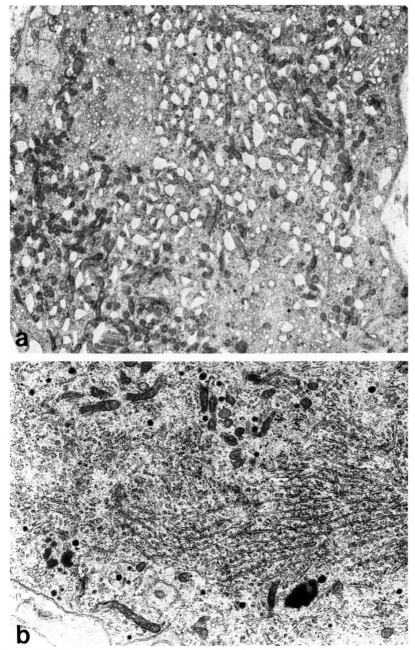

Figure 6 Feline pterygopalatine ganglion. Peripheral area of large (a) and medium-sized (b) nerve cell bodies. The cisternae of the endoplasmatic reticulum contains dilated portions in 'a' whereas in 'b' the cisternae are narrow. Electron micrograph, glutaraldehyde and OsO₄ fixation (×15 000)

portions (Fig. 6a) and lysosomes and bundles of filaments as well as polysomes are regularly encountered. Dense-cored and clear vesicles are very few. Small and medium-sized cell bodies also possess a well-developed endoplasmic reticulum, but here the cisternae are usually narrow (Fig. 6b). In addition, large (100 nm) dense-cored vesicles occur in varying numbers. These differences appear not to have been noted previously whereas the appearance of many of the other organelles is similar to what can be seen in other parasympathetic ganglia (e.g. Yoshida, 1968; Yamakado and Yohro, 1977).

Staining for acetylcholinesterase according to the method of Koelle and Friedenwald (1950) as modified by Holmstedt (1957) has revealed that some of the cell bodies are strongly acetylcholinesterase-positive and most such cells belong to the class of large neurons. After colchicine treatment virtually all cell bodies, irrespective of size, displayed intense acetylcholinesterase staining (Uddman, 1980).

Immunocytochemical and other studies (Uddman *et al.*, 1978, 1980, 1981*a*) have demonstrated that the nasal mucosa is rich in nerve fibres containing and releasing VIP. These fibres originate in the pterygopalatine ganglion (Uddman *et al.*, 1980). The ganglion harbours a large number of VIP-containing nerve cell bodies, most of which are of small or medium size (Fig. 7). These as well as other studies (cf. Fahrenkrug, 1979) support the view that VIP has a transmitter function in neurons of the pterygopalatine ganglion. Further, sequential staining for VIP and acetylcholinesterase has revealed that the VIP-immunoreactive cell bodies are distinct from those rich in acetylcholinesterase (Uddman, 1980). However, after colchicine, virtually all cell bodies are acetylcholinesterase-positive and display VIP immunoreactivity of moderate to high intensity (Fig. 7b).

In the electron microscope, immunoreactive VIP is localized within large dense-cored vesicles. Such dense-cored vesicles displaying VIP immunoreactivity occur in nerve fibres (Fig. 5b) as well as in nerve cell bodies, and after local exposure to colchicine there is a marked increase in the number of dense-cored VIP-immunoreactive vesicles in the cytoplasm of the cell bodies (Fig. 8).

Although VIP seems to be the predominating neuropeptide in the pterygopalatine ganglion, a few cell bodies of the small type have been shown to contain immunoreactive substance P (Fig. 7c). The projection of these neurons is at present unknown. After colchicine treatment also the substance P-immunoreactive cell bodies (like the ones storing VIP) contain demonstrable acetylcholinesterase activity (Uddman *et al.*, 1983). Provided the presence of acetylcholinesterase denotes the presence of acetylcholine, the substance P-containing neurons may be mixed peptidergic/cholinergic.

From the results obtained with colchicine-treated ganglia, it is evident that VIP is present in nerve cell bodies that are likely to be cholinergic. Moreover,

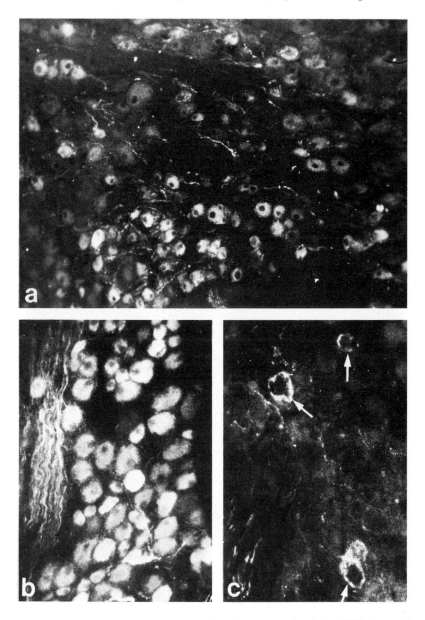

Figure 7   (a) Cat pterygopalatine ganglion immunostained for VIP (peroxidase-antiperoxidase (PAP) technique). Numerous cell bodies and fibres display VIP immunoreactivity of varying intensity (×200). (b) After local application of colchicine virtually all nerve cell bodies display VIP immunoreactivity (×300). (c) A few substance P-immunofluorescent cell bodies (arrows) can be demonstrated after local colchicine treatment (×400)

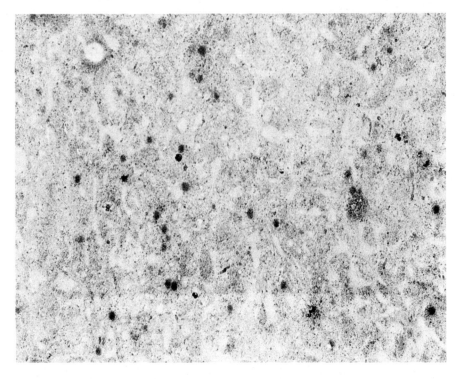

Figure 8 Immuno-electron-microscopic demonstration of VIP in nerve cell body after local application of colchicine. Detail of cytoplasm shown. VIP (dark precipitate) occurs in the dense-cored vesicles (×20 000)

in the non-treated ganglion a population of cell bodies contain VIP but no or very little acetylcholinesterase activity. The ganglion may therefore contain a population of 'genuine' VIP neurons in addition to those being mixed VIP/cholinergic. The observations add to several others (Lundberg *et al.*, 1979, 1980; Hökfelt *et al.*, 1980) indicating a coexistence of VIP and acetylcholine in certain peripheral neurons. Indeed, coexistence of conventional neurotransmitters such as noradrenaline, dopamine or serotonin and neuropeptides such as somatostatin, CCK-8 or substances P, seems to be a fairly common feature of neurons in the brain (cf. Hökfelt *et al.*, 1980).

Malm (1973) and Änggård (1974) have shown that the postganglionic mediator of secretion in the nasal mucosa is cholinergic whereas the mediator of vasodilatation is neither cholinergic nor adrenergic. Recently, it could be demonstrated (Malm *et al.*, 1980) that the neuropeptide, VIP, is capable of inducing an atropine-resistant dilatation of resistance and capacitance vessels in the cat nasal mucosa. Further, electrical stimulation of the vidian nerve evoked a dilatation of the nasal mucosa concomitantly with an increase of VIP in nasal venous blood (Uddman *et al.*, 1981). These findings make it tempting to suggest that VIP is the mediator of non-adrenergic, non-cholinergic vasodilatation in the nasal mucosa, much like in the choroid in the eye (see above).

The functional significance of the VIP in cholinergic neurons in the pterygopalatine ganglion is essentially unknown. VIP-containing and acetylcholinesterase-positive fibres are both numerous in tissues to which the ganglion projects, suggesting that both types of neurons have important functions in the peripheral tissues. Indeed, in the nasal mucosa VIP is known to have potent effects on blood flow but only little effect on seromucous secretion (Uddman *et al.*, 1980), while the reverse seems to hold for acetylcholine (Lundberg *et al.*, 1980). However, there is no information as yet on whether VIP and acetylcholine coexist in the nerve terminals as they do in the nerve cell bodies. It has been speculated (Hökfelt *et al.*, 1980) that VIP and acetycholine might occur separately in different axon branches of one and the same neuron, those terminating at blood vessels containing VIP and those innervating seromucous glands containing acetylcholine.

Nerve fibres

The preganglionic (vidian) nerve contains both cholinergic and adrenergic elements (Nomura and Matsuura, 1972). In the ganglion, adrenergic fibres are very few whereas fibres displaying VIP immunoreactivity are numerous while substance P-immunoreactive fibres are moderate in number.

Development

The pterygopalatine ganglion seems to derive mainly from the trigeminal ganglion. In very young pig or cat embryos a mass of loosely aggregated cells, identical with cells of the trigeminal ganglion, can be seen along the maxillary division of the trigeminal nerve. The cells advance along the maxillary nerve to form a close aggregate which later becomes connected with cells travelling in the greater petrosal nerve. However, this connection is not established until the pterygopalatine ganglion has formed (Kuntz, 1913; Cowgill and Windle, 1942; Pearson and Pytel, 1978). Stewart (1920), on the other hand, was unable to see any contributions to the ganglion formation from the trigeminal ganglion in rats and pigs and therefore suggested that it was mainly derived via the greater superficial petrosal nerve.

The pterygopalatine ganglion in disease

Sluder (1908, 1915) suggested that irritation of the pterygopalatine ganglion might be the cause of neuralgic pains in the lower half of the face as well as of lacrimation, hypersecretion from the nose, and nasal congestion. He proposed destruction of the ganglion as treatment. Initially his thoughts were widely accepted but later they were severely criticized by, *inter alia*, Stewart and Lambert (1930). However, as late as 1977, Ryan and Facer suggested that 'sphenopalatine neuralgia' is a distinct clinical entity, different from, for example, cluster headache. They found that extended relief was obtainable by cauterization of the pterygopalatine ganglion. The recent demonstration (Uddman *et al.*, 1980, 1981) of neuropeptides in it, of which at least substance P is known to occur in sensory fibres (Cuello *et al.*, 1976; Hökfelt *et al.*, 1977) may give reason for speculating again that the pterygopalatine ganglion is involved in sensory transmission.

Patients with severe vasomotor rhinitis resistant to other forms of therapy respond to transection of the vidian nerve (Golding-Wood 1961, 1973; Hiranandani, 1966; Chasin and Lofgren, 1967). The operation has been used with some claims of success also against recurrent polyposis nasi (Bouche *et al.*, 1971) and for perennial rhinitis (Konno and Togawa, 1979), in the latter case as an adjuvant to hyposensitization. However, the results have not been uniformly encouraging (Krant *et al.*, 1979) and the operation often gives only temporary relief against perennial rhinitis (Konno and Togawa, 1979).

ACKNOWLEDGEMENTS

This work was supported by the Swedish Medical Research Council (project number 14X-2321 and 04X-4499).

REFERENCES

Adler, R., and Varon, S. (1980). Cholinergic neuronotrophic factors: Segregation of survival- and neurite-promoting activities in heart-conditioned media. *Brain Res.*, **188**, 437–448.

Änggård, A. (1974). The effects of parasympathetic nerve stimulation on the microcirculation and secretion in the nasal mucosa of the cat. *Acta Otolaryngol.*, **78**, 277–282.

Arenson, M. S., and Wilson, H. (1971). The parasympathetic secretory nerves of the lacrimal gland of the cat. *J. Physiol. (London)*, **217**, 201–212.

Ashton, N. (1952). Observations on the choroidal circulation. *Br. J. Ophthalmol.*, **36**, 465–480.

Bill, A., Stjernschantz, J., Mandahl, A., Brodin, E., and Nilsson, G. (1979). Substance P: Release on trigeminal nerve stimulation, effects in the eye. *Acta Physiol. Scand.* **106**, 371–373.

Bouche, J., Frèche, Cr., and Fontanel, J. P. (1971). La chirurgie du nerf vidien. *Ann. Oto-laryngol.*, **88**, 529–546.

Cantino, D., and Mugnaini, E. (1974). Adrenergic innervation of the parasympathetic ciliary ganglion in the chick. *Science*, **185**, 279–282.

Cantino, D., and Mugnaini, E. (1975). The structural basis for electrotonic coupling in the avian ciliary ganglion. A study with thin section and freeze-fracturing. *J. Neurocytol.*, **4**, 505–536.

Carpenter, F. W. (1912). On the histology of the cranial autonomic ganglia of the sheep. *J. Comp. Neurol.*, **22**, 447–459.

Chasin, W. D., and Lofgren, R. H. (1967). Vidian nerve section for vasomotor rhinitis. *Arch. Otolaryngol.*, **86**, 129–135.

Chiappinelli, V. A., and Giacobini, E. (1978). Rate of appearance of alpha-bungarotoxin binding sites during development of chick ciliary ganglion and iris. *Neurochem. Res.*, **3**, 465–478.

Chiappinelli, V. A., and Zigmond, R. E. (1978). Alpha-bungarotoxin blocks nicotinic transmission in the avian ciliary ganglion. *Proc. Natl. Acad. Sci. U.S.A.*, **75**, 2999–3003.

Christensen, K. (1934). The innervation of the nasal mucosa, with special reference to its afferent supply. *Ann. Oto-laryngol.*, **43**, 1066–1083.

Ciofi-Luzzatto, A., Conti-Tronconi, B., Paggi, P., and Rossi, A. (1980). Binding of *Naja naja siamensis* alpha-toxin to the chick ciliary ganglion: a light microscopic autoradiographic study. *Neuroscience*, **5**, 313–318.

Collins, F. (1978). Induction of neurite outgrowth by a conditioned-medium factor bound to the culture substratum. *Proc. Natl. Acad. Sci. U.S.A.*, **10**, 5210–5213.

Conti-Tronconi, B., Gotti, C., Paggi, P., and Rossi, A. (1979). Acetylcholine receptors in the ciliary ganglion and in the iris muscle of the chick: specific binding and effect on the synaptic transmission of the neurotoxin from *Naja naja siamensis*. *Br. J. Pharmacol.*, **66**, 33–38.

Cowgill, E. J., and Windle, W. F. (1942). Development of the cranial sympathetic ganglia in the cat. *J. Comp. Neurol.*, **31**, 163–217.

Cuello, A. C., Polak, J. M., and Pearse, A. G. E. (1976). Substance P. A naturally occurring transmitter in human spinal cord. *Lancet*, **ii**, 1054–1056.

De Lorenzo, A. J. (1960). The fine structure of synapses in the ciliary ganglion of the chick. *J. Biophys. Biochem. Cytol.*, **7**, 31–36.

De Lorenzo, A. J. D. (1966). Electron microscopy: tight junctions in synapses of the ciliary ganglion. *Science*, **152**, 76–78.

Duke-Elder, S., and Wybar, K. (1961). *System of Ophthalmology*, Vol. II, *The Anatomy of the Visual System*, Henry Kimpton, London.

Ehinger, B. (1966a). Adrenergic nerves to the eye and to related structures in man and in the cynomolgus monkey. *Invest. Ophthalmol.*, **5**, 42–52.

Ehinger, B. (1966b). Ocular and orbital vegetative nerves. *Acta Physiol. Scand.*, **67**, 1–35.

Ehinger, B. (1967). Adrenergic nerves in the avian eye and ciliary ganglion. *Z. Zellforsch. Mikrosk. Anat.*, **82**, 577–588.

Ehinger, B., and Falck, B. (1966). Concomitant adrenergic and parasympathetic fibres in the rat iris. *Acta Physiol. Scand.*, **67**, 201–207.

Ehinger, B., and Falck, B. (1970). Uptake of some catecholamines and their precursors into neurons of the rat ciliary ganglion. *Acta Physiol. Scand.*, **78**, 132–141.

Ehinger, B., Falck, B., and Rosengren, E. (1969). Adrenergic denervation of the eye by unilateral cervical sympathectomy. *Albrecht von Graefes Arch. Ophthalmol.*, **177**, 206–211.

Ericksen, J. T., Karten, H. J., Eldred, W. D. and Brecha, N. C. (1982). Localization of substance-P-like and enkephalin-like immunoreactive within preganglionic terminals of the avian ciliary ganglion: light and electron microscopy. *J. Neurosci.*, **2**, 994–1003.

Eränkö, O., Soinila, S., and Päivärinta, H. (1980). Histochemistry and cell biology of autonomic neurons, SIF cells and paraneurons. *Adv. Biochem. Psychopharmacol.*, **25**, 1–391.

Fahrenkrug, J. (1979). Vasoactive intestinal polypeptide: measurement, distribution and putative neurotransmitter function. *Digestion*, **19**, 149–169.

Fukuda, T., and Koelle, G. B. (1959). The cytological localization of intracellular neuronal acetylcholinesterase. *J. Biophys. Biochem. Cytol.*, **5**, 433–440.

Fumagalli, L., De Renzis, G., and Miani, N. (1978). Alpha-bungarotoxin–acetylcholine receptors in the chick ciliary ganglion: effects of deafferentation and axotomy. *Brain Res.*, **153**, 87–98.

Gabella, G. (1976). *Structure of the Autonomic Nervous System*, pp. 103–116, Chapman and Hall, London.

Gangitano, C., Fumagalli, L., De Renzis, G., and Sangiacomo, C. O. (1978). Alpha–bungarotoxin–acetylcholine receptors in the chick ciliary ganglion during development. *Neuroscience*, **3**, 1101–1108.

Giacobini, E. (1959). Quantitative determination of cholinesterase in individual spinal ganglion cells. *Acta Physiol. Scand.*, **45**, 238–254.

Giacobini, E., Pilar, G., Suszkiv, J., and Uchimura, H. (1979). Normal distribution and denervation changes of neurotransmitter related enzymes in cholinergic neurons. *J. Physiol. (London)*, **286**, 233–253.

Golding-Wood, P. H. (1961). Observations on petrosal and vidian neurectomy in chronic vasomotor rhinitis. *J. Laryngol.*, **75**, 232–246.

Golding-Wood, P. H. (1973). Vidian neurectomy: its results and complications. *Laryngoscope*, **83**, 1673–1683.

Grillo, M. A., and Palay, S. L. (1962). Granule-containing vesicles in the autonomic nervous system. In *Fifth International Congress Electron Microscopy* (Ed. S. S. Breese, Jr.), Vol. 2, p. U–1, Academic Press, New York, London.

Grimes, P., and von Sallmann, L. (1960). Comparative anatomy of the ciliary nerves. *Arch. Ophthalmol.*, **64**, 81–91.

Hamburger, V., and Hamilton, H. L. (1951). A series of normal stages in the development of the chick embryo. *J. Morphol.*, **88**, 49–92.

Hámori, J., and Dyachkova, L. N. (1964). Electron microscope studies on developmental differentiation of ciliary ganglion synapses in the chick. *Acta Biol. Acad. Sci. Hung.*, **15**, 213–230.

Harriman, D. G. F., and Garland, H. (1968). The pathology of Adie's syndrome. *Brain*, **91**, 401–418.

Hess, A. (1965). Developmental changes in the structure of the synapse on the myelinated cell bodies of the chicken ciliary ganglion. *J. Cell, Biol.*, **25**, 1–19.

Hess, A., Pilar, G., and Weakly, J. N. (1969). Correlation between transmission and structure in avian ciliary ganglion synapses. *J. Physiol. (London)*, **202**, 339–354.

Hiranandani, N. L. (1966). Treatment of chronic vasomotor rhinitis with clinico-pathological study of vidian nerve section in 150 cases. *J. Laryngol. Otolaryngol.*, **80**, 902–932.

Holmstedt, B. (1957). A modification of the thiocholine method for the determination of cholinesterase. II. Histochemical application. *Acta Physiol. Scand.*, **40**, 331–357.

Huikuri, K. (1966). Histochemistry of the ciliary ganglion of the rat and the effect of pre- and postganglionic nerve division. *Acta Physiol. Scand.*, **69**, 1–83.

Huikuri, K. (1969). Electron microscopic observations on the granular vesicles in the ciliary ganglion of the rat. *Experientia*, **25**, 1067–1068.

Hökfelt, T., Johansson, O., Kellerth, J.-O., Ljungdahl, Å., Nilsson, G., Nygårds, A., and Pernow, B. (1977). Immunohistochemical distribution of substance P. In *Substance P* (Eds. U. S. von Euler and B. Pernow), pp. 117–145, Raven Press, New York.

Hökfelt, T., Johansson, O., Ljungdahl, Å., Lundberg, J. M., and Schultzberg, M. (1980). Peptidergic neurons. *Nature*, **234**, 515–521.

Jaeger, R. J., and Benevento, L. A. (1980). A horseradish peroxidase study of the innervation of the internal structures of the eye. *Invest. Ophthalmol. Visual Sci.*, **19**, 575–583.

Johnson, D. A., and Pilar, G. (1980). The release of acetylcholine from postganglionic cell bodies in response to depolarization. *J. Physiol. (London)*, **299**, 605–619.

Klepper, J. (1928). Demonstration of specimens of the sphenopalatinegasserian ganglion. *Laryngoscope*, **38**, 41–44.

Koelle, G. B. (1955). The histochemical identification of acetylcholinesterase in cholinergic, adrenergic and sensory neurons. *J. Pharmacol. Exp. Ther.*, **114**, 167–184.

Koelle, G. B., and Friedenwald, J. S. (1950). The histochemical localization of cholinesterase in ocular tissues. *Am. J. Ophthalmol.*, **33**, 253.

Koelle, W. A., and Koelle, G. B. (1959). The localization of external or functional acetylcholinesterase at the synapse of autonomic ganglia. *J. Pharmacol. Exp. Ther.*, **126**, 1–8.

Koelle, G. B., and Valk, A. de T. (1954). Physiological implications of the histochemical localization of monoamine oxidase. *J. Physiol. (London)*, **126**, 434–447.

Koenig, H. L. (1967). Quelques particularités ultrastructurales des zones synaptiques dans le ganglion ciliare du poulet. *Bull. Assoc. Anat.*, **52**, 711–719.

Kondo, H., Katayama, Y. and Yui, R (1982). On the occurrence and physiological effect of somatostatin in the ciliary ganglion of cats. *Brain Res.*, **247**, 141–144.

Konno, A., and Togawa, K. (1979). Vidian neurectomy for allergic rhinitis—Evaluation of long-term results and some problems concerning operative therapy. *Arch. Otorhinolaryngol.*, **225**, 67–77.

Krant, J. N., Wildervanck, de Blécourt, P., Dieges, P. H., and de Heer, L. J. (1979). Long-term results of vidian neurectomy. *Rhinology*, **17**, 231–235.

Kuntz, A. (1913). The development of he cranial sympathetic ganglia in the pig. *J. Comp. Neurol.*, **23**, 71–96.

Kurus, E. (1955). Uber ein Ganglienzellsystem der menschlichen Aderhaut. *Klin. Mbl. Augenheilkd.*, **127**, 198–206.

Kurus, E. (1956). Uber die Morphologie des Ganglion Ciliare. *Klin. Monatsbl. Augenheilkd.*, **129**, 183–196.

Landmesser, L., and Pilar, G. (1972). The onset and development of transmission in the chick ciliary ganglion. *J. Physiol. (London)*, **222**, 691–713.

Landmesser, L., and Pilar, G. (1974a). Synapse formation during embryogenesis on ganglion cells lacking a periphery. *J. Physiol. (London)*, **241**, 715–736.

Landmesser, L., and Pilar, G. (1974b). Synaptic transmission and cell death during normal ganglionic development. *J. Physiol. (London)*, **241**, 737–749.

Landmesser, L., and Pilar, G. (1976). Fate of ganglionic synapses and ganglion cell axons during normal and induced cell death. *J. Cell Biol.*, **68**, 357–374.

Larsell, O., and Fenton, R. A. (1928). The embryology and neurohistology of sphenopalatine ganglion connections; a contribution to the study of otalgia. *Laryngoscope*, **36**, 371–389.

Lele, P. P., and Grimes, P. (1960). The role of neural mechanisms in the regulation of intraocular pressure in the cat. *Exp. Neurol.*, **2**, 199–220.

Lele, P. P., and Weddell, G. (1959). Sensory nerves of the cornea and cutaneous sensibility. *Exp. Neurol.*, **1**, 334–359.

Lundberg, J. M., Änggård, A., Fahrenkrug, J., Hökfelt, T., and Mutt, V. (1980). Vasoactive intestinal polypeptide in cholinergic neurons of exocrine glands: Functional significance of coexisting transmitters for vasodilatation and secretion. *Proc. Natl. Acad. Sci. U.S.A.*, **77**, 1651–1655.

Macri, F. J., and Cevario, S. J. (1975a). Ciliary ganglion stimulation. I. Effects on aqueous humor inflow and outflow. *Invest. Ophthalmol.*, **14**, 28–33.

Macri, F. J., and Cevario, S. J. (1975b). Ciliary ganglion stimulation. II. Neurogenic intraocular pathways for excitatory effects on aqueous humor production and outflow. *Invest. Ophthalmol.*, **14**, 471–475.

Malcomson, K. G. (1959). The vasomotor activities of the nasal mucous membrane. *J. Laryngol. Otol.*, **73**, 73–98.

Malm, L. (1973). Vasodilatation in the nasal mucosa of the cat and the effects of parasympatholytic and beta-adrenergic blocking agents. *Acta Otolaryngol.*, **76**, 277–282.

Malm, L., Sundler, F., and Uddman, R. (1980). Effects of vasoactive intestinal polypeptide on resistance and capacitance vessels in the nasal mucosa. *Acta Otolaryngol.*, **90**, 304–308.

Malmfors, T., and Nilsson, O. (1964). Parasympathetic post-ganglionic denervation of the iris and the parotid gland in the rat. *Acta Morphol. Neerl.-Scand.*, **6**, 81–85.

Mandahl, A., Tornqvist, K., Leander, S., Lorén, I., Håkansson, R., and Sundler, F. (1981). Nerve fibres containing substance P in the anterior segment of the rabbit eye: Distribution and possible physiological significance. Submitted for publication.

Marchi, M., Giacobini, E., and Hruschak, K. (1979). Development and aging of cholinergic synapses. I. Endogenous levels of acetylcholine and choline in developing autonomic ganglia and iris of the chick. *Dev. Neurosci.*, **2**, 201–212.

Marrazzi, A. S. (1954). Ganglionic and central transmission. *Pharm. Rev.*, **6**, 105–106.

Martin, A. R., and Pilar, G. (1963a). Dual mode of synaptic transmission in the avian ciliary ganglion. *J. Physiol. (London)*, **168**, 443–463.

Martin, A. R., and Pilar, G. (1963b). Transmission through the ciliary ganglion of the chick. *J. Physiol. (London)*, **168**, 464–475.

Marwitt, R., Pilar, G., and Weakly, J. N. (1971). Characterization of two ganglion cell populations in avian ciliary ganglia. *Brain Res.*, **25**, 317–334.

Müller, L. R., and Dahl, W. (1910). Die Beteiligung des sympathischen Nervensystems an der Kopfinnervation. *Dtsch. Arch. Klin. Med.*, **10**, 48–107.

Narayanan, C. H., and Narayanan, Y. (1978). Neuronal adjustments in developing nuclear centers of the chick embryo following nuclear transplantations of an additional optic primordium. *J. Embryol. Exp. Morphol.*, **44**, 53–70.

Nishi, R., and Berg, D. K. (1977). Dissociated ciliary neurons *in vitro*: survival and synapse formation. *Proc. Natl. Acad. Sci. U.S.A.*, **74**, 5171–5175.

Nomura, Y., and Matsuura, T. (1972). Distribution and clinical significance of the autonomic nervous system in the human nasal mucosa. *Acta Otolaryngol.*, **73**, 493–501.

Okinaka, S., Yoshikawa, M., Uono, M., Muro, T., Igata, A., Tanaka, H., Veda, S., and Tomonaga, M. (1963). Uber die Cholinesterase des autonomen und peripheren Nervensystems. *Acta Neuroveg.*, **25**, 249–264.

Pearson, J., and Pytel, B. (1978). Quantitative studies of ciliary and sphenopalatine ganglia in familial dysautonomia. *J. Neurol. Sci.*, **39**, 123–130.

Perry, W. L. M., and Talesnik, J. (1953). The role of acetylcholine in synaptic transmission at parasympathetic ganglia. *J. Physiol. (London)*, **119**, 455–469.

Pilar, G., and Landmesser, L. (1976). Ultrastructural differences during embryonic cell death in normal and peripherally deprived ciliary ganglia. *J. Cell Biol.*, **68**, 339–356.

Pilar, G., and Vaughan, P. C. (1969). Electrophysiological investigations of the pigeon iris neuromuscular junctions. *Comp. Biochem. Physiol.*, **29**, 51–72.

Pilar, G., Jenden, D. J., and Campbell, B. (1973). Distribution of acetylcholine in the normal and denervated pigeon ciliary ganglion. *Brain Res.*, **49**, 245–256.

Pilar, G., Landmesser, L., and Burstein, L. (1980). Competition for survival among developing ciliary ganglion cells. *J. Neurophys.*, **43**, 233–255.

Pines, J.-L. (1927). Zur Morphologie des Ganglion ciliare beim Menschen. *Z. Mikrosk. Anat. Forsch.*, **10**, 313–380.

Prince, J. H., Diesem, C. D., Eglitis, I., and Ruskell, G. L. (1960). *Anatomy and Histology of the Eye and Orbit in Domestic Animals, Thomas Publishers, Springfield.*

Retzius, G. (1880). Untersuchungen über die Nervenzellen der cerebrospinalen Ganglien und der übrigen peripherischen Kopfganglien mit besonderer Rücksicht auf die Zellenausläufer. *Arch. Anat. Physiol. Anat. Abt.*, 369–402.

Rohen, J. W. (1964). Das Auge und seine Hilfsorgane. In *Handbuch der mikroskopischen Anatomie des Menschen* (Eds. v. Möllendorff and Bargmann), Springer-Verlag, Berlin, Göttingen, Heidelberg, New York.

Ruskell, G. L. (1964). Neurology of the orbit and globe. In *The Rabbit in Eye Research* (Ed. J. H. Prince), pp. 554–579, C. C. Thomas, Springfield.

Ruskell, G. L. (1965). The orbital distribution of the sphenopalatine ganglion in the rabbit. In *The Structure of the Eye* (Ed. J. W. Rohen), pp. 355–368, Schattauer-Verlag, Stuttgart.

Ruskell, G. L. (1970a). An ocular parasympathetic nerve pathway of facial nerve origin and its influence on intraocular pressure. *Exp. Eye Res.*, **10**, 319–330.

Ruskell, G. L. (1970b). The orbital branches of the pterygopalatine ganglion and their relationship with internal carotid nerve branches in primates. *J. Anat.*, **106**, 323–339.

Ruskell, G. L. (1971a). The distribution of autonomic post-ganglionic nerve fibres to the lacrimal gland in monkeys. *J. Anat.*, **109**, 229–242.

Ruskell, G. L. (1971b). Facial parasympathetic innervation of the choroidal blood vessels in monkeys. *Exp. Eye Res.*, **12**, 166–172.

Ruskell, G. L. (1974). Ocular fibres of the maxillary nerve in monkeys. *J. Anat.*, **118**, 195–203.

Ruskell, G. L., and Griffiths, T. (1979). Peripheral nerve pathway to the ciliary muscle. *Exp. Eye Res.*, **28**, 277.

Ruskin, A. P. (1979). Sphenopalatine (nasal) ganglion: remote effects including 'psychosomatic' symptoms, rage reaction, pain and spasm. *Arch. Phys. Med. Rehabil.*, **60**, 353–359.

Ryan, R. E., and Facer, G. W. (1977). Sphenopalatine ganglion neuralgia and cluster headache: comparisons, contrasts, and treatment. *Headache*, **17**, 7–9.

Sluder, G. (1908). The role of the sphenopalatine (or Meckle's) ganglion in nasal headaches. *N.Y. Med. J.*, 989–990.

Sluder, G. (1915). The sympathetic syndrome of sphenopalatine or nasal ganglion neurosis: together with a consideration of the neuralgic syndrome and their treatment. *Trans. Am. Laryngol. Assoc.*, **37**, 243–262.

Stewart, F. W. (1920). The development of the cranial sympathetic ganglia in the rat. *J. Comp. Neurol.*, **31**, 163–217.

Stewart, D., and Lambert, V. (1930). The spheno-palatine ganglion. *J. Laryngol. Otol.*, **45**, 753–751.

Szentágothai, J. (1964). The structure of the autonomic interneuronal synapse. *Acta Neuroveg.*, **26**, 338–359.

Takahashi, K. (1967). Special somatic spine synapses in the ciliary ganglion of the chick. *Z. Zellforsch. Mikrosk. Anat.*, **83**, 70.

Takahashi, K., and Hama, K. (1965a). Some observations on the fine structure of the synaptic area in the ciliary ganglion of the chick. *Z. Zellforsch., Mikrosk. Anat.*, **67**, 174–184.

Takahashi, K., and Hama, K. (1965b). Some observations on the fine structure on nerve cell bodies and their satellite cells in the ciliary ganglion of the chick. *Z. Zellforsch. Mikrosk. Anat.*, **67**, 835.

Taxi, J. (1961). La distribution des cholinésterases dans diverse ganglions du système nerveux autonome des Vertébrés. *Bibl. Anat.*, **2**, 73–89.

Terzuolo, C. (1951). Richerche sul gangli ciliari degli ucelli. Connesionimutamenti in relazione all'età e dopo recisione delle febre preganglionari. *Z. Zellforsch. Mikrosk. Anat.*, **36**, 255–267.

Tobari, I. (1971a). Electron microscopic study of ciliary ganglia. I. Fine structure of the ciliary ganglion cell in cat. *Acta Ophthalmol. Jpn.*, **75**, 719–727.

Tobari, I. (1971b). Electron microscopic study of ciliary ganglion. II. Fine structure of nerve endings in ciliary ganglion of adult cat. *Acta Ophthalmol. Jpn.*, **75**, 739–747.

Tschalussow, M. A. (1913). Die Innervation der Gefässe der Nasenschleimhaut. *Pflügers Arch. Gesamte Physiol.*, **151**, 523–542.

Tschernjawsky, G. J., and Pletschkowa, E. K. (1979). Morphological changes in ciliary ganglions of healthy subjects and glaucoma patients. *Albrecht von Graefe's Arch. Klin. Exp. Ophthalmol.*, **211**, 235–241.

Tum Suden, C., Hart, E. R., Lindenberg, R., and Marrazzi, A. S. (1951). Pharmacologic and anatomic indications of adrenergic neurons participating in synapses at parasympathetic ganglia (ciliary). *J. Pharmacol. Exp. Ther.*, **103**, 364–365.

Uddman, R. (1980). Vasoactive intestinal polypeptide—Distribution and possible role in the upper respiratory and digestive regions. *MD Thesis*, Lund.

Uddman, R., Alumets, J., Densert, O., Håkanson, R., and Sundler, F. (1978). Occurrence and distribution of VIP nerves in the nasal mucosa and tracheobronchial wall. *Acta Otolaryngol.*, **86**, 443–448.

Uddman, R., Malm, L., and Sundler, F. (1980a). The origin of vasoactive intestinal polypeptide (VIP) nerves in the feline nasal mucosa. *Acta Otolaryngol.*, **89**, 152–156.

Uddman, R., Alumets, J., Ehinger, B., Håkansson, R., Lorén, I., and Sundler, F. (1980b). Vasoactive intestinal peptide nerves in ocular and orbital structures of the cat. *Invest. Ophthalmol. Visual Sci.*, **19**, 878–885.

Uddman, R., Malm, L., Fahrenkrug, J., and Sundler, F. (1981). VIP increases in nasal blood during stimulation of the vidian nerve. *Acta Otolaryngol.*, **91**, 135–138.

Uddman, R., Malm, L. and Sundler, F. (1981a). Peptide containing nerves in the nasal mucosa. *Rhinology*, **19**, 75–79.

Uddman, R., Malm, L. and Sundler, F. (1983). Substance P containing nerve fibres in the nasal mucosa. *Arch. Otorhinolaryngol.*, in press.

Valu, L. (1962). Uber die Innervation des Uvea-Trabekel-Systems. *Albrecht von Graefes Arch. Ophthalmol.*, **164**, 496–502.

Walsh, F. B., and Hoyt, W. F. (1969). *Clinical Neuro-ophthalmology*, 3rd edn., William and Wilkins, Baltimore.

Warwick, R. (1954). The ocular parasympathetic nerve supply and its mesencephalic sources. *J. Anat.*, **88**, 71–93.

Warwick, R. (1956). Oculomotor organisation. *Ann. R. Coll. Surg. Engl.*, **19**, 36–52.

Watanabe, H. (1972). The fine structure of the ciliary ganglion of the guinea pig. *Arch. Histol. Jpn.*, **34**, 261–276.

Westheimer, G., and Blair, S. (1973). The parasympathetic pathways to internal eye muscles. *Invest. Ophthalmol.*, **12**, 193–197.

Wolf, G. A. (1941). The ratio of preganglionic neurons in the visual nervous system. *J. Comp. Neurol.*, **75**, 235–243.

Wolter, R. (1960). Nerves of the normal human chorioid. *Arch. Ophthalmol.*, **64**, 120–124.

Yamakado, M., and Yohro, T. (1977). Population and structure of nerve cells in mouse submandibular ganglion. *Anat. Embryol.*, **150**, 301–312.

Yoshida, M. (1968). Vergleichende elektronenmikroskopische Untersuchungen an sympathischen und parasympathischen Ganglien des Goldhamsters. *Z. Zellforsch. Mikosk. Anat.*, **88**, 138–144.

Yoshida, M. (1971). Uber die Ultrastruktur der Nervenzellen des Ganglion ciliare beim Affen (*Macacus irus* F. Cuvier). *Kobe J. Med. Sci.*, **17**, 65–73.

Autonomic Ganglia
Edited by Lars-Gösta Elfvin
© 1983 John Wiley & Sons Ltd

Pelvic Autonomic Ganglia: Structure, Transmitters, Function and Steroid Influence

CHRISTER OWMAN, PER ALM and NILS-OTTO SJÖBERG

*Departments of Histology, Pathology, and Obstetrics and Gynecology,
University of Lund, Lund, Sweden*

ORGANIZATION OF THE PELVIC AUTONOMIC INNERVATION

The pelvic organs receive nerve fibres from the sympathetic and the parasympathetic nervous systems. Sympathetic fibres reach the pelvic organs via the hypogastric nerve(s), which emanate from the inferior mesenteric ganglion (or ganglia). Some fibres also originate in the sympathetic chain. The parasympathetic innervation derives from the sacral outflow. With the exception of the macaque and man the detailed autonomic innervation pattern is very similar in the most commonly used laboratory animals (Sjöstrand, 1965). Polypeptide-containing nerves have recently been found to contribute to the autonomic innervation of the pelvic organs.

The inferior mesenteric ganglion is located close to the base of the inferior mesenteric artery. The ganglion receives fibres from the lumbar sympathetic ganglia and some fibres from the upper abdominal ganglia. One or two hypogastric nerves emerge from the ganglion. When these nerves reach the pelvic organs they split off forming a nerve plexus (pelvic plexus), which is situated in the connective tissue close to the internal genital organs, the bladder and the rectum to supply these organs. The inferior mesenteric ganglion is absent or vestigial in man. The hypogastric nerves in man are branches of the presacral nerve, which is composed of fibres from the intermesenteric and inferior mesenteric plexa, as well as fibres from the lumbar ganglia of the sympathetic chain.

Fibres from the sympathetic chain chiefly follow the arteries to the pelvic organs or join the parasympathetic fibres. The sacral parasympathetic fibres generally combine to form the two pelvic nerves (one left and one right), which intermingle with the hypogastric nerve fibres when they reach the pelvic organs.

COMPOSITION OF PELVIC AUTONOMIC GANGLIA, AND THE
CONCEPT OF SHORT ADRENERGIC NEURONS

The classical studies by Langley and Anderson (1895a, b, 1896a, b) had indicated that the peripheral ganglionic relay of the sympathetic innervation to the male and female internal genital tract was located close to the effector organs. Yet, the general opinion for a long time was that the genital organs were supplied by postganglionic fibres running in the hypogastric nerves and emanating from the inferior mesenteric ganglion. The reason for this misconcept is probably, as discussed by Sjöstrand (1965) and Sjöberg (1967), a number of studies claiming only postganglionic characteristics of the hypogastric nerves.

During the last two decades the innervation of the internal male genital organs has been the subject of renewed interest, perhaps especially because the vas deferens frequently has been used as a model organ for studies on adrenergic transmission. Sjöstrand (1962a) showed that ganglionic-blocking agents inhibit the response of the guinea-pig vas deferens to hypogastric nerve stimulation, and section and degeneration of this nerve (Sjöstrand, 1962b) does not reduce the noradrenaline content of the vas deferens and the seminal vesicle. These findings were soon confirmed by many other workers, as reviewed by Sjöstrand (1965). Simultaneously, Falck (1962) demonstrated an abundant innervation of fluorescent adrenergic nerve terminals in the vas deferens, and, consequently, the next step was the localization of the adrenergic nerve cell bodies innervating the internal male genital organs. It was found that, in the guinea-pig (Falck *et al.*, 1965), the adrenergic nerve cell bodies are located in close vicinity of the target organs. A similar arrangement was seen in several other species (Paton and Vizi, 1969). This type of adrenergic neuron, having their cell bodies in peripheral ganglia located close to the effector structures, was designated 'short adrenergic neuron' (Owman and Sjöstrand, 1965; Sjöstrand, 1965) in contrast to the ordinary 'long' adrenergic neurons, having their cell bodies located in pre- and paravertebral ganglia. Short adrenergic neurons have since been found to innervate selectively the male and female genitourinary tracts.

The general appearance of the peripheral adrenergic ganglia in the pelvic region is similar to that of the pre- and paravertebral ganglia. The ganglion cells show a varying degree of noradrenaline fluorescence, and completely non-fluorescent cells are also seen, the latter probably being cholinergic or peptidergic. Fluorescent as well as non-fluorescent nerve cell bodies may be surrounded by varicose fluorescent fibres. This is rather frequently seen in the peripheral ganglia of guinea-pig, rabbit, cat, and dog but very seldom in the rat (Owman and Sjöstrand, 1965).

Small chromaffin-like cells with an intense amine fluorescence—SIF cells— are also found in the ganglia (Falck *et al.*, 1965; Owman and Sjöstrand, 1965).

In the dog these cells probably store large amounts of adrenaline (Owman and Sjöstrand, 1965), whereas such cells in other species and in other locations seem to contain dopamine (Björklund *et al.*, 1970) or other amines (see chapter by Taxi as well as chapter by Williams and Jew). There is reason to believe that some SIF cells function as interneurons (Libet, 1976), and that at least part of the above-mentioned catecholamine-containing varicose fibres present within the ganglion are highly collateralized extensions from these SIF cells (Libet and Owman, 1974).

THE MALE GENITAL TRACT

The ganglion cells supplying the male internal genital organs with autonomic nerves (Fig. 1) are located in large clusters in the terminal parts of the hypogastric nerves, where these join the vessels close to the prostate and coagulating glands near the entrance of the vas deferens (Owman and Sjöstrand, 1965).

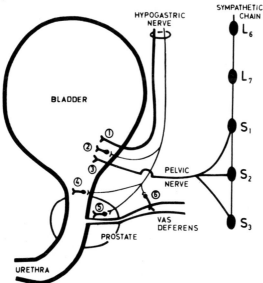

Figure 1 Sympathetic innervation of the lower urogenital tract, as studied by fluorescence microscopy of the adrenergic transmitter and by denervation. Neurons 1–3 supply the bladder trigonum. The rest of the bladder wall has only a poor adrenergic innervation. (1) Adrenergic nerves arising in inferior mesenteric ganglion (presacral plexus) to run down the hypogastric nerves. (2) Short adrenergic neurons originating in intramural ganglia. (3) Adrenergic nerves from paravertebral sympathetic ganglia S_1–S_3 to run in the pelvic nerve. (4) Intramural ganglia giving rise to short adrenergic neurons in the urethra (female). (5) Short adrenergic neurons in the prostatic smooth muscle. (6) Short adrenergic neurons arising in ganglia near accessory male genital organs and supplying vas deferens with very dense adrenergic nerve plexus

Adrenergic ganglion cells

The vast majority of neurons in the male genital ganglion are adrenergic. The ganglion cells contain a varying amount of noradrenaline as evidenced by formaldehyde histofluorescence. The cells give rise to bundles of preterminal axons which, within the genital organs, run in the connective tissue spaces of the smooth muscle coats to divide into characteristic beaded terminals located along individual smooth muscle cells. In this way the adrenergic nerves provide a well-developed motor innervation to the prostate, coagulating gland, seminal vesicle, ampullary gland, and vas deferens (Sjöstrand, 1965). It is notable that, in most sympathetically innervated tissues, several nerve terminals run together in each strand of the autonomic ground plexus, whereas in the genital structures, such as the vas deferens, most of the strands contain few or only one varicose terminal. The adrenergic nerve supply of the vas deferens is very dense, and there is reason to believe that somewhere on their surface most of the smooth muscle cells have contact with or lie in close proximity to varicosities belonging to one or more terminals.

Because of the high density of adrenergic innervation in the accessory male genital organs—in conformity with the remarkably large amounts of noradrenaline present (Sjöstrand, 1965)—these organs, particularly the vas deferens, have been subject to several ultrastructural studies in which they have served as models for investigation of the relation between autonomic nerves and smooth musculature (Burnstock, 1970; Richardson, 1962). Fluorescence histochemical studies in combination with chemical determinations of noradrenaline have shown that the short adrenergic neurons in the male genital tract have the same rate of development as the ordinary long adrenergic neurons (of pre- and paravertebral origin) that innervate other structures (Owman et al., 1971b). It is notable that, although the adrenergic nerve supply in the mouse vas deferens is well developed shortly after birth, functional transmission, as indicated by the appearance of excitatory junction potentials, does not occur until 18 days post partum (Furness et al., 1970).

The short adrenergic neurons innervating the internal male genital organs (Fig. 1) differ not only anatomically but also in several physiologic and pharmacologic properties from the conventional long adrenergic neurons (Baumgarten et al., 1975). Such peculiarities include (A) higher resistance to release of transmitter stores by repeated nerve stimulation, (B) relatively lower sensitivity to the noradrenaline-depleting effect of reserpine or α-methyl-p-tyrosine, (C) progressive reduction in noradrenaline release per volley of stimulation upon repeated electrical activation of the nerve, (D) resistance against the neurotoxic effects of 6-hydroxydopamine and 5,7-dihydroxytryptamine, (E) relatively high affinity for uptake of indoleamines, (F) a remarkable resistance to inhibition of adrenergic receptors by α-blocking agents, like phenoxybenzamine and phentolamine, or by the β-

antagonists, propranolol and dichloroisoproterenol, and (G) inhibition by exogenous noradrenaline of the twitch responses elicited from the vas deferens through electrical stimulation.

Cholinergic ganglion cells

Besides the pronounced noradrenergic input to the male internal genitals, there is also—on the basis of histologic, histochemical and electron-microscopic studies—evidence for a supplementary cholinergic motor innervation (Baumgarten *et al.*, 1975; Bell and McLean, 1967), at least in the vas deferens of the guinea-pig, dog, monkey and man. Electrophysiologic and pharmacologic investigations on the release of acetylcholine from the sympathetically denervated vas deferens and on the facilitation of transmission *in vitro* by physostigmine as well as the effect of atropine suggest that this cholinergic supply is of minor importance in the motor activity of the vas deferens. In agreement with this, the emission of sperm in pigs is little affected by atropine (Baumgarten *et al.*, 1975).

Peptidergic ganglion cells

The existence of nerves distinct from adrenergic and cholinergic nerves has been proposed on the basis of ultrastructural evidence. Such nerves have collectively been referred to as p-type: purinergic according to Burnstock (1972), peptidergic according to Baumgarten *et al.* (1970) and Sporrong *et al.* (1977). In support of this view, peptidergic nerves containing vasoactive intestinal polypeptide (VIP) were recently demonstrated in several tissues, including the genitourinary tract (Alm *et al.*, 1977). The accessory male genital organs are richly supplied with VIP nerves. Some of the nerves run within or in close association with the non-vascular smooth muscle cells. Numerous fine-varicose VIP terminals are present in the lamina propria of the mucosa, in close proximity to both blood vessels and the epithelium. There is reason to believe that the VIP fibres originate in the same ganglia as the short adrenergic and cholinergic neurons, and that they represent a separate population of nerve cells (Alm *et al.*, 1980b).

Recent reports have suggested that peptidergic nerves constitute a prominent part of the intramural or 'intrinsic' neuronal systems which seem to be present in all smooth muscle organs and in some exocrine glands as well. Of recognized peptidergic nerves, those containing VIP seem to be particularly numerous. Their physiological role is still poorly understood although their distribution suggests that they participate in regulating smooth muscle activity, local blood flow, and epithelial functions.

Enkephalin-containing nerve terminals have been found in the pelvic ganglia (Alm *et al.*, 1981). These nerves surround the adrenergic and

VIP-ergic ganglion cells. It has been suggested that they act as modulators of ganglionic functions (see chapter by Dun).

THE FEMALE REPRODUCTIVE TRACT

Adrenergic ganglionic neurons: anatomy and functional properties

In line with the findings obtained on the male genital tract and in view of the previously mentioned early observations by Langley and Anderson (1895a, b), fluorescence histochemical and fluorometric investigations on the sympathetic innervation also included the female genital tract in order to elucidate whether the organization was analogous to that found for the male (Fig. 2).

Indeed, the formaldehyde histofluorescence studies revealed the presence of large clusters of adrenergic ganglion cells situated in the upper part of the vaginal wall or in the parametrial tissue outside the uterovaginal junction (Owman and Sjöberg, 1966). Adrenergic ganglia are present at these sites also in humans (Owman *et al.*, 1967). The location corresponds to that of Frankenhäuser's paracervical ganglia. Various types of denervation experiments suggested a more complex arrangement of the adrenergic innervation than in the male (Kanerva, 1972; Thorbert *et al.*, 1977; Wakade and Kirpekar, 1972) (Fig. 2). The ovary is supplied separately, from the lumbosacral part of the paravertebral ganglia. The intraovarian adrenergic nerves innervate, for example, the follicle wall and seem to be involved in the ovulation process (Owman *et al.*, 1979). The innervation of the oviduct, uterus, and vagina is mixed—to a varying degree in different species—and originates from the paracervical ganglia (short adrenergic neurons) as well as from the prevertebral inferior mesenteric ganglia (Kanerva, 1972; Thorbert *et al.*, 1977). A small region of the uterus immediately adjacent to the tube receives a peculiar adrenergic innervation (Thorbert *et al.*, 1977), arriving from more cranial sources via the suspensory ligaments, which anchor the uterine horns to the lower ribs (Fig. 2).

In a series of pharmacological studies, mainly based on fluorometric determinations of tissue noradrenaline, it has been established that the adrenergic neurons of the reproductive tract also in the female have functional properties that differ from those of the rest of the peripheral sympathetic system (Thorbert *et al.*, 1978a). The most interesting difference in comparison with other sympathetically innervated regions is the remarkable sensitivity of the genital adrenergic neurons to sex steroids (Owman and Sjöberg, 1977). The steroid-mediated fluctuations in transmitter level of the adrenergic nerves appear to be an entirely physiological process, which takes place with a sufficiently high rate to be measureable in the course of a normal menstrual cycle (Owman *et al.*, 1976) or during the estrous cycle in the guinea-pig

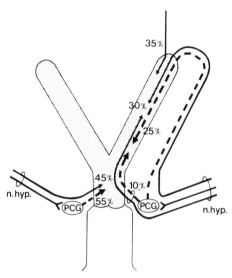

Figure 2 Schematic view of the origin and distribution of adrenergic nerves in the guinea-pig uterus, based on various denervation procedures. As shown in the left part of the figure, the cervix receives about half (55%) of its adrenergic innervation from the paracervical ganglia (PCG) by way of short adrenergic neurons (dashed) and half (45%) via the hypogastric nerves (n.hyp.), whose postganglionic fibres originate in the inferior mesenteric ganglion. The right part of the figure illustrates adrenergic supply to uterine horns; 25% of the innervation comes from short adrenergic neurons (dashed) which run from the paracervical ganglia along the uterine artery to enter the organ at the tubal end. A smaller portion of the short adrenergic neurons enter the uterus in the cervix region directly from the paracervical ganglia and run together with some postganglionic fibres from the hypogastric nerves (some 10% of innervation to uterine horns follow this course). The majority of postganglionic fibres from the hypogastric nerves enter at the tubal end via the uterine artery; this, together with the smaller, previously mentioned portion, constitutes the innervation by the hypogastric nerves, which amounts to 30%. It can be seen that 35% of the noradrenaline content in the uterine horn originates from nerves arriving via the suspensory ligament. However, these fibres are mainly restricted in their supply to the small tubal end of the uterine horn; in fact, this restricted region receives all its innervation via the ligament. Besides these major sources, a small contribution to the uterine horns by fibres running via the ovarian neurovascular pedicle may have to be taken into account

(Thorbert *et al.*, 1978b). Results on the uterus studied after early androgenization of female baby rats have directly indicated that the local adrenergic neurons constitute a separate target system for those humoral factors which determine the pattern of development of the reproductive tract by influencing the early differentiation of the hypothalamus (Broberg *et al.*, 1974).

Structural and functional changes in the short adrenergic neurons induced by pregnancy

During the early part of our studies on the adrenergic innervation of the female reproductive tract, material was collected in a rather unselected manner from various animal species under a variety of hormonal conditions. An entirely unexpected finding was the complete absence of histochemically visible adrenergic nerve fluorescence in the uterus of a cat in advanced pregnancy. This initiated a long series of studies aiming to clarify the pattern of changes in the course of pregnancy and post partum, their relationship to the location of the conceptus, and the neurobiological mechanisms underlying this pregnancy-induced complete disappearance of sympathetic neurotransmitter in the myometrium (Owman, 1981; Owman and Sjöberg, 1977; Sjöberg, 1967; Thorbert, 1978).

Pregnancy induces dramatic changes in the structure and function of the uterine adrenergic innervation, which entirely disrupts the usually constant local relationship between the amount of sympathetic innervation and the volume of the target tissue. Thus, in the course of pregnancy, there is an initial functional impairment, followed by a progressive degeneration, of the adrenergic nerve terminals so that at term the myometrium is entirely devoid of sympathetic nerves. This is a complex phenomenon probably involving at least three factors: (A) the hormonal environment of pregnancy, (B) local humoral influences from the fetus–placenta, and (C) the mechanical strain on the uterine wall produced by the growing conceptus. These assumptions are supported by, among other things, studies of the sterile horn (during unilateral pregnancy) in guinea–pigs, which is only under the influence of the first of these three factors. The changes in the adrenergic innervation of this horn are less marked and consist primarily of a functional inactivation of the nerves although, as pregnancy proceeds, a component of structural nerve degeneration is also added. At the end of pregnancy there is a pronounced transmitter decay in the cervix, too. This seems to reflect a sympathetic overactivity rather than a functional impairment of the nerves. The nerve plexus in the tubal end of the uterine horn, finally, appears to be almost entirely spared from the pregnancy-induced changes in the uterine adrenergic innervation.

The restoration post partum of the uterine adrenergic innervation shows considerable regional differences. In the cervix, the noradrenaline level becomes normalized shortly after delivery, probably reflecting a normalized functional turnover in the cervical adrenergic nerves. The restoration is slower in the sterile uterine horn following pregnancy; it is conceivably the result of 'refilling' of noradrenaline in functionally impaired but structurally intact neurons, combined to some extent with a regenerative process in the adrenergic nerve plexus. The restitution is, however, markedly slower in the sterile uterine horn than in the cervix. Prepregnancy levels of noradrenaline in this horn are not reached until three months post partum. The restitution in the uterine horn that had contained fetuses is very incomplete even half a year after pregnancy, due to the pregnancy-induced structural degeneration of the adrenergic nerves. There is reason to believe that a 'normal' neuromuscular relationship is never re-established in the main part of the uterine horn following the first pregnancy. The degree of normalization is hence much less than that following cytotoxic axon degeneration by administration of 6-hydroxydopamine or antiserum to nerve growth factor. There may be several reasons for this: (A) the pregnancy-induced degeneration is more complete and possibilities for collateral sprouting from intact axons are small, (B) the effect on the ganglion cells during pregnancy is different from that of the neurotoxic agents, or (C) the properties of the target organ have changed to such an extent that it no longer represents a natural template for the outgrowth of a dense adrenergic nerve plexus.

The guinea-pig, for example, is nevertheless highly fertile even immediately following a pregnancy. This would indicate that the extensive adrenergic innervation present in the uterus of virgin animals is not required for a pregnancy to take place, and that the small amount of innervation that does become established post partum is sufficient to fulfil the adrenergic smooth muscle control in conjunction with pregnancy. Results from the human myometrium (Thorbert *et al.*, 1979), which for practical reasons could not be obtained from nulliparous patients, suggests that a degeneration–regeneration cycle in fact takes place also in conjunction with the second and following pregnancies, but with a 'lower amplitude' than the decay occurring during the first pregnancy. This would mean that the adrenergic innervation supplying the uterus before the first pregnancy does not represent a final stage of development, and that a 'normal' degree of adrenergic innervation in the uterus is not established until after one pregnancy. It may be that the more extensive nerve supply of the myometrium already has played its main functional role during a phase preceding this first pregnancy. It is not even necessary that the uterine adrenergic nerves in these earlier phases have been involved in motor control of the smooth musculature; it may have had such functions as trophic or metabolic regulation during the differentiation, growth, or hormonal adaptation of the myometrial smooth muscle cells.

Cholinergic neurons

Although a large number of the cells in the paracervical ganglia are acetylcholinesterase-positive (Kanerva, 1972; Thorbert *et al.*, 1977), the cholinergic nerve supply to the smooth musculature in the oviduct, uterus, and vagina is very sparse (the well-developed cholinergic innervation of the ovary probably emanates from other local ganglia). The cholinergic innervation seems to be primarily related to blood vessels (Thorbert *et al.*, 1977) and glandular elements in the mucosa (Hammarström, 1980). The cholinergic nerves in the uterus appear to be unaffected by pregnancy, as evidenced by non-significant alterations in choline acetyltransferase activity measured in the human myometrium from the uterine isthmus (Thorbert *et al.*, 1979).

Peptidergic neurons

The female reproductive tract, like that of the male, is also supplied with peptidergic fibres. Primary interest has focused on VIP. The presence of VIP has been studied in rat, cat and guinea-pig, as well as in humans (Alm *et al.*, 1977, 1980a, b; Helm *et al.*, 1981; Larsson *et al.*, 1977; Walles *et al.*, 1980). VIP-immunofluorescent nerve fibres are found to a varying extent in all parts of the female reproductive tract, which has been corroborated in radioimmunological determinations of the peptide. It is notable that the highest density of VIP nerve terminals is present in the two important sphincter regions—the tubal isthmus and the uterine cervix (Alm *et al.*, 1980a; Helm *et al.*, 1981). VIP is responsible for a pronounced non-adrenergic, non-cholinergic inhibition of motor activity in the isthmus (Helm *et al.*, 1982), and it is also a potent relaxatory agent for the cervix (Walles *et al.*, 1980).

Intense VIP immunoreactivity is found in numerous nerve cells within the paracervical ganglion formations (Alm *et al.*, 1980a, b; Helm *et al.*, 1981), and denervation experiments have strongly suggested that the tubal and uterine VIP nerves (but not those in the ovary) originate from these ganglia (Alm *et al.*, 1980b), together with the short adrenergic neurons and the acetylcholinesterase-positive cells. However, it cannot be excluded that in at least some of the nerves VIP may coexist with any of the two classical autonomic transmitters. Interestingly, the level of VIP in the uterus shows a similar pattern of disappearance as the adrenergic neurotransmitter during pregnancy, but VIP normalizes rapidly after delivery, suggesting that VIP-containing nerves are not identical with the adrenergic fibres, and that the changes in the peptidergic neurons reflect functional alterations rather than axonal degeneration as found for the adrenergic system.

GANGLIA SUPPLYING URINARY BLADDER AND URETHRA

Organization of the autonomic ganglia

The lower urinary tract receives an extrinsic innervation formed by the hypogastric nerves, which intermingle with a parasympathetic component from the pelvic nerves, together forming a more or less well-developed plexus, the vesical plexus, which is located close to the urinary bladder (Kuntz and Moseky, 1935; Woźniak and Skowrońska, 1967). In addition to this, the lower urinary tract is regulated by the functionally more important intrinsic innervation. This is derived from ganglia lying close to the effector structure (Fig. 1). From histochemical studies the ganglia have been found to consist of adrenergic and cholinergic cell bodies, the latter predominating (Duarte-Escalante *et al.*, 1969; El-Badawi and Schenk, 1970; Hamberger and Norberg, 1965a, b; Hamberger *et al.*, 1964; Schulman *et al.*, 1972a, b; Sundin and Dahlström, 1973). The intrinsic adrenergic innervation of the urinary tract belongs to the system of short adrenergic neurons. The intrinsic ganglia also contain cell bodies with a positive immunohistochemical reaction for somatostatin and VIP (Alm *et al.*, 1977; Hökfelt *et al.*, 1978). The role of the somatostatin immunoreactive neuron is not known. In prevertebral ganglia, of guinea-pig and rat, somatostatin immunoreactive cells are also positive for dopamine β-hydroxylase immunoreactivity, which is a marker for adrenergic neurons, suggesting that somatostatin might be stored together with the noradrenaline transmitter within the adrenergic neuron (Hökfelt *et al.*, 1977). In view of this, it is interesting to note that not only noradrenaline (Furness and Costa, 1974) but also somatostatin has been shown to reduce the neuronal release of acetylcholine (Cohen *et al.*, 1978; Guillemin, 1976; Furness and Costa, 1979). In addition, the autonomic ganglia of the lower urinary tract also contain small, chromaffin-like cells displaying an intense amine fluorescence (SIF cells), probably acting as interneurons (see above).

Cholinergic nerve terminals with a characteristic beaded appearance enclose both the adrenergic and cholinergic cell bodies in a synaptic manner. Adrenergic nerve terminals are frequently found around and forming synapses with the cholinergic nerve cell bodies (but only occasionally with the corresponding adrenergic cells), thus offering structural possibilities for an intraganglionic adrenergic–cholinergic interaction in the regulation of bladder function (Hamberger and Norberg, 1965a; Hamberger *et al.*, 1964). Further, noradrenaline has been suggested to have a modulatory function in the presynaptic control of acetylcholine release (Knoll and Vizi, 1970; Paton and Vizi, 1969). This is in accordance with the electrophysiological observations in cats that postganglionic adrenergic stimulation can inhibit parasympathetic ganglionic transmission to the bladder (De Groat and Saum, 1971, 1972; Saum and De Groat, 1972). Immunohistochemical studies have shown that peptidergic (Leu-enkephalin immunoreactive) nerve terminals associate with a great number of the nerve cell bodies in these ganglia (Alm *et al.*, 1981) similarly to prevertebral ganglia in other locations (Schultzberg *et al.*, 1979). By electron microscopy, synaptic contacts have been demonstrated between peptidergic terminals and nerve cell bodies in cat bladder ganglia (Fehér *et al.*, 1980). In view of this and the findings by Konishi *et al.* (1979), showing presynaptic inhibition of cholinergic ganglionic transmission by Leu-enkephalin, it may be assumed that also peptidergic (Leu-enkephalin) nerves can inhibit the release of acetylcholine in the lower urinary tract.

The neurons supplying the lower urinary tract with postganglionic auto-nomic nerves are predominantly localized as a ganglionic complex at the ureter–vesical junction and the bladder base–urethral junction at the trigone area (Duarte-Escalante *et al.*, 1969; El-Badawi and Schenk, 1971; Schulman *et al.*, 1972a, b) (Fig. 1) The ganglia are mostly found in the adventitia or in the outer parts of the smooth musculature. In addition, scattered extraganglionic nerve cells are sometimes present (Duarte-Escalante *et al.*, 1969; El-Badawi and Schenk, 1966; Schulman *et al.*, 1972a, b). They are usually solitary, but sometimes an adrenergic and a cholinergic cell can be seen lying close together. The cell bodies often occur in relation to large nerve trunks and blood vessels running in the adventitia, muscularis and submucosa of the tract. Paraganglia, consisting of clusters of extra–adrenal chromaffin cells containing catecholamines, have been found in the wall of the human urinary bladder. The histochemical and structural features resemble similar cells in the carotid body (Hervonen *et al.*, 1976, 1978). Their presence in the bladder wall may suggest a local influence on the smooth muscle tone of the organ.

Adrenergic innervation

The adrenergic innervation generally displays a high density in the trigone area of the bladder base, surrounding the smooth muscle bundles of the muscularis (Alm and Elmér, 1975; El-Badawi and Schenk, 1966; Hamberger and Norberg, 1965a; Owman and Sjöberg, 1972; Sundin and Dahlström, 1973; Wakade and Kirpekar, 1972). In these locations smooth muscle α-receptors are predominant, and postganglionic adrenergic nerve stimula-tion will produce a contractile response (Edvardsen and Setekleiv, 1968; Elmér, 1974; Khanna, 1976; Raezer *et al.*, 1973). In other parts of the ureters and the urinary bladder (the detrusor muscle) the adrenergic innervation is much more sparse. Adrenergic β-receptors are predominant in the detrusor muscle, and postganglionic adrenergic nerve stimulation will evoke a relaxa-tory effect (Edwardsen and Setekleiv, 1968; Elmér, 1974; Khanna, 1976; Raezer *et al.*, 1973).

Also the urethra is supplied with adrenergic nerves surrounding smooth muscle bundles forming the internal urethral sphincter, which is primarily supplied with α-(excitatory) receptors. In contrast to the urinary bladder and the ureter there is a distinct regional variation in nerve density between species such as cat, dog, guinea-pig, and man (Benson *et al.*, 1976; Ek *et al.*, 1977; Owman *et al.*, 1971a; Owman and Sjöberg, 1972; Sundin and Dahl-ström, 1973; Ulmsten *et al.*, 1977).

Cholinergic innervation

The cholinergic innervation of the lower urinary tract is generally richer than the adrenergic, and has a more uniform distribution pattern without regional accumulations, and no overt species differences are found. The urinary bladder has a very rich supply of cholinergic nerve terminals surrounding the smooth muscle bundles in a plexiform pattern (Alm, 1978, El-Badawi and Schenk, 1966). Also the smooth musculature of the urethra and terminal ureter is innervated by cholinergic nerve terminals, though the nerve density is lower (Alm, 1978). Cholinergic nerve stimulation produces contraction of the bladder and urethral smooth musculature (Jonas and Tanagho, 1976; Kurn, 1965; Nergårdh, 1974, 1975; Nergårdh and Boréus, 1972, 1973).

Peptidergic innervation

From immunohistochemical investigations, a peptidergic (VIP) innervation, probably derived from the pelvic ganglia, is found in the lower urinary tract of various species, including man (Alm *et al.*, 1977, 1979; Larsson *et al.*, 1977). The VIP nerves are associated with the smooth musculature of the muscularis layer, and are also found around blood vessels. In cat, numerous VIP terminals occur at the ureter–vesical junction, and in the trigone area in relation to the more or less developed smooth muscle sphincters. In other parts of the urinary bladder, in the terminal ureter and proximal urethra, VIP terminals are only found occasionally. In the human lower urinary tract, VIP terminals generally have a uniform distribution. The physiological role exerted by the VIP innervation is unknown. Their rich occurrence in smooth muscle organs, particularly in sphincters, may indicate an influence on smooth muscle activity. Whether this is exerted directly on the smooth muscle cells and/or via interaction mechanisms with other nerve types, peripherally at the effector organs or at a ganglionic level, is still unknown.

SUMMARY

The male and female genitourinary tracts have a rich supply of autonomic nerves. Cholinergic neurons are collected in ganglia located in the bladder neck, as well as in the dorsal wall of the prostate and in the uterovaginal junction. Nerve cells in these locations also contain immunohistochemically demonstrable polypeptides—primary interest has so far focused on VIP, enkephalin and somatostatin—which may be involved in local reflex mechanisms regulating smooth muscle activity, local blood flow, and epithelial functions. The pelvic ganglia have a prominent adrenergic contribution forming anatomically and functionally unique 'short adrenergic neurons' innervating the well-developed smooth muscle coats of the genital organs and lower urinary tract, together with classical adrenergic fibres originating in the inferior mesenteric ganglia and running in the hypogastric nerves. In the female, the entire system of myometrial adrenergic nerves undergoes a fundamental structural and functional reorganization in the course of pregnancy, partly reflecting the peculiar sensitivity of the short adrenergic neurons to sex steroids.

ACKNOWLEDGEMENTS

Supported by grants from The Ford Foundation, World Health Organization, and the Swedish Medical Research Council.

REFERENCES

Alm, P. (1978). Cholinergic innervation of the human urethra and urinary bladder. *Acta Pharmacol. Toxicol.*, **43**, 56–62.

Alm, P., and Elmér, M. (1975). Adrenergic and cholinergic innervation of the rat urinary bladder. *Acta Physiol. Scand.*, **94**, 36–45.

Alm, P., Alumets, J., Ek, A., and Sundler, F. (1979). Peptidergic (VIP) nerves in the human urinary tract. *Proceedings of the International Continence Society, 9th Annual Meeting, Rome*.

Alm, P., Alumets, J., Håkanson, R., and Sundler, F. (1977). Peptidergic (vasoactive intestinal peptide) nerves in the genito-urinary tract. *Neuroscience*, **2**, 751–754.

Alm, P., Alumets, J., Håkanson, R., Helm, G., Owman, Ch., Sjöberg, N.-O., and Sundler, F. (1980a). Vasoactive intestinal polypeptide nerves in the human female genital tract. *Am. J. Obstet. Gynecol.*, **136**, 349–351.

Alm, P., Alumets, J., Håkanson, R., Owman, Ch., Sjöberg, N.-O., Sundler, F., and Walles, B. (1980b). Origin and distribution of VIP (vasoactive intestinal polypeptide)-nerves in the genito-urinary tract. *Cell Tissue Res.*, **205**, 337–347.

Alm, P., Alumets, J., Håkanson, R., Owman, Ch., Sjöberg, N.-O., Stjernquist, M., and Sundler, F. (1981). Enkephalin-immunoreactive nerve fibres in the feline genito-urinary tract. *Histochemistry*, **72**, 351–355.

Baumgarten, H. G., Holstein, A. F., and Owman, Ch. (1970). Auerbach's plexus of mammals and man: Electron microscopic identification of three types of neuronal processes in myenteric ganglia of the large intestine from Rhesus monkeys, guinea-pigs and man. *Z. Zellforsch. Mikrosk. Anat.*, **106**, 376–397.

Baumgarten, H. G., Owman, Ch., and Sjöberg, N.-O. (1975). Neural mechanisms in male fertility. In *Control of Male Fertility* (Eds. J. J. Sciarra, C. Markland and J. J. Speidel), pp. 26–40, Harper and Row, Hagerstown, Maryland.

Bell, Ch., and McLean, J. A. (1967). Localization of norepinephrine and acetylcholinesterase in separate neurons supplying the guinea pig vas deferens. *J. Pharmacol. Exp. Ther.*, **157**, 69–73.

Benson, G. S., Jacobowitz, D., Raezer, D. M., Corriere, J. N., and Wein, A. J. (1976). Adrenergic innervation and stimulation of canine urethra. *Urology*, **7**, 337–340.

Björklund, A., Cegrell, L., Falck, B., Ritzén, M., and Rosengren, E. (1970). Dopamine-containing cells in sympathetic ganglia. *Acta Physiol. Scand.*, **78**, 334–338.

Broberg, A., Nybell, G., Owman, Ch., Rosengren, E., and Sjöberg, N.-O. (1974). Consequence of neonatal androgenization and castration for future levels of norepinephrine transmitter in uterus and vas deferens of the rat. *Neuroendocrinology*, **15**, 308–312.

Burnstock, G. (1972). Purinergic nerves. *Pharmacol. Rev.*, **24**, 509–581.

Burnstock, G. (1970). Structure of smooth muscle and its innervation. In *Smooth Muscle* (Eds. E. Bülbring, A. F. Brading, A. W. Jones and T. Tomita), pp. 1–69, Edward Arnold, London.

Cohen, M. L., Rosing, E., Wiley, K. S., and Slater, I. H. (1978). Somatostatin inhibits adrenergic and cholinergic neurotransmission in smooth muscle. *Life Sci.*, **23**, 1659–1664.

De Groat, W. C., and Saum, W. R. (1971). Adrenergic inhibition in mammalian parasympathetic ganglia. *Nature*, **231**, 188–189.

De Groat, W. C., and Saum, W. R. (1972). Sympathetic inhibition of the urinary bladder and pelvic ganglionic transmission in the cat. *J. Physiol. (London)*, **220**, 297–314.

Duarte-Escalante, O., Labay, P., and Boyarsky, S. (1969). The neurohistochemistry of mammalian ureter: A new combination of histochemical procedures to demonstrate adrenergic, cholinergic and chromaffin structures in ureter. *J. Urol.*, **101**, 803–811.

Edvardsen, P., and Setekleiv, J. (1968). Distribution of adrenergic receptors in the urinary bladder of cats, rabbits and guinea-pigs. *Acta Pharmacol. Toxicol.*, **26**, 437–445.

Ek, A., Alm, P., Andersson, K.-E., and Persson, C. G. A. (1977). Adrenergic and cholinergic nerves of the human urethra and urinary bladder. A histochemical study. *Acta Physiol. Scand.*, **99**, 345–352.

El-Badawi, A., and Schenk, E. A. (1966). Dual innervation of the mammalian urinary bladder. A histochemical study of the distribution of cholinergic and adrenergic nerves. *Am. J. Anat.*, **119**, 405–428.

El-Badawi, A., and Schenk, E. A. (1970). Intra- and extraganglionic peripheral cholinergic neurons in the urogenital organs of the cat. *Z. Zellforsch. Mikrosk. Anat.*, **103**, 26–33.

El-Badawi, A., and Schenk, E. A. (1971). A new theory of the innervation of bladder musculature. Part 3. Postganglionic synapses in uretero-vesico-urethral autonomic pathways. *J. Urol.*, **105**, 372–374.

Elmér, M. (1974). Action of drugs on the innervated and denervated urinary bladder of the rat. *Acta Physiol. Scand.*, **91**, 289–297.

Falck, B. (1962). Observations on the possibilities of the cellular localization of monoamines by a fluorescence method. *Acta Physiol. Scand.*, **56** (Suppl. 197), 1–25.

Falck, B., Owman, Ch., and Sjöstrand, N. O. (1965). Peripherally located adrenergic neurons innervating the vas deferens and the seminal vesicle of the guinea-pig. *Experientia*, **21**, 98–100.

Fehér, E., Csányi, K., and Vajda, J. (1980). Intrinsic innervation of the urinary bladder. *Acta Anat.*, **106**, 335–344.

Furness, J. B., and Costa, M. (1974). The adrenergic innervation of the gastrointestinal tract. *Rev-. Physiol.*, **69**, 1–51.

Furness, J. B., and Costa, M. (1979). Actions of somatostatin on excitatory and inhibitory nerves in the intestine. *Eur. J. Pharmacol.*, **56**, 69–74.

Furness, J. B., McLean, J. R., and Burnstock, G. (1970). Distribution of adrenergic nerves and changes in neuromuscular transmission in the mouse vas deferens during postnatal development. *Dev. Biol.*, **21**, 491–505.

Guillemin, R. (1976). Somatostatin inhibits the release of acetylcholine induced electrically in the myenteric plexus. *Endocrinology*, **99**, 1653–1654.

Hammarström, M. (1980). Uterine secretomotor innervation. *Acta Physiol. Scand. Suppl.*, **484**, 1–24.

Hamberger, B., and Norberg, K.-A. (1965a). Studies on some systems of adrenergic synaptic terminals in the abdominal ganglia of the cat. *Acta Physiol. Scand.*, **65**, 235–242.

Hamberger, B., and Norberg, K.-A. (1965b). Adrenergic synaptic terminals and nerve cells in bladder ganglia of the cat. *Int. J. Neuropharmacol.*, **4**, 41–45.

Hamberger, B., Norberg, K.-A., and Sjöqvist, F. (1964). Evidence for adrenergic nerve terminals and synapses in sympathetic ganglia. *Int. J. Neuropharmacol.*, **2**, 279–282.

Helm, G., Håkanson, R., Leander, S., Owman, Ch., Sjöberg, N.-O., and Walles, B. (1982). Neurogenic relaxation medicated by vasoactive intestinal polypeptide (VIP) in the isthmus of the human Fallopian tube. *Regul. Peptides* **3**, 145–154.

Helm, G., Ottesen, B., Fahrenkrug, J., Larsen, J.-J., Owman, Ch., Sjöberg, N.-O., Stolberg, B., Sundler, F., and Walles, B. (1981). Vasoactive intestinal polypeptide (VIP) in the human female reproductive tract: distribution and motor effects. *Biol. Reprod.*, **25**, 227–234.

Hervonen, A., Vaalasti, A., Vaalasti, T., Partanen, M., and Kanerva, L. (1976). Paraganglia in the urogenital tract of man. *Histochemistry*, **48**, 307–313.

Hervonen, A., Vaalasti, A., and Partanen, M. (1978). Paraganglia of the bladder, *J. Urol.*, **119**, 335–337.

Hökfelt, T., Elfvin, L.-G., Elde, R., Schultzberg, M., Goldstein, M., and Luft, R. (1977). Occurrence of somatostatin-like immunoreactivity in some peripheral sympathetic noradrenergic neurons. *Proc. Natl. Acad. Sci. U.S.A.*, **74**, 3587–3591.

Hökfelt, T., Schultzberg, M., Elde, R., Nilsson, G., Terenius, L., Said, S., and Goldstein, M. (1978). Peptide neurons in peripheral tissues including the urinary tract: immunohistochemical studies. *Acta Pharmacol. Toxicol.*, **43**, 79–89.

Jonas, U., and Tanagho, E. A. (1976). Studies on vesicourethral reflexes. II. Urethral sphincteric responses to spinal cord stimulation. *Invest. Urol.*, **13**, 278–285.

Kanerva, L. (1972). Development, histochemistry and connections of the paracervical (Frankenhäuser) ganglion of the rat uterus. *Acta Inst. Anat. Univ. Helsinki Suppl.*, **2**, 1–31.

Khanna, O. P. (1976). Disorders of micturition: Neuropharmacologic basis and results of drug therapy. *Urology*, **8**, 316–328.

Knoll, J., and Vizi, E. S. (1970). Presynaptic inhibition of acetylcholine release by endogenous and exogenous noradrenaline of high rat of stimulation. *Br. J. Pharmacol.*, **40**, 554–555.

Konishi, S., Tsunoo, A., and Otsuka, M. (1979). Enkephalins presynaptically inhibit cholinergic transmission in sympathetic ganglia. *Nature*, **282**, 515–516.

Kuntz, A., and Moseky, R. L. (1935). An experimental analysis of the pelvic autonomic ganglia in the cat. *J. Comp. Neurol.*, **64**, 63–75.

Kurn, M. (1965). Nervous control of micturition. *Physiol. Rev.*, **45**, 425–494.

Langley, J. N., and Anderson, H. K. (1895a). The innervation of the pelvic and adjoining viscera. Part 4. The internal generative organs. *J. Physiol. (London)*, **19**, 122–130.

Langley, J. N., and Anderson, H. K. (1895b). The innervation of the pelvic and adjoining viscera. Part 5. Position of the nerve cells on the course of the efferent nerve fibres. *J. Physiol. (London)*, **19**, 131–139.

Langley, J. N., and Anderson, H. K. (1896a). The innervation of the pelvic and adjoining viscera. Part 6. Histological and physiological observations upon the effects of section of the sacral nerve. *J. Physiol. (London)*, **19**, 372–384.

Langley, J. N., and Anderson, H. K. (1896b). The innervation of the pelvic and adjoining viscera. Part 7. Anatomical observations. *J. Physiol. (London)*, **20**, 372–406.

Larsson, L.-I., Fahrenkrug, J., and Schaffalitzky de Muckadell, O. B. (1977). Vasoactive intestinal polypeptide occurs in nerves of the female genitourinary tract. *Science*, **197**, 1374–1375.

Libet, B. (1976). The SIF cell as a functional dopamine-releasing interneuron in the rabbit superior cervical ganglion. *Fogarty Int. Cent. Proc.*, **30**, 163–177.

Libet, B., and Owman, Ch. (1974). Concomitant changes in formaldehyde-induced fluorescence of dopamine interneurones and in slow inhibitory postsynaptic potentials of the rabbit superior cervical ganglion, induced by stimulation of the preganglionic nerve or by a muscarinic agent. *J. Physiol. (London)*, **237**, 635–662.

Nergårdh, A. (1974). The interaction between cholinergic and adrenergic receptor functions in the outlet region of the bladder. An *in vitro* study in the cat. *Scand. J. Urol. Nephrol.*, **8**, 108–113.

Nergårdh, A. (1975). Autonomic receptor functions in the lower urinary tract: a survey of recent experimental results. *J. Urol.*, **113**, 180–185.

Nergårdh, A., and Boréus, L. O. (1972). Autonomic receptor function in the lower urinary tract of man and cat. *Scand. J. Urol. Nephrol.*, **6**, 32–36.

Nergårdh, A., and Boréus, L. O. (1973). The functional role of cholinergic receptors in the outlet region of the urinary bladder. An *in vitro* study in the cat. *Acta Pharmacol.*, **32**, 467–485.

Owman, Ch. (1981). Pregnancy induces degenerative and regenerative changes in the autonomic innervation of the female reproductive tract. In *Development of the Autonomic Nervous System, Ciba Foundation Symposium 83* (Eds. K. Elliott and G. Lawrenson), pp. 252–273, Pitman, London.

Owman, Ch., and Sjöberg, N.-O. (1966). Adrenergic nerves in the female genital tract of the rabbit. With remarks on cholinesterase-containing structures. *Z. Zellforsch. Mikrosk. Anat.*, **74**, 182–197.

Owman, Ch., and Sjöberg, N.-O. (1972). The importance of short adrenergic neurons in the seminal emission mechanism of rat, guinea-pig and man. *J. Reprod. Fertil.*, **28**, 379–387.

Owman, Ch., and Sjöberg, N.-O. (1977). Influence of pregnancy and sex hormones on the system of short adrenergic neurons in the female reproductive tract. In *Endocrinology,* Vol. 1, Proceedings of the Vth International Congress of Endocrinology, Hamburg, July 18–24, 1976 (Ed. V. H. T. James), pp. 205–209, Excerpta Medica, Amsterdam and Oxford.

Owman, Ch., and Sjöstrand, N. O. (1965). Short adrenergic neurons and catecholamine-containing cells in vas deferens and accessory male genital glands of different mammals. *Z. Zellforsch. Mikrosk. Anat.*, **66**, 300–320.

Owman, Ch., Rosengren, E., and Sjöberg, N.-O. (1967). Adrenergic innervation of the human female reproductive organs: A histochemical and chemical investigation. *Obstet. Gynecol.*, **30**, 763–773.

Owman, Ch., Owman, T., and Sjöberg, N.-O. (1971a). Short adrenergic neurons innervating the female urethra of the cat. *Experientia*, **27**, 313–315.

Owman, Ch., Sjöberg, N.-O., and Swedin, G. (1971b). Histochemical and chemical studies on pre- and postnatal development of the different systems of 'short' and 'long' adrenergic neurons in peripheral organs of the rat. *Z. Zellforsch. Mikrosk. Anat.*, **116**, 319–341.

Owman, Ch., Falck, B., Johansson, E. D. B., Rosengren, E., Sjöberg, N.-O., Sporrong, B., Svensson, K.-G., and Walles, B. (1976). Autonomic nerves and related amine receptors mediating motor activity in the oviduct of monkey and man.

A histochemical, chemical and pharmacological study. In *Ovum Transport and Fertility Regulation* (Eds. M. J. K. Harper, C. J. Pauerstein, C. E. Adams, E. M. Coutinho, H. B. Croxatto and D. M. Paton), pp. 256–275, Scriptor, Copenhagen.

Owman, Ch., Sjöberg, N.-O., Wallach, E. E., Walles, B., and Wright, K. H. (1979). Neuromuscular mechanisms of ovulation. In *Human Ovulation. Mechanisms, Prediction, Detection and Induction* (Ed. E. S. E. Hafez), pp. 57–100, North-Holland, Amsterdam.

Paton, W. D. M., and Vizi, E. S. (1969). The inhibitory action of noradrenaline and adrenaline on acetylcholine output by guinea pig ileum longitudinal muscle strip. *Br. J. Pharmacol.*, **35**, 10–28.

Raezer, D. M., Greenberg, S. H., Jacobowitz, D. M., Benson, G. S., Corriere, Jr., J. N., and Wein, A. J. (1973). Autonomic innervation of canine urinary bladder. *Urology*, **2**, 211–221.

Richardson, K. C. (1962). The fine structure of autonomic nerve endings in smooth muscle of the rat vas deferens. *J. Anat.*, **95**, 427–442.

Saum, W. R., and De Groat, W. C. (1972). Parasympathetic ganglia: activation of an adrenergic inhibitory mechanism by cholinomimetic agents. *Science*, **175**, 659–661.

Schulman, C. C., Duarte-Escalante, O., and Boyarsky, S. (1972a). The ureterovesical innervation. A new concept based on a histochemical study. *Br. J. Urol.*, **44**, 698–712.

Schulman, C. C., Duarte-Escalante, O., and Boyarsky, S. (1972b). Conception nouvelle de l'innervation urétérovésicale. *Acta Urol. Belg.*, **40**, 5–17.

Schultzberg, M., Hökfelt, T., Terenius, L., Elfvin, L.-G., Lundberg, J. M., Brandt, J., Elde, R. P., and Goldstein, M. (1979). Enkephalin immunoreactive nerve fibres and cell bodies in sympathetic ganglia of guinea pig and rat. *Neuroscience*, **4**, 249–270.

Sjöberg, N.-O. (1967). The adrenergic transmitter of the female reproductive tract: Distribution and functional changes. *Acta Physiol. Scand. Suppl.*, **305**, 1–32.

Sjöstrand, N. O. (1962a). Inhibition by ganglionic blocking agents of the motor response of the isolated guinea-pig vas deferens to hypogastric nerve stimulation. *Acta Physiol. Scand.*, **54**, 306–315.

Sjöstrand, N. O. (1962b). Effect of reserpine and hypogastric denervation on the noradrenaline content of the vas deferens and seminal vesicle of the guinea-pig. *Acta Physiol. Scand.*, **56**, 376–380.

Sjöstrand, N. O. (1965). The adrenergic innervation of the vas deferens and the accessory male genital glands. *Acta Physiol. Scand.*, **65** (Suppl. 257), 1–82.

Sporrong, B., Clase, L., Owman, Ch., and Sjöberg, N.-O. (1977). Electron microscopy of adrenergic, cholinergic, and 'p-type' nerves in the myometrium and a special kind of synaptic contacts with the smooth muscle cells. *Am. J. Obstet. Gynecol.*, **127**, 811–817.

Sundin, T., and Dahlström, A. (1973). The sympathetic innervation of the urinary bladder and urethra in the normal state and after parasympathetic denervation at the spinal root level. *Scand. J. Urol. Nephrol.*, **7**, 131–149.

Thorbert, G. (1978). Regional changes in structure and function of adrenergic nerves in guinea-pig uterus during pregnancy. *Acta Obstet. Gynecol. Scand., Suppl.*, **79**, 1–32.

Thorbert, G., Alm, P., Owman, Ch., and Sjöberg, N.-O. (1977). Regional distribution of autonomic nerves in guinea pig uterus. *Am. J. Physiol.*, **233**, C25–C34.

Thorbert, G., Alm, P., Owman, Ch., and Sjöberg, N.-O. (1978a). Differential effect on the sympathetic transmitter level in uterus and other organs of guinea-pig by drugs interfering with adrenergic nerve functions. *Acta Physiol. Scand.*, **104**, 203–212.

Thorbert, G., Alm, P., and Rosengren, E. (1978b). Cyclic and steroid-induced changes in adrenergic neurotransmitter level of guinea-pig uterus. *Acta Obstet. Gynecol. Scand.*, **57**, 45–48.

Thorbert, G., Alm, P., Björklund, A., Owman, Ch., and Sjöberg, N.-O. (1979). Adrenergic innervation of the human uterus. Disappearance of the transmitter and transmitter-forming enzymes during pregnancy. *Am. J. Obstet. Gynecol.*, **135**, 223–226.

Ulmsten, U., Sjöberg, N.-O., Alm, P., Andersson, K.-E., Owman, Ch., and Walles, B. (1977). Functional role of an adrenergic sphincter in the female urethra of the guinea pig. *Acta Obstet. Gynecol. Scand.* **56**, 387–390.

Wakade, A. R., and Kirpekar, S. N. (1972). Sympathetic innervation of urinary bladder of the guinea pig. *Am. J. Physiol.*, **223**, 1477–1480.

Walles, B., Håkanson, R., Helm, G., Owman, Ch., Sjöberg, N.-O., and Sundler, F. (1980). Relaxation of human female genital sphincters by the neuropeptide vasoactive intestinal polypeptide. *Am. J. Obstet. Gynecol.*, **138**, 337–338.

Woźniak, W., and Skowrońska, U. (1967). Comparative anatomy of pelvic plexus in cat, dog, rabbit, macaque and man. *Anat. Anz.*, **120**, 457–473.

Autonomic Ganglia
Edited by Lars-Gösta Elfvin
© 1983 John Wiley & Sons Ltd

Organization and Fine Structure of Enteric Ganglia

I. J. LLEWELLYN-SMITH, J. B. FURNESS, A. J. WILSON
and M. COSTA

*Centre for Neuroscience and Departments of Human Morphology and Human Physiology,
Flinders University, Bedford Park, S.A. 5042, Australia*

INTRODUCTION

The enteric ganglia are part of the enteric nervous system, a complex nerve network that is embedded in the walls of the gastrointestinal tract, extending from the smooth muscle part of the oesophagus to the internal anal sphincter, and which includes neurons in the gall bladder, the extrahepatic biliary tract and pancreas. Langley (1900, 1921) was the first to suggest that the enteric nervous system be considered as a separate division of the autonomic nervous system and gave three reasons for distinguishing it from the sympathetic and parasympathetic divisions. First, enteric neurons were histologically different from the neurons of other autonomic ganglia. Second, the connections of enteric neurons with the central nervous system differed from those of other peripheral neurons. Third, complete reflex pathways existed in the enteric nervous system. More recent studies demonstrate that the enteric ganglia contain many different types of nerves, most of which have been distinguished by histochemical methods. The histochemically defined nerve types appear at first to be somewhat randomly distributed within either the myenteric ganglia or the submucous ganglia. However, analysis of their distributions and projections reveals that they make organized connections within the enteric plexuses and that the pattern of connections is repeated from one short segment of the digestive tube to the next. Structural studies show further differences between the enteric and other autonomic ganglia; a notable feature is that the enteric ganglia, unlike other autonomic ganglia, contain no connective tissue elements or blood vessels.

THE ENTERIC PLEXUSES AND GANGLIA

The interconnected nerve plexuses that comprise the enteric nervous system ramify in every layer of the gut wall. Their general arrangement is shown in Fig. 1 (for further details see Rintoul, 1960; Schofield, 1968; Gabella, 1976, 1979; Furness and Costa, 1980). Ganglia occur in the

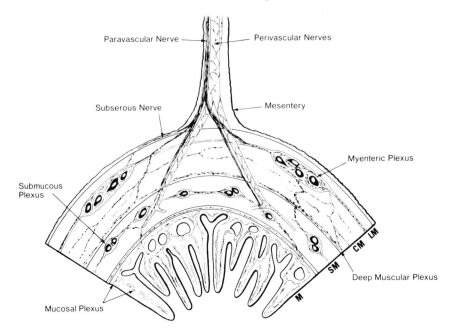

Paravascular Nerve

Perivascular Nerves

Subserous Nerve

Mesentery

Myenteric Plexus

Submucous
Plexus

CM   LM

SM

Deep Muscular Plexus

M

Mucosal Plexus

Figure 1 Diagram showing the arrangement of the enteric plexuses. The diagram was drawn for a transverse section through the small intestine of the guinea-pig. The general layout is similar in the other parts of the digestive tract, although the relative sizes and shapes of ganglia are different and the mucosa differs in organization. The deep muscular plexus is prominent in the small intestine but is not always well-delineated in other areas. LM, longitudinal muscle; CM, circular muscle; SM, submucosa; M, mucosa. Modified from Furness and Costa (1980); reproduced by permisson of Pergamon Press Ltd

myenteric plexus, which is located between the longitudinal and circular layers of the muscularis externa, and the submucous plexus, which lies in the loose connective tissue of the submucosa.

The myenteric plexus

The ganglia and interconnecting nerve strands of the myenteric plexus form a continuous meshwork with the ganglia lying at the nodes of the meshwork. The size of the ganglia and shape of the meshwork vary considerably from one part of the gastrointestinal tract to another within a species, from one species to another in the same part of the tract, from birth to maturity, and even from the mesenteric to the antimesenteric side of a single segment of intestine (Rintoul, 1960; Schofield, 1968; Gabella, 1976, 1979). Reflecting these kinds of differences, the packing density of nerve cell bodies (NCB) (i.e. NCB/cm^2 of outer surface) also varies from one part of the digestive tract to another and from one species to another (Schofield, 1968; Gabella, 1979). In most areas and species the packing density ranges from about 1000 to about 20 000 NCB/cm² (reviewed by Gabella, 1979).

The myenteric ganglia contain most of the nerve cell bodies of the enteric nervous system. The myenteric neurons, unlike other autonomic neurons, show a wide size range. In the alimentary tract of the rat, the maximal surface area of their profiles varies over at least one order of magnitude, from about 50 μm² in the small intestine to greater than 975 μm² in the caecum (Gabella, 1971a). The myenteric ganglia and the internodal strands contain the processes of intrinsic enteric neurons and glial cells and their processes. Parasympathetic, sympathetic and sensory neurons, which are called extrinsic neurons because their cell bodies lie outside the digestive tube, also contribute processes to the ganglia and their interconnecting nerve bundles (see below).

The submucous plexus

Submucous ganglia and their interconnecting nerve bundles form a meshwork in a similar way to the myenteric plexus. However, the meshes of the submucous plexus are larger and less regular than those of the myenteric plexus; the submucous ganglia are smaller, and the nerve strands linking them are finer (Henle, 1871; Goniaew, 1875). Although fewer comparative studies have been done on the submucous plexus, the arrangement of its meshes and its neuron content also appear to vary with species and region of the digestive tract (Kuntz, 1918; Ohkubo, 1936a, b; Junqueira *et al.*, 1958).

The submucous neurons are generally smaller and more homogeneous in size than myenteric neurons (Ohkubo, 1936a; Gunn, 1968). As in the myenteric plexus, submucous ganglia and internodal strands contain glial cells and their processes and the processes of intrinsic and extrinsic neurons.

MORPHOLOGICAL CLASSIFICATIONS OF ENTERIC NEURONS

Many studies have classified enteric neurons on the basis of their staining reactions with methylene blue or on their morphology after silver or gold impregnation (reviewed by Schofield, 1968; Gabella, 1976, 1979). The most widely quoted, and earliest, of these classification schemes is that of Dogiel (1895, 1896, 1899). Based on his observations of methylene blue-stained enteric ganglia from several species, Dogiel divided enteric neurons into three types (Fig. 2). *Type I cells* had many short irregular dendrites and one long slender axon which could be followed into the internodal strands; Dogiel believed that type I cells were motor. *Type II cells* had a short axon which branched within the ganglion of origin and long dendrites which extended beyond the ganglion; Dogiel thought type II cells were sensory. *Type III cells*

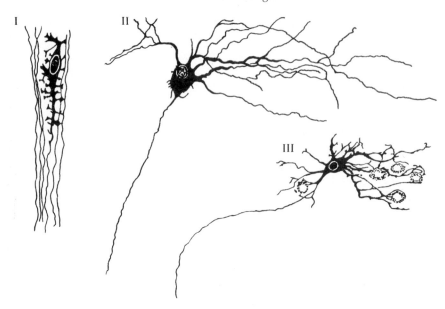

Figure 2   The three neuronal cell types described in the enteric plexuses by Dogiel, which have come to be called Dogiel type I, Dogiel type II and Dogiel type III cells. From Dogiel (1899)

had intermediate length dendrites which terminated in the same or adjacent ganglia. Many authors accepted Dogiel's classification of type I and type II cells but reported wide variations in the relative proportions of cell types between plexuses and considerable variations between regions of the gastrointestinal tract and between species. There were doubts about whether the functions ascribed to the various cell types by Dogiel were correct. Other authors proposed different classifications and even questioned whether clear-cut categories of enteric neurons existed. Nevertheless, most authors who performed these kinds of studies agreed that enteric ganglion cells had different morphologies and that cells similar to Dogiel types I and II could be recognized although other cell types were also present.

The functional significance of the morphological classifications of enteric ganglion cells proposed by these studies remains unclear. More recent work, described below, has shown that intrinsic enteric neurons can be divided into many more than three types on the basis of the active substances they contain. Thus, each morphological type of intestinal neuron probably includes several neurochemical types. When roles can be ascribed to these chemically defined classes of neurons, a correlation between morphology and function may emerge.

ORIGINS OF NERVE FIBRES IN THE ENTERIC GANGLIA

The enteric ganglia contain an extensive neuropil composed of nerve fibres that connect with or come close to the ganglion cells. Early functional and morphological studies (Langley, 1900; reviewed by Schofield, 1968; Costa and Furness, 1982) indicated that nerve cells outside the intestine contributed to the nerve fibre network in enteric ganglia, and studies with modern methods have confirmed the existence of extrinsic nerve fibres in enteric ganglia. However, many, probably most, of the nerve processes in the neuropil of enteric ganglia arise from the enteric neurons. Evidence for these intrinsic connections first came from the work of Bayliss and Starling (1900) and Langley and Magnus (1905–1906) who showed that reflexes could be elicited in isolated segments of intestine. Recent studies employing intracellular recording techniques have confirmed that intrinsic neurons receive inputs from other intrinsic neurons (Hirst and McKirdy, 1975; Hirst *et al.*, 1975). Early morphological studies also indicated the presence of connections between ganglia within a plexus and between myenteric and submucous ganglia (Auerbach, 1864; Hill, 1927). Immunohistochemistry has recently been used to provide details of these intrinsic connections. For example, enteric somatostatin-immunoreactive nerve cells appear to be interneurons connecting orally located ganglia with those situated more anally (Costa *et al.*, 1980b). Substance P-containing myenteric neurons connect one myenteric ganglion to adjacent ganglia and to submucous ganglia (Costa *et al.*, 1981b; Jessen *et al.*, 1980a, b).

AMINE-CONTAINING NERVES IN THE ENTERIC GANGLIA

Three types of amine-containing nerves can be distinguished in the enteric ganglia: noradrenergic nerves, 5-hydroxytryptamine (5-HT)-containing nerves, and enteric, non-5-HT, amine-handling nerves. The noradrenergic nerves have been studied in a variety of species and there is sufficient information for generalizations about their distribution and functions to be made. The only substantial investigations of the other two groups, however, have been made in the guinea-pig small intestine.

Noradrenergic nerves

Most light-microscope studies of the distribution of noradrenergic nerves in the gastrointestinal tract have used aldehyde-induced fluorescence to reveal the amine. Electron-microscopic studies on the identification of noradrenergic axons are described in a later section. The first fluorescence histochemical studies on the noradrenergic innervation of the gut made the striking observation that there was a dense supply of axons to the enteric ganglia (Figs. 3, 4) and a comparatively sparse supply to the non-sphincter smooth muscle (Norberg, 1964; Jacobowitz, 1965; reviewed by Furness and Costa, 1974). Noradrenergic fibres are found in both myenteric and submucous ganglia throughout the alimentary tract. Most or all enteric ganglion cells have varicose noradrenergic axons close to them but the fibres rarely form true pericellular endings in which short processes surround individual nerve cell bodies. Beaded fluorescent fibres are also observed in the internodal strands. A similar distribution of noradrenergic nerves is revealed by immunohistochemistry for dopamine β-hydroxylase (DBH), an enzyme involved in the biosynthesis of noradrenaline (Furness *et al.*, 1979). Individual varicose noradrenergic axons can be traced through the ganglia where they come close to a number of nerve cell bodies (Furness and Costa, 1974; Llewellyn-Smith, *et al.*, 1981).

Figures 3–12   These figures illustrate the three types of amine neurons that supply terminals in the intestine: noradrenergic neurons (Figs. 3, 4), 5-hydroxytryptamine (5-HT) neurons (Figs. 5–8), and intrinsic, non-5-HT, amine-handling neurons (Figs. 9–12). The noradrenergic axons were localized by the glyoxylic acid-induced fluorescence of noradrenaline and the 5-HT neurons by the immunohistochemical localization of 5-HT. The non-5-HT, amine-handling neurons were localized, after noradrenergic axons had degenerated following extrinsic denervation, by the aldehyde-induced fluorescence of dopamine: in Figs. 9 and 10 exogenously supplied dopamine was taken up by the axons and in Figs. 11 and 12 dopamine was formed by the decarboxylation of exogenously supplied *l*-DOPA. All examples are from whole mounts of the guinea-pig small intestine.

Figure 3: Noradrenergic axons in a ganglion of the myenteric plexus. The noradrenergic axons form a network of varicose fibres around the ganglion. There are no noradrenergic cell bodies in the ganglion. Calibration: 50 μm.

Figure 4: Noradrenergic axons in a submucous ganglion. Calibration: 25 μm.

Figure 5: Axons with 5-HT-like immunoreactivity in a ganglion of the myenteric plexus. Note the comparatively sparse fibre distribution compared with the non-5-HT, amine-handling axons (Fig. 9). Calibration: 50 μm.

Figure 6: Axons with 5-HT-like immunoreactivity in a submucous ganglion. Calibration: 50 μm.

Figures 7, 8: Examples of nerve cell bodies with 5-HT-like immunoreactivity in myenteric ganglia. (Such cells do not occur in submucous ganglia.) Typically, these cells have short, broad processes whereas the enteric, non-5-HT, amine-handling neurons have long fine processes (Figs. 12, 13). Calibrations: 8, 10 μm; 9, 20 μm.

Figure 9: The processes of enteric, non-5-HT, amine-handling neurons in a ganglion of the myenteric plexus. The fine processes form a dense network in the ganglion. Calibration: 50 μm.

Figure 10: Varicose processes of enteric, non-5-HT, amine-handling neurons in a submucous ganglion. Calibration: 50 μm.

Figures 11, 12: Nerve cell bodies of enteric, non-5-HT, amine-handling neurons in submucous ganglia. These cells typically have a number of fine processes. They are frequent in submucous ganglia but constitute only a small proportion of myenteric cell bodies. Calibrations: 20 μm.

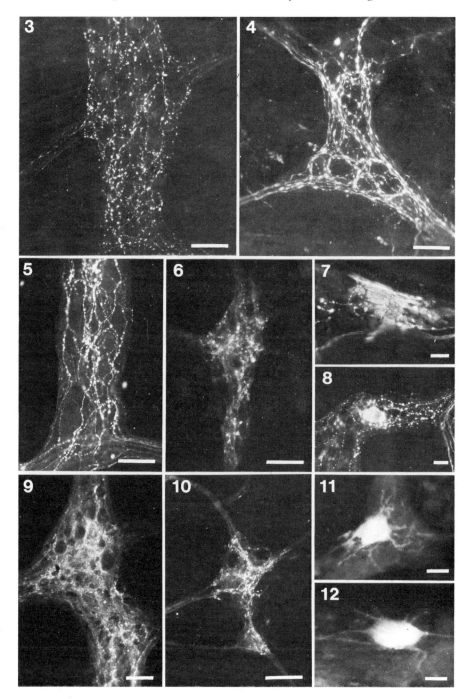

Most of the cell bodies of noradrenergic axons supplying the gut lie in the prevertebral ganglia of the coeliac, superior mesenteric, inferior mesenteric and pelvic plexuses (see Furness and Costa, 1974). In the gastrointestinal tract of mammals, only the myenteric ganglia in the proximal colon of the guinea-pig have been shown to contain significant numbers of noradrenergic nerve cell bodies (Costa, *et al.*, 1971; Furness and Costa, 1971a).

5-HT-containing neurons

Even though the fluorescence histochemical technique generally fails to detect 5-HT in intestinal nerves, evidence for the presence of nerves which contain 5-HT or a 5-HT-like substance in the gut is substantial. Gershon *et al.* (1965) showed that the myenteric plexus of mouse small intestine could take up 5-[^{3}H]hydroxytryptophan and convert it into 5-[^{3}H]HT. Robinson and Gershon (1971) were able to produce a faint yellow formaldehyde-induced fluorescence, ascribed to 5-HT, in myenteric plexus from guinea-pig small intestine by treating animals with reserpine and a monoamine oxidase inhibitor. Gershon *et al.* (1977) showed immunohistochemically that tryptophan hydroxylase occurred in enteric nerve cell bodies and processes of the rat intestine. Dreyfus *et al.* (1977a) revealed 5-HT fluorescence in myenteric nerve cell bodies from guinea-pigs given tryptophan, a monoamine oxidase inhibitor and *p*-chlorophenylalanine; and Dreyfus *et al.* (1977b) demonstrated uptake of 5-[^{3}H]HT into axons of intrinsic enteric neurons grown in explant culture.

Costa *et al.* (1981a) used an indirect immunohistochemical technique to study the distribution of intrinsic enteric nerves that contain a 5-HT-like substance. Antibodies to 5-HT bound to about 2% of nerve cell bodies in myenteric ganglia; these cells have many short thick processes and one long finer process (Figs. 7, 8) and thus resemble Dogiel type I cells. However, no immunoreactive nerve cell bodies were observed in the submucous ganglia. Varicose immunofluorescent axons with fine faint intervaricose segments wandered through each myenteric ganglion (Fig. 5) giving rise to an uneven pattern of innervation: some cell bodies were surrounded by groups of varicosities whereas others appeared to be uninnervated. In the submucous ganglia labelled varicosities were scattered among nerve cell bodies (Fig. 6). Most of the fluorescent fibres in the internodal strands of both plexuses were smooth. In the myenteric plexus the majority of the smooth 5-HT-immunoreactive fibres appeared to run over the ganglia between the plexus and the longitudinal muscle without branching, although processes arising from the smooth fibres could occasionally be seen entering the ganglia.

Furness and Costa (1981) performed operations which interrupted nerve pathways to and within the intestinal wall in guinea-pigs, and through analyses of the distributions of 5-HT-immunoreactive fibres at various times after operation were able to determine the projections of intrinsic 5-HT-containing neurons. There were no changes in the distribution of axons following extrinsic denervation. In the myenteric plexus immunofluorescent axons projected as far as 60 rows of ganglia (20–25 mm) in the anal direction. Along their course, these processes gave off small varicose branches that wound amongst nerve cell bodies in the myenteric ganglia. The varicose fibres in the submucous ganglia were derived from cell bodies in myenteric ganglia about 12 mm oral to the submucous ganglia they innervated.

Enteric, non-5-HT, amine-handling neurons

There are other neurons in the enteric ganglia which share some of the properties of 5-HT and noradrenergic nerves but which contain an amine that cannot be demonstrated with current techniques. These enteric, non-5-HT, amine-handling neurons can take up and retain catechol amines and indolamines and can decarboxylate amine precursors and store the decarboxylated product (Costa *et al.*, 1976; Furness and Costa, 1978, Costa *et al.*, 1981a). When segments of intestine in which noradrenergic nerves have degenerated are exposed to *l*-dihydroxyphenylalanine (*l*-DOPA), dopamine, 6-hydroxytryptamine or 5-hydroxytryptophan plus a monoamine oxidase inhibitor and then processed for fluorescence histochemistry, fluorescent nerve cell bodies and fluorescent varicose and non-varicose processes are observed in all parts of the myenteric and submucous plexuses (Figs. 9, 10). Most intrinsic non-5-HT, amine-handling neurons have many short or intermediate length processes and one longer process (Figs. 11, 12). Amine-handling fibres are also found in the other layers of the gut wall. The appearance of these fluorescent cells and fibres after *l*-DOPA or *l*-5-hydroxytryptophan is blocked if the intestine is exposed to an aromatic *l*-amino acid decarboxylase inhibitor.

The enteric, non-5-HT, amine-handling neurons can be distinguished from the enteric 5-HT neurons because the two nerve types have different distributions within the enteric plexuses (Costa *et al.*, 1981a). The cell bodies of 5-HT neurons are confined to the myenteric plexus. The cell bodies of neurons revealed by fluorescence histochemistry after incubation of the intestine with *l*-DOPA occur in both plexuses, and in the guinea-pig ileum constitute about 10% of submucous cell bodies and about 0.5% of myenteric cell bodies.

The nature of the transmitter of the enteric non-5-HT neurons that contain aromatic *l*-amino acid decarboxylase and monoamine oxidase is as yet unknown. However, they are unlikely to use a catecholamine as transmitter (Furness *et al.*, 1979; Howe *et al.*, 1981).

Table 1 Histochemically demonstrable nerve types in enteric ganglia

Substance localized	Myenteric ganglia	Submucous ganglia	Comment
Angiotensin-like peptide	Nerve cells and fibres		Not confirmed to be authentic angiotensin[1]
Bombesin-like peptide	Nerve cells and fibres	Nerve fibres only	Not confirmed to be authentic bombesin[2]
Cholecystokinin-like peptide	Nerve cells and fibres	Nerve cells and fibres	Probably a C-terminal octa- or tetra-peptide fragment[3]
Enkephalin	Nerve cells and fibres	Nerve fibres only	Authentic Met- and Leu- enkephalin present[4]
Motilin-like peptide			Not yet confirmed[5]
Neurotensin	Nerve fibres	Nerve fibres	Doubts have been expressed as to whether truly present[6]
Pancreatic polypeptide			Only one study[7]
Physalaemin-like peptide			Not yet confirmed[8]
Somatostatin	Nerve cells and fibres	Nerve cells and fibres	Authentic peptide, extensive studies[4]
Substance P	Nerve cells and fibres	Nerve cells and fibres	Authentic peptide, extensive studies[4]
Vasoactive intestinal polypeptide (VIP)	Nerve cells and fibres	Nerve cells and fibres	Authentic peptide or fragments, extensive studies[4]
Noradrenaline	Nerve fibres	Nerve fibres	Of extrinsic origin in most areas[9]
γ-Aminobutyric acid (GABA)	Nerve cells		Shown by uptake of [³H]GABA[10]
Monoamine oxidase	Nerve cells and fibres	Nerve cells and fibres	Not specific for aminergic neurons
Acetylcholinesterase	Nerve cells and fibres	Nerve cells and fibres	In majority of cells. Not specific for cholinergic cells
5-HT-like indolamine	Nerve cells and fibres	Fibres only	See text
Amines after uptake	Nerve cells and fibres	Nerve cells and fibres	These neurons contain no demonstrable endogenous amines (see text)[11]

Notes to Table 1

[1] Originally reported by Fuxe *et al.* (1977). Confirmed immunohistochemically by the present authors (unpublished), whose radioimmunoassay studies indicate that it may not be authentic angiotensin I or II.

[2] Dockray *et al.* (1979). The bombesin-like substance in the gut is probably closely related to amphibian skin bombesin.

[3] Different authors have different interpretations about the nature of this peptide. The predominant form in the intestine is probably CCK-8 or CCK-4 (Larsson and Rehfeld, 1979; Dockray *et al.*, 1981; see also Furness and Costa, 1982).

[4] The distributions, chemical natures and pharmacological actions of these peptides have been studied extensively in a number of species (see Furness and Costa, 1980, 1982; Schultzberg *et al.*, 1980; Furness *et al.*, 1980, 1981a; Sundler *et al.*, 1980).

[5] Reported by Chey and Lee (1980).

[6] Reported by Schultzberg *et al.* (1980), but the authenticity of this observation has yet to be confirmed (see Furness and Costa, 1982).

[7] Lorén *et al.* (1979).

[8] Lazarus *et al.* (1980).

[9] Furness and Costa (1974).

[10] Jessen *et al.* (1979).

[11] Referred to as enteric, non-5-HT, amine handling neurons (see text).

PEPTIDE-CONTAINING NEURONS IN THE ENTERIC GANGLIA

Antibodies raised against various peptides have been used histochemically to reveal nerve cell bodies and axons in enteric ganglia (Table 1). In some cases, the identity of the peptide has been confirmed by other techniques, such as amino acid sequencing or combined chromatography and radioimmunoassay (Furness and Costa, 1982). In other cases, available data only suggest that the peptide against which the antibodies were raised and the endogenous substance to which the antibodies bind are similar. Although some of the peptides have been studied extensively (reviewed by Furness and Costa, 1980, 1982; Schultzberg *et al.*, 1980; Jessen *et al.*, 1980b; Furness *et al.*, 1980; Sundler *et al.*, 1980; Furness *et al.*, 1981a) there have been few attempts to make quantitative, or even descriptive, comparisons of the distributions of the different peptides. Where this has been done, the results suggest that the peptides are in separate populations of neurons (Figs. 13–18), with the exception that some neurons may contain both somatostatin- and cholecystokinin-like peptides (Schultzberg *et al.*, 1980).

The distributions of enkephalin-, substance P-, somatostatin-, VIP- and cholecystokinin-like peptides in the various parts of the digestive tract in rats and guinea-pigs have been investigated in detail by Schultzberg *et al.* (1980) and have also been examined in a number of other studies. Some general features of the organization of these peptide-containing nerves in enteric ganglia can therefore be deduced and only these five peptides are dealt with in detail below. Observations on the other peptides listed in Table 1 are too restricted for any generalizations about their organization in the enteric ganglia to be made.

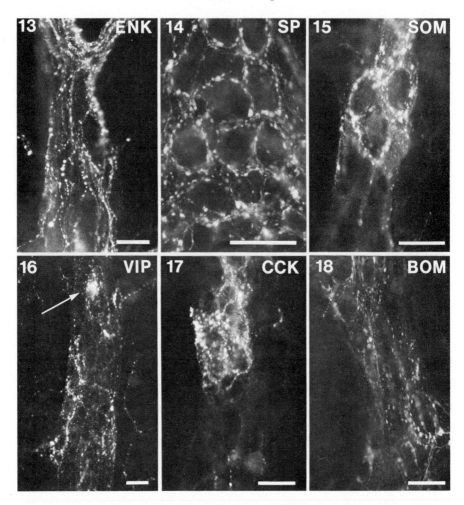

Figures 13–18 Immunohistochemical localization of neuropeptides in the myenteric plexus. The peptide-like immunoreactivity localized is indicated in each case as follows: ENK, enkephalin; SP, substance P; SOM, somatostatin; VIP, vasoactive intestinal polypeptide; CCK, cholecystokinin; BOM, bombesin. The preparations are all from the guinea-pig small intestine with the exception of Fig. 15 which is from the guinea-pig colon. A cell body positive for VIP can be seen in Fig. 16 (arrow). Enkephalin fibres form a loose plexus running through the ganglia. Substance P fibres form a dense network around all nerve cell bodies. Somatostatin and cholecystokinin fibres have very similar distributions: they form baskets around some nerve cell bodies while other cells are not supplied. VIP fibres form a sparse network with occasional nerve cell bodies being encircled by varicosities. Bar: 50 μm

Enkephalin

Enkephalin-like immunoreactivity is found in varicose fibres in the myenteric plexus of the stomach, small intestine and large intestine. The innervation is moderately dense in all these areas and the enkephalin-immunoreactive fibres appear to come close to most of the ganglion cells. Counts of immunoreactive cell bodies indicate that about 4–25% of myenteric neurons

Table 2 Percentages of peptide-containing cell bodies in the submucous and myenteric ganglia in the corpus of the stomach, the ileum and the proximal colon of rat and guinea-pig

		SP		VIP		ENK		SOM	
		s	m	s	m	s	m	s	m
Rat	Stomach	0	16.7	33.0	6.3	0	7.5	0	0
	Ileum	20.4	16.4	52.5	2.8	0	3.9	19.2	2.0
	Colon	1.7	13.0	65.9	5.6	0	4.9	3.2	14.4
Guinea-pig	Stomach	0	11.7	20.0	6.6	0	12.0	0	1.4
	Ileum	5.1	2.8	27.3	7.8	0	15.2	19.7	3.8
	Ileum*	11.3	3.5	42.3	2.4	0	24.5	17.4	4.7
	Colon	4.3	12.9	27.0	2.3	0	12.9	20.4	2.6

The proportions of peptide-containing cell bodies are given as the percentages of total numbers of nerve cell bodies counted. Abbreviations used: SP = substance P-like immunoreactivity; VIP = vasoactive intestinal polypeptide-like immunoreactivity; ENK = enkephalin-like immunoreactivity; SOM = somatostatin-like immmunoreactivity; s = submucous ganglia; m = myenteric ganglia. The figures are taken from the work of Schultzberg *et al.* (1980), except for the second group of figures for the guinea-pig ileum (*) that are from Furness and Costa (1980) with slight corrections for more recent observations. The failure to detect immunoreactive nerve cell bodies in some areas could be due to the techniques being insufficiently sensitive.

contain an enkephalin-like substance (Table 2). Enkephalin-like immunoreactivity is also found in fibres in the submucous plexus from all areas of the gut but no enkephalin-positive nerve cell bodies have yet been observed in the submucous ganglia.

Substance P

Substance P-immunoreactive fibres ramify extensively around myenteric neurons so that each neuron appears to be supplied by many fibres. This very dense investment of substance P-immunoreactive fibres around nerve cells makes it difficult to be sure of detecting all the substance P-containing cell bodies. Nevertheless, counts of substance P-immunoreactive nerve cell bodies indicate that substance P-containing neurons are present in all areas of the gastrointestinal tract and represent about 3–16% of all cell bodies. In all regions of the digestive tract there are a moderate number of substance P fibres within submucous ganglia and substance P-immunoreactive submucous

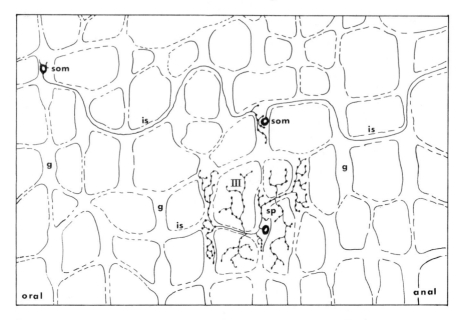

Figure 19 Diagram showing projections of two peptide-containing neurons within the myenteric plexus. Somatostatin-containing (som) neurons send processes only in the anal direction. The processes pass through several rows of ganglia before giving rise to basket-like formations of varicosities that surround either somatostatin-immunoreactive cell bodies or non-reactive cell bodies (not shown). Substance P-containing (sp) neurons have short projections to adjacent ganglia on both oral and anal sides of the ganglion of origin. They also contribute processes to the tertiary component of the myenteric plexus (III). Ganglia = g; internodal strands = is.

nerve cell bodies have been found in the small and large intestine but not in the stomach. Studies of the projections of myenteric substance P neurons in the small intestine of the guinea-pig (Costa *et al.*, 1981b) show that the majority of nerve endings in the myenteric plexus originate from cell bodies in adjacent ganglia (Fig. 19). Some of the fibres in submucous ganglia also originate from cell bdies in the myenteric ganglia. Most substance P-immunoreactive submucous neurons appear to project to the mucosa (Costa *et al.*, 1981b).

Somatostatin

Somatostatin-immunoreactive fibres have been found in myenteric ganglia of both the large and small intestine. There are fewer fibres in the stomach; in rat gastric myenteric ganglia very few or no somatostatin-containing fibres were detected (Schultzberg *et al.*, 1980). The fibres that contain a somatostatin-like substance are unevenly distributed in myenteric ganglia; they form basket-like formations around some cell bodies whereas other cells appear to be only sparsely innervated (Costa *et al.*, 1980b). No somatostatin-immunoreactive nerve cell bodies were found in the rat stomach, but in all other areas of the rat and guinea-pig digestive tracts 2–14% of neurons were somatostatin-positive (Table 2). In the guinea-pig small intestine, somatostatin-containing myenteric neurons project anally within the myenteric plexus to supply terminals around more distally located nerve cells (Fig. 19). Somatostatin-immunoreactive nerve fibres are located around nerve cell bodies in the submucous plexus of the large and small intestine but not of the stomach. In the guinea-pig small intestine the fibres in the submucous plexus appear to originate from submucous nerve cell bodies (Costa *et al.*, 1980b). In the stomach, no somatostatin-positive submucous nerve cell bodies have been found. In other areas up to about 20% of submucous neurons bind antibodies to somatostatin (Table 2).

Vasoactive intestinal polypeptide (VIP)

According to Schultzberg *et al.* (1980), VIP-immunoreactive nerve cell bodies and fibres are found in the myenteric plexus throughout the gastrointestinal tract. Jessen *et al.* (1980a), however, claimed that there were no VIP-containing cell bodies in the myenteric plexus of the guinea-pig caecum; this result implies that VIP could not be contained in the enteric inhibitory nerves that are present in the myenteric plexus. Further experiments in this laboratory (Furness *et al.*, 1981b) have confirmed the original observation of Schultzberg *et al.* (1980) so that the possibility that VIP is contained in the enteric inhibitory nerves is consistent with the immunohistochemical observations.

Within the myenteric ganglia, the VIP-containing nerve fibres form a fairly dense network with some fibres making ring-like arrangements around cell bodies (Costa *et al.*, 1980a). VIP-immunoreactive cells represent about 3–8% of all cells in the myenteric plexus (Table 2). Throughout the gastrointestinal tract submucous ganglia contain VIP-positive fibres and 25–50% of submucous neurons are found to be immunoreactive for VIP. These submucous neurons probably supply the dense VIP innervation of the mucosa.

Cholecystokinin-like peptide

A cholecystokinin-like peptide occurs in fibres in the myenteric and submucous plexuses in all regions of the digestive tract of rats and guinea-pigs with the exception of the guinea-pig stomach. Schultzberg *et al.* (1980) found cholecystokinin-immunoreactive nerve cell bodies in both plexuses in the large intestine but none in the small intestine. In our laboratory, on the other hand, cholecystokinin-immunoreactive cell bodies have been found in both plexuses in the guinea-pig small intestine (unpublished observations).

IMPLICATIONS OF IMMUNOHISTOCHEMICAL STUDIES

Some general features of the organization of the various types of neurons in the enteric ganglia are beginning to emerge from the immunohistochemical studies. In any region of the gut, each ganglion appears to represent an average of the total population of ganglia. Thus, nerve cell bodies of any particular type of peptide-containing neuron are distributed more or less randomly throughout the ganglia. Likewise, the distribution of nerve fibres immunoreactive for a particular peptide in each myenteric or submucous ganglion is similar to the distribution in every other myenteric or submucous ganglion. These immunohistochemical observations parallel those made with non-specific techniques, such as silver impregnation or methylene blue staining, which show that each ganglion has its complement of cells with different morphologies. This apparently random distribution of nerve types in enteric ganglia differs significantly from other autonomic ganglia where cells with similar functions and chemical properties appear to be grouped. In the central nervous system nerve cells also tend to be organized into morphologically or functionally similar nuclei or groups. The random distribution of peptide neurons in the enteric plexuses does not imply, however, that either myenteric or submucous ganglia are homogeneous structures. Some myenteric ganglia contain groups of pericellular fibres showing immunoreactivity for a particular peptide, while other nerve cell bodies are sparsely supplied, as is the case for somatostatin (Costa *et al.*, 1980b; Fig. 15). Several cell bodies with immunoreactivity for VIP are often grouped together in myenteric ganglia, but these groups are apparently randomly distributed throughout the ganglia (Costa *et al.*, 1980a).

Although each enteric ganglion (or group of ganglia since some cell types occur at a frequency of less than one per ganglion) represents a statistical sample of all ganglia, studies of the distributions and projections of peptide neurons in the gut indicate that the connections which the different types of neurons make within the enteric ganglia are highly ordered (Fig. 19; Furness *et al.*, 1981a). In the guinea-pig, small intestine myenteric neurons that contain a somatostatin-like substance project in the anal direction and have processes averaging 10 mm in length. Some somatostatin-immunoreactive fibres end in basket-like groups of varicosities around somatostatin-positive neurons while other fibres end around non-reactive neurons (Fig. 19). Substance P-immunoreactive myenteric neurons send processes in both oral and anal directions and end in ganglia close to (i.e. less than 1 mm from) the cell bodies of origin (Fig. 19). Likewise there is an ordered projection of neurons with 5-HT-like immunoreactivity within the myenteric plexus (see above). In the submucous plexus, some of the substance P-immunoreactive fibres arise from nerve cell bodies in the myenteric plexus (Jessen *et al.*, 1980a, b; Costa *et al.*, 1981b), and in the guinea-pig small intestine some substance P-containing fibres reach the intestine via the paravascular nerve running through the mesentery from cell bodies lying outside the gut wall. Similar studies, as yet unpublished, show that enteric neurons containing enkephalin-, VIP-, and cholecystokinin-like substances also have ordered projections within the enteric ganglia.

OTHER HISTOCHEMICAL STUDIES OF ENTERIC GANGLIA

Jessen *et al.* (1979) have found that a small number of myenteric neurons from guinea-pig taenia coli take up and retain γ-[^{3}H]aminobutyric acid (GABA). This finding suggests that some neurons in the enteric ganglia may use GABA as a transmitter.

Monoamine oxidase has been localized histochemically in nerve cell bodies in the myenteric and submucous plexuses (Koelle and Valk, 1954; Eder, 1957; Glenner *et al.*, 1957; Niemi *et al.*, 1961; Furness and Costa, 1971b; Tjälve, 1971). A large proportion of the cells contain this enzyme, many more than seem to utilize monoamines as transmitters (see section on amine-containing nerves above). This result implies that monoamine oxidase is probably contained in several types of neuron. In the guinea-pig small intestine most neurons have monoamine oxidase activity, with Dogiel type II cells being strongly reactive and Dogiel type I less reactive (Furness and Costa, 1971b).

Acetylcholinesterase activity has been localized in a high proportion of neurons in the myenteric and submucous plexuses. There is a range of intensity of activity, some cells showing strong reactivity with others being moderately or very weakly stained (Leaming and Cauna, 1961; Jacobowitz, 1965; Taxi, 1965; Gunn, 1968; McKirdy *et al.*, 1972; Van Driel and Drukker, 1973; Schardt and van der Zypen, 1974; Kyösola *et al.*, 1975). Acetylcholinesterase-positive nerve fibres are also found in enteric ganglia (Gunn, 1968, 1971; McKirdy *et al.*, 1972; Van Driel and Drukker, 1973; Schardt and van der Zypen, 1974). It is not possible to relate the presence of acetylcholinesterase to neuronal function. This enzyme would be expected to be present in both cholinergic neurons and in neurons receiving cholinergic inputs. Non-cholinergic systems may also have acetylcholinesterase associated with them (Krnjević, 1969; Silver, 1974).

FINE STRUCTURE OF THE ENTERIC GANGLIA

The ultrastructure of the enteric ganglia differs from that of other autonomic ganglia in a number of ways. Both myenteric and submucous ganglia lack internal capillaries and are surrounded only by continuous basal laminae that allow substances to penetrate into the ganglia from the extraganglionic space (Jacobs, 1977). Other autonomic ganglia have their own capillary networks and are surrounded by perineurial connective tissue capsules that isolate them, at least in part, from their immediate environment. The nerve cell bodies, nerve fibres, glial cells and glial processes that make up the enteric ganglia are tightly packed together in a way similar to the central nervous system. Other autonomic ganglia are more loosely organized and contain collagen, fibroblasts, macrophages, mast cells and chromaffin cells in addition to neurons and supporting cells. Myenteric neurons are rarely completely enclosed in glial cell processes and submucous neurons are never completely surrounded, whereas most nerve cell bodies and processes in other autonomic ganglia are almost entirely covered by satellite cell sheaths.

Fine structure of myenteric ganglia

The fine structure of the myenteric plexus has been studied in a number of laboratories and its general features appear to be consistent among the regions of the gut and the species so far investigated (Richardson, 1958; Taxi, 1959, 1965; Baumgarten *et al.*, 1970; Gabella, 1971b, c, 1972; Cook and Burnstock, 1976a, b; Yamamoto, 1977; reviewed by Gabella, 1976, 1979).

The myenteric ganglia are surrounded by a continuous basal lamina, a thin disorganized layer of collagen and the cell bodies and processes of interstitial cells, which are probably modified fibroblasts (reviewed by Gabella, 1979). Blood vessels are often found lying near the myenteric ganglia.

Myenteric ganglia are usually several cell layers thick. Glial cell bodies and neuronal and glial processes are usually interposed between nerve cell bodies with the spaces between these structures being only about 15–20 nm. The perikarya and processes of many myenteric neurons are partially covered by glial processes (Gabella, 1981). Other nerve cell bodies and processes lie directly beneath the basal lamina and some neurons at the edges of ganglia have both their serosal and luminal surfaces exposed to the extraganglionic space. Where a portion of neuronal plasma membrane is in contact with the basal lamina, the cytoplasm directly beneath often contains a band of microfilamentous material.

All nerve cell bodies in myenteric ganglia are characterized by large eccentrically placed nuclei with finely granular nucleoplasm, prominent nucleoli and sparse peripheral condensations of chromatin. In size, shape, and other aspects of fine structure, however, myenteric neurons vary widely. Many authors have discussed the great variability in the distribution of various cytoplasmic organelles among myenteric nerve cell bodies. Gabella (1972) described ultrastructural differences among large, medium and small myenteric neurons in the guinea-pig ileum. Cook and Burnstock (1976a) distinguished eight types of neuronal perikarya in guinea-pig stomach, ileum, caecum and colon; whether these categories have any functional significance is not known.

Gabella (1972) studied the processes of myenteric neurons in the guinea-pig ileum and found that the neurons gave off (1) small processes that emerged abruptly either from the cell body or from larger processes and often had synapses on them (2) broad processes that had a similar organelle content to the cell body and often lay at the surfaces of the ganglia beneath the basal laminae, (3) irregular, probably short, processes 2–4 μm in diameter with lower electron density but a similar organelle content to cell bodies, (4) thin processes 0.6–2 μm in diameter that contained many microtubules but little rough endoplasmic reticulum, and (5) variable and irregular processes that arise from cell bodies or type 3 processes and lacked organelles.

In myenteric ganglia, glial cells can outnumber neurons by more than two to one (Gabella, 1981). Glial cells in myenteric ganglia contain a protein found in the astrocytes of the central nervous system (glial fibrillary acidic protein; Jessen and Mirsky, 1980), and in some ways resemble these cells ultrastructurally (Gabella, 1971c). Glial cells have smaller and more irregular nuclei than neurons with denser more granular nucleoplasm and larger condensations of chromatin. Glial nuclei are surrounded by relatively thin rims of moderately electron-dense cytoplasm from which many thin processes containing numerous microtubules and gliofilaments arise.

Substantial portions of myenteric ganglia are occupied by neuropil which contains (1) relatively thin, electron-dense glial processes with many gliofilaments, (2) neuronal processes that have an organelle content and electron density similar to the nerve cell bodies, (3) varicose neuronal processes, which have round or fusiform dilatations and which contain variable numbers and types of vesicles but few other organelles, and (4) relatively straight neuronal processes with microtubules, microfilaments and mitochondria in an electron-lucent matrix. This last kind of process probably represents the intervaricose and non-varicose segments of axons. Since there are relatively few synapses on myenteric nerve cell bodies (see below) and there is close apposition between nerve processes in the neuropil, many of the interactions between nerves in the myenteric ganglia may occur in the neuropil.

Fine structure of the submucous ganglia

Although there are several brief references to the ultrastructure of submucous ganglia in the literature (Wong *et al.*, 1974; Fehér and Csányi, 1974; Fehér *et al.*, 1974; Oki and Daniel, 1977), the only detailed study of the fine structure of the submucous plexus is that of Wilson *et al.* (1981a) who examined ganglia in the guinea-pig ileum.

In the guinea-pig small intestine, submucous ganglia are smooth flattened

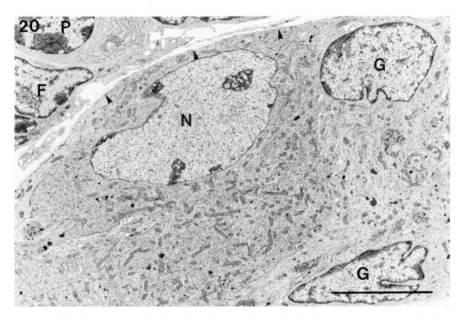

Figure 20 Electron micrograph of a portion of a submucous ganglion in the guinea-pig small intestine. The cells and processes that make up the ganglion are tightly packed together. Part of the plasmalemma (arrowheads) of a submucous nerve cell body lies directly beneath the basal lamina that surrounds the ganglion. N, neuronal nucleus; G, glial cell nucleus; F, fibroblast nucleus; P, plasma cell nucleus, Calibration: 5 μm

structures up to 200 μm long. They are surrounded by a basal lamina, a sparse layer of collagen and an incomplete irregular sheath composed of the fine processes of fibroblasts (Fig. 20), and are often located near large submucosal blood vessels.

The submucous ganglia in the guinea-pig small intestine are made up of an average of eight nerve cell bodies, arranged more or less in a monolayer, and glial cell bodies in a ratio of about 1:1 as well as the processes of these two cell types and of extrinsic nerves. The neuronal perikarya in the ganglia are tightly packed so that most nerve cell bodies are apposed to at least one other nerve cell body over part of their surface, with no intervening processes. Glial cells in the submucous plexus resemble those in the myenteric plexus and their processes rarely cover large areas of individual submucous neurons. In many cases, the plasma membranes of submucous neurons are separated from the extraganglionic space only by the basal lamina (Fig. 20). Where this occurs, the membrane has a thin dense lining of finely granular material or occasionally has a band of intracellular felt-like material running parallel to and about 100–250 nm beneath it.

Submucous neurons in the guinea-pig small intestine could not be divided into categories on the basis of either their shape, size, organelle content or the types of processes they gave off. Most submucous neurons have an irregularly oval shape with large smooth oval or round nuclei that are often eccentrically placed. The remaining neurons, primarily those lying at the edge of a ganglion along its long axis, are elongated and narrow with elongated nuclei. All neuronal perikarya have a similar, and conventional, complement of organelles whose distribution varies little from one part of the cell body to another.

Processes of several types emerge from submucous nerve cell bodies: (1) large usually straight processes up to 1.5 μm in width that contain rough and smooth endoplasmic reticulum, ribosomes, lysosome-like structures and many microtubules and often have synapses on them, (2) processes of variable length and width with fewer microtubules than the larger processes, (3) small spines, of variable shape with few organelles, that arise from either cell bodies or large processes and often have lateral synapses, and (4) cytoplasmic protrusions that are often mushroom-shaped and have an organelle content similar to the cell body and from which processes of the other three types arise.

The neuropil takes up a considerable proportion of submucous ganglia, often occupying the centre of a ganglion with nerve cell bodies arranged on either side. The submucous neuropil contains similar types of processes to those seen in the neuropil of myenteric ganglia and may also be the location for many nerve–nerve interactions.

VESICULATED NERVE PROFILES IN THE ENTERIC GANGLIA

In both myenteric and submucous ganglia vesiculated nerve profiles are round, fusiform or irregular in shape and may be up to 2 μm in length. They are often continuous at their poles with thin neuronal processes containing parallel microtubules and neurofilaments. In these cases, the profiles probably represent preterminal axonal or dendritic varicosities or boutons *en passage*. In addition to vesicles, profiles often contain mitochondria, glycogen, small cisternae of smooth endoplasmic reticulum, lysosome-like dense bodies, multivesicular bodies and, less frequently, microtubules and neurofilaments. Only a few of the vesiculated profiles in a thin section through an enteric ganglion make morphologically identifiable synaptic contacts and these show variability in the thickness of the pre- and postsynaptic thickenings with the postsynaptic densities being more prominent (Figs. 21, 24). The immediate presynaptic area is almost always occupied by small agranular vesicles.

Many of the early fine-structural studies on enteric ganglia reported the presence of various types of vesicles in enteric nerve profiles (Taxi, 1958,

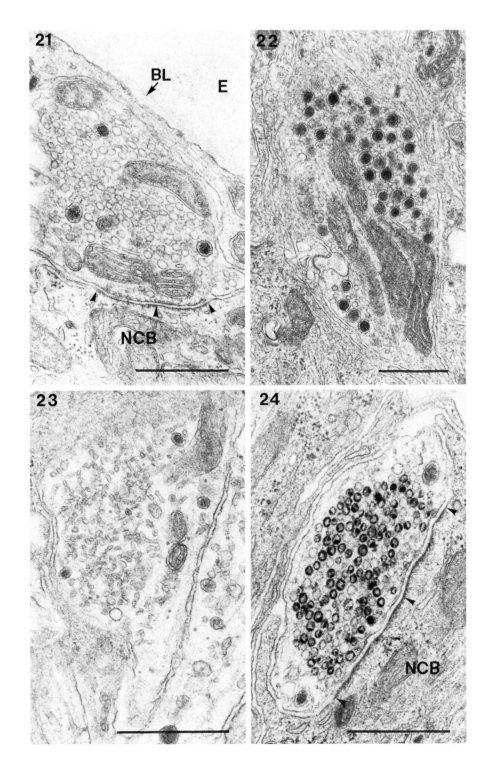

1959; Hager and Tafuri, 1959; Grillo and Palay, 1962; Tafuri, 1964; Honjin *et al.*, 1965; Honjin and Takahashi, 1966; Ono, 1967). More recently, many investigators have tried to categorize vesiculated profiles in enteric ganglia on the basis of their vesicle populations. The types of vesicle profiles and their synaptic contacts described in these studies are summarized in Table 3. The observations are difficult to compare because the preparative and analytical techniques used in the different studies vary considerably. However, some general points do emerge. The vesicle populations of the majority of profiles fall into three major classes: (1) populations consisting of variable proportions of small clear vesicles (SCV; 40–50 nm average diameter) and large granular vesicles (LGV; most ranging in diameter from about 70 nm to about 150 nm); (2) populations containing primarily small round vesicles, some of which have electron-dense cores (SGV; average diameter about 50 nm), along with a few LGV (usually 5% or less; Fig. 24); and (3) populations with a mixture of flattened vesicles, SCV and LGV (Fig. 23). The first class includes profiles in which nearly all vesicles are SCV (Fig. 21) and profiles (sometimes called 'p-type') in which up to 50% of the vesicles are LGV (Fig. 22). As explained in the next section, specific labelling methods and observations on denervated tissue have allowed the second class, enteric nerve profiles with SGV, to be subdivided into two groups—noradrenergic axons and processes of an unknown, but non-noradrenergic, intrinsic type of neuron. In guinea-pig small intestine these non-noradrenergic SGV-containing profiles have been termed ring vesicle (RV)-containing profiles because an electron-dense ring often occurs around the inner aspect of the vesicle membrane (Fig. 24).

ULTRASTRUCTURE OF CHEMICALLY IDENTIFIED NERVES IN THE ENTERIC GANGLIA

Information about the precise ways in which the many kinds of nerves in the enteric ganglia interact is difficult to obtain with conventional ultra-structural techniques. There are at least four reasons for this. (1) The cell

---

Figures 21–24   Electron micrographs of vesiculated profiles in enteric ganglia from guinea-pig small intestine. Calibrations: 0.5 μm.
Figure 21: A profile containing mostly small clear vesicles forms a synapse (arrowheads) on a nerve cell body (NCB) in a submucous ganglion. BL, basal lamina; E, extraganglionic space.
Figure 22: A profile with many large granular vesicles in addition to small clear vesicles in a submucous ganglion.
Figure 23: A profile with many flattened vesicles in a myenteric ganglion.
Figure 24: A profile that contains small round vesicles with electron-dense inclusions and electron-dense material lining the inner aspects of the vesicle membranes (ring vesicles) forms a synapse (arrowheads) on a nerve cell body (NCB) in a submucous ganglion.

Table 3 Summary of types of vesiculated profiles in enteric ganglia

| Reference | Species | Region of GIT | Ganglia | Major vesicular components of profiles (Numbers in square brackets refer to footnotes) | | | | | |
| | | | | SCV + LGV | | RV-type | SGV | Many FV | Other profiles |
				Mainly SCV	Many LGV		Others		
Baumgarten et al. (1970)	Man, monkey, guinea-pig	Large intestine	Myenteric	SCV 35–60 nm LGV 80–110 nm	LGV 85–160 nm SCV 40–60 nm		MGV 50–90 nm LGV 90–130 nm SCV 40–60 nm Few FV (man, monkey)	FV, also contains: MGV 50–90 nm LGV 90–130 nm SCV 40–60 nm (guinea-pig)	
				Axodendritic synapses	Axodendritic synapses		No synapses [1,2]	No synapses [1,2]	
Gabella (1971b, 1972)	Guinea-pig	Small intestine	Myenteric	SCV 40–60 nm also contains LGV, few FV	LGV 90–140 nm SCV 40–60 nm Also contains few FV	SGV 40–60 nm SCV 40–60 nm LGV 80–100 nm		FV 50–70 nm long Also contains SCV	Four less-common types on the basis of non-vesicular components
				Axosomatic axodendritic synapses	Axosomatic axodendritic synapses	Axosomatic axodendritic synapses [3]		Few axosomatic synapses	
Wong et al. (1974)	Rat	Small intestine	Submucous				SGV 50 nm average SCV 50 nm average [2]		
Cook and Burnstock (1976a)	Guinea-pig	Small and large intestine	Myenteric	SCV 40–60 nm LGV 80–100 nm	Three types with different distributions, LGV of different maximum diameter SCV	SGV 40–60 nm SCV 40–60 nm LGV 80–100 nm		Two types with different distributions, FV of different width, maximum diameter	Three other types on the basis of non-vesicular components

Reference	Species	Organ	Region	Axosomatic synapses	Axosomatic synapses	Axosomatic axodendritic synapses [3]		
Oki and Daniel (1977)	Dog	Stomach	Myenteric Submucous	SCV 45–70 nm LGV 70–120 nm [1]	LGV 70–140 nm SCV	SGV 40–60 nm SCV LGV	No axosomatic synapses	
Hoyes and Barber (1980)	Guinea-pig	Stomach	Myenteric	SCV 48 nm average LGV 81 nm average; Axodendritic axosomatic synapses; Some but not all small round vesicle-containing profiles [1]	LGV 96 nm average SCV 49 nm average		FV, also contains SCV LGV; No synapses; Since no FV present after 5-OHDA, probably [1]	
Llewellyn-Smith et al. (1981)	Guinea-pig	Small intestine	Myenteric	SCV 30–60 nm LGV 90–150 nm	SCV 30–60 nm LGV 90–150 nm	RV, also contain SCV, LGV; Axosomatic synapses	FV 30 × 80 nm average SCV 50 × 70 nm average Few LGV [1,2,4,5,6]	
			Submucous	Some but not all [1,4,5]	SCV 30–60 nm LGV 90–150 nm	RV, also contain SCV, LGV; Axosomatic synapses	Few with FV, SCV, LGV	
Wilson et al. (1981b)	Guinea-pig	Small intestine	Submucous		SCV 55 nm average LGV 95 nm average	RV 55 nm average SCV LGV 55–155 nm	FV 15–30 nm × up to 100 nm SCV LGV	One other type on the basis of non-vesicular components

Reference	Species	Region of GIT	Ganglia	Major vesicular components of profiles (Numbers in square brackets refer to footnotes)					Other profiles
				SCV + LGV		RV-type	SGV	Many FV	
				Mainly SCV	Many LGV		Others		
Gordon-Weeks (1981) also Gordon-Weeks and Hobbs (1979)	Guinea-pig	Large intestine	Myenteric Submucous	Axosomatic axodendritic synapses	Axosomatic axodendritic synapses	Axosomatic ax-odendritic synapses	(A) A few LGV 96 nm average SCV 50 nm average SGV 50 nm average Axosomatic axodendritic synapses [1,2] (B) Many LGV 132 nm average SCV 54 nm average SGV 54 nm average Axosomatic axodendritic synapses [7]		

FV = flattened vesicles; LGV = large granular vesicles; MGV = medium-sized granular vesicles; RV = ring vesicles (see text); SCV = small clear vesicles; SGV = small granular vesicles.

[1] loads with 5-OHDA.
[2] degenerates after 6-OHDA.
[3] presumed to be RV profiles because they look identical to RV profiles, have a similar distribution and form the same types of synapses.
[4] chromaffin-reactive.
[5] labels with horseradish peroxidase-anti-DBH.
[6] absent after extrinsic denervation.
[7] may be RV profiles.

bodies and fibres of the different nerve types are more or less randomly distributed throughout the ganglia. (2) Many neuroneuronal interactions may occur in the neuropil far from the cell soma. (3) Fewer types of enteric nerves can be identified ultrastructurally than histochemically. (4) Sites of interactions between nerves may not necessarily be marked by recognizable synapses. Some of these problems can be overcome by using electron-microscopic cytochemical and immunocytochemical techniques, which can specifically label various classes of nerves in the enteric plexuses. By studying the distributions and synaptic connections of nerves identified by these methods, insight can be gained into how they influence the functions of the gastrointestinal tract.

Noradrenergic axons

In many ultrastructural studies (Gabella, 1971b, 1972; Cook and Burnstock, 1976a; Oki and Daniel, 1977) axon profiles in enteric ganglia have been called noradrenergic because they contained SGV and therefore resembled noradrenergic profiles in other peripheral organs. More recent work (Llewellyn-Smith *et al.*, 1981; Wilson *et al.*, 1981b) has shown that this assumption is not always justified. RV profiles, which have been observed in the submucous and myenteric ganglia of the guinea-pig gut, are non-noradrenergic and yet contain small round vesicles with electron-dense inclusions. The results of studies with false transmitters (5- and 6-hydroxydopamine, 5- and 6-OHDA) can also be questioned because non-noradrenergic fibres in the enteric ganglia have been shown to take up and retain aromatic amines (see above).

Llewellyn-Smith *et al.* (1981) used a number of approaches to reinvestigate the problem of the ultrastructural identification of noradrenergic axons in the enteric plexuses. They used 5-OHDA loading (Tranzer and Thoenen, 1967), the chromaffin reaction (Tranzer and Richards, 1976) and the ultrastructural localization of DBH using an *in vivo* labelling method with horseradish peroxidase-conjugated antibodies to DBH (Rush *et al.*, 1979) to identify noradrenergic axons in the myenteric and submucous ganglia of the guinea-pig small intestine. (All of these techniques produce electron-dense deposits in the vesicles of noradrenergic axons.) The identification of noradrenergic profiles was confirmed by showing that extrinsically denervated or 6-OHDA-treated segments of intestine, in which noradrenergic nerves had degenerated (Jacobowitz, 1965; Baumgarten *et al.*, 1970; Furness and Costa, 1971a, 1974; Robinson and Gershon, 1971), contained no cytochemically labelled profiles.

Noradrenergic axons in myenteric ganglia from non-denervated experimental tissue contained many flattened vesicles in addition to oval or irregularly shaped vesicles (Fig. 25). The flattened vesicles measured about 30 nm wide and about 80–100 nm long and usually made up at least 30% of the

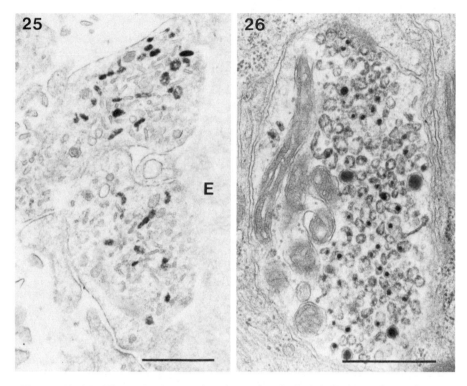

Figures 25, 26 Electron micrographs of cytochemically labelled noradrenergic axon profiles in enteric ganglia from guinea-pig small intestine. Calibrations: 0.5 μm.
Figure 25: Localization of dopamine β-hydroxylase in a noradrenergic axon profile of a myenteric ganglion. The guinea-pig had received horseradish peroxidase-conjugated antibodies to dopamine β-hydroxylase (HRP-anti-DBH) 24 hours before sacrifice. More than half the vesicles in the labelled profile are flattened (about 75 nm × 30 nm) and the rest are oval or irregularly shaped (about 60 nm × 40 nm). The profile lies directly beneath the basal lamina that surrounds the ganglion. Treatment with anti-DBH appears to increase the number of flattened vesicles in enteric ganglia. E, extraganglionic space.
Figure 26: Noradrenergic axon profile in a submucous ganglion from a segment of intestine that had been incubated with 5-hydroxydopamine (5-OHDA) contains small round vesicles (about 70 nm diameter), large round vesicles (about 110 nm diameter) and a few flattened vesicles (about 35 nm wide and very variable in length). Some vesicles contain electron-dense granules while others have electron-dense material irregularly distributed in their interiors.

total vesicle population. The oval or irregularly shaped vesicles were 40–50 nm wide and 60–70 nm long on average. Labelled noradrenergic profiles were concentrated around the edges of the myenteric ganglia with many lying directly beneath the basal lamina. Some profiles occurred near nerve cell bodies and a few in the internodal strands. Noradrenergic profiles did not form synapses on either myenteric nerve cell bodies or processes. Cytochemically labelled profiles were absent or markedly reduced in number in segments of extrinsically denervated or 6-OHDA-treated gut. Having made these observations, the authors found that it was now possible to recognize the noradrenergic profiles in conventionally fixed myenteric ganglia of guinea-pig small intestine; they contained similar types and proportions of vesicles, although without dense deposits, and had the same distribution as labelled profiles in experimental tissue. Like the cytochemically labelled profiles, these profiles also disappeared after extrinsic denervation.

The distribution of noradrenergic profiles found by Llewellyn-Smith *et al.* (1981) in the myenteric ganglia is consistent with the observations of Gabella (1979) and Manber and Gershon (1979) who showed that noradrenergic axons identified at the light-microscope level after labelling with [³H]noradrenaline or at the electron-microscope level after $KMnO_4$ fixation occurred mainly near the surfaces of the ganglia. The observed absence of synapses on myenteric nerve cell bodies is consistent with electrophysiological data indicating that noradrenergic axons have no direct actions on nerve cell bodies in the myenteric ganglia of the guinea-pig small intestine but that these axons act presynaptically (Hirst and McKirdy, 1974 see chapter by Wood).

In the submucous plexus cytochemically labelled noradrenergic axon profiles contained many small round vesicles about 50–70 nm in diameter, some large round vesicles about 90–110 nm in diameter and a few (about 9%) flattened vesicles (Fig. 26). The noradrenergic profiles were randomly distributed throughout submucous ganglia, confirming light-microscopic results on the uptake of [³H]noradrenaline in the submucous plexus (Gabella, 1979). On rare occasions labelled axons formed synapses on nerve fibres in submucous ganglia but never on nerve cell bodies. In extrinsically denervated submucous ganglia there were no noradrenergic axon profiles and their number was dramatically decreased in 6-OHDA-treated ganglia. However, in these denervated ganglia some unreactive non-noradrenergic profiles contained similar types and proportions of vesicles as the noradrenergic profiles seen in non-denervated experimental tissue. Thus, no morphological criteria for detecting submucous noradrenergic axons in conventionally processed tissue could be defined.

These recent results and those of other studies suggest that the ultrastructure of noradrenergic axons in the gastrointestinal tract can vary among plexuses, among regions of the gut and among species. Hydroxylated dopamines can probably be relied upon to label only noradrenergic nerves in the gut since no detectable loading with these drugs occurred in enteric ganglia from extrinsically denervated guinea-pig small intestine (Llewellyn-Smith *et al.*, 1981). Nevertheless, this point should be confirmed in future studies of other areas of the intestine. Thus, the profiles identified as noradrenergic with loading techniques by Baumgarten *et al.* (1970), Wong *et al.* (1974),

Hoyes and Barber (1980) and Gordon-Weeks (1981), were probably truly noradrenergic. In the guinea-pig proximal colon (Baumgarten *et al.*, 1970) profiles that had taken up 5-OHDA contained a variety of vesicle types, including flattened vesicles, and did not form synapses. In submucous ganglia of the rat duodenum (Wong *et al.*, 1974) loaded profiles contained SGV (50 nm) and did not form synapses. The presumed noradrenergic profiles of guinea-pig gastric myenteric ganglia contained SGV after 5-OHDA, although SGV profiles were not observed in tissue that was not loaded, and profiles with clear flattened vesicles disappeared after loading (Hoyes and Barber, 1980). Gordon-Weeks (1981) described profiles in myenteric ganglia of guinea-pig large intestine that contained SGV, were loaded with 5-OHDA, disappeared after extrinsic denervation and formed axosomatic and axodendritic synapses. Noradrenergic axons identified by the chromaffin reaction in rat anococcygeus muscle had flattened vesicles (Gibbins and Haller, 1979) as did the noradrenergic axons identified by Llewellyn-Smith *et al.* (1981) in the myenteric ganglia of guinea-pig small intestine. Thus, flattened vesicles may characterize noradrenergic axons in some areas of the gastrointestinal tract (Baumgarten *et al.*, 1970; Gibbins and Haller, 1979; Llewellyn-Smith *et al.*, 1981) but not in other areas. Furthermore, the shapes of the vesicles may change with experimental conditions (Hoyes and Barber, 1980; Llewellyn-Smith *et al.*, 1981). Moreover, although noradrenergic axons appear to form synapses rarely in some regions, for example the guinea-pig small intestine, noradrenergic synapses are relatively common in other regions, such as the guinea-pig distal colon (Gordon-Weeks, 1981).

Non-noradrenergic, SGV-containing profiles have now been described in a number of studies (Gordon-Weeks, 1981; Llewellyn-Smith *et al.*, 1981; Wilson *et al.*, 1981b). Comparison of these profiles with micrographs in Gabella (1971b, 1972) and Cook and Burnstock (1976a) suggests that the axons they tentatively identified as noradrenergic were in fact non-noradrenergic, SGV-containing RV profiles.

Axons that take up indolamines

Uptake of 5-[³H]HT and the degeneration caused by 5,6- and 5,7-dihydroxytryptamine have been used at the electron-microscope level to detect intrinsic non-noradrenergic axons that take up indolamines in myenteric ganglia (Rothman *et al.*, 1976; Dreyfus *et al.*, 1977b; Jonakait *et al.*, 1979; Gershon *et al.*, 1980). Both approaches show that intrinsic varicosities that take up indolamines contain a mixed population of small lucent vesicles about 70 nm in diameter and large dense-cored vesicles about 120 nm in diameter as do some other varicosities unaffected by the two treatments. The indolamine-containing axons have not been observed to form synapses. Although the degeneration studies suggest that these axons are not uniformly spread throughout myenteric ganglia, their distribution at the ultrastructural level has not been investigated in detail.

Peptide-containing axons

The only published study to date on the ultrastructural localization of peptide-containing axons in the enteric plexuses is that of Larsson (1977). Antibodies to VIP were found to bind to nerve terminals which contained large round vesicles about 120 nm in diameter in cat colonic mucosa and submucosa.

CONCLUDING REMARKS

Knowledge about the structure and organization of the enteric ganglia grew slowly from the time of the original discovery of the ganglionated plexuses in the wall of the alimentary canal (Remak, 1852; Meissner, 1857; Billroth, 1858; Auerbach, 1864) until about 20 years ago. Then ultrastructural studies began to provide insight into the morphological organization of the ganglia. However, dramatic advances in understanding have come since 1975 with the application of immunohistochemical techniques to the study of the enteric ganglia. In these few years evidence has been obtained for the presence in enteric nerves of up to eleven different peptides, most of which seem to be in separate populations of intrinsic neurons. Other histochemical techniques have revealed two types of enteric neurons that appear to contain aromatic amines. Only since 1979 have techniques become available for tracing the intrinsic pathways of these histochemically identifiable nerve types. Detailed studies of this kind have so far been confined to restricted areas of the gut in small laboratory animals. More broadly based studies are needed before general conclusions can be reached about the projections and possible roles of specific nerve types in mammals. Nevertheless, some general principles about the organization and structure of the enteric ganglia are emerging:

— The enteric ganglia contain a wide variety of nerve types. Histochemical and other studies indicate that 10, 15 or even more different kinds of nerves may exist in the enteric ganglia.
— Specific neuron types seem to be arranged in an ordered fashion in the enteric plexuses. Each type projects in defined directions for defined distances in particular layers of the gut wall.
— Many neuroneuronal interactions in the enteric ganglia probably occur in the neuropil distant from the nerve cell somata, making the physiological study of these interactions and the ultrastructural analysis of their morphological basis particularly difficult.
— There may be quite subtle regulation of reflex activity in the enteric

ganglia. Some of the enteric nerves may not be involved in direct reflex pathways but in their modulation by, for example, changing the thresholds for the activation of reflexes, delaying or hastening their effects or regulating their sequential activation.

One of the current challenges in the study of the enteric ganglia is to identify the different histochemically defined nerve cell bodies and nerve fibres at the ultrastructural level so that the synaptic relationships of nerves containing known substances can be investigated. By correlating knowledge about the ultrastructural connections of chemically defined neurons, their projections and their physiological and pharmacological properties, it may be possible to deduce the roles of the many nerve types in the enteric nervous system.

This chapter is written at a time when much new and surprising information is being gained about the nerves in the enteric ganglia. When correlated with existing knowledge, these new data may well change our concepts about the organization and roles of the nerves that make up the enteric nervous system.

ACKNOWLEDGEMENTS

Work in this laboratory was supported by the Australian Research Grants Committee, the National Health and Medical Research Council of Australia and the Flinders Medical Research Foundation. We should like to thank Pat Vilimas, Venetta Esson and Peter Hekmeijer for their technical and editorial assistance. (Manuscript completed May 1981.)

REFERENCES

Auerbach, L. (1864). Fernere vorläufige Mittheilung über den Nervenapparat des Darmes. *Arch. Pathol. Anat. Physiol. klin. Med.*, **30**, 457–460.

Baumgarten, H. G., Holstein, A.-F., and Owman, Ch. (1970). Auerbach's plexus of mammals and man: electron microscopic identification of three different types of neuronal processes in myenteric ganglia of the large intestine from Rhesus monkeys, guinea-pigs and man. *Z. Zellforsch. Mikrosk. Anat.*, **106**, 376–397.

Bayliss, W. M., and Starling, E. H. (1900). The movements and innervation of the large intestine. *J. Physiol. (London)*, **26**, 107–118.

Billroth, T. (1858). Einige Beobachtungen über das ausgedehnte Vorkommen von Nervenanastomosen im Tractus intestinalis. *Arch. Anat. Physiol. Leipzig*, 148–158.

Chey, W. Y., and Lee, K. Y. (1980). Motilin. *Clinics Gastroenterol.*, **9**, 645–656.

Cook, R. D., and Burnstock, G. (1976a). The ultrastructure of Auerbach's plexus in the guinea-pig. I. Neuronal elements. *J. Neurocytol.*, **5**, 171–194.

Cook, R. D., and Burnstock, G. (1976b). The ultrastructure of Auerbach's plexus in the guinea-pig. II. Non-neuronal elements. *J. Neurocytol.*, **5**, 195–206.

Costa, M., and Furness, J. B. (1982). Nervous control of intestinal motility. In *Handbook of Experimental Pharmacology*, **59**, 279–282.

Costa, M., Furness, J. B., and Gabella, G. (1971). Catecholamine containing nerve cells in the mammalian myenteric plexus. *Histochemie*, **25**, 103–106.

Costa, M., Furness, J. B., and McLean, J. R. (1976). The presence of aromatic *l*-amino acid decarboxylase in certain intestinal nerve cells. *Histochemistry*, **48**, 129–143.

Costa, M., Furness, J. B., Buffa, R., and Said, S. I. (1980a). Distribution of enteric nerve cell bodies and axons showing immunoreactivity for vasoactive intestinal polypeptide (VIP) in the guinea-pig intestine. *Neuroscience*, **5**, 587–596.

Costa, M., Furness, J. B., Llewellyn-Smith, I. J., Davies, B., and Oliver, J. (1980b). An immunohistochemical study of the projections of somatostatin containing neurons in the guinea-pig intestine. *Neuroscience*, **5**, 841–852.

Costa, M., Furness, J. B., Cuello, A. C., Verhofstad, A. A. J., Steinbusch, H. W. M., and Elde, R. P. (1982). Neurons with 5-hydroxytryptamine-like immunoreactivity in the enteric nervous system: their visualization and reactions to drug treatment. *Neuroscience*, **7**, 351–363

Costa, M., Furness, J. B., Llewellyn-Smith, I. J., and Cuello, A. C. (1981b). Projections of substance P neurons within the guinea-pig small intestine. *Neuroscience*, **6**, 411–424.

Dockray, G. J., Vaillant, C., and Walsh, J. H. (1979). The neuronal origin of bombesin-like immunoreactivity in the rat gastrointestinal tract. *Neuroscience*, **4**, 1561–1568.

Dockray, G. J. Vaillant, C., and Hutchison, J. B. (1981). Immunochemical characterization of peptides in endocrine cells and nerves with particular reference to gastrin and cholecystokinin. In *Cellular Basis of Chemical Messengers in the Digestive System* (Eds. M. I. Grossman, M. A. B. Brazier and J. Lechago) pp 215–230, Academic Press, New York.

Dogiel, A. S. (1895). Zur Frage über die Ganglien der Därmgeflechte bei den Säugetieren. *Anat. Anz.*, **10**, 517–528.

Dogiel, A. S. (1896). Zwei Arten sympathischer Nervenzellen. *Anat. Anz.*, **11**, 679–687.

Dogiel, A. S. (1899). Ueber den Bau der Ganglien in den Geflechten des Darmes und der Gallenblase des Menschen un der Säugethiere. *Arch. Anat. Physiol. Anat. Abt.*, 130–158.

Dreyfus, C. F., Bornstein, M. B., and Gershon, M. D. (1977a). Synthesis of serotonin by neurons of the myenteric plexus *in situ* and in organotypic tissue culture. *Brain Res.*, **128**, 125–139.

Dreyfus, C. F., Sherman, D. L., and Gershon, M. D. (1977b). Uptake of serotonin by intrinsic neurons of the myenteric plexus grown in organotypic tissue culture. *Brain Res.*, **128**, 109–123.

Eder, M. (1957). Der Histochemische nachweis des Fermentes Monoamine Oxydase. *Beitr. Pathol. Anat.*, **117**, 389–393.

Fehér, E., and Csânyi, K. (1974). Ultra-architectonics of the neural plexus in chronically isolated small intestine. *Acta Anat.*, **90**, 617–628.

Fehér, E., Csânyi, K., and Vajda, J. (1974). Comparative electron microscopic studies on the preterminal and terminal fibres of the nerve plexuses of the small intestine, employing different fixation methods. *Acta Morphol. Acad. Sci. Hung.*, **22**, 147–159.

Furness, J. B., and Costa, M. (1971a). Morphology and distribution of intrinsic adrenergic neurones in the proximal colon of the guinea-pig. *Z. Zellforsch. Mikrosk. Anat.*, **120**, 346–363.

Furness, J. B., and Costa, M. (1971b). Monoamine oxidase histochemistry of enteric neurones in the guinea-pig. *Histochemie*, **28**, 324–336.

Furness, J. B., and Costa, M. (1974). The adrenergic innervation of the gastrointestinal tract. *Ergebn. Physiol. Biol. Chem. Exp. Pharmakol.*, **69**, 1–51.

Furness, J. B., and Costa, M. (1978). Distribution of intrinsic nerve cell bodies and axons which take up aromatic amines and their precursors in the small intestine of the guinea-pig. *Cell Tissue Res.*, **188**, 527–543.

Furness, J. B., and Costa, M. (1980). Types of nerves in the enteric nervous system. *Neuroscience*, **5**, 1–20.

Furness, J. B., and Costa, M. (1982). Neurons with 5-hydroxytryptamine-like immunoreactivity in the enteric nervous system: their projections in the guinea-pig small intestine. *Neuroscience*, **7**, 341–349.

Furness, J. B., and Costa, M. (1982). Identification of gastrointestinal neurotransmitters. In *Handbook of Experimental Pharmacology* **59**, 383–460.

Furness, J. B., Costa, M., and Freeman, C. G. (1979). Absence of tyrosine hydroxylase activity and dopamine β-hydroxylase immunoreactivity in intrinsic nerves of the guinea-pig ileum. *Neuroscience*, **4**, 305–311.

Furness, J. B., Costa, M., Franco, R., and Llewellyn-Smith, I. J. (1980). Neuronal peptides in the intestine: distribution and possible functions. *Adv. Biochem. Psychopharmacol.*, **22**, 601–617.

Furness, J. B., Costa, M., Llewellyn-Smith, I. J., Franco, R., and Wilson, A. J. (1981a). Polarity and projections of peptide-containing neurons in the guinea-pig small intestine. In *Cellular Basis of Chemical Messengers in the Digestive System* (Eds. M. I. Grossman, M. A. B. Brazier and J. Lechago), Academic Press, New York.

Furness, J. B., Costa, M., and Walsh, J. (1981b). Evidence for and significance of the projection of VIP neurons from the myenteric plexus to the taenia coli in the guinea-pig. *Gastroenterology*, **80**, 1557–1561.

Fuxe, K., Hökfelt, T., Said, S. I., and Mutt, V. (1977). Vasoactive intestinal polypeptide and the nervous system: immunohistochemical evidence for localization in central and peripheral neurons, particularly intra-cortical neurons of the cerebral cortex. *Neurosci. Lett*, **5**, 241–246.

Gabella, G. (1971a). Neuron size and number in the myenteric plexus of the newborn and adult rat. *J. Anat.*, **109**, 81–95.

Gabella, G. (1971b). Synapses of adrenergic fibres. *Experientia*, **27**, 280–281.

Gabella, G. (1971c). Glial cells in the myenteric plexus, *Z. Naturforsch.*, **26b**, 244–245.

Gabella, G. (1972). Fine structure of the myenteric plexus in the guinea-pig ileum. *J. Anat.*, **111**, 69–97.

Gabella, G. (1976). *Structure of the Autonomic Nervous System*, Chapman and Hall, London.

Gabella, G. (1979). Innervation of the gastrointestinal tract. *Int. Rev. Cytol.*, **59**, 129–193.

Gabella, G. (1981). Ultrastructure of the nerve plexuses of the mammalian intestine: the enteric glial cells. *Neuroscience*, **6**, 425–436.

Gershon, M. D., Drakontides, A. B., and Ross, L. L. (1965). Serotonin: synthesis and release from the myenteric plexus of the mouse intestine. *Science*, **149**, 197–199.

Gershon, M. D., Dreyfus, C. F., Pickel, V. M., Joh, T. H., and Reis, D. J. (1977). Serotonergic neurons in the peripheral nervous system: identification in gut by immunohistochemical localization of tryptophan hydroxylase. *Proc. Natl. Acad. Sci. U.S.A.*, **74**, 3086–3089.

Gershon, M. D., Sherman, D. L., and Dreyfus, C. F. (1980). Effects of indolic neurotoxins on enteric serotonergic neurons. *J. Comp. Neurol.*, **190**, 581–596.

Gibbins, I. L., and Haller, C. J. (1979). Ultrastructural identification of non-adrenergic, non-cholinergic nerves in the rat anococcygeus muscle. *Cell Tissue Res.*, **200**, 257–271.

Glenner, G. C., Burtner, H. J., and Brown, G. W. (1957). The histochemical demonstration of monoamine oxidase activity by tetrazolium salts. *J. Histochem. Cytochem.*, **5**, 591–600.

Goniaew, K. (1875). Die Nerven des Nahrungsschlauches. Eine histologische Studie. *Arch. Mikrosk. Anat.*, **11**, 479–496.

Gordon-Weeks, P. R. (1981). Properties of nerve endings with small granular vesicles in the large bowel of the guinea-pig. *Neuroscience*, **6**, 1793–1811.

Gordon-Weeks, P. R., and Hobbs, M. J. (1979). A non-adrenergic nerve ending containing small granular vesicles in the guinea-pig gut. *Neurosci. Lett*, **12**, 81–96.

Grillo, M. A., and Palay, S. L. (1962). Granule-containing vesicles in the autonomic nervous system. In *Vth International Congress on Electron Microscopy* (Ed. S. S. Breese), Vol. 2, pp. U-1, Academic Press, New York.

Gunn, M. (1968). Histological and histochemical observations of the myenteric and submucous plexuses of mammals. *J. Anat.*, **102**, 223–239.

Gunn, M. (1971). Cholinergic mechanisms in the gastrointestinal tract. *J. Neuro-Visc. Relat.*, **32**, 224–240.

Hager, H. A., and Tafuri, W. L. (1959). Elektronenoptische Untersuchungen über die Feinstruktor des Plexus myentericus (Auerbach) in Colon des Meerschweinchens (*Cavia cobaya*). *Arch. Psychiatr. Nervenkr.*, **199**, 437–471.

Henle, J. (1871). *Handbuch der systematischen Anatomie des Menschen*, Vol. 3, Part 2, pp. 585–589, Friedrich Vieweg und Sohn, Braunschweig.

Hill, C. J. (1927). A contribution to our knowledge of the enteric plexuses. *Physiol. Trans. R. Soc.*, **215**, 355–387.

Hirst, G. D. S., and McKirdy, H. C. (1974). Presynaptic inhibition at mammalian peripheral synapse? *Nature*, **250**, 430–431.

Hirst, G. D. S., and McKirdy, H. C. (1975). Synaptic potentials recorded from neurones of the submucous plexus of guinea-pig small intestine. *J. Physiol. (London)*, **249**, 369–385.

Hirst, G. D. S., Holman, M. E., and McKirdy, H. C. (1975). Two descending nerve pathways activated by distension of guinea-pig small intestine. *J. Physiol. (London)*, **244**, 113–127.

Honjin, R., and Takahashi, A. (1966). Electron microscopy of synaptic nerve endings in the walls of digestive tract. *Symp. Cell Chem.*, **16**, 59–74.

Honjin, R., Takahashi, A., Shimasaki, S., and Maruyama, H. (1965). Two types of synaptic nerve processes in the ganglia of Auerbach's plexus of mice, as revealed by electron microscopy. *J. Electron Microsc.*, **14**, 43–49.

Howe, P. R. C., Provis, J. C., Furness, J. B., Costa, M., and Chalmers, J. P. (1981). Residual catecholamines in extrinsically denervated guinea-pig ileum. *Clin. Exp. Pharm. Physiol.*, **8**, 327–333.

Hoyes, A. D., and Barber, P. (1980). Axonal terminal ultrastructure in the myenteric ganglia of the guinea-pig stomach. *Cell Tissue Res.*, **209**, 329–343.

Jacobowitz, D. (1965). Histochemical studies of the autonomic innervation of the gut. *J. Pharmacol. Exp. Ther.*, **149**, 358–364.

Jacobs, J. M. (1977). Penetration of systemically injected horseradish peroxidase into ganglia and nerves of the autonomic nervous system. *J. Neurocytol.*, **6**, 607–618.

Jessen, K. R., and Mirsky, R. (1980). Glial cells in the enteric nervous system contain glial fibrillary acidic protein. *Nature*, **286**, 736–737.

Jessen, K. R., Mirsky, R., Dennison, M. E., and Burnstock, G. (1979). GABA may be a neurotransmitter in the vertebrate peripheral nervous system. *Nature*, **281**, 71–74.

Jessen, K. R., Polak, J. M., Van Noorden, S., Bloom, S. R., and Burnstock, G. (1980a). Peptide-containing neurones connect the two ganglionated plexuses of the enteric nervous system. *Nature*, **283**, 391–393.

Jessen, K. R., Saffrey, M. J., Van Noorden, S., Bloom, S. R., Polak, J. M., and Burnstock, G. (1980b). Immunohistochemical studies of the enteric nervous system in tissue culture and *in situ*: localization of vasoactive intestinal polypeptide (VIP), substance P and enkephalin immunoreactive nerves in the guinea-pig gut. *Neuroscience*, **5**, 1717–1735.

Jonakait, G. M., Tamir, H., Gintzler, A. R., and Gershon, M. D. (1979). Release of (^{3}H) serotonin and its binding protein from enteric neurons. *Brain Res.*, **174**, 55–69.

Junqueira, L. C. U., Tafuri, W. L., and Tafuri, C. P. (1958). Quantitative and cytochemical studies on the intestinal plexuses of the guinea-pig. *Exp. Cell Res. Suppl.*, **5**, 568–572.

Koelle, G. B., and Valk, A. T. (1954). Physiological implications of the histochemical localization of monoamine oxidase. *J. Physiol. (London)*, **126**, 434–447.

Krnjević, K. (1969). Central cholinergic pathways. *Fed. Proc.*, **28**, 113–120.

Kuntz, A. (1918). The distribution of sympathetic neurones in the myenteric and submucous plexus in the small intestine of the cat. *Anat. Rec.*, **14**, 42.

Kyösola, K., Veijola, L., and Rechardt, L. (1975). Cholinergic innervation of the gastric wall of the cat. *Histochemie*, **44**, 23–30.

Langley, J. N. (1900). The sympathetic and other related systems of nerves. In *Textbook of Physiology* (Ed. E. A. Schäfer), Vol. 2, pp. 616–696, Pentland, Edinburgh.

Langley, J. N. (1921). *The Autonomic Nervous System*, W. Heffner and Sons, Cambridge.

Langley, J. N., and Magnus, R. (1905–1906). Some observations of the movements of the intestine before and after degenerative section of the mesenteric nerves. *J. Physiol. (London)*, **33**, 34–51.

Larsson, L.-I. (1977). Ultrastructural localization of a new neuronal peptide (VIP). *Histochemistry*, **54**, 173–176.

Larsson, L.-I., and Rehfeld, J. F. (1979). Localization and molecular heterogeneity of cholecystokinin in the central and peripheral nervous system. *Brain Res.*, **165**, 201–218.

Lazarus, L. H., Linnoila, R. I., Hernandez, O., and Di Augustine, R. P. (1980). A neuropeptide in mammalian tissues with physalaemin-like immunoreactivity. *Nature*, **287**, 555–558.

Leaming, D. B., and Cauna, N. (1961). A qualitative and quantitative study of the myenteric plexus of the small intestine of the cat. *J. Anat.*, **95**, 160–169.

Llewellyn-Smith, I. J., Wilson, A. J., Furness, J. B., Costa, M., and Rush, R. A. (1981). Ultrastructural identification of noradrenergic axons and their distribution within the enteric plexuses of the guinea-pig small intestine. *J. Neurocytol.*, **10**, 331–352.

Lorén, I., Alumets, J., Håkanson, R., and Sundler, F. (1979). Immunoreactive pancreatic polypeptide (PP) occurs in the central and peripheral nervous system: preliminary immunocytochemical observations. *Histochemistry*, **78**, 179–186.

Manber, L., and Gershon, M. D. (1979). A reciprocal adrenergic-cholinergic axoaxonic synapse in the mammalian gut. *Am. J. Physiol.*, **236**, E738–E745.

McKirdy, H. C., Jones, J. V., and Ballard, K. J. (1972). Cholinesterase histochemistry of the rabbit distal colon. *Histochemie*, **29**, 287–295.

Meissner, G. (1857). Ueber die Nerven der Darmwand. *Z. Rat. Med.*, **8**, 364–366.

Niemi, M., Kouvalainen, K., and Hjelt, L. (1961). Cholinesterase and monoamine oxidase in congenital megacolon. *J. Pathol. Bacteriol.*, **82**, 363–366.

Norberg, K. A. (1964). Adrenergic innervation of the intestinal wall studied by fluorescence microscopy. *Int. J. Neuropharmacol.*, **3**, 379–382.

Ohkubo, K. (1936a). Studies on the intrinsic nervous system of the digestive tract. I. The submucous plexus of guinea-pig. *Jpn. J. Med. Sci.*, **6**, 1–20.

Ohkubo, K. (1936b). Studien über das intramurale Nervensystem des Verduungskanals. II. Die plexus myentericus und Plexus subserosus des Meerschweinchens. *Jpn. J. Med. Sci.*, **6**, 21–37.

Oki, M., and Daniel, E. E. (1977). Effects of vagotomy on the ultrastructure of the nerves of dog stomach. *Gastroenterology*, **73**, 1029–1040.

Ono, M. (1967). Electron microscopic observations on the ganglia of Auerbach's plexus and autonomic nerve endings in muscularis externa of the mouse small intestine. *Sapporo Med. J.*, **32**, 56–74.

Remak, R. (1852). Über mikroskopische Ganglien an den Ästen des N. vagus in der Wand des Magens bei Wirbeltieren. *Vers. Ges. Deut. Naturf. Aerzte.*, p. 183.

Richardson, K. C. (1958). Electronmicroscopic observations on Auerbach's plexus in the rabbit, with special reference to the problem of smooth muscle innervation. *Am. J. Anat.*, **103**, 99–135.

Rintoul, J. R. (1960). The comparative morphology of the enteric nerve plexuses. *Ph.D. Thesis*, University of St. Andrews.

Robinson, R. G., and Gershon, M. D. (1971). Synthesis and uptake of 5-hydroxytryptamine by the myenteric plexus of the guinea-pig ileum: a histochemical study. *J. Pharmacol. Exp. Ther.*, **178**, 311–324.

Rothman, T. P., Ross, L. L., and Gershon, M. D. (1976). Separately developing axonal uptake of 5-hydroxytryptamine and norepinephrine in the fetal ileum of the rabbit. *Brain Res.*, **115**, 437–456.

Rush, R. A., Millar, T. J., Chubb, I. W., and Geffen, L. B. (1979). Use of dopamine β-hydroxylase in the study of vesicle dynamics. In *Catecholamines: Basic and Clinical Frontiers* (Eds. E. Usdin, I. J. Kopin and J. Barchas), pp. 331–333, Pergamon Press, New York.

Schardt, M., and van der Zypen, E. (1974). Enzymhistochemische und quantitative Untersuchungen über regionalen Unterchiede des intramuralen Nervensystems im Magen-darm-kanal der weissen Laboratoriomsmaus. *Acta Anat.*, **90**, 403–430.

Schofield, G. C. (1968). The enteric plexuses of mammals. *Int. Rev. Gen. Exp. Zool.*, **3**, 53–116.

Schultzberg, M., Hökfelt, T., Nilsson, G., Terenius, L., Rehfeld, J. F., Brown, M., Elde, R., Goldstein, M., and Said, S. (1980). Distribution of peptide- and catecholamine-containing neurons in the gastrointestinal tract of rat and guinea-pig: immunohistochemical studies with antisera to substance P, vasoactive intestinal polypeptide, enkephalins, somatostatin, gastrin/cholecystokinin, neurotensin and dopamine β-hydroxylase. *Neuroscience*, **5**, 689–744.

Silver, A. (1974). *The Biology of Cholinesterases*, North-Holland, Amsterdam.

Sundler, F., Håkanson, R., and Leander, S. (1980). Peptidergic nervous systems in the gut. *Clinics Gastroenterol.*, **9**, 517–543.

Tafuri, W. L. (1964). Ultrastructure of the vesicular component in the intramural nervous system of the guinea-pigs intestines. *Z. Naturforsch.*, **19**, 622–625.

Taxi, J. (1958). Sur la structure du plexus d'Auerbach de la Souris, etudié au microscope électronique. *C. R. Acad. Sci.*, **246**, 1922–1925.

Taxi, J. (1959). Sur la structure des travées du plexus d'Auerbach: confrontation des données fournies par le microscope ordinaire et par le microscope électroniques. *Ann. Sci. Nat. Zool. Biol. Animal.*, *12 Ser.*, **1**, 571–593.

Taxi, J. (1965). Contribution à l'étude des connexions des neurones moteurs du système nerveux autonome. *Ann. Sci. Nat. Zool. Biol. Anim.*, *12 Ser.*, **7**, 413–674.

Tjälve, H. (1971). Catechol- and indolamines in some endocrine cell systems. An autoradiographical, histochemical and radioimmunological study. *Acta Physiol. Scand.*, **81** (Suppl. 360), 1–122.

Tranzer, J. P., and Richards, J. G. (1976). Ultrastructural cytochemistry of biogenic amines in nervous tissue: methodological improvements. *J. Histochem. Cytochem.*, **24**, 1178–1193.

Tranzer, J. P., and Thoenen, H. (1967). Electron-microscopic localization of 5-hydroxydopamine (3,4,5-trihydroxy-phenyl-ethylamine), a new 'false' sympathetic transmitter. *Experientia*, **23**, 743–745.

Van Driel, C., and Drukker, J. (1973). A contribution to the study of the architecture of the autonomic nervous system of the digestive tract of the rat. *J. Neural Transm.*, **34**, 301–320.

Wilson, A. J., Furness, J. B., and Costa, M. (1981a). The fine structure of the submucous plexus of the guinea-pig ileum. I. The ganglia, neurons, Schwann cells and neuropil. *J. Neurocytol.*, **10**, 759–784.

Wilson, A. J., Furness, J. B., and Costa, M. (1981b). The fine structure of the submucous plexus of the guinea-pig ileum. II. Description and analysis of vesiculated nerve processes. *J. Neurocytol.*, **10**, 785–804.

Wong, W. C., Helme, R. D., and Smith, G. C. (1974). Degeneration of noradrenergic nerve terminals in submucous ganglia of the rat duodenum following treatment with 6-hydroxydopamine. *Experientia*, **30**, 282–284.

Yamamoto, M. (1977). Electron microscopic studies on the innervation of the smooth muscle and the interstitial cell of Cajal in the small intestine of the mouse and bat. *Arch. Histol. Jpn*, **40**, 171–201.

Autonomic Ganglia
Edited by Lars-Gösta Elfvin
© 1983 John Wiley & Sons Ltd

The Organization and Fine Structure of Autonomic Ganglia of Amphibia

HIROSHI WATANABE

*Department of Anatomy, Yamagata University School of Medicine,
Yamagata, 990–23, Japan*

INTRODUCTION

There are several time-honoured articles on the morphology of the amphibian autonomic nervous system in which the anuran sympathetic ganglia and, to a lesser extent, parasympathetic ganglia have been elaborately discussed (Nicol, 1952; Burnstock, 1969; Pick, 1970; Taxi, 1976). In this chapter, therefore, a relatively restricted number of papers dealing with the fine structure and innervation of the principal cells of the anuran sympathetic ganglia will be reviewed.

The amphibian as well as mammalian sympathetic ganglia have been studied by a number of authors to elucidate the controversial function of small granule-containing (SGC) cells or, in other terms, small intensely fluorescent (SIF) cells or paraneurons which are located at the key stations in the autonomic nervous pathways. The present chapter will also describe some characteristic details of the fine structure of SGC cells.

ORGANIZATION OF THE AMPHIBIAN AUTONOMIC GANGLIA

Central connection of the autonomic ganglia

Cephalic outflows

The cephalic autonomic outflows in vertebrates including amphibians are usually associated with the III, VII, IX and X cranial nerves. Their preganglionic fibres may form synaptic connections with the ganglion cells in the attached autonomic (parasympathetic) ganglia. The ciliary ganglion is intercalated in the course of the III cranial nerve and is the only established autonomic ganglion in the head region of the anura. No autonomic ganglion corresponding to either the pterygopalatine, submandibular or otic ganglion in mammals has been noted in the anura. The most caudal cephalic autonomic fibres are contained in the X cranial nerve.

The vagal (X) preganglionic fibres make synaptic contact with principal cells in the parasympathetic ganglia located in or near the alimentary (Wong *et al.*, 1971; Wong, 1973)' and respiratory organs (Burnstock, 1969; Pick, 1970; Taxi, 1976). Solitary and clustered principal ganglion cells are also located in the amphibian cardiac wall apparently innervated by the preganglionic vagus fibres (Woods, 1970; McMahan and Kuffler, 1971, McMahan and Purves, 1976).

Spinal outflows

It is generally accepted that the anuran spinal autonomic outflows emerge from the spinal cord along the 2nd to 10th spinal nerves (Burnstock, 1969; Pick, 1970; Taxi, 1976). It has been suggested that the anuran preganglionic fibres may pass through the ventral and dorsal spinal roots (Pick, 1970). These anuran preganglionic fibres may form synapses with ganglion cells in the paravertebral sympathetic trunk, and also with the cells in the dorsal root ganglia (Langley and Orbeli, 1910; Bishop and O'Leary, 1938; as reviews Pick, 1970; Taxi, 1976). Pick (1970) has noted that the proportion of preganglionic fibres in the ventral root compared with those in the dorsal root is variable from segment to segment of the spinal cord. Postganglionic fibres arising from the sympathetic ganglia innervate the iris, blood vessels, glands and viscera as far as the lower colon and cloaca.

It is a most conspicuous fact that the sacral autonomic fibres arising from the most caudal (9th and 10th) spinal segments do not traverse the sympathetic trunk but pass through a nerve plexus to form eventually the rectovesical nerves (Langley and Orbeli, 1910; see also Pick, 1970). Autonomic ganglion cells located in the wall of the urinary bladder are probably innervated by such sacral preganglionic fibres (Burnstock, 1969; Taxi, 1976). This has been advocated as the first appearance of the sacral parasympathetic system in vertebrates (Burnstock, 1969). For further anatomical details, readers are referred to previous reviews (Nicol, 1952; Burnstock, 1969; Pick, 1970; Taxi, 1976).

Paravertebral sympathetic trunk

The anuran paravertebral sympathetic trunks extend from the vagal sensory ganglion (ganglion jugulare) at the base of the skull to the 9th (or 10th) spinal nerve. A series of sympathetic ganglia are formed along these trunks. The cranial part of the sympathetic trunk, from the 1st through 3rd spinal segments inclusively, is covered ventrally by muscles. The caudal part, corresponding to the 4th through 10th spinal nerves, is placed in the retroperitoneum. The most cranial parts of the bilateral sympathetic trunks are related to the ductus arteriosi; the middle and caudal parts to the dorsal aorta (Pick, 1970).

The prevertebral coeliac ganglion or plexus is located along the arteria intestinalis communis, near its origin, and is formed by the reunion of three splanchnic nerves originating from the 4th to 6th sympathetic segments. The postganglionic splanchnic nerves arising from the coeliac plexus pass to various viscera along each regional arterial supply (Pick, 1970).

LIGHT MICROSCOPY OF THE AUTONOMIC GANGLIA

A typical ganglion is composed of principal ganglion cells, pre- and postganglionic nerve fibres, satellite cells and Schwann cells, and is enclosed by a capsule which consists of several layers of fibroblasts and dense collagen bundles (Fig. 1). Mast cells and SCG cells are also present in various

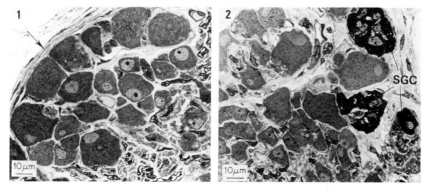

Figure 1   Light micrograph of toluidine blue-stained section of the frog, *Limnodynastes dumerili*, sympathetic ganglion. A dense connective tissue capsule ($\rightarrow$) encloses a group of principal ganglion cells. ×235

Figure 2   Clustered SGC cells (SGC) darkly stained compared with lighter principal ganglion cells in the frog sympathetic ganglion. ×235

amphibian autonomic ganglia (Fig. 2). The amphibian autonomic ganglia are as densely vascularized as those in mammals.

Principal ganglion cells

It is generally accepted that the principal ganglion cells in the anuran sympathetic ganglia are unipolar (Pick, 1970; Taxi, 1976). Similar unipolar ganglion cells have been noted in the parasympathetic ganglia in the heart of frogs (Woods, 1970; McMahan and Kuffler, 1971). The frog ciliary ganglion contains bipolar, tripolar and other multipolar cells (Stammer, 1965). In the cardiac parasympathetic ganglion of the mud puppy, 10 of 40 examined principal cells are bipolar, and the rest are unipolar (McMahan and Purves, 1976).

In the bullfrog, acetylcholinesterase-positive preganglionic fibres spiral around, arborize, and make synaptic contact with the axon hillock and initial portion of the axon of the sympathetic ganglion cells (Weitsen and Weight, 1977; Weight, this volume). In addition, a small number of synapses are formed on the rest of the somatic surface. One sympathetic ganglion cell seems to receive terminations of one, or less frequently two to three, preganglionic nerve fibres (Pick, 1963; Taxi, 1965). A similar mode of preganglionic innervation has been confirmed by some different staining techniques in the sympathetic (see Pick, 1970; Taxi, 1976) and the parasympathetic ganglion (McMahan and Kuffler, 1971) of the frog. The number of spiral turns of the preganglionic fibres before they arborize and terminate on the ganglionic cell surfaces is variable among different ganglion cells from two to 20 or more (Woods, 1970).

Based on axon conduction velocity and physiological characteristics of the neuronal membrane in the toad, sympathetic ganglion cells have been classified into B and C neurons (Nishi *et al.*, 1965). The B neuron is considered to receive preganglionic B fibres with a conduction velocity of about 5 m/sec from a single spinal root (monosegmental innervation); the C neuron receives preganglionic C fibres with a conduction velocity of 0.19 to 0.32 m/sec arising from two or three spinal roots (Nishi *et al.*, 1965).

In the toad sympathetic ganglia, large and small neurons with mean diameters of 35 μm and 18 μm, respectively, are classified (Nishi *et al.*, 1967). This has been confirmed in a serial-section study (Honma, 1970b). Similar values of diameter, 33 μm for the large and 19 μm for the small ganglion cells, have also been obtained in the frog (Watanabe and Burnstock, 1978). It seems reasonable that the large and small sympathetic ganglion cells correspond to the B and C neurons, respectively, in physiological classification (Nishi *et al.*, 1965, 1967; Honma, 1970a, b).

Recent immunohistochemical studies on the bullfrog sympathetic ganglia have suggested that peptidergic nerve endings containing luteinizing hormone releasing hormone (LHRH) immunoreactivity synapse mostly, if not only, with principal cells smaller than 30 μm in diameter (C cells) (Jan *et al.*, 1980).

Fluorescence microscopy and catecholamines

In the amphibian sympathetic ganglia, the intensity of specific fluorescence for catecholamines changes remarkably from cell to cell independently of the cell diameter. No non-fluorescent ganglion cells occur in the sympathetic ganglia. It has been generally accepted that the catecholamine contained in the amphibian sympathetic ganglion cells is adrenaline rather than noradrenaline. This has been confirmed in several anuran species (Angelakos *et al.*, 1965; Azuma *et al.*, 1965; Kojima *et al.*, 1978). Adrenaline is also contained in the postganglionic fibres and is released by sympathetic stimulation (Azuma *et al.*, 1965). Thus, adrenaline, rather than noradrenaline, is considered to be the adrenergic transmitter of the anuran sympathetic postganglionic nerves. On the other hand, it is of interest that noradrenaline is the only transmitter contained in the sympathetic ganglion cells and their processes in the newt (Angelakos *et al.*, 1965).

Parasympathetic ganglion cells that show specific fluorescence for catecholamines have never been found in the heart of the frog (Woods, 1970) or mud puppy (McMahan and Purves, 1976), the toad alimentary tract (Wong *et al.*, 1971; Wong, 1973), or the frog urinary bladder (Burnstock, 1969).

In several mammalian sympathetic ganglia, fluorescent nerve fibres with varicosities are present around or in close contact with ganglion cell bodies. They are considered to terminate upon these cells (Norberg and Sjöqvist, 1966; as reviews Jacobowitz, 1970; Matthews, 1974; Gabella, 1976a, b; Chiba, 1977). Similar preganglionic adrenergic fibres have been noted in the bullfrog sympathetic ganglia (Jacobowitz, 1970). This has been the only report on amphibians that suggests the innervation of sympathetic ganglion cells by adrenergic nerve fibres. All other previous works, however, have failed to find any fluorescent adrenergic nerve termination on the sympathetic ganglion cells in frogs, *Rana temporaria* (Norberg and McIsaac, 1967), *Limnodynastes dumerili* (Hill *et al.*, 1975), in toads, *Bufo vulgaris japonicus* (Honma, 1970a), or even in bullfrogs, *Rana catesbeiana* (Weight and Weitsen, 1977).

SGC cells

The SGC cells stain dark with toluidine blue, thereby facilitating easy identification (Fig. 2). They are mostly situated close to blood vessels, but sometimes they are closely apposed to the surface of sympathetic ganglion cells of variable size. Sometimes they appear separately in a wide connective tissue space. The SGC cells show positive chromaffin reaction in the bullfrog, *Rana catesbeiana* (Weight and Weitsen, 1977), but negative reaction in the frog, *Rana pipiens* (Pick, 1963, 1970).

The SIF cells, corresponding to the SGC cells as observed by electron microscopy, occur in variable numbers in the amphibian sympathetic ganglia (Jacobowitz, 1970; Honma, 1970a; Hill *et al.*, 1975; Weight and Weitsen, 1977; Kojima *et al.*, 1978). They are more numerous in the 5th, 6th and 7th than in the 9th and 10th paravertebral sympathetic ganglia in the frog (Hill *et al.*, 1975; as a review Taxi, 1976) and occur solitarily or more frequently in clusters (Fig. 2). Similar observations have been made in the toad and bullfrog (Piezzi and Rodriguez Echandia, 1968; Weight and Weitsen, 1977).

SIF cells have been noted also in autonomic ganglia of the urinary bladder wall in the toad, but not in the frog (Burnstock, 1969). Some SIF cells are present in the parasympathetic ganglia attached to nerve bundles in the subpleural tissue of the anuran lungs (see Burnstock, 1969). A large number of SIF cells have been observed in the parasympathetic ganglia located in the mud puppy heart (McMahan and Purves, 1976).

FINE STRUCTURE OF THE AUTONOMIC GANGLIA

Principal ganglion cells

The perikaryal cytoplasm of an anuran sympathetic ganglion cell contains well-developed rough- and smooth-surfaced endoplasmic reticulum, Golgi apparatus, and free ribosomes. Mitochondria, neurofilaments and neurotubules are also abundant. The nucleus is eccentrically placed in the periphery of the soma distant from the axon hillock. The nucleoplasm contains no peripheral dense aggregation of heterochromatin unlike the nuclei of satellite cells (Fig. 3), fibroblasts, mast cells or SGC cells. Occasionally, a large number of glycogen granules, 20 to 40 nm in diameter, are packed in the peripheral cytoplasm of the bullfrog sympathetic ganglion cell soma. A small number of granular vesicles, 80 to 120 nm in diameter, are usually observed in the perikaryon, particularly in close proximity to Golgi apparatuses (Fig. 3).

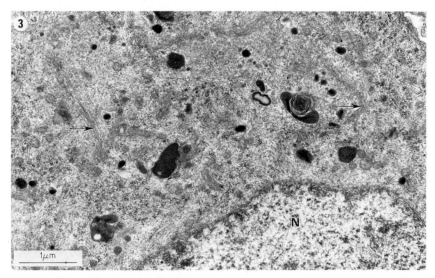

Figure 3 Note electron-dense granular vesicles, much smaller in size than dense bodies, in perikaryon of a bullfrog sympathetic ganglion cell. Arrows indicate Golgi apparatuses. N = nucleus of ganglion cell. ×7500

Most prominent in the perikaryal cytoplasm are polymorphic dense bodies with a distinct limiting membrane. Their number varies from cell to cell. They are probably lysosomal in nature (Taxi, 1965, 1976). Numbers of analogous structures, such as multivesicular bodies and lipofuscin granules, are concomitantly seen in the perikaryon (Fig. 3).

The ganglion cells are tightly and almost completely enclosed by one or several layers of attenuated processes of satellite cells (Fig. 4). The arrangement of the satellite cell sheath increases in complexity around the axon hillock and initial axoplasm (Fig. 4). This gives conspicuous features to the anuran sympathetic ganglia (Pick, 1963, 1970; Yamamoto, 1963; Uchizono, 1964; Taxi, 1976). The satellite cell cytoplasm is characterized by densely arranged microfilaments, 7.5 nm in diameter (Figs. 5–7).

Synapses

The spiral, terminal portion of the preganglionic nerve fibres is enveloped by satellite and Schwann cell sheaths surrounding also the ganglion cell bodies and axons (Fig. 4). These fibres are denuded of the Schwann cell sheath and

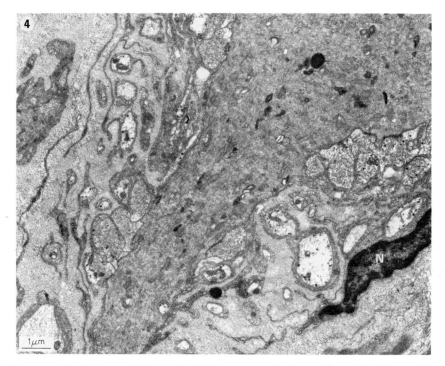

Figure 4 Typical axon hillock of a bullfrog sympathetic ganglion cell. Thin satellite cell processes cover elaborately each one of incoming preganglionic nerve fibres. Many synaptic sites can be recognized. N = nucleus of satellite cell. ×4050

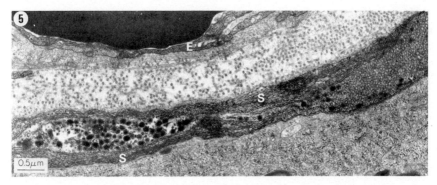

Figure 5 Two enlarged portions actually formed by one preganglionic nerve ending. The proximal portion is completely covered by a satellite sheath (S) and contains mostly large granular vesicles. The distal one is in direct contact with the principal ganglion cell and contains numerous small agranular and a few large granular vesicles. E = endothelium. ×8250

come into direct contact with the principal ganglion cells, where they form enlarged nerve endings (Fig. 5). As suggested by light microscopy, the preganglionic nerve endings are most densely distributed around the axon hillock (Fig. 4) (Weight and Weitsen, 1977; as reviews Pick, 1970; Taxi, 1976). In the toad sympathetic ganglia approximately 10% of the somatic surface is covered by such endings (Nishi *et al.*, 1967).

The nerve endings contain a great number of small agranular vesicles, 30 to 50 nm in diameter, together with a few large granular vesicles, 60 to 100 nm in diameter, mitochondria and glycogen granules. The ratio of the large granular to small agranular vesicles varies from one ending to another (Figs. 5–7). It has been found by serial thin-section studies that a single nerve ending contains remarkably different numbers of the large granular vesicles in different sections. Based on these findings of the vesicular components, it is concluded that the principal cells in the hitherto investigated amphibian sympathetic ganglia receive only one type of preganglionic nerve ending (Weitsen and Weight, 1977; Watanabe and Burnstock, 1976a, 1978).

Previous physiological studies on the frog sympathetic ganglia have revealed that acetylcholine is the synaptic transmitter released from the preganglionic nerve endings (Blackman *et al.*, 1963). This has been confirmed by a histochemical study on the localization of acetylcholinesterase (Weitsen and Weight, 1977). The nerve endings in the amphibian sympathetic ganglia seem, therefore, to be predominantly cholinergic in nature. Furthermore, the fine structure of the nerve endings cannot be altered by 5-hydroxydopamine or α-methylnorepinephrine administration (Weitsen and Weight, 1977). These findings provide additional evidence for the absence of adrenergic preganglionic fibres in the amphibian sympathetic ganglia.

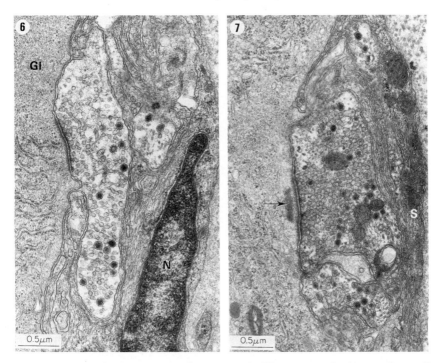

Figure 6 Preganglionic nerve ending, on a bullfrog sympathetic ganglion cell, containing numbers of small agranular vesicles and a few large granular vesicles. Pre- and postsynaptic membrane specializations and aggregation of synaptic vesicles are evident. Dense aggregation of glycogen granules (Gl) can be seen in the ganglion cell soma. The satellite cell is characterized by microfilaments. N = nucleus of satellite cell. ×11 250

Figure 7 Synapse provided with a postsynaptic bar (→) in the bullfrog sympathetic ganglion. The nerve ending contains many small agranular vesicles, a few large granular vesicles, and mitochondria. Vesicular aggregation as well as membranous density increase is seen. S = satellite sheath. ×11 250

Peptidergic nerve endings have been suggested to be present in the amphibian sympathetic ganglia (Jan *et al.*, 1980). Furthermore, Lascar *et al.* (1982) have demonstrated the subcellular distribution of an LHRH-like substance in the large granular vesicles in the nerve endings of the frog (*Rana esculenta*) sympathetic ganglia.

Postsynaptic specialization

One of the characteristic structures of the postsynaptic cytoplasm of the amphibian sympathetic ganglion cell is the postsynaptic bars or 'bandelettes soussynaptiques' (Taxi, 1967, 1976; Pick, 1970; Watanabe and Burnstock, 1978) and another is the subsurface cisterns or 'junctional subsurface organs'

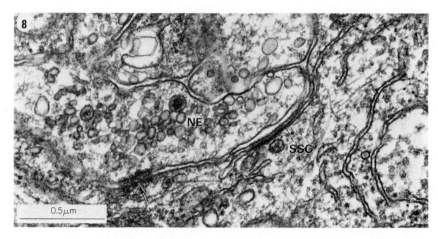

Figure 8 Postsynaptic subsurface cistern (SSC) in a frog sympathetic ganglion cell. It is continuous at both ends with lateral cisterns which are most probably a part of the rough-surfaced endoplasmic reticulum. The SSC never occurs immediately beneath the synaptic specializations. The arrow indicates a symmetrical membrane specialization. NE = preganglionic nerve ending. ×23 750

(Watanabe and Burnstock, 1976a, 1978). The postsynaptic bars (PSBs), first described by Taxi (1961) in the frog, have been found in a number of amphibian species (Taxi, 1976). The PSBs are always situated just subjacent to the postsynaptic membrane specialization (Fig. 7). In the frog, the PSBs are found in the ganglion cell somata and rarely in the axonic processes. They are usually discoid or ellipsoid in shape, 0.3 to 0.5 μm in length or in diameter, and 0.1 μm or less in thickness. The PSBs have neither limiting membrane nor special subunit structure, and consist of an aggregate of dense granular material (Fig. 7).

The PSBs occupy only a part of the total area of the specialized postsynaptic membrane, which is usually 0.4 to 0.7 μm in diameter (Watanabe and Burnstock, 1976a, 1978). The number of PSBs varies from one cell profile to another; 10 to 40% (Taxi, 1961, 1965) or 16% (Sotelo, 1968) of the specialized postsynaptic membranes are associated with the PSBs in the frog, *Rana esculenta*. Recent serial-section studies have revealed that a small ganglion cell (C cell) contains 10 to 22 PSBs, occupying 52 to 71% of the total number of postsynaptic membrane specializations (Watanabe and Burnstock, 1978). The PSBs have never been found in the large ganglion cells (B cells) in the frog. Similar findings have been obtained in *Xenopus* sympathetic ganglia. It should be noted that the PSBs are also present in a small number in the cardiac parasympathetic ganglion cells of the frog (McMahan and Kuffler, 1971).

Taxi (1979) has shown that the majority of the postsynaptic membrane specializations as well as of the PSBs disappear immediately after the section of the preganglionic fibres. These results suggest that the synaptic membrane specializations and PSBs are maintained only under the action of preganglionic nerve fibres (Taxi, 1978).

Flat and broad subsurface cisterns (SSCs) have been described in the toad (Fujimoto, 1967) and frog (Watanabe and Burnstock, 1976a) ganglion cells. In the frog the SSCs are observed most frequently in the large ganglion cells (B cells), up to 45 μm in diameter (Fig. 8) (Watanabe and Burnstock, 1978). A typical SSC is situated immediately beneath the plasma membrane of the ganglion cell, and is particularly well-developed around the axon hillock but occurs less frequently in the axon. Serial-section studies have shown that a large ganglion cell of the frog contains 8 to 16 ellipsoid SSCs, 0.4 to 0.9 μm in diameter, which mostly lie close to mitochondria and routh-surfaced endoplasmic reticulum. The SSCs are always situated opposite to the preganglionic nerve endings often with the interposition of thin satellite cell processes (Fig. 8). Less than 20% of the total 108 SSCs examined are localized subjacent to the truly postsynaptic membrane which is not covered by satellite cells (Watanabe and Burnstock, 1976a). In such relatively rare cases, neither the pre- not the postsynaptic membrane shows any remarkable membrane specialization. Neither are aggregations of synaptic vesicles formed at the presynaptic membrane (Fig. 8). The functional role of the SSCs is still uncertain. However, some previous workers have suggested that the SSCs may cause electrophysiological changes in the neuronal membrane, thereby modifying current flow through it (Rosenbluth, 1962; Watanabe and Burnstock, 1976a, 1978), while others have regarded the SSCs as special sites for metabolic exchange between neighbouring cells (Rosenbluth, 1962; Pullen and Sears, 1978).

Figure 9 illustrates in summary the characteristic features of the large and small principal cells in the anuran sympathetic ganglia.

Innervation of the parasympathetic ganglion cells

Preganglionic nerve terminals on parasympathetic ganglion cells in the frog heart are exclusively cholinergic (McMahan and Kuffler, 1971). The synaptic arrangement on the ganglion cells is similar to that in the sympathetic ganglia and is estimated to cover 3.0% of the total surface area of the soma (McMahan and Kuffler, 1971).

On the other hand, parasympathetic ganglion cells in the mud puppy heart are innervated by three different sources: preganglionic nerve fibres (cholinergic in nature) from the vagus, processes arising from intraganglionic SGC cells, and those from the fellow intraganglionic principal cells (McMahan and Purves, 1976). The parasympathetic ganglion is also characterized by occasional gap junctions formed either between the somata, the soma and a

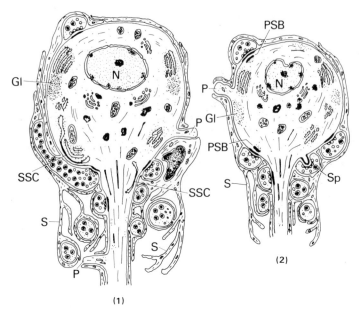

Figure 9 Schemata showing the large (1) and small (2) principal cells in the anuran sympathetic ganglia, with their innervation and satellite sheaths. Note the fact that the large cell has SSCs and the small cell PSBs. Gl = glycogen granules; N = nucleus of principal ganglion cell; PSB = postsynaptic bar; S = satellite cell; Sp = spine synapse; SSC = subsurface cistern

cytoplasmic process, or between the processes of neighbouring ganglion cells (McMahan and Purves, 1976). Electrophysiological studies have suggested the presence of electrical coupling between the principal ganglion cells in the mud puppy cardiac ganglion (Roper, 1976).

SGC cells

The SGC cells are polyhedral in shape, 10 to 20 μm in diameter, and are characterized by numerous granular vesicles with an electron-dense homogeneous matrix (Figs. 10, 11). The vesicles are considerably variable in size, ranging from 60 to 700 nm in diameter, and usually occupy the major part of the cytoplasm. All other organelles such as mitochondria, rough- and smooth-surfaced endoplasmic reticulum, and free ribosomes are apparently pushed away into limited regions. The nucleus has usually a spherical profile with an occasional indentation and contains a large amount of heterochromatin in the peripheral nucleoplasm (Figs. 10, 12).

Individual SGC cells are incompletely covered by attenuated processes of the satellite cells. Clustered SGC cells are frequently in close contact with each other without intervention of the satellite cell. Small numbers of

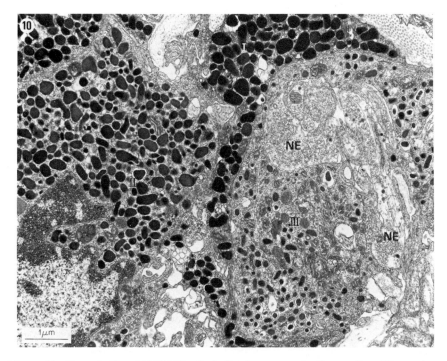

Figure 10 Type I, II and III SGC cells in the frog sympathetic ganglion. The nucleus is characterized by dense, peripheral heterochromatin. Granular vesicles are variable in size, shape and electron density between individual SGC cells. NE = presynaptic nerve ending. ×6000

attachment plaques and gap junctions are formed between these adjacent SGC cells (Watanabe, 1977).

Based on the cytoplasmic structure and the size of granular vesicles, SGC cells in the frog, *Limnodynastes dumerili*, sympathetic ganglia have been classified into four types (Hill *et al.*, 1975). These four types of amphibian SGC cells are not comparable to the type I and type II SIF cells in mammalian ganglia (see chapters by Taxi, and by Williams and Jew). Type I cells are most numerous and are characterized by larger electron-dense granular vesicles than those of the type II cells. Type I and II cells resemble noradrenaline and adrenaline cells, respectively, in the frog adrenal gland. The average diameters of the granular vesicles in both types of SGC cells are comparable to each other (Fig. 10). Type III cells are characterized by smaller (100–300 nm in diameter) vesicles with a light halo of variable width surrounding the central granule (Fig. 10). Hill *et al.* (1975) have proposed that type III cells may represent a transient functional phase of type I or type II.

Type IV cells appear separately or in small groups of 5 to 10 cells. Each cell is surrounded by a satellite cell sheath and separated from others by

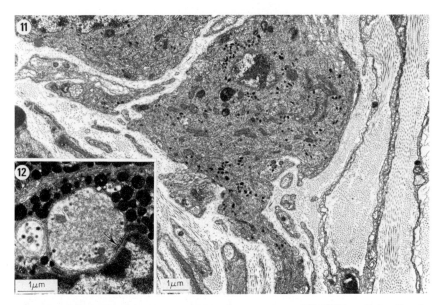

Figure 11 Cytoplasmic process arising from a type IV SGC cell in the frog sympathetic ganglion. Many granular vesicles can be seen in the cytoplasm of the soma and process. ×3250

Figure 12 Type I SGC cell in the frog sympathetic ganglion. A nerve ending is deeply invaginated forming a synaptic specialization (→) on the perikaryal cytoplasm. ×5000

intercellular connective tissue (Fig. 11). In contrast to broad and tapering extensions from types I, II and III cells, type IV projects a uniform and well-defined process and has a region comparable to the axon hillock of the principal neuron (Fig. 11). Frequently 2 to 20 processes are made up into a small bundle. The termination of the processes is uncertain. Granular vesicles characteristic of type IV cells are 100 to 150 nm in diameter. These vesicles are less in number than those of the other types of cells, but still more than those of the principal sympathetic ganglion cells. The high electron-density of the granular vesicles may imply that type IV cells contain either noradrenaline or dopamine rather than adrenaline (Hill *et al.*, 1975). The type IV cell has been considered to be a special type of adrenergic neuron rather than a kind of interneuron (Watanabe and Burnstock, 1976b).

In the bullfrog sympathetic ganglia, the SGC cells have been classified into two types based on the structure of the granular vesicles (Weight and Weitsen, 1977). They are comparable to types I and II in the frog. The majority of the SGC cells in the bullfrog seem to belong to type I or noradrenaline cells. The SGC cells in the toad pararenal ganglion exhibit similar structures to type I or noradrenaline cells (Piezzi and Rodriguez Echandia, 1968).

Innervation of the SGC cells

Regarding the innervation of the SGC cells, a remarkable variety has been described from species to species. The SGC cells in the toad, *Bufo arenarum* Hensel (Piezzi and Rodriguez Echandia, 1968), and bullfrog, *Rana catesbeiana* (Weight and Weitsen, 1977), are believed to have no innervation. On the other hand, synaptic junctions between nerve endings and SGC cells have been noted in the toad, *Bufo vulgaris japonicus* (Fujimoto, 1967).

Serial-section studies have revealed cholinergic preganglionic nerve endings terminating on the four types of SGC cells in the frog, *Limnodynastes dumerili* (Figs. 10, 12) (Hill *et al.*, 1975; Watanabe, 1977). In the frog, types I, II and III cells form 1 to 6 synaptic specializations per cell body; type IV, 6 to 8. However, there is a small number of SGC cells having no synapses in the frog (Watanabe, 1977, 1980).

Previous studies, including those with serial thin-sections, have shown that none of the principal cells in the anuran sympathetic ganglia make direct synaptic contact with SGC cells or their processes (Hill *et al.*, 1975; Watanabe, 1977, 1980). The SGC cells are mostly separated from the principal cells by a wide connective tissue space.

It seems reasonable to assume that both the innervated and non-innervated SGC cells release large amounts of catecholamines (mostly noradrenaline) in response to synaptic transmission from cholinergic nerve endings or stimulation by some fluid-dispersing mechanisms. It is also probable that the large amount of catecholamines secreted from the innervated SGC cells may affect synaptic transmission within the sympathetic ganglia. Such a function, however, seems to be less important, if any, in the ganglia containing mostly non-innervated SGC cells, since the excitation–secretion mechanism of the non-innervated SGC cells may be independent of the autonomic regulation.

A close topographical relationship between SGC cells and blood capillaries is observed in the amphibian sympathetic ganglia (Fujimoto, 1967; Watanabe, 1980). Fenestrated capillaries, which are common in the adrenal gland, are rare in the frog and *Xenopus* sympathetic ganglia. On the contrary, in the bullfrog sympathetic ganglia, the endothelium is occasionally fenestrated. However, it should also be noted that the fenestrated portions of the endothelial cells are never associated with the SGC cells in the ganglia.

These findings seem to suggest that an endocrine function of the intraganglionic SGC cells is of lower efficiency than that of the adrenal SGC cells in the amphibian (see Watanabe, 1980).

SGC cells in the parasympathetic ganglia

Although information about the fine structure of the SGC cells in the amphibian parasympathetic ganglia has been limited, 106 SGC and 250 principal cells per cardiac ganglion have been counted in the mud puppy (McMahan and Purves, 1976). The SGC cells vary in shape from round to oval, and are 15 to 30 μm in diameter. These cells appear occasionally in groups, but more often coexist with large ganglion cells, 30 to 50 μm in diameter. The granular vesicles of the SGC cells are 40 to 150 nm in size. The SGC cells receive a small number of cholinergic presynaptic nerve endings. It should be pointed out that the SGC cells and their processes in the cardiac ganglion of the mud puppy, unlike in the anuran sympathetic ganglia, make direct synapses upon the principal ganglion cell. Moreover, gap junctions are formed between the SGC and principal ganglion cells (McMahan and Purves, 1976).

These findings suggest that the SGC cells in the mud puppy cardiac ganglion may function as catecholamine-containing interneurons.

SUMMARY AND CONCLUSION

Unipolar principal ganglion cells of the amphibian, particularly anuran, sympathetic ganglia are classified into large (B) and small (C) cell types. Preganglionic nerve fibres innervating the principal cells form a spiral around the axon hillock and initial portion of the axon. Synapses are formed most numerously on the axon hillock.

A single type of nerve ending, containing numerous small agranular and less numerous large granular vesicles, is described in the sympathetic ganglia. These endings are considered to be cholinergic in nature. PSBs, SSCs and characteristic specializations of the postsynaptic membrane are frequently observed in the sympathetic ganglion cells. These structures may in some way modulate cholinergically transmitted nerve impulses.

Besides acetylcholine, polypeptides and other putative transmitter substances have been claimed to be involved in ganglionic transmission. But their real functional roles or subcellular distributions have not been completely understood (see, however, the chapters by Weight and by Dun). The catecholamine in the anuran principal ganglion cells seems to be adrenaline not noradrenaline.

The SGC cells occur separately or in clusters of variable sizes in the autonomic ganglia. They are more numerous in the 5th to 7th sympathetic ganglia than in the more caudal ganglia. Most of the SGC cells contain noradrenaline. In some anuran sympathetic ganglia, most SGC cells are innervated by what are presumed to be cholinergic nerve endings, but in other anuran species no innervation has so far been demonstrated. There has been no unequivocal evidence for the synaptic contact between SGC cells and principal ganglion cells in the amphibian sympathetic ganglia. This implies that the SGC cells in these ganglia do not play any interneuronal role. SGC cells are rarely situated opposite to the fenestrae of the capillary endothelium.

This also implies that endocrine secretion of catecholamines into the blood-stream may be less effective in the intraganglionic SGC cells than in the adrenal SGC cells.

The large amount of catecholamines secreted by innervated SGC cells may affect synaptic transmission within the anuran sympathetic ganglia. However, such a function may be insignificant in the ganglia containing mostly non-innervated SGC cells.

The functional role of the SGC cells cannot be unified by observations reported so far. It may be variable in different species, segments or in different cell types.

The principal cells of the amphibian parasympathetic ganglia are mostly unipolar in some species and bipolar or multipolar in the others. Preganglionic nerve endings on the parasympathetic ganglion cells in the frog heart are cholinergic. More complicated synaptic connections are formed in the mud puppy cardiac ganglion; the principal cells are innervated by three different sources, namely cholinergic nerve endings from the vagus nerve, SGC cells, and fellow principal ganglion cells. As distinct from those of the sympathetic ganglia, the SGC cells in the parasympathetic ganglia may function as interneurons.

ACKNOWLEDGEMENTS

The author wishes to thank Professors Toshi Yuki Yamamoto, and Akira Tonosaki, for critical reading of, and advice about, the manuscript.

REFERENCES

Angelakos, E. T., Glassman, M. P., Millard, R. W., and King, H. (1965). Regional distribution and subcellular localization of catecholamines in the frog heart. *Comp. Biochem. Physiol.*, **15**, 313–324.

Azuma, T., Binia, A., and Visscher, M. B. (1965). Adrenergic mechanisms in the bullfrog and turtle. *Am. J. Physiol.*, **209**, 1287–1294.

Bishop, G. H., and O'Leary, J. (1938). Pathways through the sympathetic nervous system in the bullfrog. *J. Neurophysiol.*, **1**, 442–454.

Blackman, J. G., Ginsborg, B. L., and Ray, C. (1963). Synaptic transmission in the sympathetic ganglion of the frog. *J. Physiol. (London)*, **167**, 355–373.

Burnstock, G. (1969). Evolution of the autonomic innervation of visceral and cardiovascular systems in vertebrates. *Pharmacol. Rev.*, **21**, 247–324.

Chiba, T. (1977). Monoamine-containing paraneurons in the sympathetic ganglia of mammals. *Arch. Histol. Jpn. Suppl.*, **40**, 163–176.

Fujimoto, S. (1967). Some observations on the fine structure of the sympathetic ganglion of the toad, *Bufo vulgaris japonicus*. *Arch. Histol. Jpn.*, **28**, 313–335.

Gabella, G. (1976a). Ganglia of the autonomic nervous system. In *The Peripheral Nerve* (Ed. D. N. Landon), pp. 335–395, Chapman and Hall, London.

Gabella, G. (1976b). *Structure of the Autonomic Nervous System*, Chapman and Hall, London.

Hill, C. E., Watanabe, H., and Burnstock, G. (1975). Distribution and morphology of amphibian extra-adrenal chromaffin tissue. *Cell Tissue Res.*, **160**, 371–387.

Honma, S. (1970a). Histochemical demonstration of catecholamines in the toad sympathetic ganglia. *Jpn. J. Physiol.*, **20**, 186–197.

Honma, S. (1970b). Functional differentiation in B and C neurons of toad sympathetic ganglia. *Jpn. J. Physiol.*, **20**, 218–295.

Jacobowitz, D. (1970). Catecholamine fluorescence studies of adrenergic neurons and chromaffin cells in sympathetic ganglia. *Fed. Proc.*, **29**, 1922–1944.

Jan, L. Y., Jan, Y. N., and Brownfield, M. S. (1980). Peptidergic transmitters in synaptic boutons of sympathetic ganglia. *Nature,* **288**, 380–382.

Kojima, H., Anraku, S., Onogi, K., and Ito, R. (1978). Histochemical studies on two types of cells containing catecholamines in sympathetic ganglia of the bullfrog. *Experientia*, **34**, 92–93.

Langley, J. N., and Orbeli, L. A. (1910). Observations on the sympathetic and sacral autonomic system of the frog. *J. Physiol. (London)*, **41**, 450–482.

Lascar, G., Taxi, J., and Kerdelhué, B. (1982). Localisation immunocytochimìque d'une substance du type gonadolibérine (LH-RH) dans les ganglions sympathiques de Grenouille. *C. R. Acad. Sci. Ser. C*, **294**, 175–179.

Matthews, M. R. (1974). Ultrastructure of ganglionic junction. In *The Peripheral Nervous System* (Ed. J. I. Hubbard), pp. 111–150, Plenum Press, New York, London.

McMahan, U. J., and Kuffler, S. W. (1971). Visual identification of synaptic boutons on living ganglion cells and of varicosities in postganglionic axons in the heart of the frog. *Proc. R. Soc. London Ser. B*, **177**, 485–508.

McMahan, U. J., and Purves, D. (1976). Visual identification of two kinds of nerve cells and their synaptic contacts in a living autonomic ganglion of the mudpuppy (*Necturus maculosus*). *J. Physiol. (London)*, **254**, 405–425.

Nicol, J. A. C. (1952). The autonomic nervous system in lower chordates. *Biol. Rev.*, **27**, 1–49.

Nishi, S., Soeda, H., and Koketsu, K. (1965). Studies on sympathetic B and C neurons and patterns of preganglionic innervation. *J. Cell. Comp. Physiol.*, **66**, 19–32.

Nishi, S., Soeda, H., and Koketsu, K. (1967). Release of acetylcholine from sympathetic preganglionic nerve terminals. *J. Neurophysiol.* **30**, 114–134.

Norberg, K.-A., and McIsaac, R. J. (1967). Cellular location of adrenergic amines in frog sympathetic ganglia. *Experientia*, **23**, 1052.

Norberg, J.-A., and Sjöqvist, F. (1966). New possibilities for adrenergic modulation of ganglionic transmission. *Pharmacol. Rev.*, **18**, 743–751.

Pick, J. (1963). The submicroscopic organization of the sympathetic ganglion in the frog (*Rana pipiens*). *J. Comp. Neurol.*, **120**, 409–462.

Pick, J. (1970). *The Autonomic Nervous System*, J. B. Lippincott, Philadelphia.

Piezzi, R. S., and Rodriguez Echandia, E. L. (1968). Studies on the pararenal ganglion of the toad *Bufo arenarum* Hensel. I. Its normal fine structure and histochemical characteristics. *Z. Zellforsch. Mikrosk. Anat.*, **88**, 180–186.

Pullen, A. H., and Sears, T. A. (1978). Modification of 'C' synapses following partial central deafferentation of thoracic motoneurones. *Brain Res.*, **145**, 141–146.

Roper, S. (1976). An electro-physiological study of chemical and electrical synapses on neurons in the parasympathetic cardiac ganglion of the mudpuppy, *Necturus maculosus*: evidence for intrinsic ganglionic innervation. *J. Physiol. (London)*, **254**, 427–454.

Rosenbluth, J. (1962). Subsurface cisterns and their relationship to the neuronal plasma membrane. *J. Cell Biol.*, **13**, 405–421.

Sotelo, C. (1968). Permanence of postsynaptic specializations in the frog sympathetic ganglion cells after denervation. *Exp. Brain Res.*, **6**, 294–305.

Stammer, A. (1965). Die mikroskopische Struktur des Ggl. ciliare der Frösche. *Acta Biol. Univ. Szeged*, **11**, 127–133.

Taxi, J. (1961). Etude de l'ultrastructure des zones synaptiques dans les ganglions sympathiques de la Grenouille. *C. R. Acad. Sci.*, **252**, 174–176.

Taxi, J. (1965). Contribution à l'étude des connexions des neurones moteurs du système nerveux autonome. *Ann. Sci. Nat. Zool. Biol. Anim.*, **7**, 413–674.

Taxi, J. (1967). Observations on the ultrastructure of the ganglionic neurons and synapses of the frog *Rana esculenta* L. In *The Neuron* (Ed. H. Hydén), pp. 221–254, Elsevier, Amsterdam, London, New York.

Taxi, J. (1976). Morphology of the autonomic nervous system. In *Frog Neurobiology* (Eds. R. Llinás and W. Precht), pp. 93–150, Springer-Verlag, Berlin.

Taxi, J. (1979). Degeneration and regeneration of frog ganglionic synapses. *Neuroscience*, **4**, 817–823.

Uchizono, K. (1964). On different types of synaptic vesicles in sympathetic ganglia of amphibia. *Jpn. J. Physiol.*, **14**, 210–219.

Watanabe, H. (1977). Ultrastructure and function of the granule-containing cells in the anuran sympathetic ganglia. *Arch. Histol. Jpn.*, **40** (Suppl.), 177–186.

Watanabe, H. (1980). Ultrastructural study of the frog sympathetic ganglia. In *Histochemistry and Cell Biology of Autonomic Neurons, SIF cells, and Paraneurons* (Eds. O. Eränkö, S. Soinila and H. Päivärinta), *Advances in Biochemical Psychopharmacology*, Vol. 25, pp. 153–157, Raven Press, New York.

Watanabe, H., and Burnstock, G. (1976a). Junctional subsurface organs in frog sympathetic ganglion cells. *J. Neurocytol.*, **5**, 125–136.

Watanabe, H., and Burnstock, G. (1976b). A special type of small granule-containing cell in the abdominal para aortic region of the frog. *J. Neurocytol.*, **5**, 465–478.

Watanabe, H., and Burnstock, G. (1978). Postsynaptic specializations at excitatory and inhibitory cholinergic synapses. *J. Neurocytol.*, **7**, 119–133.

Weight, F. F., and Weitsen, H. A. (1977). Identification of small intensely fluorescent (SIF) cells as chromaffin cells in bullfrog sympathetic ganglia. *Brain Res.*, **128**, 213–226.

Weitsen, H. A., and Weight, F. F. (1977). Synaptic innervation of sympathetic ganglion cells in the bullfrog. *Brain Res.*, **128**, 197–211.

Wong, W. C. (1973). The myenteric plexus in the oesophagus of the toad (*Bufo melanostictus*). *Acta Anat.*, **85**, 52–62.

Wong, W. C., Sit, K. H., Ng, K. K. F., and Chin, K. N. (1971). The submucous plexus in the small intestine of the toad (*Bufo melanostictus*). *Acta Anat.*, **79**, 60–69.

Woods, R. I. (1970). The innervation of the frog's heart. I. An examination of the autonomic postganglionic nerve fibers and a comparison of autonomic and sensory ganglion cells. *Proc. R. Soc. London Ser. B*, **176**, 43–54.

Yamamoto, T. (1963). Some observations on the fine structure of the sympathetic ganglion of bullfrog. *J. Cell Biol.*, **16**, 159–170.

Synapses and Neurotransmitter Functions

Autonomic Ganglia
Edited by Lars-Gösta Elfvin
© 1983 John Wiley & Sons Ltd

Transmitter Histochemistry of Autonomic Ganglia

M. SCHULTZBERG, T. HÖKFELT. J. M. LUNDBERG,
C. J. DALSGAARD and L.-G. ELFVIN

*Departments of Histology, Pharmacology and Anatomy, Karolinska Institutet,
Box 60 400, S-104 01 Stockholm, Sweden*

INTRODUCTION

There is an increasing body of evidence for the occurrence of small biologically active peptides in both the central and peripheral nervous system. In this chapter we will summarize the distribution of various neuropeptides in autonomic ganglia, and discuss the relationship between these peptides and conventional transmitters in these ganglia (for the enteric ganglia and some cranial ganglia, see chapters by Llewellyn-Smith *et al.* and by Ehinger *et al.*). These studies are based on the indirect immunofluorescence technique of Coons and collaborators (see Coons, 1958) and immunoperoxidase techniques (see Sternberger, 1974) which have been widely used, and provide convenient and sensitive methods for the detection and localization of small peptides in tissue sections. The following peptides have been found in mammalian autonomic ganglia: substance P (Hökfelt *et al.*, 1977c), vasoactive intestinal polypeptide (VIP) (Hökfelt *et al.*, 1977b), somatostatin (Hökfelt *et al.*, 1977a), methionine- and leucine-enkephalin (Schultzberg *et al.*, 1978b, 1979), cholecystokinin octapeptide (CCK-8) (Larsson and Rehfeld, 1979), neurotensin (Lundberg *et al.*, 1980c), bombesin (Schultzberg *et al.*, 1980; Schultzberg, 1982b), and pancreatic polypeptide (Lundberg *et al.*, 1980b). It has to be borne in mind that, although the antigen–antibody reaction is generally highly specific, the substance present in the tissue reacting with the antibody may not correspond to the immunogen. The antigenic determinant, in the case of peptides, is generally a sequence of four to seven amino acids. Therefore, peptides with related sequences may cross-react with the same antibodies. Hence, careful control experiments have to be carried out, and particular care has to be applied in interpretation of the results. In fact, the identity of many peptides is at present uncertain. For example, so far none of the peptides discussed in this chapter have been isolated and sequenced in any of the three species studied, namely rat, guinea pig and cat. In addition to possible species differencies, there may also exist different molecular forms, including larger precursors. Against this background it seems relevant to give a brief account of the molecular structure of the peptides dealt with and their structural relationship to other peptides. (For a detailed account of the action of peptides in sympathetic ganglia, see chapter by Dun.)

CHEMICAL CHARACTERISTICS OF NEUROPEPTIDES

Substance P was discovered in 1931 by von Euler and Gaddum as an excitatory substance different from acetylcholine in extracts of horse brain and intestine. Leeman and collaborators (Chang and Leeman, 1970; Chang *et al.*, 1971) isolated substance P from the bovine hypothalamus and characterized it as an undecapeptide. A peptide with the same amino acid sequence has also been isolated from the equine intestine (Studer *et al.*, 1973), but so far other molecular forms of substance P have not been encountered in mammalian tissues. However, substance P is structurally related to a number of other peptides, of which physalaemin (Erspamer *et al.*, 1964) and eledoisin (Erspamer and Falconieri Erspamer, 1962) are the best known. These peptides were isolated from octopus salivary gland and share the COOH-terminal sequence Leu-Met-NH_2 with substance P. Among other groups of peptides isolated from the amphibian skin, bombesin (Erspamer and Melchiorri, 1973) has the same COOH-terminal dipeptide as substance P (see below).

The octacosapeptide *VIP* was isolated from porcine duodenum by Said and Mutt (1970, 1972) and the amino acid sequence determined (Mutt and Said, 1974). There seems to be a slight variation in the amino acid sequence of VIP in different species. The chicken VIP differs in four amino acids from the porcine VIP (Nilsson, 1974), and immunochemical studies with antibodies to different portions of the peptide indicate that there are several molecular forms of VIP-like material in human and rat intestines (Dimaline and Dockray, 1978, 1979; Dimaline *et al.*, 1980). VIP is structurally related to secretin, glucagon, gastric inhibitory peptide (GIP), and a newly isolated peptide from porcine intestine (PHI) (Tatemoto and Mutt, 1980).

The *enkephalins* were first discovered as endogenous ligands for opiate receptors (see Terenius and Wahlström, 1974, 1975; Hughes, 1975) and were purified and characterized by Hughes and coworkers (Hughes *et al.*, 1975). Two pentapeptides with a similar sequence except for the COOH-terminal amino acid were found: methionine- (Met) and leucine- (Leu) enkephalin. Therefore, most enkephalin antisera that are currently used cross-react with both peptides. Moroever, a large number of peptides containing the sequence of Met- and/or Leu-enkephalin have been isolated from the adrenal glands (Lewis *et al.*, 1980; Gubler *et al.*, 1982; Noda *et al.*, 1982; see also Schultzberg, 1982a). Many of these latter peptides may represent precursors for the smaller opioid peptides.

Somatostatin, originally discovered as a factor inhibiting growth-hormone release (Krulich *et al.*, 1973), was isolated from bovine hypothalamus and characterized as a tetradecapeptide (Brazeau *et al.*, 1973). An octacosapeptide (somatostatin-28) including the somatostatin sequence at the COOH-terminus, was isolated from porcine duodenum by Pradayrol *et al.* (1978) and later also from ovine hypothalamus in addition to a smaller molecular form, somatostatin-25 (Schally *et al.*, 1980; Brazeau *et al.*, 1981).

In 1928 Ivy and Goldberg demonstrated that extracts of hog duodenum contain a substance which they called *cholecystokinin* (CCK) and which caused contraction of the gall bladder. Not until 1966 was the peptide with this property isolated and sequenced (Mutt and Jorpes, 1966), and was also shown to be identical with the substance demonstrated by Harper and Raper (1943), which stimulates pancreatic enzyme secretion. CCK-like immunoreactivity has been observed in central and peripheral neurons with antibodies to the COOH-terminus of CCK (Vanderhaeghen *et al.*, 1975; Dockray, 1976, 1979; see Rehfeld *et al.*, 1979), in which the last five amino acids are shared with gastrin (Gregory and Tracy, 1964, 1972). Biochemical studies have shown that the predominant form of the CCK-like material in brain is CCK-8 (Dockray *et al.*, 1978). This seems to be true also for the immunoreactive material in the nerve plexuses within the muscular layers in the gut (Larsson and Rehfeld, 1979; Hutchison *et al.*, 1981), but further forms may also exist (see Rehfeld *et al.*, 1979).

Neurotensin was first found by Carraway and Leeman (1973) as a factor in hypothalamic extracts causing vasodilatation and increased vascular permeability followed by cyanosis. It was isolated and sequenced from bovine hypothalamus (Carraway and Leeman, 1973, 1974, 1975), and later also from human intestine (Hammer *et al.*, 1980).

Bombesin, one of many peptides found in the skin of different species of frogs by Erspamer and coworkers (see Erspamer *et al.*, 1978), is a tetradecapeptide isolated from the frog *Bombina bombina* (Anastasi *et al.*, 1971). Recently, a mammalian counterpart called gastrin-releasing peptide (GRP), with a sequence similar to the amphibian peptide, was isolated from porcine non-antral stomach (McDonald *et al.*, 1979). The two COOH-terminal amino acids in both the amphibian and mammalian bombesin peptides are shared with substance P. Therefore, most of the available bombesin antisera cross-react to some extent with substance P in immunohistochemical studies (Schultzberg, 1982b).

Pancreatic polypeptide. A peptide with a stimulatory action on pancreatic secretion was originally isolated from the chicken pancreas by Kimmel *et al.* (1968, 1975). The human and bovine (Lin and Chance, 1974), as well as ovine, porcine and canine, homologues have since been isolated (see Lin, 1980). All these peptides have only minor differencies in the amino acid sequence, except for the avian peptide (APP) which differs from the

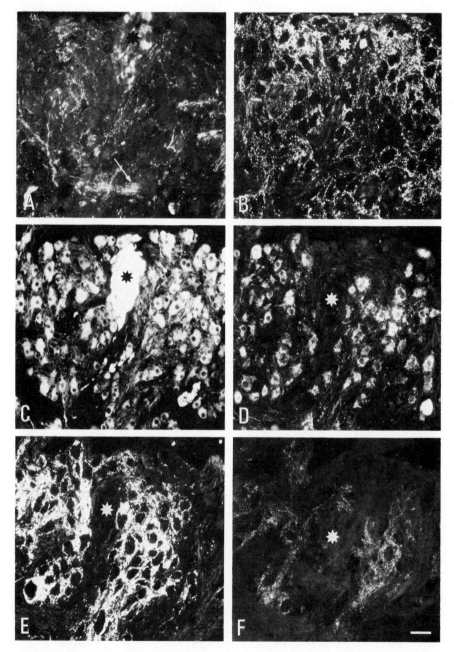

Figure 1 Immunofluorescence micrographs of semiconsecutive sections of the guinea-pig coeliac-superior mesenteric ganglion complex after incubation with anti-sera to substance P (A), enkephalin (B), dopamine β-hydroxylase (DBH) (C),

mammalian peptides in more than half of the 36 amino acids. The exact nature of the pancreatic polypeptide-like immunoreactivity in rodents and cat is still unknown.

PREVERTEBRAL GANGLIA

Distribution of neuropeptides in the inferior mesenteric ganglion and the coeliac-superior mesenteric ganglion complex

Networks of substance P (Fig. 1A) (Hökfelt *et al.*, 1977c), VIP (Fig. 1E) (Hökfelt *et al.*, 1977b), enkephalin (Fig. 1B) (Schultzberg *et al.*, 1978b, 1979), CCK (Figs. 1F, 3A) (Larsson and Rehfeld, 1979), and bombesin (Fig. 2A) (Schultzberg, 1980, 1982b) immunoreactive fibres have been observed in immunohistochemical studies of the inferior mesenteric ganglion and the coeliac-superior mesenteric ganglion complex of guinea-pig and rat. VIP, substance P, enkephalin and CCK immunoreactive fibres have been observed also in the cat prevertebral ganglia (Lundberg *et al.*, 1980c). Neurotensin immunoreactive fibres were only observed in the prevertebral ganglia of the cat (Lundberg *et al.*, 1980c). A large number of somatostatin (Figs. 1D, 3B) (Hökfelt *et al.*, 1977a) and APP (Lundberg *et al.*, 1980b) immunoreactive cell bodies have been demonstrated in the prevertebral ganglia of rat and guinea-pig, and in the cat many APP, but no somatostatin, immunoreactive cells were seen.*

The characteristics of some of the peptides found in prevertebral ganglia have been studied. The nature of the substance P and bombesin immunoreactive material in the rat and guinea-pig coeliac ganglion was studied immunochemically. The substance P-like material appeared to consist of only one molecular form corresponding to the synthetic undecapeptide (Schultzberg, 1982b), whereas the bombesin-like material appears to occur as two molecular forms, one corresponding to bombesin decapeptide and one to

somatostatin (D), vasoactive intestinal polypeptide (VIP) (E), and cholecystokinin (CCK) (F). A loose network of varicose substance P immunoreactive fibres can be seen in A. In addition bundles of smooth substance P immunoreactive fibres are observed (arrow in A). Dense networks of enkephalin (B) and VIP (E) immunoreactive fibres are observed. The VIP immunoreactive fibres appear to run in strands consisting of several varicose fibres (E). A sparse network of CCK immunoreactive fibres can be seen in F. The CCK immunoreactive fibres are varicose and seem to have a limited distribution. The principal noradrenergic ganglion cells show immunoreactivity to DBH antiserum (C). A large proportion of the ganglion cells are somatostatin immunoreactive (D). A group of small intensely fluorescent (SIF) cells, indicated by asterisks, show intense DBH immunofluorescence (C). Some SIF cells are substance P immunoreactive (A), and a few contain enkephalin-like immunoreactivity (B). Bar indicates 50 µm

---

* It should also be noted that somatostatin-like immunoreactivity has been demonstrated ultrastructurally in ganglion cells and nerve fibres of guinea pig coeliac-superior mesenteric ganglion complex and superior cervical ganglion. (Cs. Léránth, T. H. Williams, J. Y. Jew and A. Arimura, Cell Tissue Res. 1980, 212, 83–89.)

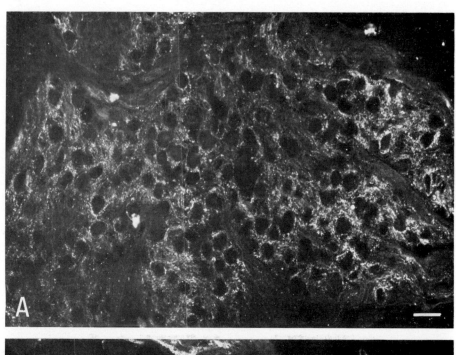

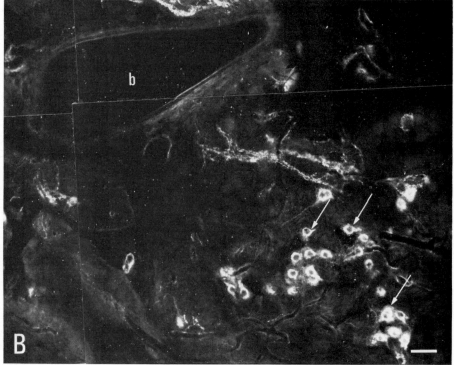

a larger molecule (Schultzberg, 1982b). The enkephalin immunoreactive material in the prevertebral ganglia was localized with antibodies to Met- and Leu-enkephalin (Schultzberg *et al.*, 1979). Both types of antisera showed the same distribution pattern of enkephalin immunoreactive structures. However, absorption experiments (Schultzberg *et al*, 1979) showed that there was a cross-reactivity of the Met-enkephalin antisera with Leu-enkephalin and *vice versa*. DiGiulio *et al.* (1978) have been able to demonstrate that both Met- and Leu-enkephalin are present in the guinea-pig prevertebral ganglia. None of the other peptides occurring in these ganglia have so far been characterized.

The distribution of the different peptides occurring in nerve fibres in the prevertebral ganglia may at first glance seem very similar. However, on closer examination the patterns of distribution are characteristic of each peptide. The VIP, enkephalin, CCK and bombesin immunoreactive fibres form dense networks (Figs. 1B, E, F, 2A), the VIP immunoreactive fibres being most numerous (Fig. 1E). The VIP immunoreactive fibres in particular often run together in strands between the principal ganglion cells (see Fig. 1E). This is true also for the enkephalin, CCK and bombesin immunoreactive fibres, although these fibres are less numerous (see Figs. 1B, F, 2A, 3A). The substance P immunoreactive fibres are considerably fewer in number and mostly run as single fibres (Fig. 1A). Like the other types of fibres, these substance P immunoreactive fibres are varicose. The intervaricose segments are, however, relatively longer. In addition, substance P-like immunoreactivity occurs in thicker, smoother fibres, probably representing axons, which are often seen in bundles of different sizes (see Fig. 1A).

The density of the different types of peptide immunoreactive fibres appears to be similar in the inferior mesenteric ganglion and the coeliac-superior mesenteric ganglion complex. However, whereas the fibres in the inferior mesenteric ganglion are fairly evenly distributed, the coeliac-superior mesenteric ganglion complex has regions which are almost devoid of fibres. This is especially the case for the VIP, bombesin and CCK immunoreactive fibres. In the case of VIP, areas with a sparse innervation of VIP immunoreactive fibres often contain VIP immunoreactive nerve cells (Fig. 2B). Usually only a small number of cells have been observed, but larger numbers of VIP immunoreactive cells can be encountered (see Fig. 2B). So far, no certain correlation between the VIP immunoreactive cells and the cells containing noradrenaline

Figure 2 Immunofluorescence micrographs of sections of the guinea-pig coeliac-superior mesenteric ganglion complex after incubation with antisera to bombesin (A) and vasoactive intestinal polypeptide (VIP) (B). Thin varicose bombesin immunoreactive fibres form a medium dense network around the principal ganglion cells (A). Many VIP immunoreactive nerve cells (arrows in B) can be seen in an area of the coeliac ganglion, which contains only a few VIP immunoreactive fibres. The immunoreactive material is present outside the nucleus and appears granular. b = blood vessel. Bars indicate 50 μm

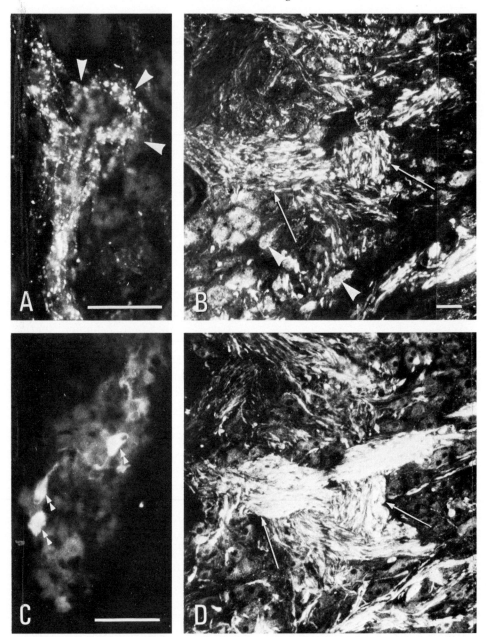

Figure 3 Immunofluorescence micrograph of a section of the guinea-pig coeliac-superior mesenteric ganglion complex after incubation with antisera to cholecystoki-nin (CCK) (A), somatostatin (B), 5-hydroxytryptamine (5-HT) (C), and dopamine β-hydroxylase (DBH) (D). The ganglion shown in B and D was treated locally with

has been observed. However, a large proportion of the dopamine β-hydroxylase (DBH)-positive ganglion cells contain somatostatin-like immunoreactivity (Hökfelt *et al.*, 1977a) (Fig. 1C, D).

Studies of consecutive sections of the guinea-pig prevertebral ganglia have shown that the somatostatin immunoreactive cells correspond to about 60% of the principal ganglion cells. However, within the coeliac-superior mesenteric ganglion complex considerable differences exist. Thus, in the posterior superior part only about 25% are somatostatin immunoreactive. The number of somatostatin immunoreactive neurons in the rat ganglia is less than in the guinea-pig. Only a very sparse network of somatostatin immunoreactive fibres have been observed in the ganglia. In cat sympathetic ganglia no somatostatin immunoreactive ganglion cells have been identified so far (Lundberg *et al.*, 1980c). Recently, studies with antibodies to APP showed immunoreactive material in a population of noradrenergic neurons in the prevertebral ganglia of rat, cat and guinea-pig, with the largest number in the coeliac ganglion (Lundberg *et al.*, 1982a). In the guinea-pig these APP immunoreactive cells seem to lack somatostatin-like immunoreactivity, suggesting that in this species at least two populations of noradrenergic cells exist, characterized by an APP- and somatostatin-like peptide, respectively (Lundberg *et al.*, 1982a).

In the coeliac-superior mesenteric ganglion of the guinea-pig, there seem to be two types of enkephalin immunoreactive fibres; namely, strongly fluorescent fibres occurring in patches together with small groups of nerve cells, and a network of less intensely fluorescent fibres which are more evenly distributed (Schultzberg *et al.*, 1979). The explanation for this phenomenon may be the presence of different amounts of enkephalin in the two types of fibres, or it may be different types of enkephalin-like peptides with varying degree of cross-reactivity with the antibodies used. DiGiulio *et al.* (1978) showed that both Met- and Leu-enkephalin occur in the guinea-pig ganglia, but there may well be other molecular forms, as in the adrenal medulla where several larger molecules containing enkephalin sequences have been found (Lewis *et al.*, 1980; Gubler *et al.*, 1982; Noda *et al.*, 1982; see also Schultzberg, 1982a). Enkephalin immunoreactive nerve fibres have also been found in human

vinblastine. The CCK immunoreactive fibres are varicose and appear to run in strands formed by two or more fibres. Sometimes ganglion cells are surrounded by basket-like formations of CCK immunoreactive fibres (arrowheads in A). The principal ganglion cells (B, D) show a medium intense immunofluorescence to DBH (D), and a population of ganglion cells are somatostatin immunoreactive (arrowheads in B). Bundles of intensely fluorescent DBH immunoreactive fibres are observed (D). Bundles of somatostatin immunoreactive fibres can be seen with a similar distribution pattern (arrows in B and D). C shows a group of small intensely fluorescent (SIF) cells. Some of the SIF cells are 5-HT immunoreactive (double arrowheads in C). Note positive processes from two of the cells. Bars indicate 50 μm

prevertebral sympathetic ganglia (Hervonen *et al.*, 1980a, b, 1981; Pelto-Huikko *et al.*, 1980), and ultrastructural studies of human ganglia showed enkephalin-like material occurring in large dense-core vesicles and some small clear vesicles (Hervonen *et al.*, 1980a).

Groups of small intensely fluorescent cells (SIF cells; Eränkö, 1976) which have high concentrations of dopamine and noradrenaline and sometimes adrenaline (Elfvin *et al.*, 1975; Verhofstad *et al.*, 1980), are often observed in the prevertebral sympathetic ganglia. Sometimes large groups of SIF cells form small paraganglia (see Fig. 1). The peptide-containing fibres within these clusters of SIF cells were few and varied with the peptide. The enkephalin immunoreactive fibres were most numerous and occurred as single fibres. A few substance P and VIP, but no CCK or bombesin immunoreactive fibres were seen.

Verhofstad and coworkers have demonstrated with antibodies to 5-hydroxytryptamine (5-HT) that some SIF cells in the superior cervical ganglion of the rat are 5-HT-containing (Vershofstad *et al.*, 1981). Similarly, some of the SIF cells in the prevertebral ganglia are 5-HT-positive (Fig. 3C) (unpublished results). Previously, it was demonstrated that an enkephalin-like peptide was present in a population of SIF cells in the prevertebral ganglia (Fig. 1B) (Schultzberg *et al.*, 1979). Recently, substance P-like immunoreactivity was also demonstrated in a number of SIF cells in prevertebral sympathetic ganglia (Schultzberg and Hökfelt (in preparation) (see Fig. 1A). At present, it is not clear whether all these substances occur in the same SIF cells or in separate cells. However, each of the populations seem to be small enough that each substance may represent a separate group of SIF cells (see Figs. 1A, B, 3C).

Origin and projections of peptidergic neurons and functional aspects

The various peptides found in nerve fibres in the prevertebral ganglia seem to have characteristic pathways (see Fig. 4). Substance P is so far the most thoroughly studied peptide with regard to origin and projections in relation to these ganglia. It was suggested by Hökfelt *et al.* (1977c) that the substance P immunoreactive fibres in the prevertebral ganglia represent projections of the substance P-containing neurons in spinal ganglia. Such projections have been demonstrated with tracing studies using horseradish peroxidase (Elfvin and Dalsgaard, 1977). Recently, retrograde tracing with fluorescent dyes, combined with immunohistochemistry showed that in fact substance P fibres in the inferior mesenteric ganglion of the guinea-pig originate in spinal ganglia (Fig. 4) (Dalsgaard *et al.*, 1981, 1982a). This is also supported by transection experiments (Baker *et al.*, 1980). Konishi *et al.* (1979a) showed that the amount of substance P-like immunoreactivity in the guinea-pig inferior mesenteric ganglion decreased after ligation or sectioning of the lumbar

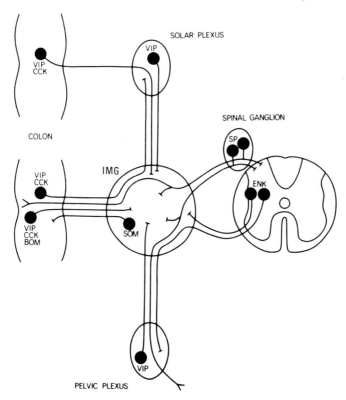

Figure 4 Schematic illustration of peptide-containing nerves in the guinea-pig inferior mesenteric ganglion (IMG), and the connections between this ganglion and the spinal cord, spinal ganglia, coeliac-superior mesenteric ganglion complex (solar plexus), pelvic plexus, and colon, which were indicated by ligation and denervation experiments and by retrograde tracing of fluorescent dyes combined with immunohistochemistry (see also Dalsgaard *et al.*, 1982a, b, c). SP = substance P; VIP = vasoactive intestinal polypeptide; ENK = enkephalin; SOM = somatostatin; CCK = cholecystokinin; BOM = bombesin

splanchnic and intermesenteric nerves. Ligation experiments in the cat also suggest that most substance P immunoreactive fibres enter the prevertebral ganglia via the splanchnic nerves (Lundberg *et al.*, 1980c), which also is the case in the guinea-pig (Dalsgaard *et al.*, 1982c). It was suggested (Hökfelt *et al.*, 1977c) that the smooth substance P immunoreactive fibres observed in the ganglia represent axons from the spinal neurons (Hökfelt *et al.*, 1975) running through the ganglia into the nerves towards the gut. In support of this hypothesis ligation of the mesenteric nerve results in an accumulation of substance P immunoreactive material on the ganglion side of these nerves (Dalsgaard *et al.*, 1982c). The functional significance of these substance P neurons innervating the prevertebral ganglia is not clear, but there is evidence for the release of substance P from the guinea-pig inferior mesenteric ganglion by high concentration of K^+ (Konishi *et al.*, 1979a). Furthermore, substance P causes an atropine-resistant depolarization of the principal ganglion cells. (For further discussion see chapter by Dun.) This is in agreement with studies on the spinal cord demonstrating an excitatory action of substance P on motoneurons (Konishi and Otsuka, 1974).

The enkephalin immunoreactive fibres in the prevertebral ganglia probably represent preganglionic nerves originating in the spinal cord (Fig. 4) (Glazer and Basbaum, 1980; Lundberg *et al.*, 1980c). Ligation of the ventral roots in both cat and guinea-pig results in accumulation of enkephalin-like material proximal to the ligation. Furthermore, retrograde tracing combined with immunohistochemistry shows the localization of fluorescent dye injected into the inferior mesenteric ganglion accumulating in enkephalin immunoreactive preganglionic neurons in the spinal cord (Dalsgaard *et al.*, 1981, 1982b). Konishi *et al.* (1979b) have shown that enkephalin inhibits cholinergic transmission in the ganglia. In addition, there is evidence which suggests that enkephalin nerves may inhibit substance P release presynaptically (Konishi *et al.*, 1979b; see also chapter by Dun).

The VIP, bombesin, and CCK immunoreactive fibres observed in the ganglia probably represent projections of enteric neurons (Fig. 4). Ligation experiments in the guinea-pig have shown that VIP, bombesin and CCK immunoreactive material accumulates on the gut side of nerves connecting the ganglia with the gut (Dalsgaard *et al.*, 1982c), and similar experiments in the cat suggest that VIP and CCK immunoreactive fibres originate in the gut via the mesenteric nerves (Lundberg *et al.*, 1979, 1980c). In agreement with this, high concentrations of VIP have been measured in the gastrointestinal tract (Bryant *et al.*, 1976; see Fahrenkrug, 1979; Said, 1981), where VIP-like immunoreactivity occurs in abundant nerve cells, especially in the submucous plexus, and in dense networks of fibres, both in the muscular and connective tissue layers and around nerve cells in the enteric plexuses (Bryant *et al.*, 1976; Larsson *et al.*, 1976; Schultzberg *et al.*, 1978a, 1980; Costa *et al.*, 1980a; Jessen *et al.*, 1980). The abundant VIP immunoreactive neurons in the gastrointestinal wall may project to the prevertebral ganglia. Ligation experiments also give evidence for a projection of VIP-containing nerves from the pelvic ganglia to the inferior mesenteric ganglion of the guinea-pig. In addition, VIP-containing nerves reach this prevertebral ganglion via the intermesenteric nerve, indicating that some ganglionic VIP fibres originate in the solar plexus ganglia and possibly also in the proximal colon (see Dalsgaard *et al.*, 1982c; Fig. 4). Such projections have been described earlier in electrophysiological (Crowcroft *et al.*, 1971; Job and Lundberg, 1952; McLennan and Pascoe, 1954; Szurszewski and Weems, 1976) and indirect anatomical (Kuntz, 1938, 1940; Kuntz and Saccomanno, 1944) studies, and have recently also been demonstrated with a tonal tracing techniques

(Dalsgaard and Elfvin, 1982). The physiological role of VIP in prevertebral ganglia is not known. However, in other tissues it has been shown that VIP meets many of the criteria for a neurotransmitter. It has been suggested as possible transmitter in non-cholinergic, non-adrenergic inhibitory neurons in the gut (Fahrenkrug *et al.*, 1978; Goyal and Rattan, 1980). It has a potent vasodilatory action as well as causing relaxation of smooth muscle in the gut and in the respiratory tract, and stimulation of bicarbonate and water secretion from the exocrine pancreas (Bodanszky *et al.*, 1976; Fahrenkrug, 1979; Said and Mutt, 1970).

The gastrointestinal tract contains numerous CCK immunoreactive neurons, possibly contributing to the nerve fibre networks in the prevertebral ganglia. The possibility has to be considered that, in addition to enteric CCK neurons projecting to the prevertebral ganglia, CCK sensory neurons (Lundberg *et al.*, 1978; Larsson and Rehfeld, 1979) in spinal ganglia also may give projections to these ganglia (Dalsgaard *et al.*, 1982c).

The bombesin immunoreactive fibres in the prevertebral ganglia represent the richest source of bombesin immunoreactive material that has been measured so far in mammals (Schultzberg, 1982b). The concentrations of bombesin-like immunoreactivity in brain and gastrointestinal tract are much lower, with the highest concentration found in stomach (Brown *et al.*, 1978; Dockray *et al.*, 1979; Moody *et al.*, 1981). The function of the rich innervation of the prevertebral sympathetic ganglia by bombesin immunoreactive neurons, presumably from the gut (Dalsgaard *et al.*, 1982c), is still unclear. However, bombesin has a number of potent biological actions, including stimulation of secretion of gastric acid, gastrin and CCK increase in blood pressure, stimulation of smooth muscle contraction and lowering of body temperature (see Erspamer and Melchiorri, 1975).   ·

The neurotensin immunoreactive nerves observed around the ganglion cells in the cat prevertebral ganglia probably represent preganglionic nerves from the thoracic spinal cord, since they disappear after section of the ventral roots (Lundberg *et al.*, 1980a, 1982b). No information on the functional role of neurotensin in sympathetic ganglia is available at present. In the gut this peptide seems to be present both in endocrine cells (see Bloom, 1978; Bloom and Polak, 1981) and in nerves (Schultzberg *et al.*, 1980). It exerts a number of actions, such as inhibition of gastric acid secretion (Andersson *et al.*, 1976), increase of glucose and glucagon in plasma (Brown and Vale, 1976; Carraway and Leeman, 1975; Nagai and Frohman, 1976) and contraction of intestinal smooth muscle (Carraway and Leeman, 1973; Rökaeus *et al.*, 1977).

The postganglionic noradrenergic neurons in the prevertebral ganglia are known to project to the gut, and it was suggested that the noradrenergic neurons also containing somatostatin-like immunoreactivity may project to the gut (Hökfelt *et al.*, 1977a). In favour of this suggestion is the fact that somatostatin-like material accumulates on the ganglion side after ligation (unpublished data). However, denervation of the guinea-pig ileum, and treatment with 6-hydroxydopamine, respectively, does not affect the number of immunofluorescent somatostatin nerves observed in the gut (Costa *et al.*, 1980b). The explanation may be that the proportion of extrinsic somatostatin fibres is too small to make a difference in the overall picture. Local application of mitotic inhibitors such as colchicine or vinblastine on the ganglia arrest the axonal transport, resulting in an accumulation of somatostatin immunoreactive material in intraganglionic axon bundles, which have a similar localization as the DBH-positive (noradrenergic) axons (see Fig. 3B, D). Somatostatin in general seems to exert inhibitory effects (see Efendić *et al.*, 1978). In the gut it has been shown to inhibit release of acetylcholine from myenteric neurons in the guinea-pig ileum (Guillemin, 1976; Cohen *et al.*, 1978). The latter effect is also an action of noradrenaline from the postganglionic sympathetic neurons projecting to the gut (Lawson, 1934; Lawson and Holt, 1937; Furness and Costa, 1974). Furthermore, Williams and North (1978) have shown that somatostatin inhibits firing of myenteric neurons, possibly by hyperpolarization.

PARAVERTEBRAL GANGLIA

Superior cervical ganglion

The innervation of the superior cervical ganglion by neuropeptide neurons is small compared to the prevertebral ganglia. Only a few scattered substance P, VIP, CCK and bombesin immunoreactive fibres have been observed. The enkephalin immunoreactive fibres are somewhat more numerous, and in the rat superior cervical ganglion a few enkephalin immunoreactive nerve cells were observed (see Fig. 5A, B) (Schultzberg *et al.*, 1979). The number of positive cells increased after treatment with colchicine, and also bundles of enkephalin immunoreactive axons could be seen (Fig. 5B). The enkephalin immunoreactive cells could be correlated to DBH-positive ganglion cells. This finding thus probably represents another case of coexistence of a peptide with noradrenaline. The somatostatin immunoreactive cells were less numerous than in the prevertebral ganglia, and only single VIP immunoreactive cells were observed. A larger number of APP immunoreactive cells that also were DBH-positive, on the other hand, were observed both in the rat, guinea-pig and cat superior cervical ganglion (Fig. 5C) (Lundberg *et al.*, 1980b, 1982a). No substance P immunoreactive cells were observed, but recent *in vitro* studies have shown that the amount of substance P increases 200-fold after three days of culture of the rat superior cervical ganglion (Kessler *et al.*, 1981), suggesting that these cells have a potential to synthesize substance P at least in these conditions. Furthermore, immunohistochemistry on these cultures has demonstrated that substance P-like immunoreactivity is

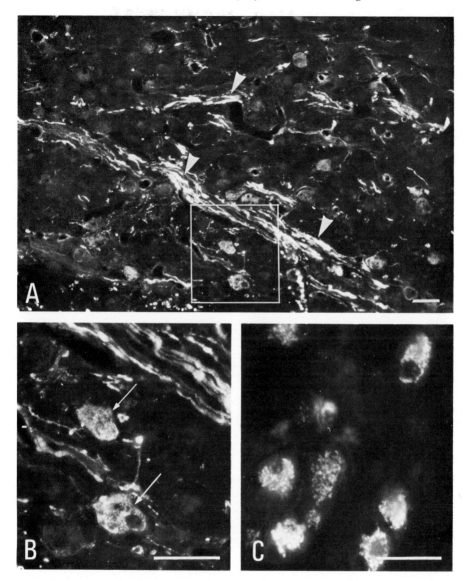

Figure 5 Immunofluorescence micrographs of a section of the rat superior cervical ganglion after incubation with antisera to enkephalin (A, B) and avian pancreatic polypeptide (APP) (C). B is a higher magnification of part of A as indicated by the rectangle. The rat (A, B) was treated locally with colchicine. Enkephalin immunoreactive material is observed in nerve cells (arrows in B), and in bundles of smooth fibres (arrowheads in A). C shows APP immunoreactive principal ganglion cells. Note the granular appearance of the APP immunoreactive material. Bars indicate 50 μm

present in principal ganglion cells. Whether or not these substance P immunoreactive cells are identical to several or any of the above-mentioned enkephalin, somatostatin and/or VIP immunoreactive neurons remains to be established.

Up until now there has been no evidence for the exact projections of the peptide nerves in the superior cervical ganglion. It is possible that the enkephalin immunoreactive fibres are preganglionic fibres and that the substance P immunoreactive fibres represent sensory nerves. The APP immunoreactive noradrenergic neurons in the superior cervical ganglion project to blood vessels (mainly arteries) in, for example, nasal mucosa and salivary glands (Lundberg *et al.*, 1980b, 1982a). Noradrenergic nerves around exocrine elements within the glands are not APP immunoreactive, suggesting that they are separate from the noradrenergic, APP-containing vascular nerves (Lundberg *et al.*, 1982a). As mentioned above, Verhofstad *et al.* (1981) have shown that some of the SIF cells in the superior cervical ganglion contain 5-HT-like immunoreactivity, in addition to the dopamine- and noradrenaline-containing cells. A few enkephalin immunoreactive SIF cells have also been observed in this ganglion (Schultzberg *et al.*, 1979).

Stellate and lumbar sympathetic ganglia

As in the superior cervical ganglion, few peptide immunoreactive fibres have been found in the stellate ganglion. The substance P immunoreactive fibres mostly occur singly and occasionally surround ganglion cell bodies (Hökfelt *et al.*, 1977c). However, many enkephalin and neurotensin immunoreactive fibres occur in the stellate ganglion and other sympathetic chain ganglia in the cat (Lundberg *et al.*, 1980c). A large proportion of the noradrenergic cells in the rat and cat stellate ganglion are APP immunoreactive (Lundberg *et al.*, 1980b, 1982a).

About 10–15% of the ganglion cells of the stellate and L-7 ganglia of the cat are non-adrenergic and VIP immunoreactive (Lundberg *et al.*, 1979; Lundberg, 1981). The VIP immunoreactive cells are also rich in acetylcholinesterase, suggesting a cholinergic nature of these neurons (Lundberg *et al.*, 1979; c.f. Sjöqvist, 1962, 1963; Holmstedt and Sjöqvist, 1959). This is also supported by the findings that about 13% of the neurons in the L-7 ganglion contain choline acetyltransferase (Buckley *et al.*, 1967). These stellate and L-7 neurons project via sciatic and brachial nerves to skeletal muscle and blood vessels as well as to sweat glands and blood vessels in the skin of the foot pads (Lundberg *et al.*, 1979).

PELVIC GANGLION

Immunohistochemical studies of the guinea-pig pelvic ganglia located at the distal end of the hypogastric nerves have shown the presence of enkephalin,

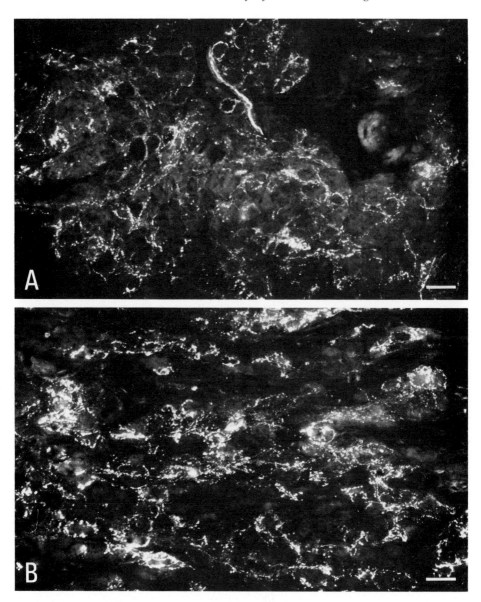

Figure 6 Immunofluorescence micrographs of sections of the guinea-pig pelvic ganglion after incubation with antisera to substance P (A) and enkephalin (B). Numerous substance P immunoreactive fibres can be seen (A). These fibres are thin and varicose and mostly run as single fibres. The enkephalin immunoreactive fibres more often run together in short strands, which often form patches. Bars indicate
50 μm

substance P, VIP, bombesin, CCK, and APP immunoreactive nerve fibres (in preparation). The substance P and enkephalin immunoreactive fibres were the most numerous (see Fig. 6A, B). As in the prevertebral ganglia, the substance P immunoreactive fibres were thin and varicose and distributed over the ganglion (Fig. 6A). The enkephalin immunoreactive fibres were also varicose, but appeared together in strands, often forming patches around a group of ganglion cells (Fig. 6B). Only few bombesin immunoreactive fibres were seen and CCK immunoreactive fibres were also sparse, mostly surrounding blood vessels. A large number of VIP, and APP immunoreactive cells were observed. When the distribution of VIP immunoreactive cells was compared with the noradrenergic cells in the ganglion, it was apparent that the two cell types were separate (see Fig. 7A, B). The relationship between the APP immunoreactive cells and the noradrenergic cells in the pelvic ganglion has not been studied, but it is conceivable that at least some of the APP immunoreactive cells are identical with the noradrenergic cells. Such a coexistence has been demonstrated in the prevertebral ganglia (Lundberg *et al.*, 1982a).

The corresponding pelvic ganglia of the cat also contain many peptide immunoreactive neurons. In the pelvic ganglia many VIP immunoreactive cell bodies are present. Many of these are acetylcholinesterase-rich (Lundberg *et al.*, 1979). There are also many substance P and enkephalin immunoreactive nerve fibres around pelvic ganglion cells. Ligation experiments suggest that substance P nerves originate from sacral and lumbar spinal ganglia, while the enkephalin nerves are of preganglionic origin from the sacral spinal cord (Lundberg *et al.*, 1980c). For further discussion on these ganglia see chapter by Owman *et al.*

OTHER PARASYMPATHETIC GANGLIA

The ciliary, pterygopalatine, otic, and submandibular ganglia contain many substance P immunoreactive fibres (Lundberg *et al.*, 1980c). Furthermore, many VIP immunoreactive cell bodies are present in the pterygopalatine, otic and submandibular ganglia (Fig. 7C) (Lundberg *et al.*, 1980a, 1981). In the pterygopalatine ganglion virtually all ganglion cells are VIP immunoreactive and are rich in acetylcholinesterase (Lundberg *et al.*, 1980a, 1981). After removal of the pterygopalatine ganglion there is a parallel loss of choline

Figure 7 Immunofluorescence micrographs of semiconsecutive sections of the guinea pig pelvic ganglion (A, B) and the cat pterygopalatine ganglion (C) after incubation with antisera to vasoactive intestinal polypeptide (VIP) (A, C) and tyrosine hydroxylase (TH) (B). A large number of VIP immunoreactive cells can be seen in the pelvic ganglion (A). The VIP immunoreactive cells appear to have a different localization than the TH-positive cells (B). b = blood vessel. All principal ganglion cells in the pterygopalatine ganglion are VIP immunoreactive (C). Bars indicate 50 μm

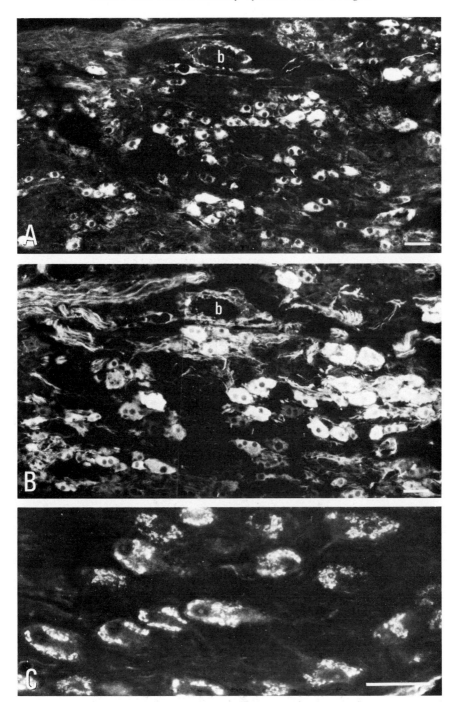

acetyltransferase and VIP in the nasal mucosa, which further supports a coexistence of VIP and acetylcholine in these nerves to exocrine elements and blood vessels (Lundberg *et al.*, 1981). Also local ganglia of the tongue, trachea and bronchi as well as in the pancreas contain many VIP immunoreactive cell bodies, many of which are acetylcholinesterase-rich (Lundberg *et al.*, 1980a, c). Functional studies (Lundberg, 1981) suggest that VIP may be responsible for the atropine-resistant part of the vasodilatation which accompanies, for example, salivary secretion and VIP potentiates the salivatory response to acetylcholine without having any secretory effect *per se*. For further discussion of the ciliary and pterygopalatine ganglion see chapter by Ehinger *et al.*

In the porcine pancreas, VIP has been suggested (Fahrenkrug *et al.*, 1979) to cause an atropine-resistant increase in water and bicarbonate secretion (Hickson, 1970). Perfusion of the porcine pancreas *in vitro* with VIP gives an increase in water and bicarbonate secretion (Lindkaer Jensen *et al.*, 1978), mimicking the response to vagal nerve stimulation (Hickson, 1970), and vagal stimulation also causes an increase of the VIP concentration in the venous outflow from the pancreas (Fahrenkrug *et al.*, 1979). In the submandibular and pancreatic ganglia there are also some enkephalin immunoreactive neurons present, which are separate from the VIP nerves. These neurons project to exocrine elements (Lundberg *et al.*, 1980c).

SUMMARY

A large number of biologically active peptides has been demonstrated in neurons in the mammalian nervous system during the last decade. Many of these neuropeptides are found in neurons both in the brain and the gastrointestinal tract, and some also occur as hormones in gut endocrine cells. Other tissues with an abundance of peptide-containing nerves are autonomic ganglia. Nerve fibres containing substance P-, VIP-, enkephalin-, CCK-, and bombesin-like immunoreactivities have been encountered in these ganglia of the rat, guinea-pig and cat. In the cat, neurotensin immunoreactive fibres have also been seen. Furthermore, noradrenergic nerve cell bodies containing somatostatin- and APP-like, and in some cases enkephalin-like, immunoreactivity have been found. The prevertebral sympathetic ganglia, such as the inferior mesenteric ganglion and the coeliac-superior mesenteric ganglion complex, are the ganglia most densely innervated by peptide-containing nerves so far observed, whereas paravertebral ganglia such as the superior cervical ganglion and the stellate ganglion are more sparsely innervated. Also, the number of somatostatin immunoreactive ganglion cells is larger in the prevertebral ganglia. The APP immunoreactive cells are, however, numerous in both types of sympathetic ganglia.

The origin and projections of peptide-containing neurons have been studied in some detail, especially the afferent and efferent connections of the inferior mesenteric ganglion of the guinea-pig. The results demonstrate that the substance P immunoreactive nerve fibres in the ganglion represent peripheral projections of primary sensory neurons, which may give off collaterals within the ganglion and continue towards the gut. The enkephalin immunoreactive fibres have been shown to originate in the spinal cord, representing preganglionic neurons. This is probably the case also for the neurotensin immunoreactive fibres in the cat prevertebral ganglia. The VIP, CCK and bombesin immunoreactive fibres appear to be projections of enteric neurons. The VIP immunoreactive neurons observed in the prevertebral ganglia may represent neurons interconnecting, for example, the coeliac ganglion with the inferior mesenteric ganglion. The somatostatin immunoreactive neurons, on the other hand, project to the gut, as the noradrenergic principal ganglion cells.

In the stellate and lumbar (L-7) sympathetic ganglia of the cat, about 10–15% of the ganglion cells are non-adrenergic and VIP immunoreactive. The VIP immunoreactive cells are also rich in acetylcholinesterase, suggesting that these neurons are cholinergic. These neurons in the L-7 ganglion project via the sciatic and brachial nerves to skeletal muscle, blood vessels and sweat glands. The pelvic and other parasympathetic ganglia, such as the pterygopalatine, otic and submandibular ganglia, also contain large numbers of VIP immunoreactive cells. Virtually all ganglion cells in the pterygopalatine ganglion appear to be VIP immunoreactive and are rich in acetylcholinesterase. These neurons innervate exocrine glands and blood vessels in the nasal mucosa. Substance P and enkephalin immunoreactive fibres are abundant in the cranial and pelvic ganglia. The substance P immunoreactive fibres in the cat pelvic ganglion seem to originate in lumbar and sacral spinal ganglia, and the enkephalin immunoreactive fibres in this ganglion are of preganglionic origin from the sacral spinal cord. Electrophysiological studies have shown actions of substance P and enkephalin in prevertebral sympathetic ganglia, and VIP in parasympathetic neurons has been suggested to be responsible for the atropine-resistant part of the vasodilatation accompanying, for example, salivary secretion.

In conclusion, mammalian autonomic ganglia are densely innervated by peptide-containing neurons, the functions of which to a large extent remain to be further investigated.

REFERENCES

Anastasi, A., Erspamer, V., and Bucci, M. (1971). Isolation and structure of bombesin and alytesin, two analogous active peptides from the skin of the European amphibians, *Bombina* and *Alytes*. *Experientia*, **27**, 166–167.

Andersson, S., Chang, E., Folkers, K., and Rosell, S. (1976). Inhibition of gastric acid secretion in dogs by neurotensin. *Life Sci.*, **19**, 367–371.

Baker, S. C., Cuello, A. C., and Matthews, M. (1980). Substance P-containing synapses in a sympathetic ganglion and their possible origin as collaterals from sensory nerve fibres. *J. Physiol. (London)*, **308**, 76–77P.

Bloom, S. R. (Ed.) (1978). *Gut Hormones*, Churchill Livingstone, Edinburgh.

Bloom, S. R., and Polak, J. M. (eds.) (1981). *Gut Hormones*, Churchill Livingstone, Edinburgh.

Bodanszky, M., Klausner, Y. S., and Said, S. I. (1976). Biological activities of synthetic peptides corresponding to fragments of and to the entire sequence of the vasoactive intestinal peptide. *Proc. Natl. Acad. Sci. U.S.A.*, **70**, 382–384.

Brazeau, P., Vale, W., Burgus, K., Ling, N., Butcher, M., Rivier, J., and Guillemin, R. (1973). Hypothalamic polypeptide that inhibits the secretion of immunoreactive pituitary growth hormone. *Science*, **179**, 77–79.

Brazeau, P., Ling, N., Esch, F., Böhlen, P., Benoit, P., and Guillemin, R. (1981). High biological activity of the synthetic replicates of somatostatin-28 and somatostatin-25. *Regul. Peptides*, **1**, 255–264.

Brown, M. R., and Vale, W. W. (1976). Effects of neurotensin and substance P on glucoregulation. *Endocrinology*, **98**, 819–822.

Brown, M., Allen, R., Villareal, J., Rivier, J., and Vale, W. (1978). Bombesin-like activity: Radioimmunologic assessment in biological tissues. *Life Sci.*, **23**, 2721–2728.

Bryant, M. G., Polak, M. M., Modlin, L., Bloom, S. R., Albuquerque, R. H., and Pearse, A. G. E. (1976). Possible dual role for vasoactive intestinal peptide as gastrointestinal hormone and neurotransmitter substance. *Lancet*, **i**, 991–993.

Buckley, G., Consolo, S., and Sjöqvist, F. (1967). Cholinacetylase in innervated and denervated sympathetic ganglia and ganglion cells of the cat. *Acta Physiol. Scand.*, **71**, 348–356.

Carraway, R., and Leeman, S. E. (1973). The isolation of a new hypotensive peptide, neurotensin, from bovine hypothalami. *J. Biol. Chem.*, **248**, 6854–6861.

Carraway, R., and Leeman, S. E. (1974). The amino acid sequence, chemical synthesis, and radioimmunoassay of neurotensin. *Fed. Proc.*, **23**, 548.

Carraway, R., and Leeman, S. E. (1975). The amino acid sequence of a hypothalamic peptide, neurotensin. *J. Biol. Chem.*, **250**, 1907–1911.

Chang, M. M., and Leeman, S. E. (1970). Isolation of a sialogogic peptide from bovine hypothalamic tissue and its characterization as substance P. *J. Biol. Chem.*, **245**, 4784–4790.

Chang, M. M., Leeman, S. E., and Niall, H. D. (1971). Amino acid sequence of substance P. *Nature*, **232**, 86–87.

Cohen, M. L., Rosing, E., Wiley, K. S., and Slater, I. H. (1978). Somatostatin inhibits adrenergic and cholinergic neurotransmission in smooth muscle. *Life Sci.*, **23**, 1659–1664.

Coons, A. H. (1958). Fluorescent antibody methods. In *General Cytochemical Methods* (Ed. J. F. Danielli), pp. 399–422, Academic Press, New York.

Costa, M., Furness, J. B., Buffa, R., and Said, S. I. (1980a). Distribution of enteric nerve cell bodies and axons showing immunoreactivity for vasoactive intestinal polypeptide in the guinea-pig intestine. *Neuroscience*, **5**, 587–596.

Costa, M., Furness, J. B., Llewellyn-Smith, I. J., Davies, B., and Oliver, J. (1980b). An immunohistochemical study of the projections of somatostatin-containing neurons in the guinea-pig intestine. *Neuroscience*, **5**, 841–852.

Crowcroft, P. J., Holman, M. E., and Szurszewski, J. H. (1971). Excitatory input from the distal colon to the inferior mesenteric ganglion in the guinea-pig. *J. Physiol. (London)*, **219**, 443–461.

Dalsgaard, C.-J., and Elfvin, L.-G. (1982) Structural studies on the connectivity of the inferior mesenteric ganglion of the guinea pig. *J. Aut. Nerv. Syst.*, **5**, 265–278.

Dalsgaard, C. J., Hökfelt, T., Elfvin, L.-G., Terenius, L., and Emson, P. (1981). Tracing of substance P and enkephalin immunoreactive neurons projecting to the guinea-pig inferior mesenteric ganglion: Immunohistochemistry combined with fluorescent retrograde labelling. *Soc. Neurosci. Abstr.*, **7**, 101.

Dalsgaard, C. J., Hökfelt, T., Elfvin, L.-G., Skirboll, L., and Emson, P. (1982a). Substance P-containing primary sensory neurons projecting to the inferior mesenteric ganglion: Evidence from combined retrograde tracing and immunohistochemistry. *Neuroscience*, **7**, 647–654.

Dalsgaard, C. J., Hökfelt, T., Elfvin, L.-G., and Terenius, L. (1982b). Enkephalin-containing sympathetic preganglionic neurons projecting to the inferior mesenteric ganglion: Evidence from combined retrograde tracing and immunohistochemistry. *Neuroscience*, **7**, 2039–2050.

Dalsgaard, C. J., Hökfelt, T., Schultzberg, M., Lundberg, J. M., Terenius, L., Dockray, G. J., Guello, C., and Goldstein, M. (1982c). Origin of peptide-containing fibres in the inferior mesenteric ganglion of the guinea pig: Immunohistochemical studies with antisera to substance P, enkephalin, vasoactive intestinal polypeptide, cholecystokinin/gastrin and bombesin. *Neuroscience*, in press.

DiGiulio, A. M., Yang, H.-Y. T., Lutold, B., Fratta, W., Hong, J., and Costa, E. (1978). Characterization of enkephalin-like material extracted from sympathetic ganglia. *Neuropharmacology*, **17**, 989–992.

Dimaline, R., and Dockray, G. J. (1978). Multiple immunoreactive forms of vasoactive intestinal peptide in human colonic mucosa. *Gastroenterology*, **75**, 387–392.

Dimaline, R., and Dockray, G. J. (1979). Molecular variants of vasoactive intestinal polypeptide in dog, rat and hog. *Life Sci.*, **25**, 1893–1900.

Dimaline, R., Vaillant, C., and Dockray, G. J. (1980). The use of region-specific antibodies in the characterization and localization of vasoactive intestinal polypeptide-like substances in the rat gastrointestinal tract. *Regul. Peptides*, **1**, 1–16.

Dockray, G. J. (1976). Immunochemical evidence of cholecystokinin-like peptides in brain. *Nature*, **264**, 568–570.

Dockray, G. J. (1979). Immunochemistry of gastrin and cholecystokinin: Development and application of region specific antisera. In *Gastrins and the Vagus* (Eds. J. F. Rehfeld and E. Amdrup), pp. 73–83, Academic Press, London.

Dockray, G. J., Gregory, R. A., Hutchinson, J. B., Harris Ieuan J., and Runswick, M. J. (1978). Isolation, structure and biological activity of two cholecystokinin octapeptides from sheep brain. *Nature*, **274**, 711–713.

Dockray, G. J., Vaillant, C., and Walsh, J. H. (1979). The neuronal origin of bombesin-like immunoreactivity in the rat gastrointestinal tract. *Neuroscience*, **4**, 1561–1568.

Efendić, S., Hökfelt, T., and Luft, R. (1978). Somatostatin. *Adv. Metab. Disord.*, **9**, 367–424.

Elfvin, L.-G., and Dalsgaard, C. J. (1977). Retrograde axonal transport of horse-radish peroxidase in afferent fibers of the inferior mesenteric ganglion of the guinea-pig. Identification of the cells of origin in dorsal root ganglia. *Brain Res.*, **126**, 149–153.

Elfvin, L.-G., Hökfelt, T., and Goldstein, M. (1975). Fluorescence microscopical, immunohistochemical and ultrastructural studies on sympathetic ganglia of the guinea pig with special reference to the SIF cells and their catecholamine content. *J. Ultrastruct. Res.*, **51**, 377–396.

Eränkö, O. (Ed.) (1976). *SIF Cells, Structure and Function of the Small Intensely Fluorescent Sympathetic Cells, Fogarty International Center Proceedings No. 30*, US Government Printing Office, Washington, DC.

Erspamer, V., and Falconieri Erspamer, G. (1962). Pharmacological actions of eledoisin on extravascular smooth muscle. *Br. J. Pharmacol.*, **19**, 337–354.

Erspamer, V., and Melchiorri, P. (1973). Active polypeptides of the amphibian skin and their synthetic analogues. *Pure Appl. Chem.*, **35**, 463–494.

Erspamer, V., and Melchiorri, P. (1975). Actions of bombesin on secretions and motility of the gastrointestinal tract. In *Gastrointestinal Hormones* (Ed. J. C. Thompson), pp. 575–589. University of Texas Press, Austin.

Erspamer, V., Anastasi, A., Bertaccini, G., and Cei, J. M. (1964). Structure and pharmacological actions of physalaemin, the main active polypeptide of the skin of *Physalaemus fuscumaculatus*. *Experientia*, **20**, 489–490.

Erspamer, V., Melchiorri, P., Falconieri Erspamer, C., and Negri, L. (1978). Polypeptides of the amphibian skin, active on the gut and their mammalian counterparts. In *Gastrointestinal Hormones and Pathology of the Digestive System* (Eds. M. Grossman, V. Speranza, N. Basso and E. Lezoche), pp. 51–64, Plenum Press, New York.

Fahrenkrug, J. (1979). Vasoactive intestinal polypeptide: Measurement, distribution and putative neurotransmitter function. *Digestion*, **19**, 149–169.

Fahrenkrug, J., Haglund, U., Jodal, M., Lundgren, O., Olbe, L., and Schaffalitzky De Muckadell, O. B. (1978). Nervous release of vasoactive intestinal polypeptide in the gastrointestinal tract of cats: Possible physiological implications. *J. Physiol. (London)*, **284**, 291–305.

Fahrenkrug, J., Schaffalitzky De Muckadell, O. B., Holst, J. J., and Lindkaer Jensen, S. (1979). Role of VIP in the vagally mediated pancreatic secretion of fluid and bicarbonate. *Am. J. Physiol.*, **237**, E535–E541.

Furness, J. B., and Costa, M. (1974). The adrenergic innervation of the gastrointestinal tract. *Ergeb. Physiol.*, **69**, 1–52.

Glazer, E. J., and Basbaum, A. I. (1980). Leucine enkephalin: Localization in and axoplasmic transport by sacral parasympathetic preganglionic neurons. *Science*, **208**, 1479–1481.

Goyal, R. K., and Rattan, S. (1980). VIP as a possible neurotransmitter of non-cholinergic non-adrenergic inhibitory neurones. *Nature*, **288**, 378–380.

Gregory, R. A., and Tracy, H. J. (1964). The constitution and properties of two gastrins extracted from hog antral mucosa. *Gut*, **5**, 103–114.

Gregory, R. A., and Tracy, H. J. (1972). Isolation of two 'big gastrins' from Zollinger-Ellison tumour tissue. *Lancet*, **ii**, 797–799.

Gubler, U., Seeburg, P., Hoffman, B. J., Gage, L. P., and Udenfriend, S. (1982). Molecular cloning establishes proenkephalin as precursor of enkephalin-containing peptides. *Nature*, **295**, 206–208.

Guillemin, R. (1976). Somatostatin inhibits the release of acetylcholine induced electrically in the myenteric plexus. *Endocrinology*, **99**, 1653–1654.

Hammer, R. A., Leeman, S. E., Carraway, R., and Williams, R. H. (1980). Isolation of human intestinal neurotensin. *J. Biol. Chem.*, **255**, 2476–2480.

Harper, A. A., and Raper, H. S. (1943). Pancreozymin, a stimulant of the secretion of pancreatic enzymes in extracts of the small intestine. *J. Physiol. (London)*, **102**, 115–125.

Hervonen, A., Pelto-Huikko, M., Helen, P., and Alho, H. (1980a). Electron-microscopic localization of enkephalin-like immunoreactivity in axon terminals of human sympathetic ganglia. *Histochemistry*, **70**, 1–6.

Hervonen, A., Pickel, V. M., Joh, T. H., Reis, D. J., Linnoila, I., Kanerva, L., and Miller, R. J. (1980b). Immunocytochemical demonstration of the catecholamine-synthesizing enzymes and neuropeptides in the catecholamine-storing cells of human fetal sympathetic nervous system. In *Histochemistry and Cell Biology of Autonomic Neurons, SIF Cells, and Paraneurons* (Eds. O. Eränkö, S. Soinila and H. Päivärinta), *Advances in Biochemical Pyschopharmacology*, Vol. 25, pp. 373–378, Raven Press, New York.

Hervonen, A., Pickel, V. M., Joh, T. H., Reis, D. J., Linnoila, I., and Miller, R. J. (1981). Immunohistochemical localization of the catecholamine synthesizing enzymes, substance P, and enkephalin in the human fetal sympathetic ganglion. *Cell Tissue Res.*, **214**, 33–42.

Hickson, J. C. D. (1970). The secretion of pancreatic juice in response to stimulation of the vagus nerves in the pig. *J. Physiol. (London)*, **206**, 275–297.

Hökfelt, T., Kellerth, J.-O., Nilsson, G., and Pernow, B. (1975). Experimental immunohistochemical studies on the localization and distribution of substance P in cat primary sensory neurons. *Brain Res.*, **100**, 235–252.

Hökfelt, T., Elfvin, L.-G., Elde, R., Schultzberg, M., Goldstein, M., and Luft, R. (1977a). Occurrence of somatostatin-like immunoreactivity in some peripheral sympathetic noradrenergic neurons. *Proc. Natl. Acad. Sci. U.S.A.*, **74**, 3587–3591.

Hökfelt, T., Elfvin, L.-G., Schultzberg, M., Fuxe, K., Said, S. I., Mutt, V., and Goldstein, M. (1977b). Immunohistochemical evidence of vasoactive intestinal polypeptide-containing neurons and nerve fibers in sympathetic ganglia. *Neuroscience*, **2**, 885–896.

Hökfelt, T., Elfvin, L.-G., Schultzberg, M., Goldstein, M., and Nilsson, G. (1977c). On the occurrence of substance P-containing fibers in sympathetic ganglia: Immunohistochemical evidence. *Brain Res.*, **132**, 29–41.

Holmstedt, B. and Sjöqvist, F. (1959). Distribution of acetylcholinesterase in the ganglion cells of various sympathetic ganglia. *Acta Physiol. Scand.*, **47**, 284–296.

Hughes, J. (1975). Isolation of an endogenous compound from the brain with pharmacological properties similar to morphine. *Brain Res.*, **88**, 295–308.

Hughes, J., Smith, T. W., Kosterlitz, H. W., Fothergill, L. A., Morgan, B. A., and Morris, H. R. (1975). Identification of two related pentapeptides from the brain with potent opiate agonist activity. *Nature*, **258**, 577–579.

Hutchison, J. B., Dimaline, R., and Dockray, G. J. (1981). Neuropeptides in the gut: Quantification and characterization of cholecystokinin octapeptide-, bombesin-, and vasoactive intestinal polypeptide-like immunoreactivities in the myenteric plexus of the guinea-pig small intestine. *Peptides*, **2**, 23–30.

Ivy, A. C., and Oldberg, E. (1928). A hormone mechanism for gall bladder contraction and evacuation. *Am. J. Physiol.*, **86**, 599–613.

Jessen, K. R., Saffrey, M. J., van Noorden, S., Bloom, S. R., Polak, J. M., and Burnstock, G. (1980). Immunohistochemical studies of the enteric nervous system in tissue culture and *in situ*: Localization of vasoactive intestinal polypeptide (VIP), substance-P and enkephalin immunoreactive nerves in the guinea-pig gut. *Neuroscience*, **5**, 1717–1735.

Job, C., and Lundberg, A. (1952). Reflex excitation of cells in the inferior mesenteric ganglion on stimulation of the hypogastric nerve. *Acta Physiol. Scand.*, **26**, 366–382.

Kessler, J. A., Adler, J. E., Bohn, M. C., and Black, I. B. (1981). Substance P in principal sympathetic neurons: regulation by impulse activity. *Science*, **214**, 335–336.

Kimmel, J. R., Pollock, H. G., and Hazelwood, R. L. (1968). Isolation and characterization of chicken insulin. *Endocrinology*, **83**, 1323–1330.

Kimmel, J. R., Hayden, L. J., and Pollock, H. G. (1975). Isolation and characterization of a new pancreatic polypeptide hormone. *J. Biol. Chem.*, **250**, 9369–9376.

Konishi, S., and Otsuka, M. (1974). Excitatory action of hypothalamic substance P on spinal motoneurones of newborn rats. *Nature*, **252**, 734–735.

Konishi, S., Tsunoo, A., and Otsuka, M. (1979a). Substance P and non-cholinergic excitatory synaptic transmission in guinea pig sympathetic ganglia. *Proc. Jpn. Acad. Ser. B*, **55**, 525–430.

Konishi, S., Tsunoo, A., and Otsuka, M. (1979b). Enkephalins presynaptically inhibit cholinergic transmission in sympathetic ganglia. *Nature*, **282**, 515–516.

Krulich, L., Dhariwal, A. P. S., and McCann, S. M. (1973). Stimulatory and inhibitory effects of purified hypothalamic extracts on growth hormone release from rat pituitary *in vitro*. *Endocrinology*, **83**, 783–790.

Kuntz, A. (1938). The structural organization of the coeliac ganglia. *J. Comp. Neurol.*, **69**, 1–12.

Kuntz, A. (1940). The structural organization of the inferior mesenteric ganglia. *J. Comp. Neurol.*, **72**, 371–382.

Kuntz, A., and Saccomanno, G. J. (1944). Reflex inhibition of intestinal motility mediated through decentralized prevertebral ganglia. *J. Neurophysiol.*, **7**, 163–170.

Larsson, L.-I., and Rehfeld, J. F. (1979). Localization and molecular heterogeneity of cholecystokinin in the central and peripheral nervous system. *Brain Res.*, **165**, 201–218.

Larsson, L.-I., Fahrenkrug, J., Schaffalitzky de Muckadell, O., Sundler, F., Håkanson, R., and Rehfeld, J. (1976). Localization of vasoactive intestinal polypeptide (VIP) to central and peripheral neurons. *Proc. Natl. Acad. Sci. U.S.A.*, **73**, 3197–3200.

Lawson, H. (1934). Role of inferior mesenteric ganglia in diphasic response of colon to sympathetic stimuli. *Am. J. Physiol.*, **109**, 257–273.

Lawson, H., and Holt, J. P. (1937). Control of large intestine by decentralized inferior mesenteric ganglion. *Am. J. Physiol.*, **118**, 780–785.

Lewis, R. V., Stein, A. S., Kimura, S., Rossier, J., Stein, S., and Udenfriend, S. (1980). An about 50.000-dalton protein in adrenal medulla: A common precursor of met- and leu-enkephalin. *Science*, **208**, 1459–1461.

Lin, T. M. (1980). Pancreatic polypeptide: Isolation, chemistry and biological function. In *Gastrointestinal Hormones* (Ed. G. B. J. Glass), pp. 275–306, Raven Press, New York.

Lin, T. M., and Chance, R. E. (1974). Bovine pancreatic polypeptide (BPP) and avian pancreatic polypeptide (APP). *Gastroenterology*, **67**, 737–738.

Lindkaer Jensen, S., Fahrenkrug, J., Holst, J. J., Vagn Nielsen, O., and Schaffalitzky de Muckadell, O. B. (1978). Secretory effects of vasoactive intestinal polypeptide (VIP) on the isolated, perfused porcine pancreas. *Am. J. Physiol.*, **235**, E387–E391.

Lundberg, J. M. (1981). Evidence for coexistence of vasoactive intestinal polypeptide (VIP) and acetylcholine in neurons of cat exocrine glands. *Acta Physiol. Scand.*, **112** (Suppl. 496), 1–57.

Lundberg, J. M., Hökfelt, T., Nilsson, C., Terenius, L., Rehfeld, J., Elde, R. P., and Said, S. (1978). Peptide neurons in the vagus, splanchnic and sciatic nerves. *Acta Physiol. Scand.*, **104**, 499–501.

Lundberg, J. M., Hökfelt, T., Schultzberg, M., Uvnäs-Wallensten, K., Köhler, L., and Said, S. (1979). Occurrence of VIP-like immunoreactivity in cholinergic neurons of the cat: Evidence from combined immunohistochemistry and acetylcholine esterase staining. *Neuroscience*, **4**, 1539–1559.

Lundberg, J. M., Änggård, A., Fahrenkrug, J., Hökfelt, T., and Mutt, V. (1980a).

Vasoactive intestinal polypeptide in cholinergic neurons of exocrine glands: Functional significance of coexisting transmitters for vasodilation and secretion. *Proc. Natl. Acad. Sci. U.S.A.*, **77**, 1651–1655.

Lundberg, J. M., Hökfelt, T., Änggård, A., Kimmel, J., Goldstein, M., and Markey, K. (1980b). Coexistence of an avian pancreatic polypeptide (APP) immunoreactive substance and catecholamine in some peripheral and central neurons. *Acta Physiol. Scand.*, **110**, 107–109.

Lundberg, J. M., Hökfelt, T., Änggård, A., Uvnäs-Wallensten, K., Brimijoin, S., Brodin, E., and Fahrenkrug, J. (1980c). Peripheral peptide neurons: Distribution, axonal transport, and some aspects on possible function. In *Neural Peptides and Neuronal Communication* (Eds. E. Costa and M. M. Trabucchi), pp. 25–36, Raven Press, New York.

Lundberg, J. M., Änggård, A., Emson, P., Fahrenkrug, J., and Hökfelt, T. (1981). Vasoactive intestinal polypeptide and cholinergic mechanisms in cat nasal mucosa: Studies on choline acetyltransferase and release of vasoactive intestinal polypeptide. *Proc. Natl. Acad. Sci. U.S.A.*, **78**, 5255–5259.

Lundberg, J. M., Hökfelt, T., Änggård, A., Terenius, L., Elde, R., Markey, K., and Goldstein, M. (1982a). Organization principles in the peripheral sympathetic nervous system: Subdivision by coexisting peptides (somatostatin, avian pancreatic polypeptide-, and vasoactive intestinal polypeptide-like immunoreactivities). *Proc. Natl. Acad. Sci. U.S.A.*, **79**, 1303–1307.

Lundberg, J. M., Rökeaus, Å., Hökfelt, T., Rosell, S., Brown, M., and Goldstein, M. (1982b). Neurotensin-like immunoreactivity in the preganglionic sympathetic nerves and in the adrenal medulla of the cat. *Acta Physiol. Scand.*, **117**, 153–155.

McDonald, T. J., Jörnvall, H., Nilsson, G., Vagne, M., Ghatei, M., Bloom, S. R., and Mutt, V. (1979). Characterization of a gastrin releasing peptide from porcine non-antral gastric tissue. *Biochem. Biophys. Res. Commun.*, **90**, 227–233.

McLennan, H., and Pascoe, J. H. (1954). The origin of certain non-medullated nerve fibres which form synapses in the inferior mesenteric ganglion of the rabbit. *J. Physiol. (London)*, **124**, 145–156.

Moody, T. W., O'Donohue, T. L., and Jacobowitz, D. M. (1981). Biochemical localization and characterization of bombesin-like peptides in discrete regions of rat brain. *Peptides*, **2**, 75–79.

Mutt, V., and Jorpes, J. E. (1966). Cholecystokinin and pancreozymin, one single hormone? *Acta Physiol. Scand.*, **66**, 196–202.

Mutt, V., and Said, S. I. (1974). Structure of the porcine vasoactive intestinal octacosapeptide: The amino acid sequence. Use of kallikrein in its determination. *Eur. J. Biochem.*, **42**, 581–589.

Nagai, K., and Frohman, L. A. (1976). Hyperglycemia and hyperglucagonemia following neurotensin administration. *Life Sci.*, **19**, 273–280.

Nilsson, A. (1974). Structure of the vasoactive intestinal octacosapeptide from chicken intestine. Amino acid sequence. *FEBS. Lett.*, **60**, 322–326.

Noda, M., Furutani, Y., Takahashi, H., Toyosato, M., Hirose, T., Inayama, S., Nakanishi, S., and Numa, S. (1982). Cloning and sequence analysis of cDNA for bovine adrenal preproenkephalin. *Nature*, **295**, 202–206.

Pelto-Huikko, M., Hervonen, A., Helen, P., Linnoila, I., Pickel, V. M., and Miller, R. J. (1980). Localization of (Met[5])- and (Leu[5])-enkephalin in nerve terminals and SIF cells in adult human sympathetic ganglia. In *Histochemistry and Cell Biology of Autonomic Neurons, SIF cells, and Paraneurons* (Eds. O. Eränkö, S. Soinila, and H. Päivärinta), *Advances in Biochemical Psychopharmacology*, vol. 25, pp. 379–383, Raven Press, New York.

Pradayrol, L., Chayville, J., and Mutt, V. (1978). Pig duodenal somatostatin: Extraction and purification. *Metabolism*, **27** (Suppl. 1), 1197–1200.

Rehfeld, J. F., Goltermann, N., Larsson, L.-I., Emson, P. M., and Lee, C. M. (1979). Gastrin and cholecystokinin in central and peripheral neurons. *Fed. Proc.*, **38**, 2325–2329.

Rökaeus, A., Burcher, E., Chang, D., Folkers, K., and Yagima, H. (1977). Actions of neurotensin and (Gln^4)-neurotensin on isolated tissues. *Acta Pharmacol. Toxicol.*, **41**, 141–147.

Said, S. I. (1982). *Vasoactive Intestinal Polypeptide, Advances in Peptide Hormone Research*, Vol. 1, Raven Press, New York.

Said, S. I., and Mutt, V. (1970). Polypeptide with broad biological activity. Isolation from small intestine. *Science*, **169**, 1217–1218.

Said, S. I., and Mutt, V. (1972). Isolation from porcine intestine of a vasoactive octacosapeptide related to secretin and glucagon. *Eur. J. Biochem.*, **28**, 199–204.

Schally, A. V., Huang, W.-Y., Chang, R. C. C., Arimura, A., Redding, T. W., Millar, R. P., Hunkapiller, M. W., and Hood, L. E. (1980). Isolation and structure of pro-somatostatin: A putative somatostatin precursor from pig hypothalamus. *Proc. Natl. Acad. Sci. U.S.A.*, **77**, 4489–4493.

Schultzberg, M. (1980). Immunohistochemical evidence for bombesin-like immunoreactivity in nerve fibres in sympathetic ganglia. *Regul. Peptides*, Suppl. 1, S101.

Schultzberg, M. (1982a). The peripheral nervous system. In *Chemical Neuroanatomy* (Ed. P. Emson), Raven Press, New York, in press.

Schultzberg, M. (1982b). Bombesin-like immunoreactivity in sympathetic ganglia. *Neuroscience*, in press.

Schultzberg, M., Dreyfus, C. F., Gershon, M. D., Hökfelt, T., Elde, R., Nilsson, G., Said, S., and Goldstein, M. (1978a). VIP, enkephalin, substance P-, and somatostatin-like immunoreactivity in neurons intrinsic to the intestine: Immunohistochemical evidence from organotypic tissue cultures. *Brain Res.*, **155**, 239–248.

Schultzberg, M., Hökfelt, T., Lundberg, J. M., Terenius, L., Elfvin, L.-G., and Elde, R. (1978b). Enkephalin-like immunoreactivity in nerve terminals in sympathetic ganglia and adrenal medulla and in adrenal medullary gland cells. *Acta Physiol. Scand.*, **103**, 475–477.

Schultzberg, M., Hökfelt, T., Terenius, L., Elfvin, L.-G., Lundberg, J. M., Brandt, J., Elde, R. P., and Goldstein, M. (1979). Enkephalin immunoreactive nerve fibers and cell bodies in sympathetic ganglia of the guinea-pig and rat. *Neuroscience*, **4**, 249–270.

Schultzberg, M., Hökfelt, T., Nilsson, G., Terenius, L., Rehfeld, J. F., Brown, M., Elde, R., Goldstein, M., and Said, S. I. (1980). Distribution of peptide- and catecholamine-containing neurons in the gastro-intestinal tract of rat and guinea-pig: Immunohistochemical studies with antisera to substance P, vasoactive intestinal polypeptide, enkephalins, somatostatin, gastrin/cholecystokinin, neurotensin and dopamine β-hydroxylase. *Neuroscience*, **5**, 689–744.

Sjöqvist, F. (1962). Morphological correlate to a cholinergic sympathetic function. *Nature*, **194**, 298.

Sjöqvist, F. (1963). The correlation between the occurrence and localization of acetylcholinesterase-rich cell bodies in the stellate ganglion and the outflow of cholinergic sweat secretory fibres to the fore paw of the cat. *Acta Physiol. Scand.*, **57**, 339–351.

Sternberger, L. A. (1974). *Immunocytochemistry*, Prentice-Hall, Englewood Cliffs, NJ.

Studer, R. O., Trazeciak, H., and Lergier, W. (1973). Isolierung und Aminosäurese-
quenz von Substanz P aus Pferdedarm. *Helv. Chim. Acta*, **56**, 860–866.
Szurszewski, J. H., and Weems, W. A. (1976). Control of gastrointestinal motility by
prevertebral ganglia. In *Physiology of Smooth Muscle* (Eds. E. Bülbring and M. F.
Shuba), pp. 313–379, Raven Press, New York.
Tatemoto, K., and Mutt, V. (1980). Isolation of two novel candidate hormones using a
chemical method for finding naturally occurring polypeptides. *Nature*, **285**, 417–418.
Terenius, L., and Wahlström, A. (1974). Inhibitor(s) of narcotic receptor binding in
brain extracts and cerebrospinal fluid. *Acta Pharmacol. Toxicol.*, **35** (Suppl. 1), 55.
Terenius, L., and Wahlström, A. (1975). Search for an endogenous ligand for the
opiate receptor. *Acta Physiol. Scand.*, **94**, 78–81.
Vanderhaeghen, J. J., Signeau, J. C., and Gepts, W. (1975). New peptide in the
vertebrate CNS reacting with gastrin antibodies. *Nature*, **257**, 604–605.
Verhofstad, A. A. J., Steinbusch, H. W. M., Penke, B., Varga, J., and Joosten, H.
W. J. (1980). Use of antibodies to norepinephrine and epinephrine in immunohis-
tochemistry. In *Histochemistry and Cell Biology of Autonomic Neurones, SIF cells,
and Paraneurons* (Eds. O. Eränkö, S. Soinila and H. Päivärinta), *Advances in
Biochemical Psychopharmacology*, Vol. 25, pp. 185–193, Raven Press, New York.
Verhofstad, A. A. J., Steinbusch, H. W. M., Penke, B., Varga, J., and Joosten, H.
W. J. (1981). Serotonin-immunoreactive cells in the superior cervical ganglion of
the rat. Evidence for the existence of separate serotonin- and catecholamine-
containing small ganglionic cells. *Brain Res.*, **212**, 39–49.
von Euler, U. S., and Gaddum, J. H. (1931). An unidentified depressor substance in
certain extracts. *J. Physiol. (London)*, **72**, 74–87.
Williams, J. T., and North, R. A. (1978). Inhibition of firing of myenteric neurons by
somatostatin. *Brain Res.*, **155**, 165–168.

ACKNOWLEDGEMENTS

The present studies were supported by the Swedish Medical Research
Council (projects 04X-2887; 12X-5189), the Magnus Bergvall Foundation,
the Knut and Alice Wallenberg Foundation and funds from the Karolinska
Institutet.

Note

After the manuscript for this chapter was submitted, several research reports
have appeared in which immunoreactivity for substance P, vasoactive intestinal polypeptide (VIP) and enkephalin has been demonstrated at the
ultrastructural level in nerve fibers of prevertebral sympathetic ganglia of the
guinea pig:

H. Kondo and R. Yui, Brain Res. 1981, 222, 134–137; M. R. Matthews and
A. C. Cuello, Proc.Natl.Acad.Sci. USA 1982, 79, 1668–1672 (Substance P).

H. Kondo and R. Yui, Brain Res. 1982, 237, 227–231 (VIP).

H. Kondo and R. Yui, Brain Res. 1982, 252, 142–145 (Enkephalin).

Monoamine Connections in Sympathetic Ganglia

TERENCE WILLIAMS and JEAN JEW

Department of Anatomy, University of Iowa,
College of Medicine, Iowa 52242, USA

INTRODUCTION

The molecular, biostructural and physiological aspects of neuronal information processing are different parts of the same subject and each part is vital to understanding the transfer of information in a sympathetic ganglion. Although synapses are the most clearly identifiable communication sites, additional less easily observed binding sites for monoamines and other transmitters may influence ganglionic components to alter the propagation of signals to the output.

The preganglionic output was first seen to be connected to the postganglionic input in a beautifully simple way. In the beginning, it was envisioned that all sympathetic efferent pathways consist of two neurons (Sherrington, 1906), the presence of a nicotinic cholinergic synapse between preganglionic and postganglionic (Langley, 1893) neurons having been established by showing that intravenous administration of curare can cause interruption of ganglionic transmission (Langley and Dickinson, 1889). Subsequently, morphological, physiological and biochemical evidence emerged which seemed to indicate that the basic two neuron effector chain is only a foundation for a much more complex mechanism.

Since the discovery of chromaffin cells in sympathetic ganglia of many species including man (Smirnow, 1890; Kohn, 1902, 1903), the properties of these cells have been studied extensively. In spite of efforts using a variety of methods (see Coupland, 1965, for details) the chromaffin reaction is still not fully understood. Experiments on extraganglionic chromaffin tissue (Oliver and Schafer, 1894; Biedl and Wiesel, 1902) provided early indications that pressor substances were present and the active principle was named 'adrenaline' (Takamine, 1901) or 'epinephrine' (Aldrich, 1901). Iwanow (1932) conjectured that ganglionic chromaffin cells might secrete a substance that could act at sympathetic synapses, thereby enhancing transmission and, subsequently, Marazzi (1939) and Bulbring (1944) reported inhibition, in some cases followed by facilitation, by adrenaline. Later, a slow inhibitory postsynaptic potential (s-IPSP) was recorded in rabbit superior cervical ganglion (SCG) by Eccles and Libet (1961) and this appeared compatible with the view that the chromaffin cells release a catecholamine which diffuses to principal ganglionic neurons (PGNs), making them refractory to preganglionic stimulation.

What are the precise mechanisms for monoamine-induced effects on transmission through a sympathetic ganglion? Theoretically, monoamines may act at various intraganglionic sites (Black *et al.*, 1979), including preganglionic terminals, PGNs, small intraganglionic blood vessels and possibly Schwann cells, operating through different biochemical mechanisms, presumably by binding on to and activating receptors with different properties. The occurrence of many species and regional variations in these mechanisms, together with the failure of many scientists to recognize the full extent of these differences, has undoubtedly delayed our understanding of these mechanisms despite the accumulation of a large body of data generated from morphological studies, electrophysiological observations and biochemical/pharmacological experiments. The newer methods of immunocytochemistry will enable localization of various putative transmitters, such as serotonin (Verhofstad *et al.*, 1981), and establish which monoamines and neuropeptides are present in various ganglia. Electron microscopy should make it possible to demonstrate with precision the sites of release and, eventually, the specific receptor sites for these chemical mediators. Our present report addresses monoamine transmission in ganglia: in particular, interneuronal connections, the apparent transport from paraneurons (Heym and Williams, 1979) and the hypothesized existence of dendrodendritic connections between PGNs (Jacobowitz, 1970).

SIF CELLS AND GANGLIONIC TRANSMISSION

Much of the interest in SIF cells (for definition, see below) has arisen from a need to provide a structural basis for special features of synaptic transmission observed in various sympathetic ganglia (Fig. 1). In sympathetic ganglia of mammals and other vertebrates, the most regular and reproducible synaptic potential observed in the PGNs is a fast excitatory postsynaptic potential (f-EPSP) brought about by stimulation of the preganglionic fibres. In some PGNs of certain vertebrate sympathetic ganglia, the f-EPSP may be followed by slow potentials. The routes by which catecholamine travels from SIF cell to its sites of action is a question which remains partially unresolved. Another partially resolved question concerns the chemical identities of the SIF cell transmitters and/or modulators, indications being that they include catecholamines, serotonin and peptides and that a number of these may be present in a particular ganglion (Table 1). The slow postsynaptic potentials which have been attributed to the actions of catecholamines are of two types: (1) hyperpolarization expressed in the generation of an s-IPSP, and (2)

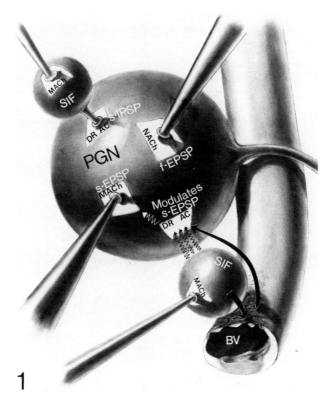

Figure 1 Schematic drawing representing some biochemical and physiological hypotheses for the roles of SIF cells in ganglionic transmission. Preganglionic fibres synapse on principal ganglionic neurons (PGNs) and SIF cells, releasing acetylcholine. *On the PGN*, acetylcholine binds to nicotinic receptors (NACh) to mediate the f-EPSP. *On the SIF cell*, it binds to muscarinic receptors (MACh) resulting in release of dopamine at the SIF cell efferent synapse (in the case of SIF cell interneurons) or into the ganglionic portal system or extracellular space (in the case of SIF cell paraneurons). At the SIF cell efferent synapse, dopamine release results in generation of a cyclic AMP mediated s-IPSP in the PGN. Dopamine reaching the PGN via portal vessels or the extracellular space may be responsible for enhancement of the s-EPSP. Other abbrev: DR AC = dopamine receptor–adenylate cyclase complex; BV = blood vessel

modulation expressed as a long-lasting enhancement of the s-EPSP (see below).

An indication that neuronal activity might regulate the sensitivity of the PGNs was provided by physiological and pharmacological experiments carried out in cat stellate ganglia (Eccles, 1943). Experiments by Libet and coworkers (see Libet, 1980, for review) suggested that release of a non-cholinergic transmitter is required to elicit the s-IPSP response in PGNs of

Table 1 Presumptive SIF cell transmitters

	Species	Ganglion	Reference
Dopamine	Rabbit	Superior cervical	Libet and Tosaka, 1970; Libet and Owman, 1974; Libet, 1979a; Kalix *et al.*, 1974
	Rat	Superior cervical	Rybarcyzk *et al.*, 1976; Björklund *et al.*, 1970; Lu *et al.*, 1976; Koslow, 1976
	Cat	Cervical; thoracic	Björklund *et al.*, 1970
	Guinea-pig	Superior cervical	König, 1979
	Pig	Cervical; thoracic	Björklund *et al.*, 1970
	Monkey	Superior cervical	Chiba *et al.*, 1977
Norepinephrine	Rat	Superior cervical	König and Heym, 1978; Eränkö and Eränkö, 1971; Lever *et al.*, 1976
		Paracervical	Rybarcyzk *et al.*, 1976
	Guinea-pig	Superior cervical	Elfvin *et al.*, 1975; König, 1979; Wamsley *et al.*, 1978
	Human	Superior cervical	Hervonen *et al.*, 1980
Epinephrine	Rat	Superior cervical	Koslow, 1976; Ciaranello *et al.*, 1973; Saavedra and Liuzzi, 1976
Serotonin	Rat	Superior cervical	Saavedra and Liuzzi, 1976; Verhofstad *et al.*, 1981; Eränkö and Härkönen, 1965
	Rabbit	Superior cervical	Dun *et al.*, 1980; Hertzler, 1961; Wallis and Woodward, 1974
Enkephalin	Guinea-pig	Superior cervical; coeliac-superior mesenteric; inferior mesenteric	Hökfelt, 1979; Schultzberg *et al.*, 1979

The pharmacological, physiological and morphological studies cited provide direct or indirect evidence for presumptive SIF cell neurotransmitters.

rabbit ganglia. They found that muscarinic agonists elicit a biphasic response: an initial hyperpolarization (s-IPSP) followed by a more prolonged depolarization (s-EPSP). When they stopped presynaptic release of transmitters by lowering the calcium/magnesium ratio, the s-IPSP was no longer elicited by muscarinic agonist stimulation. It was inferred that intraganglionic release of a second neurotransmitter is necessary for production of the s-IPSP and, in rabbit SCG, dopamine (DA) was believed to be this second transmitter.

However, in the same ganglion, DA may have an additional action as a modulator. The term 'modulation' as applied to synaptic actions has been defined as alteration of effective synaptic transmission by mechanisms other than changes in postsynaptic potentials or direct changes in excitatory level that may be produced by a transmitter (Libet, 1980). According to this definition, the observed DA-induced, long-lasting enhancement of the s-EPSP response to acetylcholine in the rabbit SCG is a modulatory effect.

While the physiologists were hypothesizing that mediation of the s-IPSP might be attributed to release of catecholamine by ganglionic chromaffin cells (Eccles and Libet, 1961), morphologists studying ganglia in cat (Hamberger *et al.*, 1963) and rat (Eränkö and Härkönen, 1963; Norberg and Sjöqvist, 1966) were describing cells which, with histochemical fluorescence techniques for monoamines, fluoresced strongly and were named small, intensely fluorescent (SIF) cells (Norberg and Sjöqvist, 1966). Using the electron microscope, Siegrist *et al.* (1966) and Grillo (1966) found groups of small cells containing granular vesicles in the rat SCG. Williams (1967) observed that these small granule-containing (SGC) cells in the rat SCG possess both afferent and efferent synapses and from this concluded that they were sympathetic ganglionic interneurons, making synaptic contact with processes which were presumed to be dendrites of PGNs. This view was confirmed by further ultrastructural studies (Siegrist *et al.*, 1968; Williams and Palay, 1969; Matthews and Raisman, 1969; Yokota, 1973). An indication that the SGC cells were ultrastructural counterparts of (at least some of) the SIF cells in rat SCG was obtained using fluorescence microscopy in conjunction with electron microscopy (Grillo *et al.*, 1974; Williams *et al.*, 1975, 1976b).

Although SIF cells have been found in SCG of all species studied so far, including rat, cat, mouse, rabbit, guinea-pig, ox, monkey, galago, hamster, and human (see Taxi, 1979, for review), efferent synapses have been reported only in certain ganglia of a few species. In addition to the rat, SIF cell efferent synapses have been described in SCG of monkey (Chiba *et al.*, 1977), rabbit and guinea-pig (Jew, 1980). Demonstration of SIF cell afferent and efferent synapses provided morphological evidence for an adrenergic interneuron in sympathetic ganglia.

This interneuron theory was supported by physiological and biochemical studies. Libet (1970) postulated that activation (by preganglionic afferents) of the muscarinic cholinergic receptor on the SIF cell leads to release of DA (in the rabbit SCG) from SIF cell efferents, causing the generation of an s-IPSP. It was found that preganglionic stimulation of rabbit SCG produced a 372% increase in cyclic AMP levels over control values, whereas postganglionic stimulation was without effect (McAfee *et al.*, 1971). When the rabbit SCG was stimulated physiologically with a single supramaximal stimulus (in the presence of hexamethonium to abolish f-EPSPs), theophylline potentiated the hyperpolarization produced by this stimulus and, in addition, DA and monobutyryl cyclic AMP each caused hyperpolarization of the resting membrane potential—an action potentiated by theophylline. Therefore, Greengard and his colleagues hypothesized that preganglionic stimulation of the muscarinic cholinergic receptor on the SIF cell leads to release of DA at the efferent synapse between the SIF cell and the PGN. DA binds to a DA receptor, activating an adenylate cyclase to cause increased cyclic AMP synthesis within the PGN. The increase in cyclic AMP leads to hyperpolarization of the PGN, resulting in generation of an s-IPSP (Greengard, 1976) (Fig. 1). Whether or not the s-IPSP is mediated by cyclic AMP is discussed in detail in the chapter by Kobayashi and Tosaka. A search for a DA receptor–adenylate cyclase complex in other species revealed its presence in the cow (Kebabian and Greengard, 1971; Black *et al.*, 1978), small amounts in the cat (Black *et al.*, 1978) and none in the rat (Cramer *et al.*, 1973; Lindl and Cramer, 1975) or guinea-pig (Wamsley *et al.*, 1978). However, the cow and guinea-pig possess β-adrenergic receptor–adenylate cyclase complexes (Kebabian and Greengard, 1971; Wamsley *et al.*, 1978, 1980), whereas the cat SCG has none.

Whereas some SIF cells seem to fulfil the classical morphological criteria of interneurons, other SIF cells seem to lack 'axonal' projections and may not engage in classical-type chemical efferent synapses. Such SIF cells could release their transmitters into intraganglionic (portal) blood vessels and/or into the extracellular space to act on PGNs located some distance away. The longer time required for these transport mechanisms would be compatible with the second action of DA described for rabbit SCG by the physiologists: modulation by enhancement of the s-EPSP.

The extraordinary species differences in the small, monoamine-containing intraganglionic cells of sympathetic ganglia have been the subject of numerous biostructural, biochemical and electrophysiological reports and, until we have more complete knowledge, extrapolations and broad generalizations across species lines has little to commend it.

MORPHOLOGICAL FEATURES OF SIF CELLS

In the majority of species studied, SIF cells of the SCG are rather sparse; in the order of 2 to 7 cells per mg of tissue (Table 2). The rat and guinea-pig ganglia stand apart, being rich in SIF cells (one or two orders of magnitude more in guinea-pig and rat, respectively). We have found that SIF cells are numerous also in the hamster. This suggests that the mechanisms for intraganglionic modulation may be either quantitatively or qualitatively different in rodents.

In most species studied it is possible to distinguish, on the basis of morphological characteristics, two categories of SIF cell in the SCG (Williams *et al.*, 1976b). We designated as type I SIF cells those which have long varicose processes extending among ganglionic neurons. Type II SIF cells, on the other hand, are intimately related to subcapsular or stromal blood vessels: an arrangement reminiscent of some endocrine glands. As a general rule,

Table 2 SIF cells in the superior cervical sympathetic ganglia of different species

Species	Total No. of cells	No. of cells per mg tissue	No. of ganglia examined
Cow	6480 ± 150[a]	5.2 ± 0.1[a]	3
Cat	104	4.1	1
Monkey	68.8 ± 19[a]	2.3 ± 0.7[a]	4
Rabbit	284 ± 110[a]	6.9 ± 0.5[a]	3
Rat	368 ± 12[a]	280 ± 30[a]	3
Guinea-pig	372 ± 103[a]	76 ± 20[a]	4

[a] Mean ± S.E.M.
Taken from Williams *et al.*, 1977.

type I SIF cells are solitary whereas type II SIF cells are found in clusters. The rat and guinea-pig break this rule, however, since in both cases fairly long varicose fluorescent processes can be observed arising from the clustered SIF cells. In both these rodents, small clusters of SIF cells are located among ganglionic neurons. Therefore we speculated that type I and type II SIF cells form intermingled clusters in some ganglia, such as in rat and guinea-pig SCG. For this reason no attempt was made to differentiate type I and type II SIF cells in either of these species. It should be noted that a number of authors (Watanabe, 1971; Heym and Williams, 1979; Taxi, 1979) have designated SIF cell types on the basis of their granules.

In semithin sections stained with toluidine blue, SIF cells appear much smaller than PGNs, with diameters approximately 10–25 μm. Compared to PGNs and Schwann cells, SIF cell cytoplasm and nuclei are pale. The nuclei are round or oval, with chromatin condensations along the periphery (Fig. 2). In electron micrographs, the most conspicuous feature of SIF cells is the presence of dense-cored vesicles which may vary in size, shape, and electron density according to species, fixation and different physiological states (see Taxi, 1979, and chapter by Taxi for review). Although SIF cell processes are also characterized by the presence of dense-cored vesicles in their cytoplasm, it has been claimed that they cannot be distinguished conclusively from other nerve processes (Siegrist *et al.*, 1968; Watanabe, 1971). The SIF cell efferent synapse in the rat SCG shows the following features which distinguish it from other synapses in the ganglion: (1) a presynaptic cluster of vesicles, with patches of electron-dense material apposed to the membrane; (2) a synaptic cleft containing a moderately electron-dense substance after osmic acid fixation; (3) a postsynaptic web which in some cases is unevenly developed in different parts of the contact zone. As in the SIF cell perikarya and their processes, the most striking feature of efferent synapses is the presence of large granule-containing presynaptic vesicles (LGVs).

Yokota (1973) made a careful three-dimensional analysis of a cluster of four SIF cells in rat SCG. All four of these cells received afferent synapses. So

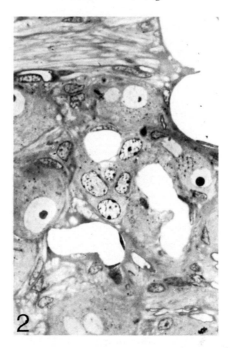

Figure 2 Typical arrangement of SIF cells from rabbit SCG seen in a plastic-embedded 0.5 μm section stained with toluidine blue. The cluster of five SIF cells resembles in size an average ganglion cell and, as is typically the case, the cluster lies in apposition to blood capillaries. Most of the chromatin of the nucleus is distributed in clumps against the nuclear membrane. ×675

far as she could determine, only two of them made efferent somatodendritic synapses with presumed PGNs. The other two cells were naked (i.e. without Schwann cell sheath covering) over a greater area than those which possessed efferent synapses. A direct diffusion of the SIF cells' secretory products within the rat ganglion was discussed by Taxi (1979), and Yokota's findings support the view that there may be two modes of distribution of transmitter from SIF cells.

MONOAMINERGIC TRANSMISSION VIA SYNAPTIC INTERACTIONS

The sympathetic ganglia contain the synapses between preganglionic and postganglionic neurons, the latter referred to as PGNs in this chapter. In addition, many believe that sensory axons are also found in sympathetic ganglia, conveying signals via dorsal root ganglia to the central nervous system (Léránth *et al.*, 1970, 1980a). Each preganglionic fibre synapses with more than one PGN, Billingsley and Ranson (1918) having claimed a ratio of approximately one preganglionic fibre to 32 PGNs in cat SCG while Wolf (1941) estimated a ratio between 1:11 and 1:17. It was also suggested by Billingsley and Ranson (1918) that connector neurons form the linkages between preganglionic axons and PGNs; and Lawrentjew (1924) deduced— from persistence of pericellular plexuses in the SCGs of cats and rabbits after complete preganglionic and postganglionic transection—that intraganglionic connector neurons must exist. Although Samuel (1951) concluded after experimental studies in rat SCG that such intraganglionic connector neurons were unlikely, later electro-microscopic work demonstrated the presence of SGC cells in rat SCG (Siegrist *et al.*, 1966; Grillo, 1966) and provided direct evidence for the interneuronal nature of these cells (Williams, 1967).

Yokota's (1973) study of four granule-containing cells in rat SCG under-lined the possibility that different SIF cell types may coexist in a single cluster. On this basis, the proposal that some granule-containing cells of a cluster may be interneurons and the others paraneurons appears to have achieved wide acceptance (but the possibility must be entertained that some synapses could be missed using thin-section sampling at 0.5 μm intervals). According to Verhofstad *et al.* (1981), some SIF cell groups in rat SCG (presumptive serotonin-containing granule-containing cells) are provided with clearly observable processes whereas other groups (presumptive catecholamine-containing) are generally without processes. The former may make inter-neuronal connections and the latter may be less likely to form axosomatic synapses on PGNs. To recognize that the members of any SIF cell cluster may differ so widely from those of other clusters opens up a new range of potential interpretations of SIF cell function, and it should be emphasized that the problems of interpretation call for caution.

Recent findings indicate that SIF cell clusters may be quite dissimilar in (1) the nature of their monoamine transmitter(s), (2) their action(s) upon other ganglionic cells and (3) the biostructurally describable aspects of transmis-sion, for example by synaptic or endocrine (paraneuronal) communication or both. Although the same considerations apply to other species, we have noted (Williams *et al.*, 1976b, 1977) that the SIF cells of the rat SCG have a different distribution pattern from those seen in some other species. To the extent that basic properties of SIF cells vary between species and between individual ganglia, information obtained about any one sympathetic ganglion (e.g. rat SCG) can only provide indications of the kinds of intraganglionic monoaminergic interactions that may exist within other ganglia. In the rabbit, we observed SIF efferent terminals (identifiable by proximity to SIF cells and their similar vesicle appearances to the latter cells), making synaptic contacts with presumed PGN dendrites and dendritic spines. Thus, as in rat SCG (Williams, 1967) we hypothesize that in the rabbit these granule-containing cells are interneurons interposed between the preganglionic and postganglionic elements. In the guinea-pig SCG, the nature of the postsynaptic element usually observed is different. In our experience the efferent synaptic contacts made by SIF cells in the guinea-pig were restricted to soma-to-soma, soma-to-process, process-to-soma and process-to-process contacts between granule-containing cells. Presumably, the modifier processes in ganglia differ widely because they bring about divergent and unique responses in a range of organs and animals that are as varied behaviourally as taxonomically. Thus it needs to be recognized that synaptic relationships in any one ganglion need not be identical, or even necessarily similar, to those found in another ganglia, and this opens up a wide range of potential possibilities.

Based on the presence of small, dense-cored vesicles in postsynaptic elements, Yokota (1973) made the suggestion that, in rat SCG, granule-containing cell efferents may synapse with recurrent collateral axons, but it has been noted (Taxi, 1965, 1973, 1979) that it is not unusual to find small, dense-cored vesicles within the dendrites of PGNs. Despite the generally accepted view that synapses between granule-containing cells do not occur (Siegrist *et al.*, 1968) or are rare except in axotomized ganglia (Matthews, 1976), our recent data from guinea-pig SCG (see below) make it more difficult to deny the possibility that SIF to SIF contacts may occur in normal rat ganglia also. But we have observed no clear example of such a connection.

SIF cell or PGN regulation by axon collaterals from PGNs is another possibility to be considered. Dail and Evan (1978) have asked whether a presynaptic element can always be identified as belonging to a SIF cell and indeed there could be other sources for some of the catecholaminergic terminals observed in sympathetic ganglia. The electron microscope does not always differentiate with certainty between a process of a SIF cell (in which small granule-containing vesicles may be present) and an axon collateral from a PGN. It is also necessary to determine whether or not SIF cells and/or PGNs make synaptic contacts with preganglionic cholinergic axons, since there is evidence (Nishi, 1979) that the latter may possess α_2-receptors and that transmission can be blocked by an α_2-agonist. In monkey SCG, Chiba *et al.* (1977) observed presynaptic elements (which contained large dense-cored as well as other vesicles) making synaptic contact with presumed cholinergic elements (see Fig. 8 in Chiba *et al.*, 1977). Also, Elfvin (1971) reported that the cat inferior mesenteric ganglion contains a large number of apparent axoaxonic synapses between preganglionic axons.

It is possible that dendrodendritic interactions may significantly influence ganglionic transmission. Various writers (Dogiel, 1895, 1896, 1899; Ramon y Cajal, 1911; De Castro, 1932) have studied dendritic forms in ganglia in great detail and have noted that, while some dendrites taper until they are almost invisible, others end in small swellings. De Castro (1932) referred to dendritic 'receptor plates' and Mitchell (1953) has remarked that, in the prevertebral ganglia, dendrites are sometimes spread out at their terminations like small brushes. The possible existence of associative connections between PGNs (Elfvin, 1971; Jacobowitz, 1970; Kondo *et al.*, 1980) deserves further study. In rabbit and guinea-pig SCG (Jew, 1980), as in the rat, dense-cored vesicles are sometimes found clustered against regions of the plasma membranes of unidentified nerve processes. This occurs at sites where such a process is separated from another nerve fibre profile by a gap not exceeding 200 Å, or where the plasma membrane is in direct continuity with the extracellular space.

MONOAMINERGIC TRANSMISSION VIA PARANEURONS

The electron-microscopic evidence that there is an interneuron in the rat SCG has now become well accepted. In the SCG of the monkey, morphological and biochemical observations have provided supporting, though so far inconclusive, evidence for the presence of interneurons (Chiba *et al.*, 1977); and some, at least, of the SGC cells in guinea-pig and rabbit superior ganglia meet the ultrastructural criteria for interneurons (Jew, 1980). However, the generalization cannot be made that all small monoamine-storing cells are interneurons. Some SIF cells may share the properties of both interneurons and paraneurons. One of the more interesting elaborations of the accepted views on transmission is the concept of an intraganglionic portal system for distributing the monoamine from ganglionic paraneurons.

Paraneurons are cells of neuroectodermal origin, produce peptide hormones and/or substances related to or identical with a monoamine transmitter, and form neurosecretory-like granules which are released in response to membrane depolarization (Fujita, 1976). Paraneurons secreting into an intraganglionic portal circulation could influence a very large number of PGNs. Capillary fenestrations observed in some species near groups of SGC cells (Siegrist *et al.*, 1968; Williams *et al.*, 1976a) may facilitate entry of the monoamine or peptide into the capillaries.

In the small arboreal shrew *Tupaia glis*, a primate at the lowest stage of phylogeny (Noback and Moskowitz, 1963), large clusters of small cells were observed in the SCG (Heym and Williams, 1979). As many as 300 SIF cells were counted in a single cluster. Large aggregates of SIF cells were also a feature of the *Tupaia* sellate ganglia examined in the same study. In *Tupaia*, two main vessels generally enter the SCG at its inferior pole in association with the preganglionic trunk. Thin-walled vascular channels resembling glomeruli arise from the main vessels and these glomeruli are interconnected by long narrow channels (Fig. 3). The small cells, corresponding to the SIF cells of fluorescence microscopy, are located adjacent to the curled capillaries of the glomeruli.

In preparations made with the glyoxylic acid method for catecholamine fluorescence, the SIF cells can be distinguished by their relatively bright

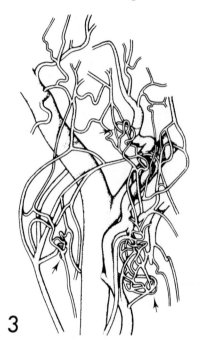

3

Figure 3 Reconstruction drawing made from 80 1 µm plastic-embedded sections of *Tupaia* SCG, stained with toluidine blue. It illustrates blood vessels found near the caudal pole of the ganglion, with glomerulus-like loops of small vessels (arrows). From Heym and Williams, 1979, *Evidence for autonomic paraneurons in sympathetic ganglia of a shrew (Tupaia glis)*, in Journal of Anatomy. Reproduced by permission of Cambridge University Press

fluorescence, which varies from bright yellow to green. The SIF cell clusters in *Tupaia* SCG are very unevenly dispersed (Heym and Williams, 1979), and the cells of these clusters are devoid of processes or else possess only short ones mainly directed towards the blood vessels. The relatively few solitary SIF cells possess long, varicose processes which sometimes ramify between principal ganglionic neurons and are indistinguishable from type I SIF cells (presumptive interneurons) of other species (Williams *et al.*, 1976b). On the basis of vesicle criteria alone, two populations of SGC cells were distinguished within the cluster. Some contain 'type A' spherical vesicles averaging 60–80 nm in size, enclosing cores of intermediate electron density. Other SGC cells contain 'type B' vesicles of greater size (ranging from 100 to 200 nm in diameter) and electron density. Both varieties of SGC cells were encountered in the same cell cluster. Our type A granules resemble in electron density the epinephrine-containing granules of rat adrenal medulla (Coupland and Hopwood, 1966). The hypothesis that different catecholamines are associated with type A or B granules in *Tupaia* may be ascertainable using immuno-cytochemical methods.

The vascular path for transportation of the SIF cell transmitter(s) is rather clearly defined in *Tupaia*, providing new morphological evidence for the existence of a portal system for conveying monoamines from clusters of paraneurons to PGNs. Where they approach the basal membrane of blood capillary endothelium, SGC cells often lack a covering sheath, an arrangement that could facilitate the transport of monoamines into the blood vessels, as was inferred also by Elfvin *et al.* (1975) who were studying SGC cells in the mesenteric ganglion of the guinea-pig. On the basis of fluorescence microscopy, the relatively small number (14.3% of total SIF cells) of solitary SIF cells in *Tupaia* SCG may be interneurons because, although there has been no electron-microscopic identification of efferent synapses, their processes are much longer than those of the paraneurons and wind among PGNs.

MONOAMINERGIC CONNECTIONS AND GANGLIONIC FUNCTION AS CONTRASTED IN RABBIT, GUINEA-PIG AND HAMSTER

SIF cells have been identified in every sympathetic ganglion examined and exhibit considerable variations in their numbers, specific catecholamines, and morphological characteristics (see Williams *et al.*, 1976a, b, 1977, for review). Arguments for specific functional roles for SIF cells have been strongest when supported by a combination of biochemical, physiological and morphological data, and such studies have been most extensive in the rabbit SCG.

Rabbit

Libet and his co-workers described two postsynaptic actions, an s-IPSP (Kobayashi and Libet, 1970; Libet, 1970) and s-EPSP (Libet and Tosaka, 1970) in PGNs of rabbit SCG. They concluded that intraganglionic release of a second, non-cholinergic transmitter is required between preganglionic release of acetylcholine and the s-IPSP response and that the transmitter is DA. The SIF cell seemed a likely candidate to fulfil the role of the adrenergic interneuron hypothesized to mediate the s-IPSP (Eccles and Libet, 1961). The fluorophore in rabbit SCG SIF cells is DA; and either orthodromic, preganglionic nerve impulses or direct action by a muscarinic agonist releases DA from SIF cells (Libet and Owman, 1974). It was shown that depletion of DA content in SIF cells was accompanied by a reduction in the s-IPSP response and that a complete loss of the s-IPSP response occurred when total DA concentration was lowered by about 50% (Libet and Owman, 1974). When depleted SIF cells took up exogenous DA, a partial restoration of the s-IPSP response was noted. Biochemical studies by Greengard and his colleagues (McAfee and Greengard, 1972; McAfee *et al.*, 1971; Greengard,

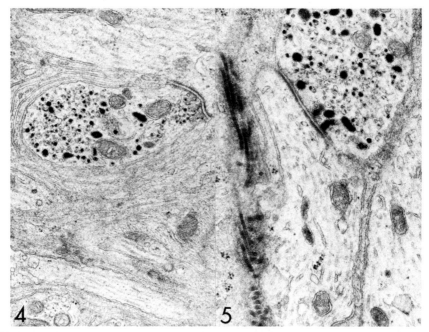

Figures 4, 5 Electron micrographs of SCG from rabbits treated with the monoamine marker analog 5-OHDA.
Figure 4: A presumed SIF cell process (containing large and small granular vesicles) is in synaptic contact with a presumed dendrite of a PGN. ×27 000.
Figure 5: A nerve process found near a SIF cell cluster and containing large and small granular vesicles makes an efferent contact with a presumed PGN dendrite. In the latter is an elongated profile containing material of moderate electron density. ×30 750.

1976) demonstrated a DA-activated DA receptor–adenylate cyclase complex in the rabbit SCG and this led them to conclude that the s-IPSP is generated by SIF cell activation of an adenylate cyclase to cause increased cyclic AMP synthesis by the PGN. The increase in cyclic AMP leads to hyperpolarization of the PGN, resulting in the generation of an s-IPSP.

Ultrastructural evidence for SIF cell interneurons in rabbit SCG has been provided (Jew, 1980). After 5-hydroxydopamine (5-OHDA) pretreatment to mark monoamine-containing vesicles, the ganglia were processed for light and electron microscopy. Thin sections containing SIF cells were surveyed to locate catecholaminergic synapses and nerve cell bodies and processes containing the electron-dense marker. SIF cells occurred doth singly and in clusters adjacent to blood vessels and contained large granular vesicles (LGVs) 1800 to 3000 Å in diameter. Terminals of cholinergic type (Matthews and Raisman, 1969) containing agranular vesicles together with some granular vesicles devoid of the 5-OHDA marker made synaptic contact with SIF cells and processes of PGNs. Nerve processes containing LGVs were, with few exceptions (which may have arisen from SIF cells outside the plane of the section), found within 150 μm of SIF cell bodies, and some of these processes were traced back to their SIF cell bodies of origin. SIF cell processes containing LGVs made synaptic contacts with presumed PGN dendrites (Figs. 4, 5) or dendritic spines. For the time being, it must suffice to indicate that the postsynaptic elements have the morphological features of dendrites and dendritic spines (of PGNs) since we did not trace them back to their somata of origin. This interpretation seems inherently reasonable, since these presumed PGN dendrites were devoid of the LGVs found in SIF cells.

The 5-OHDA marker was also found in small granular vesicles (SGVs) of PGNs and their processes and in nerve processes whose cells of origin were unknown. However, synaptic terminals containing marked granular vesicles were not observed in areas distant from the SIF cells, so we obtained no support for the suggestion that PGNs may give rise to feedback collaterals (Jacobowitz, 1970). Some of the presumed PGN dendrites were observed to have clusters of SGVs along portions of the plasma membrane that were devoid of Schwann cell sheath (Fig. 6).

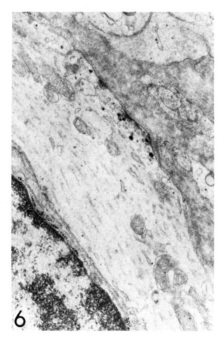

Figure 6 Electron micrograph of rabbit SCG treated with the monamine marker analog 5-OHDA. A number of small and intermediate vesicles, some containing the monoamine marker, lie adjacent to the plasma membrane of the presumed PGN dendrite which, at this point, has no sheath cell covering. ×22 000

Therefore, it seems that, in the rabbit, SIF cells fulfil the morphological criteria of interneurons. However, some problems arise in designating the SIF cell as the direct and only mediator for the s-IPSP in all PGNs.

(1) In the first place, the numbers of SIF cells are quite small in SCG of rabbit as well as of other species compared to the numbers of PGNs and reportedly an s-IPSP can be elicited from virtually all PGNs (Kobayashi and Libet, 1970; Libet, 1970). Figure 7, representing surveys of SIF cells and processes containing LGVs and SGVs and PGN cell bodies in a single section of rabbit ganglion, is provided to address what we believe is an important question. Although some of the LGV-containing processes may arise from SIF cells in other sections, processes containing LGVs are present in significant numbers only in the vicinity of the SIF cells. It can be argued that the smaller and more peripheral processes of SIF cells may contain only SGVs. However, our fluorescence-microscopic preparations show that SIF cell processes seldom exceed 200 μm in length and have only modest numbers of branches (in contrast to axons from locus coeruleus cells whose small numbers belie the extent of their widespread innervation). How extensive are the synaptic fields of the ganglionic SIF cells? Libet and Owman (1974) reported that the fluorescent fibre network surrounding nearly all of PGNs contains DA. When horseradish peroxidase was applied to the postganglionic nerve, no label was found in 'adrenergic terminals' in the SCG (Dail and Evan, 1978), leading the investigators to conclude that the terminals were not of PGN origin. From these and other studies (Dail and Wood, 1977) it is suggested that the adrenergic terminals around the PGNs are of intraganglionic origin and represent ubiquitous DA-releasing sites by which SIF cells might elicit s-IPSPs in most or all of the PGNs. From our surveys of sections from rabbit SCG we can make no claim that all PGNs receive direct synaptic input from a SIF cell. 5-OHDA-labelled processes observed in more distant areas of the section contained SGVs.

Figure 7   Reconstruction of part of an ultrathin section of rabbit SCG. The only group of SIF cells found in this section is enclosed within the rectangle. The solid squares indicate locations of nerve processes which contain large granular vesicles (LGVs). It is inferred that these are SIF cell processes and they are located preferentially close to the SIF cell group. Others many have arisen from SIF cells outside the plane of section. Solid triangles represent nerve processes containing small granular vesicles (SGVs)

Figure 8   Reconstruction from a part of an ultrathin section of guinea-pig SCG. The only two SIF cell bodies in the plane of section are enclosed in the rectangle. As in Fig. 7, solid squares represent profiles containing large granular vesicles (LGVs). Groups of these profiles are located near the SIF cells as well as in two locations at the upper and lower parts of the right side of the field. Again, it is inferred that they represent SIF cell processes although some of the presumed SIF cells clusters are presumed to be outside the plane of section. Profiles containing small granular vesicles (SGVs) are distributed evenly across the section

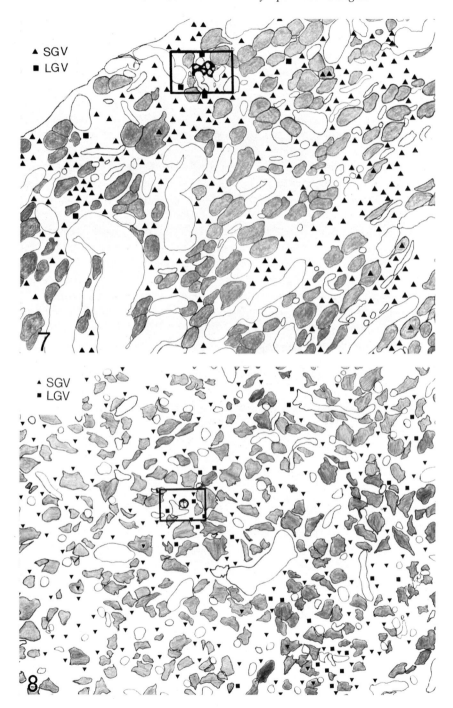

(2) As seen in thin sections of rabbit SCG, SIF cell efferent synapses are not abundant. Our observations lead us to hypothesize that the basic requirements for direct synaptic communication from SIF cells to PGNs are clearly only present in relatively small zones around SIF cells. 'Long-calls', conveying hypothesized messages from SIF cells to more distant PGNs, would appear to call for one or more of a number of alternative mechanisms: (a) dendrodendritic (or axodendritic) connections between PGNs, (b) transport of the transmitter(s) through intraganglionic blood vessels, or (c) diffusion through intercellular spaces. It has been hypothesized that the relatively long synaptic delay preceding the s-IPSP could be accomplished by a close proximity of the s-IPSP receptors to DA-releasing sites (Libet, 1979b); i.e. classical type synapses may not be necessary. Although our own work in the rabbit SCG and that of others (Dail and Evan, 1978) showed nerve processes with labelled granular vesicles close to portions of 'unsheathed' plasma membrane, as yet there is no morphological evidence for release of the transmitter from these processes into the extracellular space. Libet (1980) has reported an s-IPSP response in the rabbit SCG which is mediated by a norepinephrine (NE)-releasing intraganglionic structure which is non-muscarinically activated. This type of s-IPSP could be generated by elements other than SIF cells and is compatible with the dendrodendritic communication model proposed by investigators of ganglia of other species (Elfvin, 1971; Jacobowitz, 1970; Kondo *et al.*, 1980).

Many SIF cells including their processes are located close to intraganglionic blood vessels. This applies to many species. The frequent absence of a Schwann cell sheath around these processes coupled with fenestrations in the vascular endothelium supports the hypothesis that the SIF cells may engage in vascular secretion. This would be compatible with the other observed postsynaptic action by DA in rabbit SCG, that of modulatory enhancement of the s-EPSP. Therefore, morphological and physiological observations indicate that SIF cells may act both as interneurons and paraneurons.

Guinea-pig

In the guinea-pig SCG, the SIF cell circuitry differs from that of the rabbit, in terms of morphology, biochemistry and physiology. As in the rabbit ganglion, SIF cells were arranged in clusters adjacent to blood vessels (Fig. 8) and were characterized by the presence of many LGVs, approximately 2000 Å in diameter, which contained the 5-OHDA marker. Some SIF cell processes have been found in close relationship to capillary walls. SIF cell processes contain LGVs and some SGVs (Fig. 9) and synapse with SIF cell bodies and SIF cell processes (Figs. 10–12). The synaptic specializations include presynaptic vesicles, presynaptic dense patches (presumptively related to a vesicle release phenomenon) (Taxi, 1979), a clear synaptic gap and a fine postsynaptic web. To be sure, it is quite possible that there may be exceptions but it appears clear that, in guinea-pig SCG, SIF cells make direct associative connections with other SIF cells. As in the rabbit, we found sites on unidentified neurites where the plasma membrane was in direct continuity with the extracellular space, and dense-cored vesicles labelled with 5-OHDA were clustered against the plasma membranes at these sites.

In contrast to the rabbit, an s-IPSP has not been found in the guinea-pig SCG (Libet, 1970). In addition, biochemical studies indicate that the DA/NE ratio of this ganglion was only 1/8 of that in rabbit SCG (Black *et al.*, 1979). It is possible that this small amount of DA (in the guinea-pig) is present merely as an NE precursor. Whereas the rabbit SCG contains a DA receptor–adenylate cyclase complex, the guinea-pig ganglion contains a β-adrenergic receptor adenylate cyclase complex (Wamsley *et al.*, 1980). Although pre-ganglionic stimulation elevated cyclic AMP levels in rabbit SCG, this effect was completely lacking in the guinea-pig. Immunohistochemical studies have demonstrated that SIF cells contain dopamine β-hydroxylase (but not pheny-lethanolamine-*N*-methyltransferase), providing additional evidence that NE is a transmitter in SIF cells of the guinea-pig SCG. Since the s-IPSP is absent in the guinea pig SCG, the effect, if any, of the β-adrenergic receptor–adenylate cyclase complex is not known.

The presence of associative synapses between SIF cells, the absence of the DA receptor complex and the lack of an s-IPSP, all indicate that the mechanism of SIF cell action in the guinea-pig SCG differs from that in the rabbit SCG. The versatility of monoaminergic ganglionic communication is well expressed in the differences between SIF cell morphology and transmitter biochemistry in the rabbit versus guinea-pig SCG. Although it appears that, in the rabbit some PGNs could respond to synaptic input on the SIF cells, the finding of SIF to SIF synapses in the guinea-pig strengthens the case for a transmitter portal pathway perhaps with assistance from transmitter diffusing through the intracellular space. In *Tupaia* we have provided evidence for such a pathway (Heym and Williams, 1979).

Hamster

Some preliminary work has been carried out on another rodent, the hamster (Black *et al.*, 1979). Isoproterenol, a β-adrenergic agonist, increases cyclic AMP levels in the hamster SCG; DA produces no cyclic AMP response. Therefore, as in rat and guinea-pig SCG, hamster SCG contains a β-adrenergic receptor adenylate cyclase complex, but lacks a DA receptor–adenylate cyclase complex. Also, the low DA/NE ratio suggests that NE may be a SIF cell transmitter. Electron microscopy (unpublished observations) showed that SIF cells of the hamster SCG receive afferent input from presumed preganglionic cholinergic fibres (Fig. 13). In close proximity to SIF

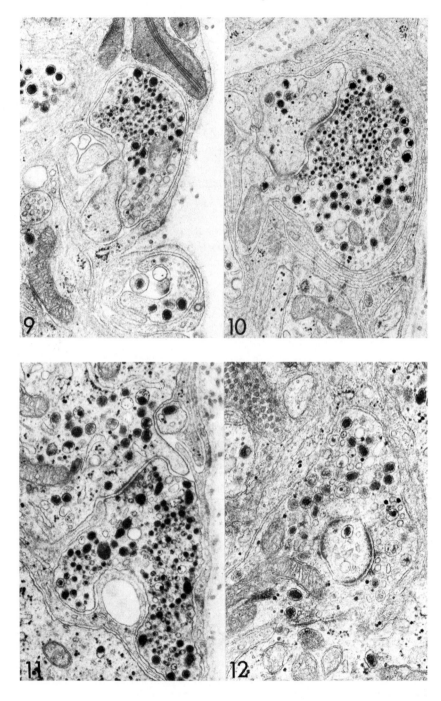

cell bodies, SIF cell processes can be seen making synaptic contact with neurite processes (Fig. 14). The neurite processes we have observed do not contain the LGVs characteristic of SIF cells processes, but it is still necessary to seek confirmation that the SIF cell processes are synapsing with PGNs.

The three species cited above exemplify the complexities surrounding the role of the SIF cell in ganglionic transmission. The SIF cell appears to fit quite well the roles of the adrenergic interneuron which might, in some ganglia, produce the s-IPSP and the paraneuron which might account for the enhanced s-EPSP, although questions regarding the number, distribution and mechanisms by which SIF cells might mediate the s-IPSP of PGNs remain to be resolved. Other mammalian species in which the s-IPSP has been identified in the SCG are cat and rat (Libet, 1970). SCGs of both species contain a DA receptor–adenylate cyclase complex (Black *et al.*, 1974, Cramer *et al.*, 1973; Williams *et al.*, 1975) and their SIF cells reportedly contain DA (see section above on SIF cell transmitters). Libet (1970) postulated that the s-IPSP represents an independent and specific synaptic transmitter effect of DA in the rabbit SCG. An analogous role for certain NE-containing SIF cells (e.g. guinea-pig and hamster), activated by a nicotinic–type of cholinergic action, remains an untested possibility. Also, the possible role of NE in mediating the long-lasting modulatory synaptic action on the s-EPSP—as DA-containing SIF cells do according to the hypothesis of Kobayashi and Libet (1970)—has not been tested in ganglia with NE-containing SIF cells. Finally, it should be emphasized that although much morphological, physio-logical, and biochemical data point to the likelihood that SIF cells mediate presynaptic inhibition by catecholamines, the depression of presynaptic function by applied exogenous catecholamines is presently classified as a pharmacological rather than a physiological phenomenon (Libet, 1980). Indeed, the complexity and variability of the SIF cell transmitters and their connections would suggest multiple mechanisms for their regulatory actions in ganglionic transmission.

Figures 9–12   Electron micrographs from guinea-pig SCG. The animals were treated with the monoamine analog marker 5-OHDA.
Figure 9: SIF cell processes including a terminal packed with vesicles of different sizes lie in the neuropil, covered with thin sheaths of Schwann cell cytoplasm. ×29 250.
Figure 10: A large SIF cell terminal makes efferent synaptic contact with a smaller profile containing large dense-cored vesicles. ×27 350.
Figure 11: Typical SIF to SIF synaptic contact as seen in guinea-pig SCG. Vesicles and presynaptic dense projections are seen on one side of the contact site, and a postsynaptic web is present on the other. In the region of the contact site, it is possible to see electron-dense material in the synaptic gap. ×34 100.
Figure 12: An SIF cell terminal surrounds and synapses with a presumed SIF cell spinous process. ×31 500.

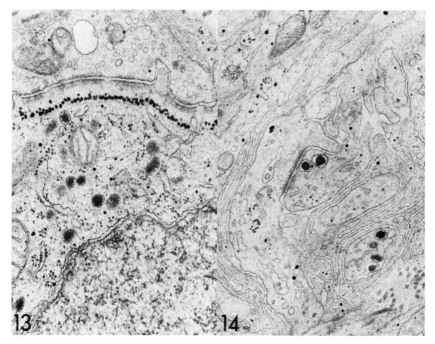

Figures 13, 14   Electron micrographs of hamster SCG. The animals were treated with the monoamine analog marker 5-OHDA.
Figure 13: The presumed preganglionic axon terminal forms a connection with the soma of a SIF cell. Note the line of presumed glycogen particles neatly arranged parallel to the contact site, within the SIF cell cytoplasm. ×33 750.
Figure 14: A SIF cell process makes an efferent contact with a presumed PGN dendrite. ×28 200.

SUMMARY

Figure 15 provides a summary of the monoaminergic connections in sympathetic ganglia as proposed by morphological findings. This diagram is actually a composite of observations by several investigators in several species (*vide supra*). It is proposed that monoaminergic transmission occurs via interneurons, whereby the preganglionic fibre synapses on a monoaminergic interneuron (the SIF cell), which in turn synapses with the PGN (a). The monoaminergic SIF cell has also been observed making another type of connection—SIF cell to SIF cell (b). Preganglionic axons may also synapse with SIF cells which act as paraneurons, releasing their transmitter into extracellular space or into intraganglionic portal vessels (c), thereby influencing a large pool of PGNs. It has also been suggested that SIF cells may make synaptic contact with cholinergic preganglionic fibres (d) (Chiba *et al.*, 1977). Monoaminergic transmission within the ganglion may also be effected via

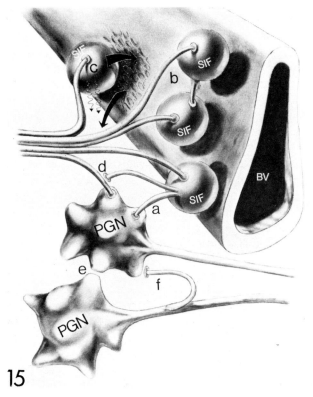

Figure 15 Schematic drawing illustrating morphological features of monoaminergic transmission that have been claimed for sympathetic ganglia. SIF cells receive preganglionic cholinergic inputs and (a) send efferents to synapse on principal ganglionic neurons (PGNs), (b) synapse with other SIF cells, (c) transport their transmitter substance presumably to PGNs via portal vessels (BV) or through the extracellular space, (d) influence PGN firing by acting on the preganglionic axon. Reportedly, PGNs may influence other PGNs via (e) dendrodendritic connections and (f) axon collaterals. BV =

PGNs, which may communicate with and influence firing of other PGNs via dendrodendritic or dendrosomatic connections (e) (Elfvin, 1971; Kondo *et al.*, 1980) or via recurrent collaterals (f) (Grillo, 1966). Although supporting morphological data are thus far lacking, other types of monoaminergic connections have been hypothesized including axoaxonic connections between PGNs, between PGNs and preganglionics and between PGNs and SIF cells (see Williams *et al.*, 1976a, for review).

Regarding monoaminergic transmission in sympathetic ganglia, the mechanisms are still far from clear. The messages that the ganglia eventually transmit to the viscera and blood vessels have far-reaching and important consequences, and it appears that the nature of the messages is influenced by numerous modifying mechanisms within the ganglion. The SIF cell appears to be a major modifying mechanism, perhaps, as hypothesized, by being responsible for s-IPSPs and modulation of s-EPSPs in some cases and operating via different mechanisms in others. Indeed, it has been speculated that 'the particular effects of the (SIF) cells may prove to be at least as numerous as the various methods of recruitment, types of transmitter or neurohumoral secretion, postsynaptic sites or neuroendocrine targets, and varieties of receptor mechanisms would permit' (Matthews, 1980). Although the connections and transmitters and therefore the mechanisms by which SIF cells operate may differ in different species, one consistent feature is their presence in every sympathetic ganglion of every species studied, including man.

Although SIF cells which act as interneurons may have been demonstrated only in certain ganglia of certain species, it may be that they are few in number in some ganglia and difficult to discover. Since in some ganglia the number of SIF cells and efferent synapses is small relative to the number of PGNs, SIF cells may be involved only to a limited extent as local circuit neurons. In any event, the proximity of SIF cells, including some of those identified as interneurons, to blood vessels would support the concept of a dual role for SIF cells—paraneuronal and interneuronal. Whether their function is inhibitory (Libet, 1980; Siegrist *et al.*, 1968) or facilitatory (Libet, 1980), or both, the SIF cells would influence the messages ultimately generated by the PGN. That SIF cells have this ability and that SIF cell dysfunctions may be related to dysfunctions in the organism's homeostatic mechanisms, have been hinted at by studies in the spontaneously hypertensive rat. Lütold *et al.* (1979) found that dihydroxyphenylacetic acid levels, a relative measure of DA release and metabolism, were lower than normal in the coeliac ganglion of spontaneously hypertensive rats at a stage when hypertension is developing, where NE levels were above normal. In addition, Saavedra (personal communication) has observed elevated DA levels in the stellate ganglion of spontaneously hypertensive rats. Further dynamic studies are needed to elucidate the physiological role of SIF cells within ganglia.

Exogenous monoamines are able to effect ganglionic transmission (Marazzi, 1939; see Libet, 1980, for review; Dun *et al.*, 1980) but studies are not yet sufficient to support the contention that exogenous monoamines have a major physiological role in transmission. Further investigations of monoaminergic connections and other sites of release of monoamines and peptides would be of prime importance in determining the sites of action of these transmitters within the ganglia and their roles in he regulation of transmission.

REFERENCES

Aldrich, T. B. (1901). A preliminary report on the active principle of the suprarenal gland. *Am. J. Physiol.*, **5**, 457–461.

Biedl, A., and Wiesel, J. (1902). Ueber die functionelle Bedeutung der Nebenorgane des Sympathicus (Zuckerkandl) und der chromaffinen Zellgruppen. *Pflügers Arch. Gesamte Physiol.*, **91**, 434–461.

Billingsley, P. R., and Ranson, S. W. (1918). On the number of nerve cells in the ganglion cervicale and of nerve fibers in the cephalic end of the truncus sympathicus in the cat, and on the numerical relations of the preganglionic and postganglionic neurones. *J. Comp. Neurol.*, **29**, 359–384.

Björklund, A., Cegrell, L., Falck, B., Ritzen, M., and Rosengren, E. (1970). Dopamine-containing cells in sympathetic ganglia. *Acta Physiol. Scand.*, **78**, 334–338.

Black, A. C., Jr., Bhalla, R. C., and Williams, T. H. (1974). Mechanisms of neural transmission in the superior cervical ganglia of the cat and rabbit: morphological and biochemical correlates. *Anat. Rec.*, **178**, 311.

Black, A. C., Jr., Chiba, T., Wamsley, J. K., Bhalla, R. C., and Williams, T. H. (1978). Interneurons of sympathetic ganglia: Divergent cyclic AMP responses and morphology in cat and cow. *Brain Res.*, **148**, 389–398.

Black, A. C., Jr., Jew, J. Y., West, J. R., Wamsley, J. K., Sandquist, D., and Williams, T. H. (1979). Catecholamines and cyclic nucleotides in the modulation of superior cervical ganglia. *Neurosci. Biobehav. Rev.*, **3**, 125–135.

Bülbring, E. (1944). Action of adrenaline on transmission in the superior cervical ganglion. *J. Physiol. (London)*, **103**, 55–67.

Chiba, T., Black, A. C., Jr., and Williams, T. H. (1977). Evidence for dopamine-storing interneurons and paraneurons in rhesus monkey sympathetic ganglia. *J. Neurocytol.*, **6**, 441–453.

Ciaranello, R. D., Jacobowitz, D., and Axelrod, J. (1973). Effect of dexamethasone on phenylethanolamine *N*-methyltransferase in chromaffin tissue of the neonatal rat. *J. Neurochem.*, **20**, 799–805.

Coupland, R. E. (1965). *The Natural History of the Chromaffin Cell*, Longmans, Green and Co., London.

Coupland, R. E., and Hopwood, D. (1966). The mechanism of differential staining reaction for noradrenalin- and adrenalin-storing granules in tissues fixed in glutaraldehyde. *J. Anat.*, **100**, 227–243.

Cramer, H., Johnson, D. G., Hanbauer, I., Silberstein, S. D., and Kopin, I. J. (1973). Accumulation of adenosine 3′,5′-monophosphate induced by catecholamines in rat superior cervical ganglion *in vitro*. *Brain Res.*, **53**, 97–104.

Dail, W. G., and Evan, A. P. (1978). Ultrastructure of adrenergic terminals and SIF cells in the superior cervical ganglion of the rabbit. *Brain Res.*, **148**, 469–477.

Dail, W. G., and Wood, J. (1977). Studies on the possibility of an extraganglionic source of adrenergic terminals to the superior cervical ganglion. *Soc. Neurosci. Abstr.*, **3**, 248.

De Castro, F. (1932). Sympathetic ganglia: normal and pathological. In *Cytology and Cellular Pathology of the Nervous System* (Ed. W. Penfield), pp. 319–379, Hoeber, New York.

Dogiel, A. S. (1895). Zur Frage über den feineren Bau des sympathischen Nervensystems bei den Saugenthieren. *Arch. Mikrosk. Anat.*, **46**, 305–344.

Dogiel, A. S. (1896). Zwei arten sympathischer Nervenzellen. *Anat. Anz.*, **11**, 679–687.

Dogiel, A. S. (1899). Ueber den Bau der Ganglien in den Geflechten des Darmes und der Gallenblase des Menschen und der Säugenthiere. *Arch. Anat. Physiol. Anat. Abt.*, 130–158.

Dun, N. J., Ingerson, A., and Karczmar, A. G. (1980). A neurochemical and neurophysiological study of serotonin in the superior cervical ganglia of the rabbit. *Society for Neuroscience 10th Annual Meeting*, Vol. 6, p. 216.

Eccles, J. C. (1943). Synaptic potentials and transmission in sympathetic ganglia. *J. Physiol. (London)*, **101**, 465–483.

Eccles, R. M., and Libet, B. (1961). Origin and blockade of the synaptic responses of curarized sympathetic ganglia. *J. Physiol. (London)*, **157**, 484–503.

Elfvin, L. G. (1971). Ultrastructural studies on the synaptology of the inferior mesenteric ganglion of the cat. III. The structure and distribution of the axodendritic and dendrodendritic contacts. *J. Ultrastruct. Res.*, **37**, 432–448.

Elfvin, L. G., Hökfelt, T., and Goldstein, M. (1975). Fluorescence microscopical, immunohistochemical and ultrastructural studies on sympathetic ganglia of the guinea pig, with special reference to the SIF cells and their catecholamine content. *J. Ultrastruct. Res.*, **51**, 377–396.

Eränkö, L., and Eränkö, O. (1971). Effect of guanethidine on nerve cells and small intensely fluorescent cells in sympathetic ganglia of new born and adult rats. *Acta Pharmacol. Toxicol.*, **30**, 403–416.

Eränkö, O., and Härkönen, M. (1963). Histochemical demonstration of fluorogenic amines in the cytoplasm of sympathetic ganglion cells of the rat. *Acta Physiol.*, **58**, 285–286.

Eränkö, O., and Härkönen, M. (1965). Monoamine-containing small cells in the superior cervical ganglion of the rat and an organ composed of them. *Acta Physiol. Scand.*, **63**, 511–512.

Fujita, T. (1976). The gastro-enteric endocrine cell and its paraneuronic nature. In *Chromaffin, Enterochromaffin and Related Cells* (Eds. R. E. Coupland and T. Fujita), pp. 191–208, Elsevier, Amsterdam.

Greengard, P. (1976). Possible role for cyclic nucleotides and phosphorylated membrane proteins in postsynaptic actions of neurotransmitters. *Nature*, **260**, 101–108.

Grillo, M. A. (1966). Electron microscopy of sympathetic tissues. *Pharmacol. Rev.*, **18**, 387–399.

Grillo, M. A., Jacobs, L., and Comroe, J. H., Jr. (1974). A combined fluorescence histochemical and electron microscopic method for studying special monoamine-containing cells (SIF cells). *J. Comp. Neurol.*, **153**, 1–14.

Hamberger, B., Norberg, K. A., and Sjoqvist, F. (1963). Cellular localization of monoamines in sympathetic ganglia of the cat. A preliminary report. *Life Sci.*, **9**, 659–661.

Hertzler, E. C. (1961). 5-Hydroxytryptamine and transmission in sympathetic ganglia. *Br. J. Pharmacol. Chemother.*, **17**, 406–413.

Hervonen, A., Pickel, V. M., Joh, T. H., Reis, D. J., Linnoila, I., Kanerva, L., and Miller, R. J. (1980). Immunocytochemical demonstration of the catecholamine-synthesizing enzymes and neuropeptides in the catecholamine-storing cells of human fetal sympathetic nervous system. In *Histochemistry and Cell Biology of Autonomic Neurons, SIF Cells and Paraneurons* (Eds. O. Eränkö, S. Soinila and H. Päivärinta), *Advances in Biochemical Psychopharmacology*, Vol. 25, pp. 373–378, Raven Press, New York.

Heym, C., and Williams, T. H. (1979). Evidence for autonomic paraneurons in sympathetic ganglia of a shrew (*Tupaia glis*). *J. Anat.*, **129**, 151–164.

Hökfelt, T. (1979). Polypeptides: Localization. *Neurosci. Res. Prog. Bull.*, **17**, 424–443.

Iwanow, G. (1932). Das chromaffine und interreale System des Menschen. Ergeb. *Anat. Entwicklungsgesch.*, **29**, 87–280.

Jacobowitz, D. (1970). Catecholamine fluorescence studies of adrenergic neurons and chromaffin cells in sympathetic ganglia. *Fed. Proc.*, **29**, 1929–1944.

Jew, J. Y. (1980). Connections of local circuit neurons in guinea pig and rabbit superior cervical ganglia. In *Histochemistry and Cell Biology of Autonomic Neurons, SIF Cells, and Paraneurons* (Eds. O. Eränkö, S. Soinila and H. Päivä-rinta), *Advances in Biochemical Psychopharmacology*, Vol. 25, pp. 119–125, Raven Press, New York.

Kalix, P., McAfee, D. A., Schorderet, M., and Greengard, P. (1974). Pharmaco-logical analysis of synaptically mediated increase in cyclic adenosine monophos-phate in rabbit superior cervical ganglion. *J. Pharmacol. Exp. Ther.*, **188**, 676–687.

Kebabian, J. W., and Greengard, P. (1971). Dopamine-sensitive adenyl cyclase: Possible role in synaptic transmission. *Science*, **174**, 1346–1349.

Kobayashi, H., and Libet, B. (1970). Actions of noradrenaline and acetylcholine on sympathetic ganglion cells. *J. Physiol. (London)*, **208**, 353–372.

Kohn, A. (1902). Das Chromaffin Gewebe. *Ergeb. Anat. Entwicklungsgesch.* **12**, 253–348.

Kohn, A. (1903). Die paraganglion. *Arch. Mikrosk. Anat.*, **62**, 263–365.

Kondo, H., Dun, N. J., and Pappas, G. D. (1980). A light and electronmicroscopic study of the rat superior cervical ganglion cells by intracellular HRP-labelling. *Brain Res.*, **197**, 193–199.

König, R. (1979). Consecutive demonstration of catecholamines and dopamine-β-hydroxylase within the same specimen. *Histochemie*, **61**, 301–305.

König, R., and Heym, C. (1978). Immunofluorescence localization of dopamine-β-hydroxylase in small intensely fluorescent cells of the rat superior cervical ganglion. *Neurosci. Lett.*, **10**, 187–191.

Koslow, S. H. (1976). Mass fragmentographic analysis of SIF cell catecholamines of normal and experimental rat sympathetic ganglia. *Fogarty Int. Cent. Proc.*, **30**, 82–88.

Langley, J. N. (1893). Preliminary account of the arrangement of the sympathetic nervous system based chiefly on observations upon pilomotor nerves. *Proc. R. Soc. London Ser. B.*, **52**, 547–556.

Langley, J. N., and Dickinson, W. L. (1889). On the local paralysis of peripheral ganglia, and on the connection of different classes of nerve fibres with them. *Proc. R. Soc.*, **46**, 423–431.

Lawrentjew, B. J. (1924). Zur Morphologie des Ganglion cervicale super. *Anat. Anz.*, **58**, 529–539.

Léránth, Cs., and Ungvary, Gy. (1970). Axon terminals of spinal ganglia and terminal ganglion cells in the prevertebral ganglia. *Septième Congres International de Microscopie Electronique* (Ed. P. Favard), pp. 741–742, Grenoble.

Léránth, Cs., and Ungvary, Gy. (1980a). Axon types of irevertebral ganglia and the peripheral autonomic reflex arc. *J. Autonom. Nerv. Syst.*, **1**, 265–281.

Léránth, Cs., Williams, T. H., Jew, J. Y., and Arimura, A. (1980b). Immunoelec-tron-microscopic identification of somatostatin in cells and axons of guinea pig sympathetic ganglia. *Cell Tissue Res.*, **212**, 83–89.

Lever, J. D., Santer, R. M., Lu, K. S., and Presley, R. (1976). Electron probe X-ray microanalysis of small granulated cells in rat sympathetic ganglia after sequential aldehyde and dichromate treatment. *J. Histochem. Cytochem.*, **25**, 275–279.

Libet, B. (1970). Generation of slow inhibitory and excitatory postsynaptic potentials. *Fed. Proc.*, **29**, 1945–1956.

Libet, B. (1979a). Dopaminergic synaptic processes in the superior cervical ganglion: models for synaptic actions. In *The Neurobiology of Dopamine* (Eds. A. Horn, J. Korf and B. H. C. Westerink), Academic Press, London.

Libet, B. (1979b). Slow postsynaptic actions in ganglionic functions. In *Integrative Functions of the Autonomic Nervous System* (Eds. C. M. Brooks, K. Koizumi and A. K. Sato), pp. 197–222, University of Tokyo Press and Elsevier/North-Holland Biomedical Press, Amsterdam.

Libet, B. (1980). Functional roles of SIF cells in slow synaptic actions. In *Histochemistry and Cell Biology of Autonomic Neurons, SIF Cells and Paraneurons* (Eds. O. Eränkö, S. Soinila and H. Päivärinta), *Advances in Biochemical Psychopharmacology*, Vol. 25, pp. 111–118, Raven Press, New York.

Libet, B., and Owman, C. (1974). Concomitant changes in formaldehyde-induced fluorescence of dopamine interneurons and in slow inhibitory postsynaptic potentials of the rabbit superior cervical ganglion, induced by stimulation of the preganglionic nerve or by a muscarinic agent. *J. Physiol. (London)*, **237**, 635–662.

Libet, B., and Tosaka, T. (1970). Dopamine as a synaptic transmitter and modulator in sympathetic ganglia: a different mode of synaptic action. *Proc. Natl. Acad. Sci. U.S.A.*, **67**, 667–673.

Lindl, T., and Cramer, H. (1975). Evidence against dopamine as the mediator of the rise in cyclic AMP in the superior ganglion of the rat. *Biochem. Biophys. Res. Commun.*, **65**, 731–739.

Lu, K. S., Lever, J. D., Santer, R. M., and Presley, R. (1976). Small granulated cell types in rat superior cervical and cardiac-mesenteric ganglia. *Cell Tissue Res.*, **172**, 331–343.

Lütold, B. E., Karoum, F., and Neff, N. H. (1979). Deficient dopamine metabolism in the celiac ganglion of spontaneously hypertensive rats. *Circ. Res.*, **44**, 467–471.

Marazzi, A. S. (1939). Electrical studies on the pharmacology of autonomic synapses. II. The action of a sympathetic drug (epinephrine) on sympathetic ganglia. *J. Pharmacol. Exp. Ther.*, **65**, 395–404.

Matthews, M. R. (1976). Synaptic and other relationships of small granule-containing cells (SIF cells) in sympathetic ganglia. In *Chromaffin, Enterochromaffin and Related Cells* (Eds. R. E. Coupland and T. Fujita), pp. 131–146, Elsevier, Amsterdam.

Matthews, M. R. (1980). Ultrastructural studies relevant to the possible functions of small granule-containing cells in the rat superior cervical ganglion. In *Histochemistry and Cell Biology of Autonomic Neurons, SIF Cells and Paraneurons* (Eds. O. Eränkö, S. Soinila and H. Päivärinta), *Advances in Biochemical Psychopharmacology*, Vol. 25, pp. 77–86, Raven Press, New York.

Matthews, M. R., and Raisman, G. (1969). The ultrastructure and somatic efferent synapses of small granule-containing cells in the superior cervical ganglion. *J. Anat.*, **105**, 255–282.

McAfee, D. A., and Greengard, P. (1972). Adenosine 3′,5′-monophosphate: electrophysiological evidence for a role in synaptic transmission. *Science*, **178**, 310–312.

McAfee, D. A., Schorderet, M., and Greengard, P. (1971). Adenosine 3′,5′-monophosphate in nervous tissue: Increase associated with synaptic transmission. *Science*, **171**, 1156–1158.

Mitchell, G. A. G. (1953). *Anatomy of the Autonomic Nervous System*, E. and S, Livingstone, Edinburgh and London.

Nishi, S. (1979). The catecholamine-mediated inhibition in ganglionic transmission. In *Integrative Functions of the Autonomic Nervous System* (Eds. C. M. Brooks, K. Koisumi and A. Sato), pp. 223–233, University of Tokyo Press and Elsevier/North-Holland Biomedical Press, Amsterdam.

Noback, C., and Moskowitz, N. (1963). The primate nervous system: functional and structural aspects. In *Evolutionary and Genetic Biology of Primates* (Ed. J. Buettner-Janusch), Vol. 1, pp. 131–177, Academic Press, New York.

Norberg, K. A., and Sjöqvist, F. (1966). New possibilities for adrenergic modulation of ganglionic transmission. *Pharmacol. Rev.*, **18**, 743–751.

Oliver, G., and Schäffer, E. A. (1894). The physiological effects of extracts of the suprarenal capsules. *J. Physiol. (London)*, **18**, 230–276.

Ramon y Cajal (1911). *Histologie du Systeme Nerveux de l'Homme et des Vértebrés*, Edition Française, traduite de l'espagnol par le Dr. L. Azoulay. A. Marloine, Paris.

Rybarczyk, K. E., Baker, H. A., Burke, J. P., Hartman, B. K., and Van Orden, L. S., III. (1976). Histochemical and immunocytochemical identification of catecholamines, dopamine-β-hydroxylase and phenylethanolamine-N-methyltransferase. *Fogarty Int. Cent. Proc.*, **30**, 68–81.

Saavedra, J. M., and Liuzzi, A. (1976). Nerve growth factor: effects on 5-hydroxytryptamine and phenylethanolamine-N-methyltransferase in the superior cervical ganglion of the rat. *Fogarty Int. Cent. Proc.*, **30**, 124–131.

Samuel, E. P. (1951). *Anatomy of the Autonomic Nervous System* (Ed. G. A. G. Mitchell), E. and S. Livingstone, Edinburgh and London.

Schultzberg, M., Hökfelt, T., Terenius, L., Elfvin, L.-G., Lundberg, J. M., Brandt, J., Elde, R., and Goldstein, M. (1979j'. Enkephalin immunoreactive nerve terminals and cell bodies in sympathetic ganglia of the guinea-pig and rat. *Neuroscience*, **4**, 249–270.

Sherrington, C. S. (1906). *Integrative Action of the Nervous System*, Yale University Press, New Haven.

Siegrist, G., de Ribaupierre, F., Dolivo, M., and Rouiller, C. (1966). Les cellules chromaffin des ganglions cervicaux superieurs du rat. *J. Microsc. (Paris)*, **5**, 791–794.

Siegrist, G., Dolivo, M., Dunanat, Y., Foroglou-Kerameus, C., de Ribaupierre, F., and Rouiller, Ch. (1968). Ultrastructure and function of the chromaffin cells in the superior cervical ganglion of the rat. *J. Ultrastruct. Res.*, **25**, 381–407.

Smirnow, A. E. von (1890). Die Struktur der Nervenzellen im Sympathiens der Amphibien. *Arch. Mikrosk. Anat.*, **35**, 407–424.

Takamine, J. (1901). Adrenaline, the active principle of the suprarenal glands and its mode of preparation. *Am. J. Pharm.*, **73**, 523–531.

Taxi, J. (1965). Contribution á l'étude des connexions des neurones moteurs du système nerveux autonome. *Ann. Sci. Nat. Zool.*, **7**, 413–674.

Taxi, J. (1973). Observations complementaires sur l'ultrastructure des ganglions sympathiques des mammiféres. *Trab. Inst. Cajal Invest. Biol.*, **65**, 9–40.

Taxi, J. (1979). The chromaffin and chromaffin-like cells in the autonomic nervous system. *Cytologia*, **56**, 283–343.

Verhofstad, A. A. J., Steinbusch, H. W. M., Penke, B., Varga, J., and Joosten, H. W. J. (1981). Serotonin-immunoreactive cells in the superior cervical ganglion of the rat. Evidence for the existence of separate serotonin- and catecholamine-containing small ganglionic cells. *Brain Res.*, **212**, 39–49.

Wallis, D. I., and Woodward, B. (1974). The facilitatory actions of 5-hydroxytryptamine and bradykinin in the superior ganglion of the rabbit. *Br. J. Pharmacol.*, **51**, 521–531.

Wamsley, J. K., Black, A. C., Jr., Redick, A., West, J. R., and Williams, T. H. (1978). SIF cells, cyclic AMP responses and catecholamines of the guinea pig superior cervical ganglion. *Brain Res.*, **156**, 75–82.

Wamsley, J. K., Black, A. C., Jr., West, J. R., and Williams, T. H. (1980). Cyclic AMP synthesis in guinea pig superior cervical ganglia: response to pharmacological and preganglionic physiological stimulation. *Brain Res.*, **182**, 415–421.

Watanabe, H. (1971). Adrenergic nerve elements in the hypogastric ganglion of the guinea pig. *Am. J. Anat.*, **130**, 305–330.

Williams, T. H. (1967). Electron microscopic evidence for an autonomic neuron. *Nature*, **214**, 309–310.

Williams, T. H., and Palay, S. L. (1969). Ultrastructure of the small neurons in the superior cervical ganglion. *Brain Res.*, **15**, 17–34.

Williams, T. H., Black, A. C., Chiba, T., and Bhalla, R. C. (1975). Morphology and biochemistry of small, intensely fluorescent cells of sympathetic ganglia. *Nature*, **256**, 315–317.

Williams, T. H., Black, A. C., Jr., Chiba, T., and Jew, J. (1976a). Interneurons/SIF cells in sympathetic ganglia of various mammals. In *Chromaffin, Enterochromaffin and Related Cells* (Eds. R. E. Coupland and T. Fujita), pp. 95–116, Elsevier, Amsterdam.

Williams, T. H., Chiba, T., Black, A. C., Jr., Bhalla, R. C., and Jew, J. (1976b). Species variation in SIF cells of superior cervical ganglia: are there two functional types? *Fogarty Int. Cent. Proc.*, **30**, 143–162.

Williams, T. H., Black, A. C., Jr., Chiba, T., and Jew, J. Y. (1977). Species differences in mammalian SIF cells. In *SIF Cells* (Eds. E. Costa and G. L. Gessa), *Advances in Biochemical Psychopharmcology*, Vol. 16, pp. 505–511, Raven Press, New York.

Wolf, G. A., Jr. (1941). The ratio of preganglionic neurons to postganglionic neurons in the visceral nervous system. *J. Comp. Neurol.*, **75**, 235–243.

Yokota, R. (1973). The granule-containing cell somata in the superior cervical ganglion of the rat, as studied by a serial sampling method for electron microscopy. *Z. Zellforsch. Mikrosk. Anat.*, **141**, 331–345.

Autonomic Ganglia
Edited by Lars-Gösta Elfvin
© 1983 John Wiley & Sons Ltd

Fast Synaptic Transmission in Autonomic Ganglia

V. I. SKOK

Bogomoletz Institute of Physiology, Bogomoletz Street, Kiev 24, USSR

Neurons in autonomic ganglia respond by changes in their membrane potential to the action of various neurotransmitters and hormones which alter the ionic permeability of the cell membrane through the activation of appropriate membrane receptors (see reviews by, for example, Skok, 1973, 1980a, b; Kuba and Koketsu, 1978). In particular, nicotinic cholinergic receptors (AChRs) are responsible for a fast excitatory postsynaptic potential (f-EPSP) that triggers the initiation of the postsynaptic spike. Activation of other receptors is usually followed by slow changes in the membrane potential that do not trigger spike initiation but play a modulatory role only. Some studies indicate that synaptic transmission through sympathetic ganglia may occur via non-nicotinic mechanisms (Jänig *et al.*, 1979). However, the evidence for this is still scarce.

There are autonomic ganglia where the postsynaptic spike is triggered by electrical transmission. In this case the action current of the preganglionic fibre directly stimulates the postsynaptic neuron causing the fast post-junctional potential. Only fast transmission, i.e. nicotinic and electrical, is discussed in this review.

NEURONAL ORGANIZATION OF THE FAST PATHWAY

Types of pathways

There are three types of pathways in autonomic ganglia: centrifugal, peripheral reflex and intrinsic. Centrifugal pathways exist in all autonomic ganglia; they comprise preganglionic fibres and the neurons that receive preganglionic innervation. Peripheral reflex pathways are present only in a few extramural ganglia (solar plexus and inferior mesenteric ganglia), but they are common for intramural ganglia, for example for the myenteric plexus. Peripheral reflex pathways are composed of afferent fibres of peripheral origin and neurons that receive afferent innervation through nicotinic synapses (see Skok, 1973, p. 35). Instrinsic pathways are present exclusively in intramural ganglia. Besides the above neurons, they include spontaneously active neurons and interneurons (Hirst *et al.*, 1972; Nishi and North, 1973; Wood, 1975; Wood and Mayer, 1979; Hirst, 1979; Furnes and Costa, 1980). A detailed analysis of fast transmission only in the centrifugal pathway will be presented here since it has been studied better than other pathways.

Centrifugal pathway

There are no internuncial neurons in centrifugal pathways in either sympathetic or extramural parasympathetic ganglia. The evidence for this has been obtained mainly from morphological studies: no intact presynaptic terminals have been observed in the ganglia following degeneration of their preganglionic fibres (Lakos, 1970; see Gabella, 1976, p. 27).

The results of early electrophysiological studies were confusing: the delay in transmission through some pathways in mammalian sympathetic ganglia was much longer than in other pathways of the same ganglia suggesting involvement of the internuncial neurons in the transmission (see Skok, 1973, p. 70). However, according to recent results, such long delays are due to low conduction velocities in preganglionic terminals that extend over long distances inside the ganglion. Their conduction velocities range from 2 to 10% of the conduction velocities in corresponding preganglionic fibres. If this is taken into account, the mean value of true synaptic delay is 1.6 msec (Skok and Heeroog, 1975), which is similar to the value found in amphibian sympathetic ganglia (1.5–2.0 msec: Christ and Nishi, 1971), a value much longer than that found in neuromuscular junctions, (0.22 msec: Hubbard and Schmidt, 1963).

There is evidence that transmission through the centrifugal extramural pathway may be more complex than the above simple scheme. In amphibian sympathetic ganglion the spike evoked by direct stimulation is followed by the appearance of a low calcium- and *d*-tubocurarine-sensitive local response suggesting that there are recurrent pathways which operate through nicotinic transmission (Minota and Koketsu, 1978). Nicotinic transmission has also been found between the neurons in amphibian parasympathetic ganglia (Roper, 1976) and between cultured mammalian sympathetic neurons (O'Lague *et al.*, 1978), in addition to their contacts with preganglionic neurons (Ko *et al.*, 1976). The physiological role of such interneuronal contacts remains unknown.

Conduction velocities in preganglionic and postganglionic fibres range from 0.4 m/sec (Blackman *et al.*, 1969) to 35 m/sec (Skok and Heeroog, 1975) and from 0.2 m/sec to 9 (Melnichenko and Skok, 1969), respectively.

A single preganglionic fibre may establish contacts with as many as 240 neurons of the ganglion (Wallis and North, 1978). On the other hand, each neuron may receive innervation from only one preganglionic fibre, while other neurons are multiply innervated. According to electrophysiological results, the former group includes the neurons of mammalian ciliary (Martin and Pilar, 1963), and submandibular ganglia (Lichtman, 1980), the neurons in amphibian intracardial ganglia (Dennis and Sargent, 1978) and the B group neurons in amphibian sympathetic ganglia (Nishi *et al.*, 1965). At birth each neuron in the submandibular ganglion receives an average of five preganglionic fibres, while in maturity their number is reduced to one (Lichtman, 1977). In singly innervated neurons the EPSP evoked by a single preganglionic stimulus has a simple shape and is suprathreshold for spike initiation.

Most of the neurons in mammalian sympathetic ganglia belong to the latter group, i.e. are multiply innervated. A suprathreshold orthodromic stimulus evokes in each neuron a multiple EPSP, each component of which is either related to a certain group of preganglionic fibres or to a single fibre (Fig. 1A). The number of preganglionic fibres (or their groups with identical thresholds within the group) connected to a single neuron in some mammalian sympathetic ganglia is two to seven (Skok and Heeroog, 1975), or ten (Njå and Purves, 1977), while in others the number may reach 40 (Crowcroft and Szurszewski, 1971).

In contrast to singly innervated neurons, those multiply innervated respond to the stimulation of a single preganglionic fibre with a small EPSP of an

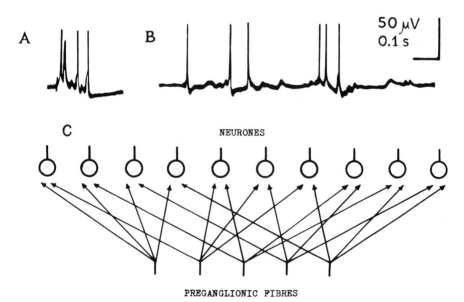

Figure 1 Complex electrical response of a neuron from the rabbit superior cervical ganglion to a single preganglionic stimulus (A), and natural activity recorded in the same neuron when the preganglionic fibres are intact (B). A scheme at the bottom (C) explains the appearance of 'non-effective' EPSPs in B. For details see text

amplitude that is much lower than the threshold for spike initiation. To trigger a postsynaptic spike, synchronous firing of several preganglionic fibres converging upon that neuron is needed. In the natural activity of a sympathetic neuron evoked by spontaneous firing of intact preganglionic fibres the subthreshold EPSPs can be observed among the large ones that trigger spikes (Fig. 1B). Blockade of conduction in preganglionic fibres immediately abolishes all EPSPs and postsynaptic spikes. When the block is applied only to some groups of preganglionic fibres, a decrease in the rate of EPSPs and postsynaptic spikes is observed, indicating that the normal activity of a postsynaptic neuron is triggered by more than one group of spontaneously active preganglionic fibres (Mirgorodski and Skok, 1970). Such multiple innervation is typical for vasomotor neurons to skeletal muscles (Lebedev *et al.*, 1978).

Two questions arise: (1) What is the physiological significance of the convergence of preganglionic fibres? (2) Why in some neurons (multiply innervated) is synchronous firing of several preganglionic fibres needed to evoke a postsynaptic spike, while in others (single innervated) this can be done by the firing of a single preganglionic fibre?

The ganglia with preganglionic convergence differ from those without convergence by having a much higher ratio between postganglionic neurons and preganglionic fibres: from 11:1 to 196:1 in the former group (see Skok, 1973, p. 8, and Gabella, 1976, p. 39), and only 1:1 (Martin and Pilar, 1963) or 2:1 (Wolf, 1941) in the latter group.

A concept, based upon this correlation, has been developed (Skok 1974) that convergence of preganglionic fibres provides a possibility to evoke spikes selectively in certain neurons within their large population using a strongly limited total number of preganglionic fibres. To make this point clear, suppose that each neuron receives innervation from two preganglionic fibres (Fig. 1C), and responds with a discharge only in the case of their synchronous firing, while a separate firing of each fibre evokes only subthreshold EPSP. It is easy to calculate that, for example, ten such neurons need only five preganglionic fibres to discharge each of them independently of all others (the number of combinations of two from the total five, $C_5^2 = 10$), instead of ten preganglionic fibres in singly innervated neurons. In this example each preganglionic fibre has contact with four neurons.

In the model just described two preganglionic fibres that evoke a discharge in one particular neuron should evoke subthreshold EPSPs ('odd EPSPs') in six other neurons. In support of the concept presented such subthreshold EPSPs have actually been observed during the natural activity of sympathetic ganglia (Fig. 1B).

In the complexity of their organization the autonomic ganglia resemble the central nervous system. However, in contrast to the central nervous system, no direct inhibition similar to fast excitation in its time course has been found in autonomic ganglia (see Skok, 1973, pp. 104, 127); only the slow inhibitory postsynaptic potentials (s-IPSIs) have been observed in untreated intramural neurons (Hartzell *et al.*, 1977; Wood and Mayer, 1979).

It has been widely accepted that the function of nicotinic transmission is to evoke postsynaptic discharge. However, section of preganglionic fibres or long-lasting blockade of nicotinic transmission is followed by a decrease in the activity of tyrosine hydroxylase in sympathetic ganglion neurons (Purves and Lichtman, 1978), and this effect cannot be prevented by antidromic stimulation of the ganglion (Chalazonitis and Zigmond, 1980). Therefore, it seems possible that nicotinic transmission fulfils one more function—a direct trans-synaptic regulation of the cell metabolism.

This suggests an alternative explanation for the physiological significance of preganglionic convergence and for naturally occurring subthreshold EPSPs: the activation of nicotinic receptors in addition to those evoking a postsynaptic spike.

MECHANISMS OF FAST SYNAPTIC TRANSMISSION

Release of acetylcholine from preganglionic nerve terminals

Spontaneous quantal release of acetylcholine (ACh) evokes miniature EPSPs of subthreshold amplitude in the neurons of isolated autonomic ganglia; the rate of their appearance is usually less than a few per minute (Nishi and Koketsu, 1960; Blackman *et al.*, 1963; McLachlan, 1975). A preganglionic stimulus triggers quantal release of ACh (Blackman *et al.*, 1963; Sacchi and Perri, 1971), with quantal numbers of 129 and 79 corresponding to B and C types of neurons in amphibian sympathetic ganglia (Nishi *et al.*, 1967). The release of ACh is due to calcium entry into the preganglionic terminal which increases the number of release sites (Bennett *et al.*, 1976).

According to recent models (for details see reviews by Skok, 1973; Kuba and Koketsu, 1978), ACh released by preganglionic stimulation is either newly synthesized from choline supplied by hydrolysis of previously released ACh (Collier, 1969; Bennett and McLachlan, 1972), or it is taken from preformed stocks (Birks and Fitch, 1974) which can be effectively modulated by patterns of preganglionic activity (Birks, 1978).

Repetitive stimulation of preganglionic fibres increases ACh output compared with that produced by a single stimulus. This effect can be explained by summation of individual facilitatory effects of each impulse (McLachlan, 1975). It has been suggested that facilitation is due to the activation of 'residual' calcium remaining in the terminal from previous impulses; in addition, a depression caused by depletion of ACh stores has been observed (Tashiro *et al.*, 1976).

Binding of acetylcholine to nicotinic cholinergic receptors

As in neuromuscular junctions and electroplax, ACh binds to AChRs in
autonomic ganglia in at least two sites of the receptor molecule: in the anionic
site and in the site of hydrophobic interactions (see reviews by Michelson and
Zeimal, 1970; Anichkov, 1974; Vulfius, 1978). Reduction of disulphide bonds
in AChR protein to free sulphydryl groups by dithiothreitol makes AChR
insensitive to nicotinic agonists. Thus, disulphide bonds are important for the

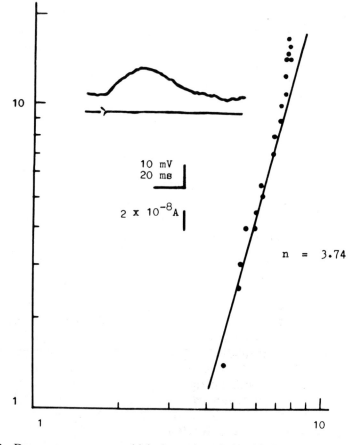

Figure 2   Dose–response curve which shows the relationship in a single neuron of the
rabbit superior cervical ganglion between the iontophoretic charge used to release
acetylcholine from a micropipette and the amplitude of the potential evoked by
acetylcholine. Double logarithmic scale. Hill number calculated as the slope of the
straight line is, in this case, 3.74. Inset illustrates the time course of the potential
(upper trace) evoked by the iontophoretic pulse (lower trace). Modified from
Selyanko and Skok, (1979); reproduced by permission of Elsevier/North-Holland
Biomedical Press

normal functioning of an AChR protein molecule (Brown and Kwiathkowski, 1976; Trinus and Skok, 1979); the same has been found in other types of nicotinic synapses (Karlin, 1969; Vulfius, 1978). ACh or tetramethylammonium protect AChR against the action of dithiothreitol, indicating that functionally important disulphide bonds are located in the vicinity of the anionic site of the AChR molecule (Trinus and Skok, 1979).

There is evidence that two ACh molecules bind to one AChR molecule. This follows from the mean value of the Hill coefficient equal to 2.4 if measured as the slope in the relationship between the amount of the iontophoretically applied ACh and the resulting depolarization of the membrane in a mammalian sympathetic ganglion neuron (Fig. 2; Selyanko and Skok, 1979). Similar values of the Hill coefficient have been obtained in other nicotinic synapses (Ziskind and Werman, 1975; Dreyer *et al.*, 1976a; Peper *et al.*, 1976).

A potent neuromuscular blocker, α-bungarotoxin (α-BTX). which probably binds to the recognition component of the AChR molecule (Katz and Miledi, 1978; Colquhoun, 1979; O'Brien *et al.*, 1979; Fumagalli and De Renzis, 1980), does not block transmission through the sympathetic ganglion (Magazanik *et al.*, 1974; Brown and Fumagalli, 1977) or through some pathways in parasympathetic ganglia (see Luzzatto *et al.*, 1980). At the same time, α-BTX binds to AChRs in these ganglia (Brown and Fumagalli, 1977). This paradox is now close to being explained. Recently it has been found that in sympathetic neurons α-BTX blocks the depolarizing effect of exogenous ACh (Dun and Karczmar, 1980), and, in contrast to the neuro-muscular junction, the number of AChR–α-BTX binding sites is not affected by denervation (Fumagalli *et al.*, 1978). These results suggest that those sympathetic AChRs which bind to α-BTX are not important for nicotinic transmission through the ganglion (probably they are extrasynaptic).

Unlike α-BTX, surugatoxin has a high affinity for ganglionic nicotinic AChRs but not for neuromuscular AChRs; there is also a marked difference between these two types of nicotinic receptors in their sensitivities to other blocking agents (see Brown, 1980).

Properties of the ionic channels in nicotinic cholinergic receptors

The reversal potential of EPSP or of excitatory postsynaptic current (EPSC) in the autonomic ganglia neurons is a few millivolts below zero (Nishi and Koketsu, 1960; Dennis *et al.*, 1971; Selyanko and Skok, 1979; Selyanko *et al.*, 1979) as shown in Fig. 3A, B. The reversal potential has not been changed by the removal of chloride ions from the perfusion medium. It is shifted towards the resting potential level by a decrease in either the external sodium or potassium concentration and shifted towards the zero level by an increase in the external potassium concentration. Increase or decrease in the external

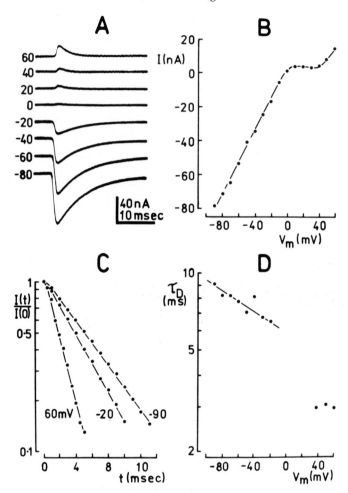

Figure 3 The effect of membrane potential on EPSC. (A) The EPSC recorded at different membrane potential levels indicated in millivolts. (B) The relationship between the peak amplitude of the EPSC and membrane potential level; negative values correspond to inward current. (C) The time course of decay of the EPSC recorded at three different membrane potential levels indicated in millivolts (semi-logarithmic scale). (D) The relationship between the time constant of the EPSC decay and membrane potential level (semilogarithmic scale). All data presented have been obtained from the same neuron of the rabbit superior cervical ganglion

calcium concentration shifts the reversal potential for EPSP towards the resting potential level or to the zero level, respectively. It has been concluded that the binding of ACh to AChR increases membrane permeability to sodium and potassium ions, and the ratio between these two processes depends upon the external concentration of calcium (see Koketsu, 1969;

Selyanko and Skok, 1979). The ionic mechanisms of nicotinic transmission in sympathetic ganglia appear to be similar to those observed in the neuromuscular junction (Takeuchi and Takeuchi, 1960). The effect of calcium on the membrane permeability increase caused by ACh is apparently due to changes in membrane surface charge (see Van der Kloot and Cohen, 1979).

In approximately one half of the neurons in mammalian sympathetic ganglion a depolarization with a reversal potential similar to that in EPSP can be evoked by a transmitter quite distinct from ACh, by 5-hydroxytryptamine (5-HT). It is not yet clear whether these neurons possess, besides their nicotinic receptors, 5-HT receptors with identical ionic mechanisms, or whether 5-HT can activate some nicotinic receptors (Skok and Selyanko, 1979).

The iontophoretic application of ACh to the postsynaptic membrane evokes fluctuations of the membrane current (Fig. 4); they are due to the continuous fluctuation of the AChRs ionic channels which open and close in a random manner. The analysis of these fluctuations allows an estimate of the mean channel lifetime τ (the mean time the channel stays open) as the time constant of the ACh fluctuation autocorrelation function (Fig. 4), and the mean conductance γ of one open channel (Katz and Miledi, 1972; Anderson and Stevens, 1973). The value of τ initially obtained with the use of

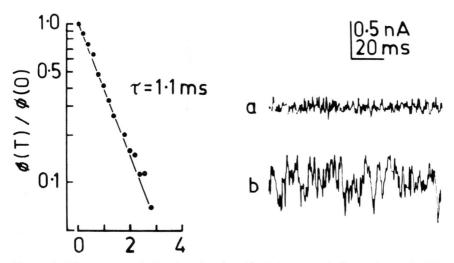

Figure 4 The autocorrelation function (a.c.f.) of the acetycholine noise evoked by the iontophoretic application of acetylcholine in the neuron of rabbit superior cervical ganglion. The curve shown is a result of subtracting the a.c.f. in the absence of acetylcholine from the a.c.f. in the presence of acetylcholine. The time constant of the a.c.f. (1.1 msec) corresponds to the mean lifetime of the ionic channel opened by acetylcholine. The inset traces are digitized records of filtered (1–500 Hz) voltage-clamp currents recorded before (a) and during (b) iontophoretic application of acetylcholine at a membrane potential of −80 mV and a temperature of 33–37 °C

fluctuation analysis (see Neher and Sakmann, 1976) from the neurons of the rabbit superior cervical ganglion at a membrane potential of -80 mV and a temperature of 34–37 °C was 1.1 msec (Derkach *et al.*, 1981). This channel lifetime is longer than that found in the mammalian neuromuscular junction at the same membrane potential and temperature (0.3 msec: Dreyer *et al.*, 1976b). A channel lifetime much longer than that in sympathetic neurons has been found in mammalian parasympathetic neurons (Ascher *et al.*, 1979).

The decay of EPSC in the neurons of autonomic ganglia is exponential and becomes longer with membrane hyperpolarization (Fig. 3C, D); the voltage dependence is higher in mammalian (Selyanko *et al.*, 1979) than in amphibian ganglia (Kuba and Nishi, 1979; MacDermott *et al.*, 1980). This effect of hyperpolarization is probably due to prolongation of the lifetime in the channel opened by ACh as was first suggested for the end-plate current (Stevens, 1976). Thus, the decay of EPSC reflects the closing of channels opened by ACh during its brief presence, and this provides another method for measuring mean channel lifetime as the time constant of EPSC decay (Anderson and Stevens, 1973). Using this method, the mean channel lifetime in AChRs of mammalian sympathetic ganglion neurons was found to be 3.6 msec (Selyanko *et al.*, 1979), which is longer than that obtained using fluctuation analysis*. The difference suggests that there exist two populations of channels with different lifetimes. In amphibian sympathetic neurons the mean time constant of EPSC decay is 4.3 msec (Kuba and Nishi, 1979) or 5.3 msec (MacDermott *et al.*, 1980), suggesting that their AChR channel lifetime does not differ essentially from that in mammalian sympathetic neurons. Mean conductance of the open AChR channel in the mammalian sympathetic neuron is close to that in mammalian parasympathetic ganglion neuron and in neuromuscular junction (Dreyer *et al.*, 1976a; Ascher *et al.*, 1979).

Electrical transmission

Electrical transmission occurs in addition to chemical (nicotinic) transmission in the neurons of avian ciliary ganglia that innervate the ciliary muscle (Martin and Pilar, 1963; Landmesser and Pilar, 1972). Electrical transmission is due to the unique structure of the interneuronal contact, particularly to the plasma membranes that cover both the presynaptic terminal and the post-synaptic neuron and make the portion of presynaptic action current that penetrates the postsynaptic membrane strong enough to evoke a postsynaptic

---

* Since the manuscript was presented, two populations of AChRs have been found using another method (fluctuation power spectra analysis), with fast- and slow-operating channels ($\tau_f = 1.1 \pm 0.1$ msec, and $\tau_s = 5.6 \pm 0.6$ msec correspondingly) of the identical conductance (36 ± 3 pS); τ_s approaches the time constant of the EPSC decay in pooled results (Skok, V. I., *et al.*, 1982)

spike (Hess *et al.*, 1969; Marwitt *et al.*, 1971). Amphibian parasympathetic (Roper, 1976) and cultured mammalian parasympathetic (O'Lague *et al.*, 1978) neurons can establish electrical contacts with neighbouring neurons. The physiological significance of these contacts remains unknown.

CONCLUSIONS

Fast (nicotinic) transmission in autonomic ganglia differs essentially from nicotinic transmission in skeletal muscles and transmission in the electric organ both in its organization at the cellular level and in molecular mechanisms. Multiple innervation of each neuron provides the possibility for the activity of the ganglion to be viewed as a complex integrative centre rather than the simple multiplicatory relay station postulated in classical concepts. However, in contrast to central integrative mechanisms, autonomic ganglia operate without direct inhibition similar to fast excitation in its time course, only s-IPSPs have been found.

The physiological significance of nicotinic transmission in autonomic ganglia is not limited to the transfer of excitation from preganglionic fibres to postganglionic ones, but includes trans-synaptic control of the postsynaptic cell metabolism.

Molecular mechanisms underlying nicotinic transmission in autonomic ganglia have the following unique features: (1) the recognition site of AChR activated by endogenous ACh is insensitive to α-BTX (2) the sensitivity of AChR to various blockers differs markedly from that in other types of nicotinic AChRs; (3) the AChR ionic channel lifetime is much longer than in other types of nicotinic AChRs and this correlates with a much longer synaptic delay.

REFERENCES

Anderson, C. R., and Stevens, C. F. (1973). Voltage clamp analysis of acetylcholine produced end-plate current fluctuations at frog neuromuscular junction. *J. Physiol. (London)*, **235**, 655–691.

Anichkov, S. V. (1974). *Selective Action of Mediator Drugs*, Medicine, Leningrad (in Russian).

Ascher, P., Large, W. A., and Rang, H. P. (1979). Studies on the mechanism of action of acetylcholine antagonists on rat parasympathetic ganglion cells. *J. Physiol. (London)*, **295**, 139–170.

Bennett, M. R., and McLachlan, E. M. (1972). An electrophysiological analysis of the synthesis of acetylcholine in preganglionic nerve terminals. *J. Physiol. (London)*, **221**, 669–682.

Bennett, M. R., Florin, T., and Pettigrew, A. G. (1976). The effect of calcium ions on the binomial statistics parameters that control acetylcholine release at preganglionic nerve terminals. *J. Physiol. (London)*, **257**, 597–620.

Birks, R. I. (1978). Regulation by patterned preganglionic neural activity of transmitter stores in a sympathetic ganglion. *J. Physiol. (London)*, **280**, 559–572.

Birks, R. I., and Fitch, S. J. G. (1974). Storage and release of acetylcholine in a sympathetic ganglion. *J. Physiol. (London)*, **240**, 125–134.

Blackman, J. G., Ginsborg, B. L., and Ray, C. (1963). On the quantal release of the transmitter at a sympathetic synapse. *J. Physiol. (London)*, **167**, 402–415.

Blackman, J. G., Crowcroft, P. J., Devine, C. E., Holman, M. E., and Yonemura, K. (1969). Transmission from preganglionic fibres in the hypogastric nerve to peripheral ganglia of male guinea-pigs. *J. Physiol. (London)*, **201**, 723–743.

Brown, D. A. (1980). Locus and mechanism of action of ganglion-blocking agents. In *Pharmacology of Ganglionic Transmission* (Ed. D. A. Kharkevich), pp. 185–236, Springer-Verlag, Berlin, Heidelberg, New York.

Brown, D. A., and Fumagalli, L. (1977). Dissociation of α-bungarotoxin binding and receptor block in the rat superior cervical ganglion. *Brain Res.*, **129**, 165–168.

Brown, D. A., and Kwiatkowski, D. (1976). A note on the effect of dithiothreitol (DTT) on the depolarization of isolated sympathetic ganglia by carbachol and bromoacetylcholine. *Br. J. Pharmacol.*, **56**, 128–130.

Chalazonitis, A., and Zigmond, R. E. (1980). Effects of synaptic and antidromic stimulation on tyrosine hydroxylase activity in the rat superior ganglion. *J. Physiol. (London)*, **300**, 525–538.

Christ, D. D., and Nishi, S. (1971). Effects of adrenaline on nerve terminals in the superior cervical ganglion of the rabbit. *Br. J. Pharmacol.*, **41**, 331–338.

Collier, B. (1969). The preferential release of newly synthesized transmitter by sympathetic ganglion. *J. Physiol. (London)*, **205**, 341–353.

Colquhoun, D. (1979). The link between drug binding and response: theories and observations. In *The Receptors. A Comprehensive Treatise* (Ed. R. D. O'Brien), Vol. 1, pp. 93–142, Plenum Press, New York.

Crowcroft, P. J., and Szurszewski, J. H. (1971). A study of the inferior mesenteric and pelvic ganglia of guinea-pigs with intracellular electrodes. *J. Physiol. (London)*, **219**, 421–441.

Dennis, M. J., and Sargent, P. B. (1978). Multiple innervation of normal and re-innervated parasympathetic neurones in the frog cardiac ganglion. *J. Physiol. (London)*, **281**, 63–76.

Dennis, M. J., Harris, A. J., and Kuffler, S. W. (1971). Synaptic transmission and its duplication by focally applied acetylcholine in parasympathetic neurons of the heart of the frog. *Proc. R. Soc. London Ser. B*, **177**, 509–539.

Derkach, V. A., Selyanko, A. A., and Skok, V. I. (1981). Analysis of acetylcholine noise in mammalian sympathetic ganglion neurones. Dokladi Akaderuiji Nauk SSSR, **259**, 981–984 (in Russian).

Dreyer, F., Müller, K. D., Peper, K., and Sterz, R. (1976a). The m. omohyoideus of the mouse as a convenient mammalian muscle preparation. *Pflügers Arch.*, **367**, 115–122.

Dreyer, F., Walter, C., and Peper, K. (1976b). Junctional and extrajunctional acetylcholine receptors in normal and denervated frog muscle fibres: noise analysis experiments with different agonists. *Pflügers Arch.*, **366**, 1–9.

Dun, N. J., and Karczmar, A. G. (1980). Blockade of ACh potentials by α-bungarotoxin in rat superior cervical ganglion cells. *Brain Res.*, **196**, 536–540.

Fumagalli, L., and De Renzis, G. (1980). α-Bungarotoxin binding sites in the rat superior cervical ganglion are influenced by postganglionic axotomy. *Neuroscience*, **5**, 611–616.

Fumagalli, L., De Renzis, G., and Miami, N. (1978). α-Bungarotoxin–acetylcholine receptors in the chick ciliary ganglion: effects of deafferentation and axotomy. *Brain Res.*, **153**, 87–98.

Furnes, J. B., and Costa, M. (1980). Types of nerves in the enteric nervous system. *Neuroscience*, **5**, 1–20.

Gabella, G. (1976). *Structure of the Autonomic Nervous System*, Chapman and Hall, London.

Hartzell, H. C., Kuffler, S. W., Stickgold, R., and Yoshikami, D. (1977). Synaptic excitation and inhibition resulting from direct action of acetylcholine on two types of chemoreceptors on individual amphibian parasympathetic neurons. *J. Physiol. (London)*, **271**, 817–846.

Hess, A., Pilar, G., and Weakly, J. N. (1969). Correlation between transmission and structure in avian ciliary ganglion synapses. *J. Physiol. (London)*, **202**, 339–354.

Hirst, G. D. S. (1979). Mechanisms of peristalsis. *Br. Med. Bull.*, **35**, 263–268.

Hirst, G. D. S., Holman, M. E., Prosser, C. L., and Spence, I. (1972). Some properties of the neurons of Auerbach's plexus. *J. Physiol. (London)*, **225**, 60–61.

Hubbard, J. I., and Schmidt, R. F. (1963). An electrophysiological investigation of mammalian motor nerve terminals, *J. Physiol. (London)*, **166**, 145–167.

Jänig, W., Krauspe, R., and Wiedersatz, G. (1979). Reflex activation of post-ganglionic neurons supplying skeletal muscle via non-nicotinic synaptic mechanisms in sympathetic ganglia. *Pflügers Arch.*, **382** (Suppl.), R43.

Karlin, A. (1969). Chemical modification of the active site of the acetylcholine receptor. *J. Gen. Physiol.*, **54**, 245–254.

Katz, B., and Miledi, R. (1972). The statistical nature of the acetylcholine potential and its molecular components. *J. Physiol. (London)*, **224**, 665–699.

Katz, B., and Miledi, R. (1978). A re-examination of curare action at the motor endplate. *Proc. R. Soc. London Ser. B.*, **203**, 119–133.

Ko, C. P., Barton, M., Johnson, M. I., and Bunge, R. P. (1976). Synaptic transmission between rat superior cervical ganglion neurons in dissociated cell cultures. *Brain Res.*, **117**, 461–486.

Koketsu, K. (1969). Cholinergic synaptic potentials and the underlying ionic mechanisms. *Fed. Proc.*, **28**, 101–131.

Kuba, K., and Koketsu, K. (1978). Synaptic events in sympathetic ganglia. *Prog. Neurobiol.*, **11**, 77–169.

Kuba, K., and Nishi, S. (1979). Characteristics of the fast excitatory postsynaptic current in bullfrog sympathetic ganglion cells. *Pflügers Arch.*, **378**, 205–212.

Lakos, I. (1970). Ultrastructure of chronically denervated superior cervical ganglion in the cat and rat. *Acta Biol. Sci. Hung.*, **21**, 425–427.

Landmesser, L., and Pilar, G. (1972). The onset and development of transmission in the chick ciliary ganglion. *J. Physiol. (London)*, **222**, 691–713.

Lebedev, V. P., Syromyatnikov, A. V., and Skok, V. I. (1978). Convergence of preganglionic fibres on vasomotor neurons of the sympathetic ganglia in cats. *Neurophysiology (Consultants Bureau, New York)*, **9**, 448–451.

Lichtman, J. W. (1977). The reorganization of synaptic connections in the rat submandibular ganglion during post-natal development. *J. Physiol. (London)*, **273**, 155–177.

Lichtman, J. W. (1980). On the predominantly single innervation of submandibular ganglion cells in the rat. *J. Physiol. (London)*, **302**, 121–130.

Luzzatto, A. C., Tronconi, B. C., Paggi, P., and Possi, A. (1980). Binding of *Naja naja siamensis* α-toxin to the chick ciliary ganglion: a light-microscopy autoradiographic study. *Neuroscience*, **5**, 313–318.

MacDermott, A. B., Connor, E. A., Dionne, V. E., and Parsons, R. L. (1980). Voltage clamp study of fast excitatory synaptic currents in bullfrog sympathetic ganglion cells. *J. Gen. Physiol.*, **75**, 39–60.

Magazanik, L. G., Ivanov, A. Y., and Lukomskaya, N. Y. (1974). Inability of snake venom polypeptides to block the cholinoreception in the isolated sympathetic ganglion of rabbit. *Neurophysiology (Consultants Bureau, New York)*, **6**, 652–654.

Martin, A. R., and Pilar, G. (1963). Dual mode of synaptic transmission in the avian ciliary ganglion. *J. Physiol. (London)*, **168**, 443–463.

Marwitt, R., Pilar, G., and Weakly, J. N. (1971). Characterization of two ganglion cell populations in avian ciliary ganglion. *Brain Res.*, **25**, 317–334.

McLachlan, E. M. (1975). An analysis of the release of acetylcholine from pre-ganglionic nerve terminals. *J. Physiol. (London)*, **245**, 447–466.

Melnichenko, L. V., and Skok, V. I. (1969). Electrophysiological investigation of the cat ciliary ganglion. *Neurophysiology (Consultants Bureau, New York)*, **1**, 79–84.

Michelson, M. Y., and Zeimal, E. V. (1970). *Acetylcholine*, pp. 94–120, Nauka, Leningrad (in Russian).

Minota, Sh., and Koketsu, K. (1978). Recurrent synaptic activation of the bullfrog sympathetic ganglion cells by direct intracellular stimulation. *Jpn. J. Physiol.*, **28**, 799–806.

Mirgorodsky, V. N., and Skok, V. I. (1970). The role of different preganglionic fibres in tonic activity of the mammalian sympathetic ganglion. *Brain Res.*, **22**, 262–263.

Neher, E., and Sakmann, B. (1976). Noise analysis of drug induced voltage clamp currents in denervated frog muscle fibres. *J. Physiol. (London)*, **258**, 705–729.

Nishi, S., and Koketsu, K. (1960). Electrical properties and activities of single sympathetic neurons in frog. *J. Cell. Comp. Physiol.*, **55**, 15–30.

Nishi, S., and North, A. (1973). Intracellular recordings from the myenteric plexus of the guinea-pig ileum. *J. Physiol. (London)*, **231**, 471–491.

Nishi, S., Soeda, H., and Koketsu, K. (1965). Studies on sympathetic B and C neurons and patterns of preganglionic innervation. *J. Cell. Comp. Physiol.*, **66**, 19–32.

Nishi, S., Soeda, H., and Koketsu, K. (1967). Release of acetylcholine from sympathetic preganglionic nerve terminals. *J. Neurophysiol.*, **30**, 114–134.

Njå, A., and Purves, D. (1977). Specific innervation of guinea-pig superior cervical ganglion cells by preganglionic fibres arising from different levels of the spinal cord. *J. Physiol. (London)*, **264**, 565–583.

O'Brien, R. D., Gibson, R. E., and Sumikawa, K. (1979). The nicotinic acetylcholine receptor from *Torpedo* electroplax. In *The Cholinergic Synapse* (Ed. S. Tuček), *Progress in Brain Research*, Vol. 49, pp. 279–292, Elsevier, Amsterdam.

O'Lague, P. H., Furshpan, E. J., and Potter, D. D. (1978). Studies on rat sympathetic neurons developing in cell culture. *Dev. Biol.*, **67**, 404–423.

Peper, K., Dreyer, F., and Müller, K.-D. (1976). Analysis of cooperativity of drug–receptor interaction. *Cold Spring Harbor Symp. Quant. Biol.*, **40**, 187–192.

Purves, D., and Lichtman, J. W. (1978). Formation and maintenance of synaptic connection in autonomic ganglia. *Physiol. Rev.*, **58**, 821–862.

Roper, S. (1976). An electrophysiological study of chemical and electrical synapses on neurons in the parasympathetic cardiac ganglion of the mudpuppy, *Necturus maculosus*: evidence for intrinsic ganglionic innervation. *J. Phyiol. (London)*, **254**, 427–454.

Sacchi, O., and Perri, V. (1971). Quantal release of acetylcholine from the nerve endings of the guinea-pig superior cervical ganglion. *Pflügers Arch.*, **329**, 207–219.

Selyanko, A. A., and Skok, V. I. (1979). Activation of acetylcholine receptors in mammalian sympathetic ganglion neurons. In *The Cholinergic Synapse* (Ed. S. Tuček), *Progress in Brain Research*, Vol. 49, pp. 241–252, Elsevier, Amsterdam.

Selyanko, A. A., Derkach, V. A., and Skok, V. I. (1979). Fast excitatory postsynaptic currents in voltage-clamped mammalian sympathetic ganglion neurons. *J. Autonom. Nerv. Syst.*, **1**, 127–137.

Skok, V. I. (1973). *Physiology of Autonomic Ganglia*, Igaku Shoin Ltd., Tokyo.

Skok, V. I. (1974). Convergence of preganglionic fibres in autonomic ganglia. In *Mechanisms of Neuronal Integration in Nervous Center* (Ed. P. G. Kostyuk), pp. 27–34, Nauka, Leningrad (in Russian).

Skok, V. I. (1980a). Ganglionic transmission: morphology and physiology. In *Pharmacology of Ganglionic Transmission* (Ed. D. A. Kharkevich), pp. 9–39, Springer-Verlag, Berlin, Heidelberg, New York.

Skok, V. I. (1980b). Introductory remarks. In *Transmission in Autonomic Ganglia*, Symposium, XXVIII International Congress of Physiological Sciences, Budapest.

Skok, V. I., and Heeroog, S. S. (1975). Synaptic delay in superior cervical ganglion of the cat. *Brain Res.*, **87**, 343–353.

Skok, V. I., and Selyanko, A. A. (1979). Acetylcholine and serotonin receptors in mammalian sympathetic ganglion neurons. In *Integrative Functions of the Autonomic Nervous System* (Eds. Ch. McC. Brooks, K. Koizumi and A. Sato), pp. 248–253, University of Tokyo Press and Elsevier/North Holland Biomedical Press, Amsterdam.

Skok, V. I., Selyanko, A. A., and Derkach, V. A. (1982). Two modes of activity of nicotinic acetylcholine receptor channels in sympathetic neurons. *Brain Res.*, **238**, 480–483.

Stevens, Ch. F. (1976). Molecular basis for postjunctional conductance increases induced by acetylcholine. *Cold Spring Harbor Symp. Quant. Biol.*, **40**, 169–173.

Takeuchi, A., and Takeuchi, N. (1960). Further analysis of relationship between end-plate potential and end-plate current. *J. Neurophysiol.*, **23**, 397–402.

Tashiro, N., Gallagher, J. P., and Nishi, S. (1976). Facilitation and depression of synaptic transmission in amphibian sympathetic ganglia. *Brain Res.*, **118**, 45–62.

Trinus, K. F., and Skok, V. I. (1979). Disulfide bonds found in the cholinoreceptors of the frog sympathetic ganglion neurons. *Neurophysiology (Consultants Bureau, New York)*, **11**, 445–451.

Van der Kloot, W. G., and Cohen, I. (1979). Membrane surface potential changes may alter drug interactions: an example, acetylcholine and curare. *Science*, **203**, 1351–1353.

Vulfius, E. A. (1978). Study of cholinergic receptors with chemical modification method. In *Itogy Nauki i Tekchniki; Biofizika* (Ed. B. N. Veprintsev), Vol. 8, pp. 97–202, Moscow (in Russian).

Wallis, D. I., and North, R. A. (1978). Synaptic input to cells of the rabbit superior cervical ganglion. *Pflügers Arch.*, **374**, 145–152.

Wolf, G. A. (1941). The ratio of preganglionic neurons to postganglionic neurons in the visceral nervous system. *J. Comp. Neurol.*, **75**, 235–243.

Wood, J. D. (1975). Neurophysiology of Auerbach's plexus and control of intestinal motility. *Physiol. Rev.*, **55**, 307–324.

Wood, J. D., and Mayer, C. J. (1979). Serotonergic activation of tonic-type enteric neurons in guinea pig small bowel. *J. Neurophysiol.*, **42**, 582–593.

Ziskind, L., and Werman, R. (1975). At least three molecules of carbamylcholine are needed to activate a cholinergic receptor. *Brain Res.*, **88**, 177–180.

Autonomic Ganglia
Edited by Lars-Gösta Elfvin
© 1983 John Wiley & Sons Ltd

Slow Synaptic Actions in Mammalian Sympathetic Ganglia, with Special Reference to the Possible Roles Played by Cyclic Nucleotides

HARUO KOBAYASHI and TSUNEO TOSAKA

Department of Physiology, Tokyo Medical College, 1-1 Shinjuku-6-chome,
Shinjuku-ku, Tokyo 160, Japan

INTRODUCTION

General features of slow synaptic responses

In mammalian sympathetic ganglia, particularly in the superior cervical ganglion (SCG) of the rabbit, three types of postsynaptic potentials can be elicited in response to suitable preganglionic stimuli: a fast excitatory one (fast or f-EPSP), a slow inhibitory one (slow or s-IPSP) and a slow excitatory one (slow or s-EPSP) (Libet, 1970, 1979a) (see also the inset of Fig. 1). Each ganglion cell can exhibit all of these three responses in the above-stated sequence. An even more slowly occurring EPSP component, which was originally reported for amphibian sympathetic ganglia (and termed 'late slow EPSP') (Nishi and Koketsu, 1968), appears also to exist in mammalian ganglia. These postsynaptic potentials (PSPs) can otherwise be distinguished pharmacologically: the f-EPSP is obviously elicited by nicotinically acting acetylcholine (ACh), whereas the s-IPSP and s-EPSP components are elicited by muscarinically acting ACh. Additional evidence has been accumulated, suggesting that the synaptic pathway for the s-IPSP (at least in the rabbit SCG) includes the activity of intervening adrenergic cells (termed 'small intensely fluorescent', or 'SIF', cells) (Eränkö and Härkönen, 1963) between the preganglionic input and the production of s-IPSP in the ganglion cells: the SIF cell releases, in response to muscarinic activation, the secondary neurotransmitter dopamine (DA) (Libet and Owman, 1974) which in turn hyperpolarizes the ganglion cell (Eccles and Libet, 1961; Dun and Karczmar, 1978). (The functional significance of the adrenergic SIF interneuron for the mediation of mammalian s-IPSP will be discussed more fully later.) DA has another novel mode of action in the ganglion: it brings about a modulatory augmentative change selectively in the s-EPSP and this effect lasts for several hours (Libet and Tosaka, 1970). The postulated synaptic relationship between the involved cellular elements for the production of these ganglionic

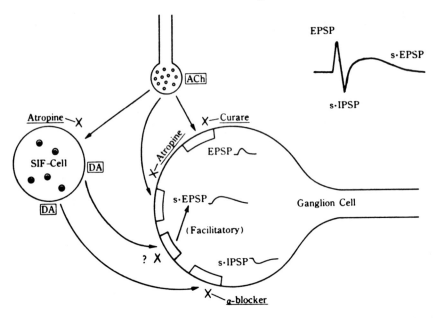

Figure 1 Diagram illustrating the synaptic relationship between the intraganglionic elements for the generation of f-EPSP, s-IPSP amd s-EPSP as shown in the inset. Rabbit SCG. The substances in the boxes are the neurotransmitters and those underlined are the specific antagonists. From Tosaka and Kobayashi (1977), modified from the original figure in Libet (1970); reproduced by permission of *Archivum Histologicum Japonicum*

responses is illustrated in Fig. 1. The transmitter for the late s-EPSP in amphibian sympathetic ganglia has now been shown probably to be a luteinizing hormone releasing factor (LHRF)-like peptide (Jan *et al.*, 1979), thus raising the possibilities for the involvement of peptides in general in ganglionic transmission. Mammalian ganglion cells are also shown depolarized by substance P (Dun and Karczmar, 1979). Further detail of the action of peptides in the ganglion is described in the chapter by Dun.

The s-PSPs are unique in their extraordinarily delayed onset and long duration, as compared with the classically known f-PSPs (Libet, 1967, 1970). Synaptic delays for the s-IPSP are about 25 msec and those for s-EPSP are 200–300 msec in the rabbit SCG. Durations are of the order of seconds, rather than of milliseconds. With a single preganglionic volley, the s-PSPs are relatively small, while they are effectively built up on repetition at appropriate frequencies. Moreover, the electrogenic mechanisms for the s-PSPs appear strikingly different in principle from those for the classical f-PSPs: they do not require any increase in membrane conductance to certain ion species (Kobayashi and Libet, 1968, 1970). Selective sensitivity of the s-EPSP to oxidative metabolic inhibitors points to a metabolically based electrogenic mechanism rather than one simply involving the opening and closing of ionic channels (Kobayashi and Libet, 1968; Libet, 1970). The additional time presumed to be required for such an electrogenic mechanism, for example, the time required for the production and subsequent actions by cyclic GMP as the probable intracellular mediator (see further below), may help to explain the extraordinarily long synaptic delay and duration of the s-EPSP.

Evidence for disynaptic mediation, by acetylcholine and dopamine, for the mammalian s-IPSP

As described previously, it has been postulated that the s-IPSP in the rabbit SCG is a response to DA released from an interneuron on its cholinergic activation. This 'disynaptic hypothesis', however, has recently been challenged by Gallagher and others (1980) who suggest that the s-IPSP may be a direct cholinergic (muscarinic) hyperpolarizing response. A similar kind of argument has also been presented for the amphibian s-IPSP (Weight and Smith, 1980). In these circumstances, it may be worthwhile at this stage to review in full the experimental evidence accumulated in relation to the possibility of disynaptic mediation, which is in question now.

The following lines of evidence may provide the support to the concept of disynaptic mediation for the mammalian s-IPSP.

(1) In the rabbit SCG, some preganglionic fibres, which do not directly innervate a given postganglionic neuron, appeared to be still able to produce a small but distinct s-IPSP in that cell without eliciting any f-EPSP in it (Libet and Tosaka, 1969). This can be best explained by assuming that such preganglionic fibres would innervate an interneuron releasing secondary transmitter which in turn produces s-IPSP in the adjacent postganglionic neurons.

(2) A low Ca^{2+}–high Mg^{2+} medium abolished the hyperpolarizing (but not depolarizing) component present in the diphasic response of ganglion to muscarinic agents such as bethanechol, (BCh) (Libet, 1970; Dun and Karczmar, 1978). This also suggests that the release of secondary transmitter from an intervening element is necessary for the hyperpolarizing response.

(3) The intraganglionic SIF cell might be the most probable candidate for an interneuron which contains the secondary transmitter directly eliciting the s-IPSP. By fluorescence analysis DA was identified and found to be plentiful in the rabbit SIF cells (Libet and Owman, 1974). After specifically designed treatment of the ganglion, such as prolonged exposure to BCh or long-term conditioning stimulation of preganglionic nerves, there was an indication that the functionally releasable DA in the SIF cells was effectively depleted. This

observation could be coupled with a selective and persisting reduction of subsequent s-IPSP. Further, both the reduced s-IPSP and the DA content in the depleted SIF cells were restored to the original levels by treating the ganglion with DA, but not any other species of catecholamine, for a period; during that time the depleted SIF cells might take up DA and refill themselves. (For experimental details, see Libet and Tosaka, 1970).

(4) Evidence was presented for the occurrence of the metabolites closely related to DA in the porcine SCG after orthodromic simulation (Pearson and Sharman, 1974). This result can be interpreted as further confirming, though indirectly, an intraganglionic release of DA following preganglionic activity.

(5) All three species of natural catecholamines—epinephrine (E), nore-pinephrine (NE) and dopamine (DA)—could directly hyperpolarize the postganglionic neurons (for rabbits: Libet, 1970; Kobayashi, 1976; Cole and Shinnick-Gallagher, 1979. For rats: Brown and Caulfield, 1979). Hyperpolar-ization by catecholamines could occur even in the low Ca^{2+} medium. Although DA was always equally found by the above investigators to be the least potent of the three catecholamines, there is no reason to assume that the strongest must be the actual transmitter substance (Gallagher *et al.*, 1980). It should be most emphasized that the catecholamine-induced hyperpolarizing responses appeared to be generated by the membrane mechanism identical to that for the s-IPSP: there is no increase in the ionic conductance of neuronal membrane (for rabbits: Kobayashi and Libet, 1968, 1970; Dun and Nishi, 1974; Dun and Karczmar, 1978. For rats: Brown and Caulfield, 1979).

A recent report by Ivanov and Skok (1980) showed that in the rabbit SCG the cells responding with the s-IPSP to orthodromic activation could be classified into two categories according to the membrane characteristics of their s-IPSPs: in one of these two groups the s-IPSP was accompanied by an increase in membrane conductance (probably of K^+ ions) and in the second group the s-IPSP was generated in association with virtually no change in conductance. NE, on the other hand, was shown by them to be able to induce hyperpolarizing responses in some, but not all, of the cells with no change in conductance. They subsequently suggested that the s-IPSP in the second group of cells was mediated by NE. This idea is acceptable, but, in order to conclude this more adequately, they should hopefully demonstrate ex-perimentally that the cells responding to NE (with no change in conductance) actually belonged to the second group with respect to the nature of their orthodromic s-IPSP.

(6) Adrenergic antagonists, such as dibenamine, phenoxybenzamine, phen-tolamine and dihydroergotamine, could suppress the s-IPSP as well as the catecholamine-induced hyperpolarizations (Eccles and Libet, 1961; Libet and Tosaka, 1970). As a matter of fact, the effectiveness of those antagonists on the s-IPSP was always less marked than that on the hyperpolarizations induced by extrinsically applied catecholamines, in the range of doses in

which non-selective depression of all the PSPs did not occur (Libet, 1970). This might be explained by supposing that catecholamine transmitter would be highly concentrated at the specific synaptic sites where it was released on preganglionic activities, and its strong action there could not be easily antagonized by the drugs at doses as indicated above. Perhaps such considerations may explain the relative inability of anti-adrenergic agents for depressing the s-IPSP in the reports of others (Cole and Shinnick-Gallagher, 1980).

(7) An inhibitor of catechol *O*-methyltransferase (COMT) which is responsible for the enzymatic inactivation of catecholamine transmitters at the corresponding synaptic sites, U-0521 (3′, 4′-dihydroxy-2-methylpropiophenone, Upjohn) was shown to augment the s-IPSP (Libet and Tosaka, 1971). The significance of the action of this drug can be regarded as equivalent to that of physostigmine, at the cholinergic synaptic sites, inhibiting acetylcholine esterase (Ashe and Libet, 1981). (Morphological aspects on the function of SIF cells are extensively discussed elsewhere by several other authors in this book.)

The argument about the requirement of interneuronal mediation for the amphibian s-IPSP is not within the scope of our present article. But we wish to add briefly here that the initial experiments by Weight and Padjen (1973), showing that low Ca^{2+}–high Mg^{2+} medium did not block or eliminate the hyperpolarizing response to ACh, were carried out with nicotinized frog ganglia. Libet and Kobayashi (1974) later confirmed the above observation by Weight and Padjen, but they additionally showed that, in curarized ganglia, the low Ca^{2+}–high Mg^{2+} condition did in fact depress the hyperpolarizing response induced by muscarinically acting agents. Apparently nicotine appeared to introduce some sort of pharmacological peculiarity to produce an additional type of response. Furthermore, in the report by Weight and Smith (1980), it was clearly shown that the hyperpolarizing response to methacholine (MCh) in the curarized frog ganglion was effectively eliminated by 'zero' calcium condition for 30 min. Curiously, some hyperpolarizing component reappeared after the prolonged soaking (for 60 min) of the ganglion in the 'zero' calcium medium. Obviously the issue about the necessity (or non-necessity) of the interneuronal step for the amphibian s-IPSP is still in a somewhat confused state. There is a more recent paper by Horn and Dodd (1981), in which they legitimately showed that the hyperpolarizing response induced by ACh in the C-type neuron in the curarized frog ganglion was not eliminated by low Ca^{2+}–high Mg^{2+} treatment. It would be interesting if they were to test the effect of catecholamine (preferably E) on this C neuron to see whether it could induce any hyperpolarizing response. Actually there is a component, in the s-IPSP response of the whole frog ganglion, which appears sensitive to α-adrenergic antagonists and COMT inhibitor (Libet and Kobayashi, 1974). (For further discussion on transmission in frog ganglia see chapter by Weight).

POSSIBILITY FOR THE INVOLVEMENT OF CYCLIC NUCLEOTIDES IN GANGLIONIC TRANSMISSION

An idea similar to the well-known 'intracellular second messenger concept' for hormonal action on target cells was first introduced by Greengard and his group into the understanding of the mechanism of chemical synaptic transmission in the nervous system (Greengard and Kebabian, 1974; Greengard, 1976). In this idea, hormones and neurotransmitters are considered to be functionally analogous in their roles as the first messenger molecules conveying certain biological information from one cell to the others, and cyclic nucleotides are synthesized within the receiving cells in response to the actions of those messengers, causing the cells to produce their specific cellular reactions.

In sympathetic ganglion cells in particular, the above idea can be paraphrased into a simple statement that adenosine 3', 5'-cyclic monophosphate (cyclic AMP) mediates the dopaminergic s-IPSP, while guanosine 3', 5'-cyclic monophosphate (cyclic GMP) mediates the muscarinic s-EPSP (McAfee and Greengard, 1972). However, the experimental results on which this hypothesis is based have been extensively criticized in recent years by many investigators through their electrophysiological and biochemical analyses. Therefore, it would be worthwhile at this stage to re-evaluate the validity of this hypothesis by way of precisely examining the factual evidence available so far.

Does cyclic AMP mediate the DA-induced s-IPSP?

According to Greengard and his group, the evidence on which their hypothesis is based can be summarized in the following four points (McAfee *et al.*, 1971; Kebabian and Greengard, 1971; McAfee and Greengard, 1972; Kalix *et al.*, 1974). (1) Intraganglionic cyclic AMP content is increased either by stimulation of preganglionic nerves or by application of muscarinic cholinergic agents and various catecholamines. (2) s-IPSP, as well as DA-induced hyperpolarization, can be augmented by a phosphodiesterase (PDE) inhibitor—theophylline. (3) Prostaglandin E_1 (PGE_1) depresses the s-IPSP, as well as DA-induced hyperpolarization. (4) Externally applied cyclic AMP (mono or dibutyryl derivatives) causes ganglionic hyperpolarization.

Intraganglionic increases in cyclic AMP (point 1) has been generally confirmed by many other investigators, but the results are variable, depending on the animal species used and on the type of stimulation. In response to DA, the increases were most prominent in bovine ganglia (Kebabian and Greengard, 1971; Roch and Kalix, 1975; Williams *et al.*, 1975, 1976, 1977; Black *et al.*, 1978). Increases in rabbit and rat were meagre (Kalix *et al.*, 1974; Cramer *et al.*, 1973; Lindl and Cramer, 1975), and those in cat were almost undetectable (Williams *et al.*, 1975, 1976, 1977). In rabbit SCG, however, increases of about 60–100% over the control level were recently reported either by application of DA or by preganglionic nerve stimulation (Wamsley *et al.*, 1980; Williams *et al.*, 1980). A similar increase was also confirmed by us (Mochida *et al.*, 1981a, 1981b), provided the penetration of externally applied DA into the whole ganglion tissue was further ensured by a prolonged incubation time (30 min) and the possible enzymatic breakdown of DA during such a relatively long incubation time was prevented by the concomitant use of a COMT inhibitor U-0521 (see also Ashe and Libet, 1981). An attempt was made to relate the observed variability in the extent of DA-induced increases in cyclic AMP to that in the population density of the morphologically identified subclasses of SIF cells in the ganglion (Williams *et al.*, 1976, 1977; Black *et al.*, 1978), but the results appear to be not quite conclusive. A large increase in cyclic AMP mediated by the activity of β-adrenergic receptors has been reported in the SCG of several animal species (for cow: Kebabian and Greengard, 1971. For rat: Cramer *et al.*, 1973; Lindl and Cramer, 1975; Quenzer *et al.*, 1978; Brown *et al.*, 1979; Lindl, 1979. For guinea-pig: Wamsley *et al.*, 1980; Williams *et al.*, 1980). In the rabbit SCG, we found in the present study that there was a relatively small but significant β-type increase, contrary to previous reports (for example, Williams *et al.*, 1980) of its absence. In our experimental conditions, as described previously, cyclic AMP increase by DA was in fact suppressed in part (about a half) by propranolol (5×10^{-6} M). The residual portion of increase was blocked by specific DA-receptor antagonists. It thus appears that two different types of receptors are involved in cyclic AMP increase in the rabbit SCG: one is DA-specific and another is β-type. Considerations about the physiological significance of each type of increase will be made later.

The effects of theophylline (point 2 above) should be carefully evaluated. Assuming that theophylline would prevent enzymatic hydrolysis of cyclic AMP by PDE, the actions of DA should be enhanced by theophylline if they are mediated by cyclic AMP. Apparently such an enhancing effect on the s-IPSP was reconfirmed (Libet, 1979b). A more potent and selective PDE inhibitor, RO-20-1724 (4-[3-butoxy-4-methoxybenzyl]-2-imidazolidinone; see Sheppard and Wiggan, 1971), however, was found to produce no significant change at a dose which certainly induced a promoted accumulation of cyclic AMP (Kalix *et al.*, 1974), while it brought about a notable increase in the depolarizing s-EPSP response. Theophylline, on the other hand, has an augmentative effect on another type of hyperpolarizing response, after-spike hyperpolarization in the presence of atropine and phenoxybenzamine, hence being unrelated to the dopaminergic s-IPSP. A similar kind of effect was also reported by others (Dun and Karczmar, 1977b). Obviously the effects of theophylline are diverse, and may include non-specific side-effects in addition to its simply inhibiting PDE. Therefore, the observed augmentation of s-IPSP by theophylline may not be evidence to support unequivocally the hypothesis that the s-IPSP is mediated by cyclic AMP.

Prostaglandins are known either to stimulate or inhibit effectively the adenyl cyclase system in various tissues (Horton, 1969). On the assumption that PGE_1 in particular would antagonize DA-induced activation of adenyl cyclase in the ganglion, its marked depressant action (point 3 above) on the s-IPSP, as well as on DA-induced hyperpolarization, has been taken as the supporting evidence for the hypothesis in question now. Later PGE_1 was shown, however, to be unable to suppress ganglionic adenyl cyclase, but rather to augment it (for cow: Tomasi et al., 1977. For rat: Lindl, 1979). These electrophysiological and biochemical data regarding PGE_1 have thus been shown to be inconsistent with the proposed hypothesis.

Finally, in direct tests on the ability of cyclic AMP to produce hyperpolarizing responses, the original observation by Greengard and his group (point 4 above) was not confirmed in various different ways of applying the agents and recording the electrical potential changes. With extracellular (sucrose-gap) recordings, hyperpolarization in the rabbit SCG was not observed in response to either cyclic AMP or to its dibutyryl derivative (up to 2.5 mM) added to the perfusate (Dun and Karczmar, 1977b). We ourselves were also unable to obtain any consistent hyperpolarizing response using a similar but more sensitive recording technique (see Libet, 1979b). With intracellular recordings, cyclic AMP failed to elicit any hyperpolarizing response in rabbit and rat SCG when applied externally (in the form of butyryl derivatives) (Kobayashi et al., 1977; Dun et al., 1977a; Hsu and McIsaac, 1978) or internally by means of iontophoretic injections (Gallagher and Shinnick-Gallagher, 1977; Kobayashi et al., 1977, 1978). In their tests, depolarizing, rather than hyperpolarizing, responses were sometimes obtainable when the amount of cyclic AMP applied was relatively high. Recently Brown and his group proposed that the apparent hyperpolarization inducible in the rat SCG by externally applied cyclic AMP and related nucleotides was due to an action on the adenosine receptors on the cell sursface, not via intracellular mediation as originally thought (Brown et al., 1979).

All in all, it seems very difficult to approve, with appropriate satisfaction, the cyclic AMP hypothesis for the s-IPSP on the basis of the evidences initially presented. It is still true, however, that cyclic AMP is accumulated within the ganglion in response to preganglionic nerve stimulation or to the application of catecholamines, especially DA (point 1). This leaves us a big question: To what kind of cellular function, other than hyperpolarization, is this increase in cyclic AMP related in sympathetic ganglia?

At this point, it is worth noting that catecholamine receptors responsible for ganglionic hyperpolarization appeared to be of a type classified as α_2. This was first proposed for rat (Brown and Caulfield, 1979) and was suggested also for rabbit (Cole and Shinnick-Gallagher, 1979). In our own studies in the rabbit SCG with sucrose-gap and other techniques (Mochida *et al.*, 1981a, 1981b), we found that (1) ganglionic hyperpolarizations were inducible, in addition to DA, NE and E, by clonidine, which was regarded as relatively selective to α_2 receptors, and even by phenylephrine (rather selective to α_1 receptors) and isoproterenol (selective to β receptors), at the transient peak concentrations in the chamber, shortly after brief single injections into the perfusate, above 10^{-6} M (for clonidine) and 10^{-5} M (for phenylephrine and isoproterenol). (2) Phentolamine and dihydroergotamine, antagonists which could not clearly distinguish α_1 and α_2 receptors, were able to suppress hyperpolarizing responses to the above catecholamines and related compounds. Prazosin, known as being selective to α_1 receptors, was unable to antagonize at doses up to 10^{-5} M, while yohimbine, selective to α_2 receptors, effectively antagonized at doses below 10^{-6} M. β-Antagonists were incapable of suppressing hyperpolarization, but they showed rather an augmentative effect at higher concentrations (2×10^{-4} M or more). Antagonists known as being specific to DA receptors, including some phenothiazines and haloperidol, were also found ineffective against hyperpolarizing responses (see also Nakamura, 1978). (3) Cyclic AMP synthesis in response to extrinsically applied DA was not antagonized by α-blockers, such as dihydroergotamine, at doses which effectively antagonized hyperpolarizing responses, in contrast to the previous reports (Kebabian and Greengard, 1971; Kalix *et al.*, 1974) that cyclic AMP synthesis in ganglia was suppressed by α-adrenergic antagonists.

Through the above analyses of pharmacological characteristics, the catecholamine receptors responsible for hyperpolarization and cyclic AMP synthesis thus appear to be different. This observation may also provide additional evidence against the cyclic AMP hypothesis for ganglionic hyperpolarization by catecholamines.

Cyclic AMP is involved in the DA-induced modulatory enhancement of s-EPSP

In addition to eliciting the hyperpolarizing response, DA was found to exert another new type of action on the postsynaptic neurons in the ganglion, namely 'the long-lasting enhancing effect on the muscarinic slow depolarizing response' (Libet and Tosaka, 1970). As shown in Fig. 2, the muscarinic slow depolarizing response, equivalent to the s-EPSP, induced by the application of an agonist (MCh), was enhanced (usually by 50–100%) after a brief exposure of the ganglion to DA. It should be noted (1) that this effect was selective for the s-EPSP or equivalent muscarinic slow depolarization, but not for any other type of postsynaptic responses, and (2) that only DA was able to produce this effect, while the other catecholamines were virtually ineffective. (3) The muscarinic depolarization remained enhanced for several hours

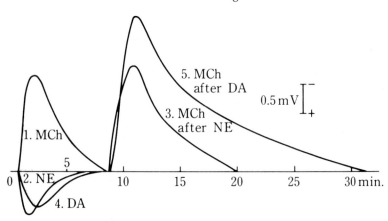

Figure 2 Modulatory enhancement by DA of slow muscarinic depolarization induced by MCh. Surface (sucrose-gap) recordings from rabbit SCG at 22 °C. Ganglion was pretreated by BCh to deplete endogenous DA so as to eliminate the initial hyperpolarizing component normally elicitable by MCh (see Libet and Owman, 1974). Trace 1: control response to a single, quick injection of 1 μmole of MCh into the perfusate. Trace 2: response to NE, 1 μg dose. Trace 3: MCh response repeated shortly after (2). Trace 4: response to DA, 1 μg dose. Trace 5: MCh response repeated after (4). Note the substantial increase in amplitude and duration of MCh response in (5), but virtually not in (3). From Libet (1979a), based on reports in Libet and Tosaka (1970); reproduced by permission of University of Tokyo Press

following DA treatment even though no further DA was applied; then it gradually decayed and finally returned to the control level.

All of the above-described characteristics of the enhancing effect of DA on the muscarinic slow depolarization by extrinsically applied MCh can be fully mimicked by cyclic AMP, as shown in Fig. 3, when administered externally in the form of butyryl derivatives (Libet *et al.*, 1975). Intracellular iontophoretic injection of cyclic AMP was also found capable of producing the enhancing effect, as seen in Fig. 4 (Kobayashi *et al.*, 1977, 1978). In this experiment, injected cyclic AMP was shown to affect the s-EPSP responses elicited by the orthodromic stimulation of the ganglion. Similarly, the test spike responses of postganglionic nerve in the posttetanic facilitatory phase were subjected to lasting augmentation following exposure to theophylline or cyclic AMP (dibutyryl form) (Hsu and McIsaac, 1978). The enhancing effect can be demonstrated even by an action of physiological origin: the s-EPSP responses were enhanced, in a similar manner to that after DA treatment, following a conditioning train of volleys applied to the preganglionic nerves (Tosaka and Kobayashi, 1977; Kobayashi *et al.*, 1977, 1978). In ganglia presumed to have been at least partially depleted of endogenous DA judging from the relative disappearance of s-IPSP (Libet and Owman, 1974), such an enhancing effect could not be induced by preganglionic conditioning (except for much briefer

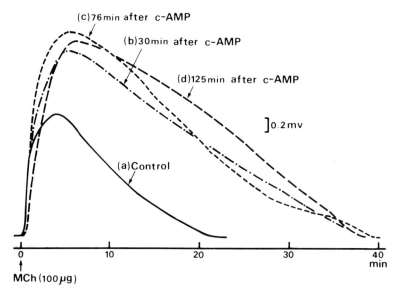

Figure 3 Modulatory enhancement by cyclicAMP of slow muscarinic depolarization induced by MCh. Surface (sucrose-gap) recordings from rabbit SCG at 22 °C. Ganglion was pretreated as in Fig. 2. (a) Control MCh response, 100 μg dose. (b) MCh response repeated 30 min after the brief exposure of ganglion to dibutyryl cyclicAMP (1 mM for 10 min). (c) and (d) MCh responses repeated 76 min and 125 min, respectively, after cyclicAMP treatment. Note that the MCh responses stay enhanced with almost no decay even at 2 hours after cyclicAMP. Unpublished figure, based on reports in Libet *et al.* (1975)

ordinary posttetanic potentiation of all the PSPs). These results can be interpreted as that preganglionic conditioning might release endogenous DA from the SIF cells and produce the enhancing effect by increasing cyclic AMP in the postsynaptic neurons. Evidence of a similar nature, though indirect, for the enhancement of physiological s-EPSP was available: the atropine-sensitive after-discharge recordable in the postganglionic nerve, which would be a reflection of firing due to the underlying s-EPSP in the ganglion cells, was found to be augmented for a prolonged period after preganglionic conditioning (Volle, 1962; McIsaac, 1977). The results thus accumulated appear to support the presence of the aforementioned enhancing effect as a physiological regulatory mechanism.

We have now a novel mode of transmitter action which is more commonly termed 'modulatory' (Libet and Tosaka, 1970; Kupfermann, 1979; Libet, 1979d). This concept of 'neuromodulators', different from conventional 'neurotransmitters', is that one synaptic mediator (DA in the particular case of sympathetic ganglia of some mammalian species) does not simply excite (or inhibit) postsynaptic cells by way of directly eliciting in them the changes in

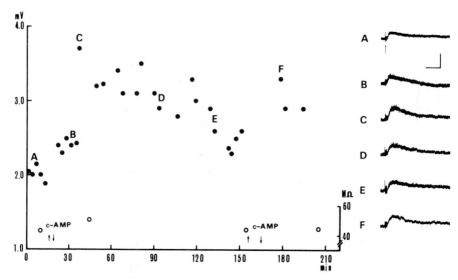

Figure 4 Modulatory enhancement of the s-EPSP responses by intracellularly injected cyclicAMP. Intracellular recordings from rabbit SCG cells at 34 °C. Ganglion was pretreated as in Fig. 2 and moderately curarized (dtc 20 μg/ml). Each s-EPSP, as shown in the inset on the right, was evoked at 3–10-min intervals by a train of preganglionic supramaximal stimuli (20 per sec for 1 sec). Records A–F correspond to the lettered points on the graph. Calibration: 5 mV and 5 sec. Iontophoretic injections of cAMP were made between arrows with the current of 0.5 nA. Note that the enhanced state lasts for almost 90 min or more after a brief injection of cyclicAMP, and it can be repeated by a second injection after the effect due to the first injection has subsided. The enhancement occurs with no significant changes in resting membrane potential or resistance. From Kobayashi *et al.* (1978). Reprinted by permission from *Nature*, Vol. 271, pp. 268–270. Copyright © 1978 Macmillan Journals Limited

membrane potential or conductance, but rather is involved in affecting the events induced by the other transmitters or those due to the endogenous properties of the cells. The 'modulator' concept can be traced back to Florey (1967) who suggested that it may be comparable with the mode of action of hormones. It should be noted, in contrast to the classically known transmitter actions, that hormonal actions are not limited to the locally specialized (synaptic) regions of neurons; their effects are more prolonged and may involve an intracellular mechanism for the production of the final cellular reactions. This mode of action appears to be adequately applicable to that found for DA showing a lasting enhancing effect on the s-EPSP, or muscarinic slow depolarization, in sympathetic ganglia. Following a brief treatment by either DA or cyclic AMP, the modulatory enhancing effect usually lasts for many hours, during the early part of that period the initially applied agents have, of course, been thoroughly washed out. While DA or cyclic AMP is still present, the enhancing effect is invisible and all the PSPs are rather decreased in amplitude, possibly due to the depressant effect of DA or cyclic AMP on the release of transmitter from the presynaptic terminals (Dun and Nishi, 1974; Dun and Karczmar, 1977a; Nishi, 1970, 1974, 1979, Hsu and McIsaac, 1978). The occurrence of the enhancing effect of DA appears to be eliminated by the specific DA antagonists butaclamol and spiroperidol (Ashe and Libet, 1981; Mochida *et al.*, 1981a, 1981b), but cyclic AMP is still able to produce the enhancing effect in the presence of those antagonists. Furthermore, the enhanced state of the muscarinic response, once having been induced either by DA or cyclic AMP, can no longer be affected by later application of DA antagonists (Libet, 1979c). The enhancing effect is produced with no accompanying change in membrane potential or resistance (Kobayashi *et al.*, 1978). All these findings strongly suggest that the enhancing effect itself would be an enduring neuronal change in an intracellular mechanism at least more than one step beyond the DA receptor. This change may primarily include an increased synthesis of cyclic AMP, in response to the activation of DA receptor, and a sequence of subsequent physicochemical changes which finally affect in a lasting fashion the molecular mechanism for the generation of muscarinic depolarization. This sequence of changes may obviously take a substantial length of time for its completion. The time required for any detectable rise of ganglionic cyclic AMP appears to be in the range of several minutes following either preganglionic nerve stimulation (Aleman *et al.*, 1974; Kalix *et al.*, 1974) or DA treatment (Roch and Kalix, 1975). The further possible sequence of biochemical changes (which would involve an activation of protein kinase and subsequent phosphorylation of specific proteins) may take additional time. Such a total length of time for the completion of an adequate sequence of biochemical reactions would be regarded as properly corresponding to the observed latency of 15–20 min in the full development of the enhancing effect in a ganglion cell (Kobayashi *et al.*, 1978; Libet, 1979c). The detailed nature of this change at the molecular level, whose development is initiated by the DA receptor, and the exact cellular site at which the control of the amplitude and duration of muscarinic slow depolarization is operated, need to be clarified.

    The DA receptor for the production of the enhancing effect appears to be one that is specific for DA, in contrast to the one for hyperpolarization being found to be more related to the so-called α_2 type (for rat: Brown and Caulfield, 1979. For rabbit: Mochida *et al.*, 1981a, 1981b). (1) α-Adrenergic antagonists were mostly ineffective against the enhancing effect. The previous report that they could antagonize the enhancing effect (Libet and Tosaka, 1970) was later withdrawn (Libet, 1979c), as this conclusion was based on the use of phenoxybenzamine which would have some considerable side-effect later shown as antagonizing the DA stimulation of adenyl cyclase, an action regarded as unrelated to the α-adrenergic blocking (Walton *et al.*, 1978). The competitive type α antagonist dihydroergotamine, which must be much better for the present experimental purpose, did not antagonize the enhancing effect at all, at concentrations completely eliminating the DA-induced hyperpolarizing response. β-Adrenergic antagonists (such as propranolol) were also without effect on the enhancement. (2) The enhancing effect could be effectively antagonized by a known DA blocker haloperidol (10^{-5} M) and a neuroleptic butaclamol (both *d*- and *l*-form at 10^{-6} to 10^{-7} M), in contrast to their inability at these concentrations to block the hyperpolarization induced by DA and other catecholamines. Sulpiride and metoclopramide, known as D_2-receptor antagonists (Kebabian and Calne, 1979), did not show any antagonism. Metoclopramide, in fact, produced some enhancing effect by itself. (3) Agents which potently antagonized the DA-induced enhancing effect were also shown to have a similarly potent depressant action on DA-stimulated cyclic AMP synthesis in the ganglion. Apomorphine, an agent which did produce a marked enhancing effect (Libet *et al.*, unpublished results, see Libet, 1979c), was also found to be able to stimulate cyclic AMP synthesis in the rat ganglion (Lindl, 1979).

Thus it seems likely that both the DA-induced enhancing effect and the increase in cyclic AMP synthesis are commonly related to the one and the same DA receptor which may be referred to as D_1 type (Kebabian and Calne, 1979). It may be reasonable to assume that the activated DA receptor first induces an increased synthesis of cyclic AMP which further stimulates the production of the enhancing effect on the muscarinic slow depolarizing response. The finding that DA, applied after maximum enhancement had already been produced by cyclic AMP, never produced any further enlargement of already enhanced muscarinic response, which suggests that the actions by both agents converge on the same mechanism (Libet *et al.*, 1975), may also provide additional support for cyclic AMP as an intracellular mediator for the production of DA-induced enhancement.

As described previously, there appear to be the β-type receptors which are responsible in part for the increase of cyclic AMP in the ganglion. However, this β-type increase might not be related to the enhancing effect, probably because such β-receptors would be non-neuronal, but would more likely be glial in origin. In fact, it has been demonstrated that glial cells of the rat in culture have β-receptors linked with adenyl cyclase, which can also be activated partially by DA (Premont *et al.*, 1975). Our result that the combined use of propranolol and butaclamol suppressed almost completely the cyclic AMP increase in the presence of DA in our experimental conditions may further support the above idea.

Dual role of cyclic GMP. A: The direct mediation of the s-EPSP

Cyclic GMP was proposed as mediating intracellularly the production of s-EPSP response (Greengard, 1976) on the basis of the evidence (1) that a slow depolarizing response could be elicited in the rabbit SCG by externally applied dibutyryl cyclic GMP (McAfee and Greengard, 1972), and (2) that a substantial increase in cyclic GMP could be induced in bovine SCG in response to muscarinic agonists (Kebabian *et al.*, 1975). Increases in cyclic GMP were later confirmed by us (unpublished data by Kobayashi and Ushiyama, cited in Hashiguchi *et al.*, 1978) in the rabbit SCG either by preganglionic stimulation or by application of the muscarinic agonist BCh. Ganglionic depolarization by cyclic GMP was also unfailingly recorded using the sucrose-gap technique. Although the proposed hypothesis thus appears plausible, it is crucial that the observed depolarization should somehow be proved to be developed with membrane changes identical to those accompanying the s-EPSP itself. This crucial test could primarily be done by measuring the change in membrane resistance (r_m) associated with any depolarization induced by cyclic GMP.

Intracellular tests have revealed that externally applied cyclic GMP (dibutyryl form) can elicit two kinds of depolarizing response in the rabbit SCG cells depending on the different ranges of concentration. With lower concentrations (about 10^{-4} M or less), cyclic GMP produced a distinct depolarization, as shown in Fig. 5A, which was not associated with either increase or a decrease in membrane conductance (reciprocal of r_m) (Kobayashi *et al.*, 1977; Hashiguchi *et al.*, 1978). This feature of depolarization is fundamentally in accord with that of the s-EPSP (or equivalent muscarinic depolarizing response). Often, a small decrease in conductance is observed in association with the s-EPSP (Kobayashi and Libet, 1968, 1970; Kobayashi *et al.*, 1977; Hashiguchi *et al.*, 1978). This point will further be discussed later in terms of the suppression of the 'M current' (Brown and Adams, 1980) which appears to be unrelated to the action of cyclic GMP.

With relatively higher concentrations (more than about 2.5×10^{-4} M), cyclic GMP produced a larger depolarization which was usually accompanied by a marked increase in membrane conductance (Kobayashi *et al.*, 1977; Hashiguchi *et al.*, 1978). Similar types of depolarizing responses by cyclic GMP in sympathetic neurons were reported by others (Dun *et al.*, 1977b, 1978; Gallagher and Shinnick-Gallagher, 1977). This second type of depolarization would conceivably be a non-specific one due to an excessive concentration of cyclic nucleotides built up inside the cell, as even cyclic AMP could also induce such a type of potential changes when injected intracellularly in a large amount (Gallagher and Shinnick-Gallagher, 1977). Similarly, mammalian spinal motoneurons also responded to injected cyclic GMP with depolarization accompanied by an increase in conductance (Krnjevic *et al*, 1976; Krnjevic and van Meter, 1976). Even in a non-synaptic membrane like that of peripheral nerves, higher doses of cyclic GMP produced a depolarizing potential change (McAfee and Greengard, 1972). When evaluating the

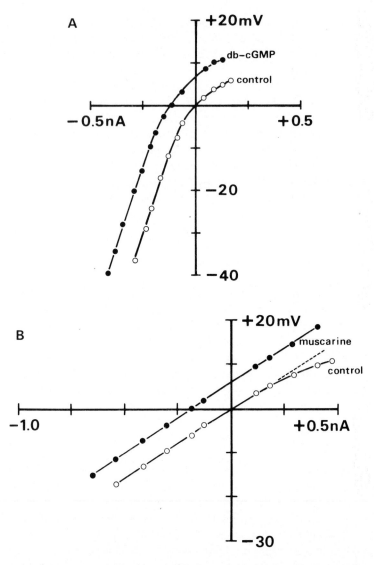

Figure 5 Effects of cyclicGMP (lower concentration) and muscarinic agonist on the rabbit SCG cell membrane. Voltage–current (V–I) analysis was made before (open circles) and after (filled circles) the application of agents. Current pulses of 1-sec duration were passed across the membrane and corresponding electrotonic potentials were recorded, at the steady levels of which the amplitudes of voltage shifts were measured and plotted. Data in A and B were obtained from the different cells with resting potentials (zero level of the ordinates) of $-51\,mV$ (A) and $-61.5\,mV$ (B), respectively. (A) dibutyryl cyclicGMP (db-cGMP; $10^{-4}\,M$). Note that the essentially parallel shift of the V–I curve toward the depolarizing direction at all levels of membrane potential in the presence of cyclicGMP indicates the depolarization is

physiological role of cyclic GMP, this apparently non-specific type of depolarization should cautiously be excluded in order to avoid any further confusion.

As described previously, the s-EPSP (or equivalent muscarinic depolarization) in sympathetic neurons is often associated with a small decrease in membrane conductance. This was first reported by Kobayashi and Libet (for both frogs and rabbits: Kobayashi and Libet, 1968, 1970), and was later confirmed by others (mainly for frogs: Weight and Votava, 1970; Kuba and Koketsu, 1976a, b). Muscarinic responses with similar membrane characteristics were reported also for mammalian central neurons (Krnjevic *et al.*, 1971; Dingledine *et al.*, 1977). In sympathetic neurons, this characteristic was often used as one of the criteria to discriminate the s-EPSP from the action of cyclic GMP, leading to the conclusion that they were unrelated to each other (Gallagher and Shinnick-Gallagher, 1977; Dun *et al.*, 1978). Recently it was reported by Brown and Adams (1980) that a voltage-sensitive steady outward K^+ current (termed 'M current') developed in frog sympathetic neurons in a certain range (-60 to $-20\,mV$) of membrane potential, and that the suppression of this M current by muscarinic agents could account for the observed muscarinic decrease in conductance. A similar persistent outward current has now been confirmed by us (Kobayashi *et al.*, 1981) also in rabbit SCG cells. It should be noted, however, that, unlike the condition for frog neurons, muscarinic agents could evoke in the rabbit neurons an additional depolarization with no change in membrane conductance at all levels of membrane potential including those more negative than $-60\,mV$ (Fig. 5B). This type of depolarization could not be accounted for by any change in the M current, but could more reasonably be attributable to the depolarizing action of cyclic GMP (at lower concentrations). Therefore, it can be proposed that two types of muscarinic action may contribute to the production of s-EPSP in the mammalian sympathetic neurons: (1) A depolarization occurs with no change in membrane conductance through an as yet unknown cellular mechanism; it is producible independently of membrane potential levels and may be mediated intracellularly by cyclic GMP. (2) An additional depolarization occurs with a decrease in membrane conductance, due to the suppression

produced with no change in membrane conductance. In some cases the recovery of the control condition after washing out of the agent was in fact confirmed, eliminating the possibility of an artefactual shift of the curves. From Hashiguchi *et al.* (1978). Reprinted by permission from *Nature*, Vol. 271, pp. 267–268. Copyright © 1978 Macmillan Journals Limited. (B) DL-Muscarine chloride ($10^{-5}\,M$). Note that the rectification (due to the M current) in the depolarized range of the control curve was found to be antagonized in the presence of muscarine, and additional depolarization with no change in conductance was induced at all levels of membrane potential. From Kobayashi *et al.* (1981) and Hashiguchi *et al* (1982)

of the M current, only at a range of membrane potential more positive than about $-60\,mV$, and would not involve cyclic GMP mediation.

In most of the experiments using intracellular recording by means of microelectrodes, it is inevitable to introduce some leaky injury when impaling the cells. Therefore, although it is difficult to tell accurately how much the normal resting potential is of unimpaled cells, most reported records (in intracellular studies) of about $-50\,mV$ would presumably be in a somewhat depolarized range. In the physiological condition, the resting potential of the cells must be more negative than $-60\,mV$ and type 1 depolarization may first occur in response to the muscarinic action, and, when the membrane potential has eventually been brought into the working range of the M current, the type 2 action may become manifest. These two mechanisms may function cooperatively to increase the efficacy of synaptic transmission (because of the sustained depolarization and associated decrease in shunting conductance of the membrane adjacent to the synaptic region) and may thereby favour the maintenance of repetitive firing in sympathetic neurons.

Frog sympathetic neurons appear to lack the type 1 mechanism, as cyclic GMP does not produce any depolarization in the postsynaptic cells of this species (Suria, 1976; Busis et al., 1978; Weight et al., 1978). This is in accordance with our recent observation (Hashiguchi et al., 1982) that muscarinic agents can only produce in the frog neurons an antagonism of the steady outward (M) current in the depolarized range of membrane potential, without bringing about any potential change in the range more negative than $-60\,mV$. In fact, very little or almost no s-EPSP is recordable from the unimpaled (therefore non-depolarized) neurons of curarized frog sympathetic ganglia (Libet, 1979a).

Dual role of cyclic GMP. B: The disruptive regulation of modulatory enhancement by DA and/or cyclic AMP

In addition to possibly mediating a component of the s-EPSP, cyclic GMP has another kind of postsynaptic effect in the ganglion: it antagonizes the development of the long-term modulatory change in the muscarinic depolarizing response either by DA or cyclic AMP (Libet et al., 1975). Its most remarkable feature lies in its striking time-dependency: treatment of the ganglion with cyclic GMP (usually $5 \times 10^{-5}\,M$ for 6 min at $22\,°C$) within 4–5 min immediately after brief exposure to DA (or cyclic AMP) can fully prevent the expected later occurrence of modulatory enhancement of the muscarinic depolarizing response (Fig. 6). If cyclic GMP treatment is delayed for more than 10–15 min after DA (or cyclic AMP), it is found to be ineffective in preventing the modulatory enhancement (Fig. 7). These experimental observations may lead us to conceive that some time-requiring neuronal change (which may involve the formation of cyclic AMP as the

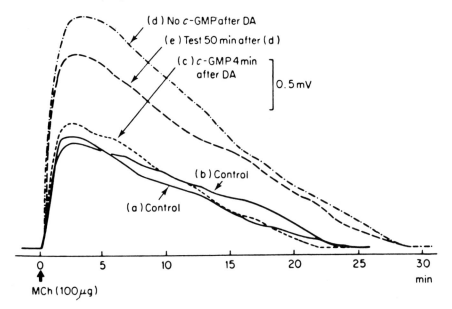

Figure 6 Time-dependent disruptive action of cyclicGMP against the development of modulatory enhancement of slow muscarinic depolarization by DA. Surface (sucrose-gap) recordings from rabbit SCG. Experimental conditions are as in Figs. 2 and 3. (a, b) Control MCh responses. Then ganglion was briefly exposed to DA, and a subsequent cyclicGMP treatment was made within *4 min* after DA. (c) MCh response at 35 min after DA, with an interposed cyclicGMP treatment as described above. (d) MCh response at 35 min after a second dose of DA, but with no interposed cyclicGMP treatment this time. (e) MCh response at 50 min after that in (d). Note that the normally expected occurrence of enhanced MCh response in (c) was prevented, in contrast to the enhanced state of MCh responses in (d) and (e). From Libet *et al.* (1975). Reprinted by permission from *Nature*, Vol. 258, pp. 155–157. Copyright © 1975, Macmillan Journals Limited

initial part of a process consisting of sequential physicochemical changes) starts to develop in the ganglion cell after the DA action (Aleman *et al.*, 1974; Libet *et al.*, 1975). Cyclic GMP has a time-dependent disruptive capability against the development of this neuronal change while the initial part of the process for the development takes place. When this has been fully developed, however, without suffering any disruptive influence before its completion, cyclic GMP can no longer affect its capability to alter the s-EPSP response, and the enhanced state lasts for many hours until it gradually decays to the original level. Some preliminary evidence is reported to be available that, not only exogenously applied cyclic GMP, but also cylic GMP produced endogenously by a strong muscarinic action on ganglion cells may also be capable of producing a disruptive effect on the modulatory change by DA (Libet, 1979a). Based on the evidence of the DA-induced, cyclic AMP-mediated

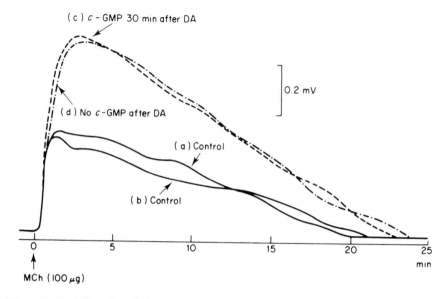

Figure 7 Inability of cyclicGMP, depending on the timing of treatment, to disrupt the development of DA-induced modulatory enhancement of the slow muscarinic depolarization. Preparation and other experimental conditions are as in Fig. 6. (a, b) Control MCh responses. (c) MCh response at about 60 min after a brief exposure to DA, with an interposed cyclicGMP treatment which was made 30 min after DA. (d) MCh response at 60 min after a second dose of DA, with no interposed cyclicGMP treatment. Note that MCh response in (c) was enhanced, in contrast to (c) in Fig. 6, in spite of the interposed cyclicGMP treatment after DA. From Libet *et al.* (1975). Reprinted by permission from *Nature*, Vol. 258, pp. 155–157. Copyright © Macmillan Journals Limited

production of the modulatory enhancement of the s-EPSP and the intracellular cyclic GMP mediation of the s-EPSP response itself, it can be assumed that cyclic AMP and cylic GMP may synergize physiologically in mammalian sympathetic ganglia. An additional fact of the capability of cyclic GMP to disrupt the development of DA modulatory action, however, may further provide an idea that both nucleotides also work antagonistically. It is worth noting that cyclic GMP may thus play a significant key physiological role in the ganglion cell by being synergistic to cyclic AMP on the one hand, but may sometimes be antagonistic, on the other hand, in a kind of negative-feedback fashion, depending on the various different conditions.

GENERAL CONCLUSIONS

It is still true and acceptable even today that the transmission of electrical signals in mammalian sympathetic ganglia can be achieved primarily by a

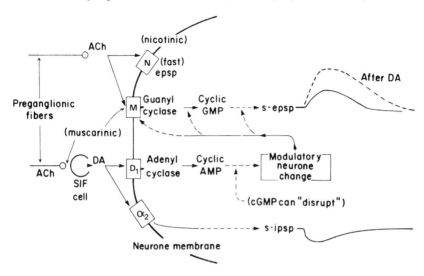

Figure 8 Proposed schema of postsynaptic intracellular pathways for responses to ACh and DA in the rabbit SCG. Muscarinic receptors responsible for the antagonism of M current, not via cyclicGMP mediation, is not shown. The existence of separate receptors corresponding to two different actions of DA has been demonstrated recently (Mochida *et al.*, 1981a, b). The general possible routes for the intracellular processes to lead the specific cellular reactions are indicated by dashed lines, though most of these need to be substantiated in future studies. From Libet *et al.* (1975), with some modifications. Reprinted by permission from *Nature*, Vol. 258, pp. 155–157. Copyright © Macmillan Journals Limited. See also Libet (1979a, c)

nicotinic action of preganglionically released ACh which gives rise to the f-EPSP response in the postganglionic neurons. However, recent development in our knowledge about the slow synaptic processes further elucidates the physiological significance of the mechanisms which regulate (or modulate) the mode of electrical signalling of the ganglion cells in the background, rather than directly conveying each signal itself. In this regulatory mechanism the contribution of cyclic nucleotides has now been largely substantiated. Their roles can be summarized as follows: (1) Cyclic AMP is not involved in the production of the DA-induced slow hyperpolarizing postsynaptic response (s-IPSP), but it certainly mediates a long-term modulatory enhancement of the muscarinic slow depolarizing responses (s-EPSP). (2) Cyclic GMP directly mediates at least a component of the mechanisms underlying the production of the s-EPSP itself. (3) Cyclic GMP may also regulate, in a disruptive manner depending on the conditions, the development of DA-induced modulatory change in the s-EPSP. This wide range of functions is schematized in Fig. 8 (showing mainly the intracellular pathways).

The confirmation of the involvement of cyclic nucleotides in ganglionic transmission has long been a subject of serious controversy. But no simple agreement can be reached unless the enormous diversity of neurotransmitter actions in the ganglion, as revealed in recent years, is taken into consideration. Most of the detailed cellular mechanisms in the diverse actions of neurotransmitters are not fully clarified as yet, but the possible involvement of cyclic nucleotides in some of them may provide useful clues for further analysis in future.

Finally, the slow synaptic processes bear apparent functional similarities to enduring changes in the activities of the brain. Particularly they may at least present a prototype model for synaptic coupling into the production of a neuronal memory trace (Libet *et al.*, 1975) in terms of synaptic plasticity.

ACKNOWLEDGEMENTS

The authors express their sincere gratitude to Professor Benjamin Libet of the University of California, San Francisco, for his constant encouragement and valuable advice throughout this research over a long span of years. Thanks also to Drs T. Tanaka and T. Hashiguchi, and Ms N. S. Ushiyama, S. Mochida and J. Tasaka of Tokyo Medical College for their collaboration with the authors in carrying out this work. The authors also wish to thank the Upjohn Company, Michigan, for the kind supply of the useful test chemical U-0521. This research was partly supported by a grant to HK from the Ministry of Education, Culture and Science of Japan.

REFERENCES

Aleman, V., Bayon, A., and Molina, J. (1974). Functional changes of synapses. *Adv. Behav. Biol.*, **10**, 115–124.

Ashe, J. H., and Libet, B. (1981). Modulation of slow postsynaptic potentials by dopamine, in rabbit sympathetic ganglia. *Brain Res.*, **217**, 93–106.

Black, A. C., Jr., Chiba, T., Wamsley, J. K., Bhalla, R. C., and Williams, T. H. (1978). Interneurons of sympathetic ganglia: Divergent cyclic AMP responses and morphology in cat and cow. *Brain Res.*, **148**, 389–398.

Brown, D. A., and Adams, P. R. (1980). Muscarinic suppression of a novel voltage-sensitive K^+ current in a vertebrate neurone. *Nature*, **283**, 673–676.

Brown, D. A., and Caulfield, M. P. (1979). Hyperpolarizing α_2-adrenoceptors in rat sympathetic ganglia. *Br. J. Pharmacol.*, **65**, 435–445.

Brown, D. A., Caulfield, M. P., and Kirby, P. J. (1979). Relation between catecholamine-induced cyclic AMP changes and hyperpolarization in isolated rat sympathetic ganglia. *J. Physiol. (London)*, **290**, 441–451.

Busis, N. A., Weight, F. F., and Smith, P. A. (1978). Synaptic potentials in sympathetic ganglia: Are they mediated by cyclic nucleotides? *Science*, **200**, 1079–1081.

Cole, A. E., and Shinnick-Gallagher, P. (1979). Characterization of a post-ganglionic catecholamine-receptor in the rabbit superior cervical ganglion. *Soc. Neurosci. Abstr.*, **5**, 738.

Cole, A. E., and Shinnick-Gallagher, P. (1980). Alpha-adrenoceptor and dopamine receptor antagonists do not block the slow inhibitory postsynaptic potential in sympathetic ganglia. *Brain Res.*, **187**, 226–230.

Cramer, H., Johnson, D. G., Hanbauer, I., Silberstein, S. D., and Kopin, I. J. (1973). Accumulation of adenosine 3',5'-monophosphate induced by catecholamine in the rat superior cervical ganglion *in vitro*. *Brain Res.*, **53**, 97–104.

Dingledine, R., Dodd, J., and Kelly, J. S. (1977). ACh-evoked excitation of cortical neurones. *J. Physiol. (London)*, **273**, 79–80p.

Dun, N. J., and Karczmar, A. G. (1977a). The presynaptic site of action of norepinephrine in the superior cervical ganglion of guinea-pig. *J. Pharmacol. Exp. Ther.*, **200**, 328–335.

Dun, N. J., and Karczmar, A. G. (1977b). A comparison of the effect of theophylline and cyclic adenosine 3',5'-monophosphate on the superior cervical ganglion of the rabbit by means of the sucrose-gap method. *J. Pharmacol. Exp. Ther.*, **202**, 89–96.

Dun, N. J., and Karczmar, A. G. (1978). Involvement of an interneuron in the generation of slow inhibitory postsynaptic potential in mammalian sympathetic ganglia. *Proc. Natl. Acad. Sci. U.S.A.*, **75**, 4029–4032.

Dun, N. J., and Karczmar, A. G. (1979). Actions of substance P on sympathetic neurons. *Neuropharmacology*, **18**, 215–218.

Dun, N. J., and Nishi, S. (1974). Effect of dopamine on the superior cervical ganglion of rabbit. *J. Physiol. (London)*, **239**, 155–164.

Dun, N. J., Kaibara, K., and Karczmar, A. G. (1977a). Dopamine and adenosine 3',5'-monophosphate responses of single mammalian sympathetic neurons. *Science*, **197**, 778–780.

Dun, N. J., Kaibara, K., and Karczmar, A. G. (1977b). Direct postsynaptic membrane effect of dibutyryl cyclic GMP on mammalian sympathetic neurons. *Neuropharmacology*, **16**, 715–717.

Dun, N. J., Kaibara, K., and Karczmar, A. G. (1978). Muscarinic and cGMP-induced membrane potential changes: Differences in electrogenic mechanisms. *Brain Res.*, **150**, 658–661.

Eccles, R., and Libet, B. (1961). Origin and blockade of the synaptic responses of curarized sympathetic ganglia. *J. Physiol. (London)*, **157**, 484–503.

Eränkö, O., and Härkönen, M. (1963). Histochemical demonstration of the fluorogenic amines in the cytoplasm of sympathetic ganglion cells of the rat. *Acta Physiol. Scand.*, **58**, 285–286.

Florey, E. (1967). Neurotransmitters and modulators in the animal kingdom. *Fed. Proc.*, **26**, 1164–1178.

Gallagher, J. P., and Shinnick-Gallagher, P. (1977). Cyclic nucleotides injected intracellularly into rat superior cervical ganglion cells. *Science*, **198**, 851–852.

Gallagher, J. P., Shinnick-Gallagher, P., Cole, A. E., Griffith, W. H. III, and Williams, B. J. (1980). Current hypotheses for the slow inhibitory postsynaptic potential in sympathetic ganglia. *Fed. Proc.*, **39**, 3009–3015.

Greengard, P. (1976). Possible role for cyclic nucleotides and phosphorylated membrane proteins in postsynaptic actions of neurotransmitters. *Nature*, **260**, 101–108.

Greengard, P., and Kebabian, J. W. (1974). Role of cyclic AMP in synaptic transmission in the mammalian peripheral nervous system. *Fed. Proc.*, **33**, 1059–1067.

Hashiguchi, T., Kobayashi, H. Tosaka, T. and Libet, B. (1982) Two muscarinic depolarizing mechanisms in mammalian sympathetic neurons. *Brain Res.*, **242**, 378–382.

Hashiguchi, T., Ushiyama, N. S., Kobayashi, H., and Libet, B. (1978). Does cyclic GMP mediate the slow excitatory synaptic potential in sympathetic ganglia? *Nature*, **271**, 267–268.

Horn, J. P., and Dodd, J. (1981). Monosynaptic muscarinic activation of K^+ conductance underlies the slow inhibitory postsynaptic potential in sympathetic ganglia. *Nature*, **292**, 625–627.

Horton, E. W. (1969). Hypotheses on physiological roles of prostaglandins. *Physiol. Rev.*, **49**, 122–161.

Hsu, S. Y., and McIsaac, R. J. (1978). Effects of theophylline and N^6, O^2-dibutyryl adenosine $3',5'$-monophosphate on sympathetic ganglionic transmission in rats. *J. Pharmacol. Exp. Ther.*, **205**, 91–103.

Ivanov, A. Y., and Skok, V. I. (1980). Slow inhibitory postsynaptic potentials and hyperpolarization evoked by noradrenaline in the neurones of mammalian sympathetic ganglion. *J. Autonom. Nerv. Syst.*, **1**, 255–263.

Jan, Y. N., Jan, L. Y., and Kuffler, S. W. (1979). A peptide as a possible transmitter in sympathetic ganglia of the frog. *Proc. Natl. Acad. Sci. U.S.A.*, **76**, 1501–1505.

Kalix, P., McAfee, D. M., Schorderet, M., and Greengard, P. (1974). Pharmacological analysis of synaptically mediated increase in cyclic adenosine monophosphate in rabbit superior cervical ganglion. *J. Pharmacol. Exp. Ther.*, **188**, 676–687.

Kebabian, J. W., and Calne, D. B. (1979). Multiple receptors for dopamine. *Nature*, **277**, 93–96.

Kebabian, J. W., and Greengard, P. (1971). Dopamine-sensitive adenyl cyclase: Possible role in synaptic transmission. *Science*, **174**, 1346–1349.

Kebabian, J. W., Steiner, A. L., and Greengard, P. (1975). Muscarinic cholinergic regulation of cyclic guanosine $3',5'$-monophosphate in autonomic ganglia: Possible role in synaptic transmission. *J. Pharmacol. Exp. Ther.*, **193**, 474–488.

Kobayashi, H. (1976). On the slow synaptic responses in autonomic ganglia. *Adv. Neurol. Sci.*, **20**, 186–198 (in Japanese).

Kobayashi, H., and Libet, B. (1968). Generation of slow postsynaptic potentials without increases in ionic conductance. *Proc. Natl. Acad. Sci. U.S.A.*, **60**, 1304–1311.

Kobayashi, H., and Libet, B. (1970). Actions of noradrenaline and acetylcholine on sympathetic ganglion cells. *J. Physiol. (London)*, **208**, 353–372.

Kobayashi, H., Ushiyama, N. S., and Hashiguchi, T. (1977). Intracellular study of the effects of cyclic nucleotides in the mammalian sympathetic ganglion cells. *Proc. 27th Int. Congr. Physiol. Sci., Paris*, **13**, 394.

Kobayashi, H., Hashiguchi, T., and Ushiyama, N. S. (1978). Postsynaptic modulation of excitatory process in sympathetic ganglia by cyclic AMP. *Nature*, **271**, 268–270.

Kobayashi, H., Hashiguchi, T., Tosaka, T., and Mochida, S. (1981). Muscarinic antagonism of a persistent outward current in sympathetic neurons of the rabbits and its partial contribution to the generation of the slow EPSP. *Neurosci. Lett. Suppl.*, **6**, S–64.

Krnjevic, K., and van Meter, W. G. (1976). Cyclic nucleotides in spinal cells. *Can. J. Physiol. Pharmacol.*, **54**, 416–421.

Krnjevic, K., Pumain, R., and Renaud, L. (1971). The mechanism of excitation by acetylcholine in the cerebral cortex. *J. Physiol. (London)*, **215**, 247–268.

Krnjevic, K., Puil, E., and Werman, R. (1976). Is cyclic guanosine monophosphate the internal 'second messenger' for cholinergic actions on central neurons ? *Can. J. Physiol. Pharmacol.*, **54**, 172–176.

Kuba, K., and Koketsu, K. (1976a). Analysis of the slow excitatory postsynaptic potential in bullfrog sympathetic ganglion cells. *Jpn. J. Physiol.*, **26**, 651–669.

Kuba, K., and Koketsu, K. (1976b). The muscarinic effects of acetylcholine on the action potential of bullfrog sympathetic ganglion cells. *Jpn. J. Physiol.*, **26**, 703–716.

Kupfermann, I. (1979). Modulatory actions of neurotransmitters. *Annu. Rev. Neurosci.*, **2**, 447–465.

Libet, B. (1967). Long latent period and further analysis of slow synaptic responses in sympathetic ganglia. *J. Physiol. (London)*, **30**, 494–514.

Libet, B. (1970). Generation of slow inhibitory and excitatory postsynaptic potentials. *Fed. Proc.*, **29**, 1945–1956.

Libet, B. (1979a). Slow postsynaptic actions in ganglionic functions. In *Integrative Function of the Autonomic Nervous System* (Eds. C. M. Brooks, K. Koizumi and A. Sato), pp. 197–222, University of Tokyo Press and Elsevier/North-Holland Biomedical Press, Amsterdam.

Libet, B. (1979b). Which postsynaptic action of dopamine is mediated by cyclic AMP? *Life Sci.*, **24**, 1043–1058.

Libet, B. (1979c). Dopaminergic synaptic processes in the superior cervical ganglion: Models for synaptic actions. In *The Neurobiology of Dopamine* (Eds. A. Horn, J. Korf and B. H. C. Westerink), pp. 453–474, Academic Press, London.

Libet, B. (1979d). Neuronal communication and synaptic modulation: experimental evidence vs. conceptual categories. *Behav. Brain Sci.*, **2**, 431–432.

Libet, B., and Kobayashi, H. (1974). Adrenergic mediation of slow inhibitory postsynaptic potential in sympathetic ganglia of the frog. *J. Neurophysiol.*, **37**, 805–814.

Libet, B., and Owman, Ch. (1974). Concomitant changes in formaldehyde-induced fluorescence of dopamine interneurones and in slow inhibitory postsynaptic potentials of the rabbit superior cervical ganglion, induced by stimulation of the preganglionic nerve or by a muscarinic agent. *J. Physiol. (London)*, **237**, 635–662.

Libet, B., and Tosaka, T. (1969). Slow inhibitory and excitatory postsynaptic responses in single cells of mammalian sympathetic ganglia. *J. Neurophysiol.*, **32**, 43–50.

Libet, B., and Tosaka, T. (1970). Dopamine as a synaptic transmitter and modulator in sympathetic ganglia: A different mode of synaptic action. *Proc. Natl. Acad. Sci. U.S.A.*, **67**, 667–673.

Libet, B., and Tosaka, T. (1971). Dopaminergic synaptic actions in sympathetic ganglia. *Fed. Proc.*, **30**, 323.

Libet, B., Kobayashi, H., and Tanaka, T. (1975). Synaptic coupling into the production and storage of a neuronal memory trace. *Nature*, **258**, 155–157.

Lindl, T. (1979). cAMP and its relation to ganglionic transmission. A combined biochemical and electrophysiological study of the rat superior cervical ganglion *in vitro. Neuropharmacology*, **18**, 227–235.

Lindl, T., and Cramer, H. (1975). Evidence against dopamine as the mediator of the rise of cyclic AMP in the superior cervical ganglion of the rat. *Biochem. Biophys. Res. Commun.*, **65**, 731–739.

McAfee, D. M., and Greengard, P. (1972). Adenosine 3′,5′-monophosphate: Electrophysiological evidence for a role in synaptic transmission. *Science*, **178**, 310–312.

McAfee, D. M., Schorderet, M., and Greengard, P. (1971). Adenosine 3′,5′-monophosphate in nervous tissue: Increase associated with synaptic transmission. *Science*, **171**, 1156–1158.

McIsaac, R. J. (1977). After discharge on postganglionic sympathetic nerves following repetitive stimulation of the rat superior cervical ganglion *in vitro. J. Pharmacol. Exp. Ther.*, **200**, 107–116.

Mochida, S., Kobayashi, H., Tosaka, T., and Tasaka, J. (1981a). Dopamine receptors mediating two different synaptic actions in the rabbit sympathetic ganglia. *J. Physiol. Soc. Jpn.*, **43**, 298.

Mochida, S., Kobayashi, H., Tosaka, T., Ito, J., and Libet, B. (1981b). Specific dopamine receptor mediates the production of cyclic AMP in the rabbit sympathetic ganglia and thereby modulates the muscarinic postsynaptic responses. *Adv. Cyclic Nucleotide Res.*, **14**, 685.

Nakamura, J. (1978). The effect of neuroleptics on the dopaminergic and cholinergic systems in sympathetic ganglia. *Kurume Med. J.*, **25**, 241–253.

Nishi, S. (1970). Cholinergic and adrenergic receptors at sympathetic preganglionic nerve terminal. *Fed. Proc.*, **29**, 1957–1965.

Nishi, S. (1974). Ganglionic transmission. In *The Peripheral Nervous System* (Ed. J. I. Hubbard), pp. 225–255, Plenum Press, New York, London.

Nishi, S. (1979). The catecholamine-mediated inhibition in ganglionic transmission. In *Integrative Function of the Autonomic Nervous System* (Eds. C. M. Brooks, K. Koizumi and A. Sato), pp. 223–233, University of Tokyo Press and Elsevier/North-Holland Biomedical Press, Amsterdam.

Nishi, S., and Koketsu, K. (1968). Early and late after-discharge of amphibian sympathetic ganglion cells. *J. Neurophysiol.*, **31**, 33–42.

Pearson, J. D. M., and Sharman, D. F. (1974). Increased concentration of acidic metabolites of dopamine in the superior cervical ganglion following preganglionic stimulation *in vivo*. *J. Neurochem.*, **22**, 547–550.

Premont, J., Benda, P., and Jard, S. (1975). ^{3}H-Norepinephrine binding by rat glial cells in culture: lack of correlation between binding and adenylate cyclase activation. *Biochim. Biophys. Acta*, **381**, 368–376.

Quenzer, L., Yahn, D., Alkadhi, K. and Volle, R. L. (1978). Transmission blockade and stimulation of ganglionic adenylate cyclase by catecholamines in rat superior cervical ganglia. *Fed. Proc.*, **37**, 538.

Roch, Ph., and Kalix, P. (1975). Effects of biogenic amines on the concentration of adenosine $3',5'$-monophosphate in bovine superior cervical ganglion. *Neuropharmacology*, **14**, 21–24.

Sheppard, H., and Wiggan, G. (1971). Analogues of 4-(3,4-dimethoxybenzyl)-2-imidazolidinone as potent inhibitors of rat erythrocyte adenosine cyclic $3',5'$-phosphate phosphodiesterase. *Mol. Pharmacol.*, **7**, 111–115.

Suria, A. (1976). Cyclic GMP modulates the intensity of post-tetanic potentiation in bullfrog sympathetic ganglia. *Neuropharmacology*, **15**, 11–16.

Tomasi, V., Biondi, C., Trevisani, A., Martini, M., and Perri, V. (1977). Modulation of cyclic AMP levels in the bovine superior cervical ganglion by prostaglandin E_1 and dopamine. *J. Neurochem.*, **28**, 1289–1297.

Tosaka, T., and Kobayashi, H. (1977). The SIF cell as a functional modulator of ganglionic transmission through the release of dopamine. *Arch. Histol. Jpn.*, **40** (Suppl), 187–196.

Volle, R. L. (1962). Enhancement of postganglionic responses to stimulating agents following repetitive preganglionic stimulation. *J. Pharmacol. Exp. Ther.*, **136**, 68–74.

Walton, K. G., Liepmann, P., and Baldessarini, R. J. (1978). Inhibition of dopamine-stimulated adenylate cyclase activity by phenoxybenzamine. *Eur. J. Pharmacol.*, **52**, 231–234.

Wamsley, J. K., Black, A. C., Jr., West, J. R., and Williams, T. H. (1980). Cyclic AMP synthesis in guinea-pig superior cervical ganglia: Response to pharmacological and preganglionic physiological stimulation. *Brain Res.*, **182**, 415–421.

Weight, F. F., and Padjen, A. L. (1973). Acetylcholine and slow synaptic inhibition in frog sympathetic ganglion cells. *Brain Res.*, **55**, 225–228.

Weight, F. F., and Smith, P. A. (1980). Small intensely fluorescent cells and the generation of slow postsynaptic inhibition in sympathetic ganglia. In *Histochemistry and Cell Biology of Autonomic Neurons, SIF Cells, and Paraneurons* (Eds. O. Eränkö, S. Soinila and H. Päivärinta), *Advances in Biochemical Psychopharmacology*, Vol. 25, pp. 159–171, Raven Press, New York.

Weight, F. F., and Votava, J. (1970). Slow synaptic excitation in sympathetic ganglion cells: Evidence for synaptic inactivation of potassium conductance. *Science*, **170**, 755–758.

Weight, F. F., Smith, P. A., and Schulman, J. A. (1978). Postsynaptic potential generation appears independent of synaptic elevation of cyclic nucleotides in sympathetic neurons. *Brain Res.*, **158**, 197–202.

Williams, T. H., Black, A. C., Jr., Chiba, T., and Bhalla, R. C. (1975). Morphology and biochemistry of small intensely fluorescent cells of sympathetic ganglia. *Nature*, **256**, 315–317.

Williams, T. H., Chiba, T., Black, A. C., Jr., Bhalla, R. C., and Jew, J. Y. (1976). Species variation in SIF cells of superior cervical ganglia: Are there two functional types? *Fogarty Int. Cent. Proc.*, **30**, 143–162.

Williams, T. H., Black, A. C., Jr., Chiba, T., and Jew, J. Y. (1977). Species differences in mammalian SIF cells. In *SIF Cells* (Eds. E. Costa and G. L. Gessa), *Advances in Biochemical Psychopharmacology*, Vol. 16, pp. 505–511, Raven Press, New York.

Williams, T. H., Black, A. C., Jr., West, J. R., Sandquist, D., and Gluhbegovic, N. (1980). Biochemical aspects of SIF cell function in guinea-pig and rabbit superior cervical ganglia. In *Histochemistry and Cell Biology of Autonomic Neurons, SIF Cells and Paraneurons* (Eds. O. Eränkö, S. Soinila and H. Päivärinta), *Advances in Biochemical Psychopharmacology*, Vol. 25, pp. 127–131, Raven Press, New York.

Autonomic Ganglia
Edited by Lars-Gösta Elfvin
© 1983 John Wiley & Sons Ltd

Synaptic Mechanisms in Amphibian Sympathetic Ganglia

FORREST F. WEIGHT

*Laboratory of Preclinical Studies,
National Institute on Alcohol Abuse and Alcoholism,
Rockville, Maryland 20852, USA*

INTRODUCTION

Amphibian sympathetic ganglia have several features that make them particularly well suited for investigations on membrane and synaptic mechanisms in vertebrate neurons. These features include: (1) accessibility; (2) simplicity of the synaptic organization; (3) postsynaptic potentials of different types that can be elicited by stimulation of separate preganglionic nerves; (4) neurons without dendrites of sufficient size for intracellular electrophysiological investigation; (5) synapses located on the neuronal soma; and (6) physiological stability *in vitro* for long periods of time. This paper will review our current state of knowledge of the synaptic organization, the identification of the neurotransmitters, and the mechanisms involved in the generation of postsynaptic potentials in amphibian sympathetic ganglia. The review will focus particularly on the IXth and Xth paravertebral sympathetic ganglia of the bullfrog, since most recent studies have been conducted on those ganglia.

SYNAPTIC ORGANIZATION

The structure of the frog autonomic nervous system was described by nineteenth century anatomists and summarized in the classic work of Ecker and Wiedersheim, revised by Gaupp (1899). The sympathetic ganglia are numbered sequentially from rostral to caudal on the basis of the spinal nerve to which they are connected (Fig. 1A). The IXth and Xth ganglia receive two systems of preganglionic fibres that make synaptic contact with neurons in the ganglia (Fig. 1B) (Skok, 1965; Nishi *et al.*, 1965; Libet *et al.*, 1968; Tosaka *et al.*, 1968; Weight and Votava, 1970; Weight and Padjen, 1973a). One has a low threshold for electrical excitation and a B fiber conduction velocity (1–14 m/sec). The preganglionic B fibers enter the sympathetic chain via the IVth to VIth spinal nerves and descend in the chain to the IXth and Xth ganglia. The second system has a high threshold for electrical excitation and a

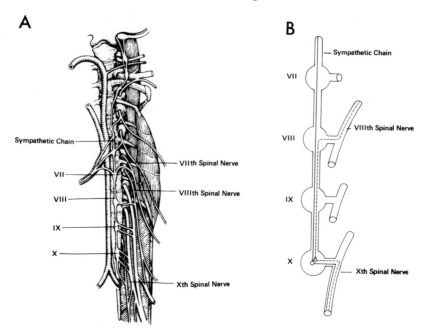

Figure 1 Anatomy and pathways of frog sympathetic nervous system. (A) Diagram of the sympathetic nervous system of the frog. Sympathetic ganglia VII to X are indicated by Roman numerals (after Gaupp, 1899). (B) Schematic diagram of pathways in Xth paravertebral sympathetic ganglion of frog. Solid lines represent axons with B fibre conduction velocity. Preganglionic B fibres in the sympathetic chain make synaptic connection with postganglionic B neurons. Dashed lines represent axons with C fibre conduction velocity. Preganglionic C fibres enter the sympathetic chain via the VIIth and VIIIth spinal nerves and make synaptic connection with postganglionic C neurons. After Skok (1965), Libet *et al.* (1968)

C fiber conduction velocity (0.2–0.8 m/sec). The preganglionic C fibres enter the sympathetic chain via the VIIth and VIIIth spinal nerves, and descend in the chain to the IXth and Xth ganglia. Intracellular recording has revealed two types of neurons in the IXth and Xth ganglia—one with a B fibre conduction velocity axon (B neurons), and the other with a C fibre conduction velocity axon (C neurons) (Fig. 1B). The postganglionic axons of B and C neurons exit via the IXth or Xth ramus communicans and course posteriorly in the distal portion of the spinal nerve (Fig. 1B). The B neurons receive synaptic connections from preganglionic B fibres, whereas the C neurons receive innervation primarily from preganglionic C fibres. In general, a single preganglionic B fibre makes synaptic connection with a B neuron, and the majority of C neurons are innervated by a single preganglionic C fibre. In addition, some C neurons receive a convergence of synaptic connections from

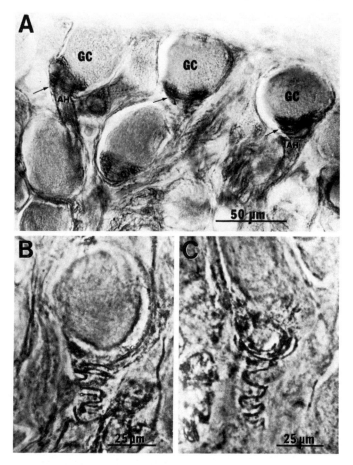

Figure 2 Morphologic appearance of bullfrog sympathetic neurons. (A) Bright-field micrograph of sympathetic neurons in the Xth paravertebral ganglion showing localization of acetylcholinesterase (AChE). The AChE reaction product is primarily in the preganglionic axons and the synaptic boutons (arrows) on the soma and the axon hillock (AH) region of the ganglion cells (GC). (B, C) Phase-contrast micrographs of individual ganglion cells showing localization of AChE in the preganglionic axon that spirals around the axon hillock. From Weitsen and Weight (1977)

more than one preganglionic C fibre, and on occasion a C neuron receives a synaptic connection from a preganglionic B fibre (Smith and Weight, 1981).

The cellular morphology of amphibian sympathetic neurons was investigated extensively in the nineteenth century using light-microscopic techniques (for review see Huber, 1900). The neurons are unipolar with a cell body that is more or less round or oval. The presynaptic fibre forms a spiral around the axon hillock region before arborizing to make synaptic contact with the neuron (Fig. 2). Recent electron-microscopic studies have revealed that most synapses are located on the soma and axon hillock region of the neuron (Nishi et al., 1967; Taxi, 1976; Weitsen and Weight, 1977; see also chapter by Watanabe).

IDENTIFICATION OF SYNAPTIC EVENTS

Early electrophysiological studies using surface recording electrodes identified three types of synaptic responses in curarized sympathetic ganglia. A surface negative potential (N wave) is elicited by a single preganglionic stimulus (Eccles, 1943). With repetitive preganglionic stimuli, the N wave is followed by a positive (P) wave and a late-negative (LN) wave (Laporte and Lorente de Nó, 1950). The sequence of N, P, and LN waves can be recorded in reptilian (Laporte and Lorente de Nó, 1950), mammalian (Eccles, 1952), and amphibian (Libet et al., 1968; Nishi and Koketsu, 1968a) sympathetic ganglia. More recent experiments, using intracellular recording techniques, have identified three types of synaptic potentials in both mammalian and amphibian ganglia—a fast EPSP (excitatory postsynaptic potential), a slow IPSP (inhibitory postsynaptic potential), and a slow EPSP, referred to as f-EPSP, s-IPSP and s-EPSP, respectively. Comparison of the surface potentials with the intracellularly recorded synaptic potentials has shown that the N wave corresponds to the f-EPSP, the P wave to the s-IPSP, and the LN wave to the s-EPSP (Nishi and Koketsu, 1960, 1968a; Libet, 1967; Tosaka et al., 1968). In addition, in amphibian ganglia, a surface late-late negative (LLN) wave is also recorded and corresponds to a fourth type of postsynaptic potential, the late-slow EPSP (ls-EPSP) (Nishi and Koketsu, 1968a).

THE FAST EXCITATORY POSTSYNAPTIC POTENTIAL (f-EPSP)

In 1960, Nishi and Koketsu reported their pioneering intracellular investigation in frog sympathetic ganglia. They found that a single electrical stimulus to preganglionic fibres elicits an EPSP that usually initiates the generation of an action potential in the ganglion cell. In cells uncomplicated by action potential generation, the EPSP has a rapid time course, rising to a peak in about 3–4 msec and decaying exponentially with a duration of 30–50 msec (Fig. 3). The rapid time course of this synaptic event, in comparison with other types of long-duration postsynaptic potentials in sympathetic ganglia, led to its subsequent designation of f-EPSP.

The transmitter mediating the f-EPSP has been identified as acetylcholine (ACh) acting on nicotinic postsynaptic receptors on the basis of the following evidence: (1) nicotinic antagonists such as tubocurarine and hexamethonium significantly reduce the amplitude of the f-EPSP (Blackman et al., 1963; Nishi and Koketsu, 1968a; Tosaka et al., 1968); (2) ACh depolarizes the neurons (Blackman et al., 1963), with the ACh-depolarization having essentially the

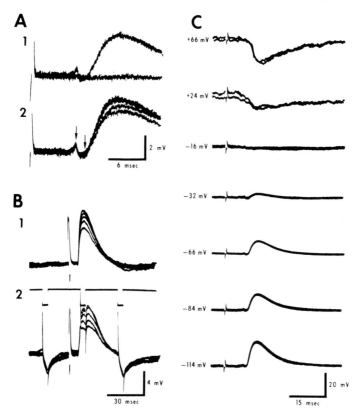

Figure 3 f-EPSPs recorded with an intracellular microelectrode. (A) 1: Stimulation of the preganglionic axon at threshold. 2: Stimulation of the preganglionic axon with a supramaximal stimulus of constant strength. Three superimposed traces. The small deflection preceding the EPSP (first arrow) is the electrical pick-up of the action potential in the preganglionic axon. The second arrow indicates the beginning of the EPSP. (B) 1: Five superimposed EPSPs elicited by supramaximal stimulation of the preganglionic axon. 2: Hyperpolarizing constant current pulses—one preceding, one at the peak of, and one following the EPSP. The top record shows the current trace; the current pulse was −0.2 nA. (C) Amplitude of f-EPSP as a function of membrane potential. Resting membrane potential was −66 mV. Recorded from a B neuron in the Xth paravertebral ganglion of bullfrog. From Weitsen and Weight (1977)

same reversal potential as the f-EPSP (Nishi *et al.*, 1969; Dennis *et al.*, 1971); (3) nicotine depolarizes the neurons (Ginsborg and Guerrero, 1964), and with continuous nicotine superfusion there is repolarization within 30 min, and the f-EPSP is totally blocked (Nishi and Koketsu, 1968a; Kobayashi and Libet, 1970; Weight and Votava, 1970; Weight and Padjen, 1973a); (4) cholinesterase inhibitors potentiate the f-EPSP (Blackman *et al.*, 1963); and (5) ACh is released by preganglionic stimulation (Nishi *et al.*, 1967). In addition, the preganglionic fibres that make synaptic contact with both the large (B) and the small (C) neurons stain for acetylcholinesterase (Fig. 2), providing histochemical data consistent with the identification of the preganglionic fibres as cholinergic (Weitsen and Weight, 1977).

The nature of the postsynaptic action of the transmitter underlying the generation of the f-EPSP in sympathetic neurons is similar in many respects to the action of the transmitter at the neuromuscular junction (see Steinback and Stevens, 1976; Takeuchi, 1977). Two types of evidence indicate that membrane permeability (conductance) is increased during the f-EPSP: (1) an action potential superimposed on the f-EPSP is reduced in amplitude (Nishi and Koketsu, 1960; Blackman et al., 1963); (2) the voltage deflection produced by a hyperpolarizing constant current pulse (i.e. membrane resistance) is markedly reduced at the peak of the f-EPSP (Fig. 3B) (Weitsen and Weight, 1977). The permeability change during the f-EPSP has been found to involve an increased conductance to both Na^+ and K^+ on the basis of the following observations: (1) the f-EPSP has a reversal potential at a membrane potential between -8 and $-20\,mV$ (Fig. 3C) (Nishi and Koketsu, 1960; Weitsen and Weight, 1977); and (2) the reversal potential for the f-EPSP is changed by altering the extracellular concentration of Na^+ and K^+ in a manner consistent with an increased conductance to Na^+ and K^+ (Koketsu, 1969). The kinetics and properties of the conductance change underlying the generation of the f-EPSP have recently been investigated using the voltage-clamp technique (Kuba and Nishi, 1979; MacDermott et al., 1980). The synaptic currents at these neuronal synapses are similar qualitatively to the end-plate currents at the neuromuscular junction (see Steinback and Stevens, 1976; Takeuchi, 1977). However, quantitatively the decay of the fast excitatory postsynaptic current (EPSC) is slower and less voltage-dependent than the decay of the end-plate current. For further discussion of the f-EPSP, see Skok (this volume).

THE SLOW EXCITATORY POSTSYNAPTIC POTENTIAL (s-EPSP)

In addition to the f-EPSP elicited by a single preganglionic stimulus, repetitive preganglionic stimuli result in the generation of long-lasting or slow postsynaptic potentials. Repetitive stimulation of preganglionic B fibres in the sympathetic chain leads to the generation of a s-EPSP in B neurons (Nishi and Koketsu, 1968a; Tosaka et al., 1968; Weight and Votava, 1970). The s-EPSP has a time course that is of the order of a thousand times longer than the f-EPSP, rising to a peak in several seconds and having a duration of 30–60 sec (Fig. 4). The transmitter mediating the s-EPSP has been identified as ACh acting on muscarinic postsynaptic receptors on the basis of the following observations: (1) the same preganglionic fibre appears to be responsible for generating both the f-EPSP and the s-EPSP, since both responses are

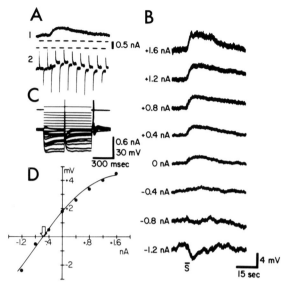

Figure 4 s-EPSP recorded intracellularly in a B neuron of bullfrog sympathetic ganglion. (A) 1: s-EPSP at resting membrane potential. 2: Upper record = hyperpolarizing constant current pulses of −0.5 nA. Lower = bridge balanced before stimulation such that current pulses produced no voltage deflection. Note that during EPSP the −0.5 nA current pulses produced a hyperpolarizing voltage deflection of 1 mV, indicating that the membrane resistance increased by 2 megaohms. (B) Amplitude of s-EPSP in A as a function of depolarizing (+) and hyperpolarizing (−) current. (C) Amplitude of antidromic spike after-hyperpolarization as a function of membrane potential. Upper record monitors current. Lower record shows antidromic spike after-hyperpolarization superimposed at various levels of membrane potential. (D) Graphic relationship of amplitude of s-EPSP (in B) to current. The reversal potential of s-EPSP is the point at which the curve crosses the abscissa. Arrow indicates the reversal potential of antidromic spike after-hyperpolarization shown in C. Note that the reversal potential of after-hyperpolarization (arrow) coincides with the reversal potential of s-EPSP (curve intercept). The Ringer's solution contained 30 μm nicotine to antagonize the f-EPSP. From Weight and Votava (1970)

all-or-none, and the threshold stimulus for activating both responses is the same (Tosaka *et al.*, 1968); (2) nicotinic antagonists such as *d*-tubocurarine or nicotine do not reduce the s-EPSP (Nishi and Koketsu, 1968a; Tosaka *et al.*, 1968; Weight and Votava, 1970); (3) the s-EPSP can be selectively antagonized by low concentrations of the muscarinic antagonist atropine (Nishi and Koketsu, 1968a; Tosaka *et al.*, 1968; Weight, unpublished observations); and (4) the s-EPSP can be mimicked by the iontophoretic application of ACh or the muscarinic agonist methacholine (MCh) (Koketsu *et al.*, 1968; Schulman and Weight, 1976).

The electrophysiological properties of the s-EPSP differ from those of the f-EPSP. The s-EPSP is usually associated with an increase in membrane resistance and it can be reversed with membrane hyperpolarization (Kobayashi and Libet, 1970; Weight and Votava, 1970). Weight and Votava (1970) have proposed that the primary mechanism involved in the electrogenesis of the s-EPSP is a decrease in K^+ conductance. That hypothesis was based on the following observations in nicotinized ganglia: (1) membrane conductance decreased (resistance increased) during the s-EPSP (Fig. 4A); (2) membrane depolarization increased the amplitude of the s-EPSP; (3) progressive membrane hyperpolarization decreased and then reversed the s-EPSP (Fig. 4B); (4) the s-EPSP reversed near the potassium equilibrium potential, E_k (Fig. 4C, D); and (5) extracellular Cl^- removal had no significant effect on the s-EPSP or its reversal potential. In addition, in a number of cells, more notably in curarized preparations, there is a later phase that is augmented by hyperpolarization and appears to be due to an increased conductance, probably to Na^+ and Ca^{2+} (Weight and Votava, 1971; Kobayashi and Libet, 1974; Kuba and Koketsu, 1976).

The proposal that the s-EPSP involves predominantly a decreased K^+ conductance has received strong support from recent voltage-clamp experiments (Brown and Adams, 1980; MacDermott and Weight, 1980; Weight and MacDermott, 1981). Analysis of the ionic current(s) involved in s-EPSP generation is considerably more complex than such an analysis of the f-EPSP, because the various K^+ currents of the membrane must be characterized in order to determine the K^+ current or currents that are decreased during the s-EPSP. The voltage-clamp analysis suggests that there are at least three different types of K^+ currents in the membrane. One type is activated by membrane depolarization and is blocked by tetraethylammonium chloride (TEA)—a voltage-activated or delayed rectifier current. The second type is dependent upon depolarization-induced influx of Ca^{2+} and is blocked by Co^{2+}—a Ca^+-activated K^+ current. The third type appears to be a slow voltage-dependent current that is blocked by both Ba^{2+} and muscarinic receptor activation (Brown and Adams, 1980; MacDermott and Weight, 1980; Constanti *et al.*, 1981; Weight and MacDermott, 1981) (Fig. 5). Brown and Adams (1980) have called this third type the 'M' current, and suggested that suppression of this voltage-dependent K^+ current by muscarinic receptor activation may be the ionic mechanism underlying the generation of the s-EPSP.

THE SLOW INHIBITORY POSTSYNAPTIC POTENTIAL (s-IPSP)

Studies on the pathway and neurotransmitter mediating the s-IPSP

The s-IPSP is generated in C neurons by repetitive stimulation of preganglionic C fibres in the VIIth or VIIIth spinal nerves (Fig. 6) (Tosaka *et al.*, 1968; Weight and Padjen, 1973a). The s-IPSP attains maximal amplitude in

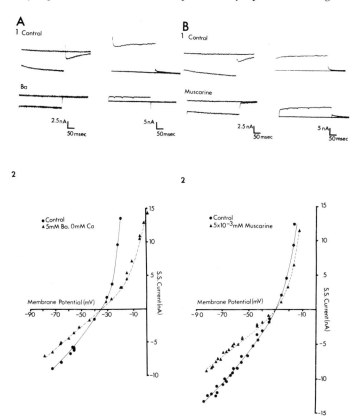

Figure 5 Effect of barium (Ba) and muscarine on membrane currents in bullfrog sympathetic neurons. (A) 1: Currents recorded from a neuron voltage clamp at a holding potential of −35 mV, and stepped to −57 mV (left) and to −19 mV (right). The bottom records show the currents recorded in a Ringer's solution containing 0 mM CaCl₂ and 5 mM BaCl₂. 2: Steady-state current–voltage relationship in normal Ringer's and in the Ringer's solution with BaCl₂. From the same experiment as A1. (B) 1: Currents recorded from a different neuron clamped at a holding potential of −30 mV, and stepped to −55 mV (left) and −16 mV (right). The bottom records show the currents recorded in 10 μM muscarine. 2: Steady-state current–voltage relationship in normal Ringer's solution, and in the Ringer's solution containing 5 μM muscarine. From the same experiment as the records illustrated in B1. Records obtained from B neurons using two-electrode voltage clamp. From Weight and MacDermott (1981)

about 1–2 sec, and has a duration lasting 4–20 sec. Two hypotheses have been proposed for the pathway and neurotransmitter mediating the s-IPSP. One proposes that the s-IPSP is mediated by a disynaptic pathway involving an adrenergic interneuron. That hypothesis was first advanced by Eccles and Libet (1961) to explain pharmacological observations in rabbit superior cervical ganglion. They found that atropine blocks and that dibenamine

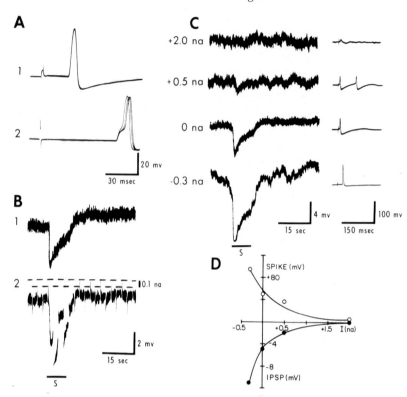

Figure 6 s-IPSP recorded intracellularly in a C neuron in the Xth sympathetic ganglion of bullfrog. (A) 1: Antidromic action potential. Antidromic conduction velocity of 0.24 m/sec identifies the neuron as a C cell. 2: f-EPSP initiates action potential; f-EPSP elicited by stimulation of preganglionic C fibres in the VIIIth spinal nerve. (B) 1: s-IPSP elicited in the same C cell by stimulation of preganglionic C fibres in the VIIIth nerve at a frequency of 50 Hz after nicotinic blockade (30 μM nicotine). 2: Upper record = hyperpolarizing constant-current pulses of −0.1 nA. Lower record = resistance change during s-IPSP. The bridge was balanced before stimulation such that current pulses produced no voltage deflection. Note that during the s-IPSP the current pulse produced a hyperpolarizing voltage deflection of 2 mV, indicating a resistance increase of 20 megaohms. Resting input resistance of this cell, determined from I–V curves, was 78 megaohms. (C) Effect of membrane polarization by a steady d.c. current. Left: Ampliude of s-IPSP as a function of depolarizing (+) and hyperpolarizing (−) current. Right: Amplitude of antidromic spike recorded during the same polarizing current. (D) Amplitude of s-IPSP (filled circles) and antidromic spike (open circles) in C, represented graphically as a function of the polarizing current. From Weight and Padjen (1973a)

partially reduces the P wave. They proposed that ACh released from preganglionic fibres stimulates muscarinic receptors on chromaffin cells; these cells in turn release a catecholamine that acts on adrenergic receptors on the ganglion cells to generate the P wave (s-IPSP). In the frog ganglia, atropine also blocks the s-IPSP, but the s-IPSP is only weakly depressed by dibenamine (Libet *et al.*, 1968). Nevertheless, Tosaka *et al.* (1968) proposed that the s-IPSP in frog ganglia is also mediated by a disynaptic pathway involving an adrenergic interneuron.

It should be noted, however, that dibenamine and other similar adrenergic antagonists can also block muscarinic (Stone and Loew, 1952, Furchgott, 1954, 1955; Benfey and Grillo, 1963; Boyd *et al.*, 1963; Furchgott, 1966; Beddoe *et al.*, 1971), as well as histamine (Loew and Micetich, 1948; Graham and Lewis, 1953) and serotonin (Freyburger *et al.*, 1952; Gaddum *et al.*, 1955; Gyermek, 1966) receptors. Consequently, Boyd *et al.* (1963) concluded that such antagonists cannot be used to distinguish conclusively between adrenergic and other types of transmitters. It should also be noted that, although catecholamines can hyperpolarize frog ganglion cells, they hyperpolarize B as well as C neurons (Tosaka *et al.*, 1968). Consequently, if chromaffin (or small intensely fluorescent [SIF] cells) mediate the s-IPSP, they must be either immediately adjacent to or make synaptic connection with C neurons, since the s-IPSP is generated only in C neurons. However, morphological studies have revealed that there are very few chromaffin/SIF cells in the IXth and Xth ganglia of bullfrogs, and those present are not selectively localized in the vicinity of the small (C) neurons (Weight and Weitsen, 1977). Moreover, specific synaptic connections from chromafin/SIF cells to neurons in the IXth and Xth ganglia have not been observed. In fact, in frog ganglia, the chromaffin/SIF cells do not appear to have any efferent processes or synapses (Weight and Weitsen, 1977; Watanabe, 1980; see chapter by Watanabe).

The second hypothesis for the transmitter and pathway mediating the s-IPSP was advanced by Weight and Padjen (1973b). They proposed that the s-IPSP is a direct muscarinic postsynaptic response mediated by ACh released from cholinergic preganglionic fibres. That hypothesis was based on the following observations: (1) cholinergic preganglionic C fibres make synaptic contact with C neurons (see above); (2) the s-IPSP is elicited by stimulation of the same preganglionic C fibres that innervate the C neurons (Tosaka *et al.*, 1968); (3) atropine blocks the s-IPSP (Nishi and Koketsu, 1968a; Tosaka *et al.*, 1968; Weight and Padjen, unpublished); (4) ACh administered iontophoretically to C cells hyperpolarizes those neurons with a time course similar to that of the s-IPSP (Weight and Padjen, 1973b); (5) the electrophysiological properties of the ACh-hyperpolarization appear to be identical to the properties of the s-IPSP (Weight and Padjen, 1973b); (6) the ACh-hyperpolarization is not reduced in a Ringer's solution containing high magnesium (Mg^{2+}) and low calcium (Ca^{2+}) in nicotinized ganglia, indicating that the hyperpolarization is a direct muscarinic postsynaptic response of ganglion cells.

The observation that a high Mg^{2+}–low Ca^{2+} Ringer does not reduce the

ACh-hyperpolarization in nicotinized ganglia was confirmed by Libet and Kobayashi (1974). However, they reported that in curarized ganglia the ACh- or MCh-hyperpolarization was abolished by a low Ca^{2+}–high Mg^{2+} Ringer, and concluded that, in curarized ganglia, the s-IPSP is mediated by a disynaptic pathway involving an adrenergic interneuron. That conclusion was supported by the following observations: (1) the s-IPSP was enhanced by U-0521, an inhibitor of catechol O-methyltransferase (COMT); and (2) the s-IPSP was partially depressed by the α-adrenergic antagonists dihydroergotamine and phentolamine. There are, however, several problems with the observations on which that conclusion is based.

First, the adrenergic interneuron hypothesis was based primarily on the observation that low Ca^{2+}-high Mg^{2+} Ringer abolished the ACh- or MCh-hyperpolarization in curarized ganglia. However, extensive recent experiments have failed to substantiate that observation; viz. it has been found that a MCh-hyperpolarization can be elicited in curarized ganglia when transmitter release is inhibited by a Ringer's solution containing: (1) tetrodotoxin (10^{-5} M); (2) 4 mM cobalt; (3) Ca^{2+}-free (no Ca^{2+} added); (4) Ca^{2+}-free with 10^{-4} M EGTA; or (5) Ca^{2+}-free with 10 mM Mg^{2+} (Fig. 7B, C) (Weight and Smith, 1980; Smith and Weight, 1981). The observation that the muscarinic hyperpolarization can be elicited in curarized ganglia under a variety of conditions that prevent transmitter release indicates that the response is a direct muscarinic postsynaptic hyperpolarization of ganglion cells.

Second, it is unlikely that the effect of U-0521 is due to the assumed inhibition of COMT for several reasons. (1) The primary mechanism for transmitter removal at adrenergic synaptic junctions is uptake, not enzymatic destruction (see Kopin, 1972; Axelrod, 1973; Iversen, 1975). (2) COMT is not a surface membrane enzyme like acetylcholinesterase at cholinergic junctions; it is located intracellularly being confined largely to the soluble cytoplasmic fraction (see Axelrod, 1966, 1973; Kopin, 1972). Consequently, inhibition of COMT would not be expected to potentiate an adrenergic synaptic response. (3) If U-0521 enhanced the s-IPSP by inhibition of COMT, it would be expected to potentiate hyperpolarizations resulting from the administration of catecholamines; however, U-0521 had little effect on the hyperpolarizations elicited by the direct application of catecholamines.

Third, the depressant actions of the α-adrenergic antagonists dihydroergotamine and phentolamine on the s-IPSP may be due to non-specific depressant effects of those drugs. Dihydroergotamine in a concentration of 10 μM effectively antagonizes adrenergic hyperpolarizations (produced by the administration of epinephrine, norepinephrine and dopamine), but does not affect either the s-IPSP or the ACh-hyperpolarization in either nicotinized or curarized ganglia (Fig. 7A) (Weight, 1973; Weight and Smith, 1980). In addition, phentolamine in concentrations greater than 10 μM has non-

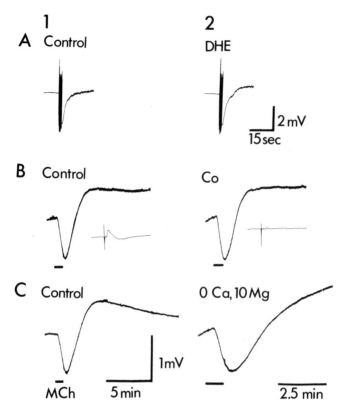

Figure 7 Effect of α-adrenergic antagonist on s-IPSP, and inhibition of transmitter release on muscarinic hyperpolarization. (A) 1: s-IPSP in normal Ringer containing 70 μM *d*-tubocurarine. 2: Effect of 10 μM dihydroergotamine on the s-IPSP in A1. (B) 1: Methacholine (MCh) response in normal Ringer containing 70 μM *d*-tubocurarine. Inset: f-EPSP elicited by stimulation of VIIIth nerve. 2: MCh-response after superfusion for 15 min with Ringer's solution containing 4 mM cobalt chloride (Co). Note abolition of f-EPSP (inset). (C) 1: MCh-response in normal Ringer containing 70 μM *d*-tubocurarine. 2: MCh-response in a Ca^{2+}-free (90 min)–10 mM Mg^{2+} (15 min) Ringer's solution. Note that time-base in C2 is twice that in C1. Records in A, B and C are from different experiments. Records were obtained from the IXth or Xth ganglia of bullfrog using the sucrose-gap method. From Weight and Smith (1980)

specific depressant effects on synaptic transmission in frog ganglia (Yavari and Weight, 1981). The concentrations of dihydroergotamine and phentolamine used by Libet and Kobayashi (1974) were 40 and 200 μM. It has also been reported that in mammalian sympathetic ganglia the α-adrenergic antagonists dibenamine, phenoxybenzamine, phentolamine, and yohimbine do not appreciably affect the s-IPSP in concentrations less than 10 μM; however, in higher concentrations they non-selectively depress all ganglionic responses (Cole and Shinnick-Gallagher, 1980, 1981; Dun and Karczmar, 1980).

In view of the preceding discussion, there appear to be few substantiated data to support the adrenergic interneuron hypothesis for mediation of the s-IPSP in frog sympathetic ganglia. On the other hand, the observation that ACh or MCh produces a direct muscarinic hyperpolarization of ganglion cells, in curarized as well as nicotinized ganglia, provides strong support for the proposal that the s-IPSP is mediated by a muscarinic postsynaptic action of ACh on C neurons.

It should be noted that, at the present time, the synaptic pathway and the neurotransmitter involved in the generation of the s-IPSP in mammalian sympathetic ganglia is uncertain (see Nakamura, 1978; Cole and Shinnick-Gallagher, 1980, 1981; Dun and Karczmar, 1980; Libet, 1980; Gallagher *et al.*, 1980). In both amphibian and mammalian parasympathetic ganglia, evidence has recently been presented that the mediation of the s-IPSP is by a direct muscarinic action of ACh (Hartzell *et al.*, 1977; Griffith *et al.*, 1980). (For further discussion on the slow synoptic actions in mammalian sympathetic ganglia see chapter by Kobayashi and Tosaka.)

Studies on the mechanism of s-IPSP generation

The ionic mechanism involved in the electrogenesis of the s-IPSP has been the subject of a number of investigations in recent years. The electrophysiological properties of the s-IPSP differ from the properties of IPSPs generated by increases in membrane conductance (see Eccles, 1964). Weight and Padjen (1973a) proposed that the s-IPSP involves a decrease in resting Na^+ conductance. That hypothesis was based on the following observations in nicotinized ganglia: (1) membrane conductance decreased (resistance increased) during the s-IPSP (Fig. 6B); (2) moderate hyperpolarization of the membrane increased the amplitude of the s-IPSP; (3) progressive depolarization of the membrane decreased and then annulled the s-IPSP (Fig. 6C); (4) removing extracellular Na^+ decreased or abolished the hyperpolarization elicited by the iontophoretic administration of ACh.

On the other hand, Nishi and Koketsu (1967, 1968b) proposed that the s-IPSP is generated by the synaptic activation of the electrogenic Na^+ pump. That hypothesis was based primarily on the observation in nicotinized ganglia that the s-IPSP was abolished by ouabain, a cardiac glycoside that selectively inhibits the electrogenic Na^+ pump. In addition, Koketsu and Yamamoto (1974) concluded that the Na^+ pump hypothesis was supported by the observation that replacing extracellular Na^+ by lithium ions (Li^+) markedly depressed or abolished the s-IPSP, because Li^+ is not extruded by the Na^+ pump (Maizels, 1954; Zerahn, 1955; Keynes and Swan, 1959). However, the hypothesis that the s-IPSP is generated by the synaptic activation of the electrogenic Na^+ pump does not appear to provide a satisfactory explanation of either the voltage dependence of the s-IPSP or the increased membrane resistance during the s-IPSP observed in nicotinized preparations, since in most cells the electrogenic Na^+ pump is voltage independent and is not associated with a change in membrane resistance (see Thomas, 1972). It should also be noted that the effects of ouabain and Li^+ on the s-IPSP can also be explained in terms of the decreased Na^+ conductance hypothesis as follows. (1) An IPSP generated by a decrease in Na^+ conductance depends on the electrochemical gradient for Na^+. Since ouabain inhibits the extrusion of intracellular Na^+, treatment with ouabain could lead to an intracellular accumulation of Na^+ (see Thomas, 1972) that would decrease the Na^+ gradient, thus reducing or abolishing an IPSP generated by a Na^+ conductance decrease. (2) Since Li^+ is not extruded by the Na^+ pump yet enters through Na^+ channels, replacing extracellular Na^+ by Li^+ would result in an intracellular accumulation of Li^+. This would decrease the electrochemical gradient for Li^+ and thereby decrease or abolish an IPSP generated by a decrease in Li^+ conductance. In addition, since membrane permeability to Li^+ is less than that to Na^+ (Armett and Ritchie, 1963), an IPSP generated by a decrease in Na^+ conductance would be decreased in amplitude in a Ringer in which Na^+ is replaced by Li^+, by virtue of the diminished resting Li^+ conductance.

The role of the electrogenic Na^+ pump in the generation of the s-IPSP was re-evaluated by Smith and Weight (1977). They first demonstrated that both the K^+-free Ringer and $1\,\mu M$ ouabain effectively inhibit potential changes resulting from activity of the electrogenic Na^+ pump. They concluded that the s-IPSP does not involve the synaptic activation of the electrogenic Na^+ pump on the basis of the following observations: (1) K^+-free Ringer rapidly and persistently increased the amplitude of the s-IPSP (Fig. 8A); (2) $1\,\mu M$ ouabain did not reduce the amplitude of the s-IPSP in curarized ganglia; and (3) although $1\,\mu M$ ouabain partially reduced the s-IPSP in nicotinized ganglia, the s-IPSP in ouabain was potentiated by K^+-free Ringer (Fig. 8B).

Recently, the electrogenic Na^+ pump hypothesis has been modified to a proposal that the s-IPSP is generated by two components: (1) the synaptic activation of the electrogenic Na^+ pump; and (2) an increase of K^+ conductance (Akasu and Koketsu, 1976; Akasu *et al.*, 1978). That hypothesis is based primarily on the observations in curarized ganglia that, in ouabain, the s-IPSP reverses near the reversal potential for the spike after-hyperpolarization, and that the reversal potential shifts in K^+-rich solutions. In terms of that proposal, if a component of the s-IPSP is due to synaptic activation of the electrogenic Na^+ pump, one would expect that inhibiting the Na^+ pump would reduce the amplitude of the s-IPSP to the extent that the Na^+ pump contributes to its generation. However, as noted above, in curarized ganglia the s-IPSP is not reduced by $1\,\mu M$ ouabain (Smith and Weight, 1977). On the

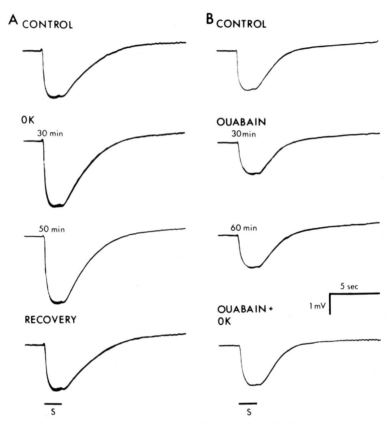

Figure 8 Effects of K⁺-free Ringer and ouabain on the s-IPSP. (A) Effect of K⁺-free Ringer. Top: control record of slow IPSP. Middle: s-IPSPs recorded 30 and 50 min after beginning superfusion of ganglion with K⁺-free Ringer. Bottom: recovery of s-IPSP recorded 25 min after return to normal Ringer. (B) Effect of ouabain. Top: control record of a s-IPSP. Middle: s-IPSPs recorded 30 and 60 min after beginning superfusion with Ringer's solution containing ouabain (10^{-6} M). Bottom: s-IPSP after 20 min superfusion with K⁺-free Ringer containing ouabain (10^{-6} M) (record taken after 90 min in 10^{-6} M ouabain shown above). Records in A and B are from different experiments. Records were obtained from IXth or Xth ganglia of bullfrog using sucrose gap method. The f-EPSP was antagonized by 30 μM nicotine throughout each experiment. From Smith and Weight (1977)

basis of that observation, it would appear that the Na⁺ pump does not contribute, even in part, to the generation of the s-IPSP. Furthermore, if the Na⁺ pump does not contribute to the generation of the s-IPSP, then, in terms of the two component proposal of Akasu and Koketsu (1976) and Akasu *et al.* (1978), the s-IPSP would be generated by a K⁺ conductance alone. However, as discussed below, the s-IPSP does not have the electrophysiological properties of a K⁺ conductance alone. These observations do not appear to be compatible with the hypothesis that s-IPSP is generated by the synaptic activation of the electrogenic Na^+ pump either alone or combined with an increased K^+ conductance.

The electrophysiological properties of the s-IPSP in curarized ganglia have recently been investigated further by Weight and Smith (1981). That analysis shows: (1) the s-IPSP can have a reversal potential that is significantly more negative than the potassium equilibrium potential, E_K (Fig. 9A); and (2) the reversal potential for the s-IPSP is sensitive to extracellular K^+ (Fig. 9B). The latter observation suggests the involvement of an increased K^+ conductance in the generation of the s-IPSP. However, the observation that the reversal potential is more negative than E_K suggests that the generation of the s-IPSP cannot be explained by an increased K^+ conductance alone, since an IPSP generated by a K^+ conductance alone would reverse at E_K (see Katz, 1966; Weight, 1974). In 1971, Brown *et al.* predicted, on theoretical grounds, that a PSP can be generated by an increased permeability to one ion combined with a decreased permeability to another ion. In their mathematical analysis, they showed that if a PSP is generated by changes in the conductances to Na^+ and K^+, and if one of those conductances is increased and the other is decreased, the reversal potential of the PSP can be negative to the K^+ equilibrium potential (E_K). Based on the observation that the s-IPSP has a K^+-dependent reversal potential that is negative to E_K, as well as the previous observations on the s-IPSP, Weight and Smith (1981) have proposed that the s-IPSP is generated by a combined Na^+ conductance decrease and K^+ conductance increase.

The proposal that the s-IPSP is generated by a simultaneous decreased Na^+ and increased K^+ conductance appears to account for most, if not all, of the observed electrophysiological properties of the s-IPSP. The generation of a PSP by opposite conductance changes to two different ions can result in a response with unusual electrophysiological properties that are dependent upon the ratio of the conductance changes involved. First, a PSP can be generated with no demonstratable reversal potential. As noted previously, in investigations on the s-IPSP in nicotinized ganglia, a reversal of the s-IPSP has not been demonstrated. Second, it is possible to have a PSP in which there is no significant change in input membrane resistance. In this regard, a significant resistance change was usually not observed during the s-IPSP in curarized ganglia (Smith and Weight, unpublished observations), in contrast to an increase in membrane resistance observed in nicotinized ganglia (Weight and Padjen, 1973a). It is of interest to note that it has been reported that there is no detectable resistance change during the s-IPSP in rabbit superior cervical ganglion (Kobayashi and Libet, 1968).

It is apparent that certain differences have been observed in electrophysiological properties of the s-IPSP depending on whether nicotine or *d*-tubocurarine was used to antagonize the f-EPSP. In addition to being an

A. dTC

B. dTC 6K

antagonist, nicotine can also increase steady-state Na^+ conductance in a dose-dependent manner (Wang and Narahashi, 1972). In terms of the proposed combined conductance mechanism for generation of the s-IPSP, a nicotine-induced increase in Na^+ conductance could increase the number of open Na^+ channels available for closing by activation of the s-IPSP mechanism. In this way, nicotine could increase the Na^+ inactivation component of a s-IPSP generated by a combined conductance mechanism. This would account for most, if not all, of the differences in the properties of the s-IPSP observed in nicotine- and *d*-tubocurarine-treated preparations. For example, it explains the increase in membrane resistance observed during the s-IPSP in nicotine-treated preparations (Weight and Padjen, 1973a). It also accounts for the observation that in nicotine-treated preparations there is a greater potentiation of s-IPSP amplitude by moderate hyperpolarization (Nishi and Koketsu, 1968b; Smith and Weight, unpublished observations) as well as the observation that a reversal of the s-IPSP has not been observed in nicotine-treated preparations (Nishi and Koketsu, 1968b; Smith and Weight, unpublished observations). A nicotine-induced dose-dependent increase in Na^+ conductance would also account for the different effects of ouabain observed in different concentrations of nicotine. Since ouabain inhibits the extrusion of Na^+, in the presence of ouabain a greater membrane Na^+ conductance would result in a greater intracellular accumulation of Na^+. Moreover, since the amplitude of an IPSP involving a decreased Na^+ conductance is dependent upon the electrochemical gradient for Na^+ (see Weight, 1974), an accumulation in intracellular Na^+ would result in a proportional decrease in the amplitude of the IPSP. In the presence of ouabain, one would therefore expect that increasing the concentration of nicotine would result in a greater reduction in the amplitude of the s-IPSP. Such an effect on the amplitude of the s-IPSP has in fact been observed. In the presence of $1 \mu M$ ouabain, the s-IPSP is abolished in $100 \mu M$ nicotine (Nishi and Koketsu, 1967; Smith and Weight, unpublished), whereas it is only partially (10–40%) reduced in $30 \mu M$ nicotine (Smith and Weight, 1977). On the other hand, *d*-tubocurarine does not increase resting Na^+ conductance (Jenkinson, 1960), and the s-IPSP is not reduced in $1 \mu M$ ouabain in curarized preparations (Smith and Weight, 1977). It thus appears that many, if not all, of the diverse observations on the s-IPSP

Figure 9 Effect of membrane potential on the s-IPSP in curarized sympathetic ganglion of bullfrog. The effect of depolarizing current (DI) and hyperpolarizing current (HI) on 'B' f-EPSP (left), s-IPSP (middle) and antidromic spike after-hyperpolarization (right) in (A) normal Ringer's solution (containing $2 \, mM \, K^+$), and in (B) high K^+ Ringer's solution (containing $6 \, mM \, K^+$). The magnitude of the polarizing current is indicated to the left of each set of records; the units are $\times 10^{-7} \, A$. The experiments were performed on the IXth or Xth paravertebral ganglion using the sucrose gap technique. The Ringer's solution contained $70 \, \mu M$ *d*-tubocurarine (dTC). From Weight and Smith (1981)

can be accounted for by the proposal that the s-IPSP involves a Na^+ conductance decrease combined with a K^+ conductance increase. However, the combined conductance mechanism should not be considered as established until additional experiments demonstrate the appropriate quantitative relationship between the reversal potential of the s-IPSP and changes of extracellular Na^+ and K^+.

Atypical observations related to the s-IPSP

A few atypical observations related to the s-IPSP have been reported and should be briefly commented upon. (1) A small hyperpolarization preceding the s-EPSP has been recorded in a few B cells in the presence of very high nicotine concentrations (Kobayashi and Libet, 1974; Kuba and Koketsu, 1978). The absence of reports of this phenomenon in experiments using either *d*-tubocurarine or low concentrations of nicotine suggests that the response is induced by the high concentrations of nicotine. It has also been reported that in very high nicotine concentrations, the initial portion of the s-EPSP can reverse at a membrane potential between resting potential and E_K (Kobayashi and Libet, 1974; Kuba and Koketsu, 1978). This contrasts with the observation that in low concentrations of nicotine the reversal potential for the s-EPSP is near E_K (Weight and Votava, 1970). This difference suggests that high concentrations of nicotine may shift the reversal potential for the s-EPSP to a more positive membrane potential. (2) In sucrose-gap experiments, stimulation of preganglionic B fibres elicits a s-IPSP in either nicotine- or curare-treated ganglia. That observation has been interpreted as evidence that B fibres result in the generation of a s-IPSP in B neurons (see Koketsu, 1969; Kuba and Koketsu, 1978). However, there are no known reports of intracellular experiments in which such a s-IPSP has been observed in B neurons using either low concentrations of nicotine or curare. On the other hand, stimulation of preganglionic B fibres in the sympathetic chain can elicit a f-EPSP in a small percentage of C neurons. Moreover, stimulation of the same preganglionic B fibre, after nicotinic blockade, can elicit a s-IPSP in the same C neuron (Smith and Weight, 1981). In view of these observations, the author feels that there is not sufficient evidence to support the opinion that the s-IPSP is generated in B neurons. (3) Koketsu and Yamamoto (1975) have reported that ACh can elicit a small hyperpolarization in a Ringer's solution containing both nicotine and atropine. They concluded that the ACh-hyperpolarization was produced by a specific ACh action that was neither a nicotinic nor a muscarinic response. It should be noted, however, that the concentration of ACh usually applied in those experiments was 0.1 M, which is extremely high, and was more than 700 times greater than the concentration of atropine. This raises the question of whether the high concentration of ACh might partially overcome the atropine antagonism of muscarinic receptor activation.

THE LATE-SLOW EPSP (ls-EPSP)

The late-slow EPSP (ls-EPSP) is a very long-lasting depolarization that is elicited by repetitive stimulation of preganglionic C fibres (Nishi and Koketsu, 1968a). With a 2-sec train of stimuli, the ls-EPSP reaches maximal amplitude in 1–2 min and lasts as long as 5–10 min (Fig. 10A). The ls-EPSP

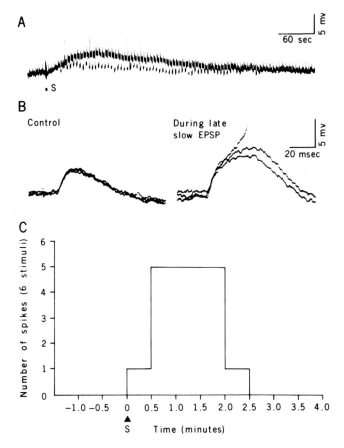

Figure 10 Postsynaptic potentiation of f-EPSPs. (A) ls-EPSP elicited by repetitive stimulation (S) of VIIIth nerve for 2 sec at a frequency of 50 Hz. Constant-current pulses across membrane indicate that membrane resistance increased by 19.5 megaohms during the ls-EPSP. (B) Monosynaptic f-EPSPs elicited by stimulation of the sympathetic chain. Left: records of f-EPSPs prior to the ls-EPSP. Right: records of f-EPSPs during the ls-EPSP. (C) Effect of ls-EPSP on spike generation by f-EPSPs. The graph divides the experimental period into 30-sec segments. Each segment records the number of action potentials initiated by six f-EPSPs. Note that during the 4.5-min control period, no f-EPSPs fired spikes. However, after stimulation (S) of the VIIIth nerve, the enlarged f-EPSPs initiated the generation of action potentials for a period of 2.5 min. From Schulman and Weight (1976)

can be recorded intracellularly in both B and C neurons (Nishi and Koketsu, 1968a; Schulman and Weight, 1976). The C fibres that elicit this long-lasting PSP enter the sympathetic chain via the VIIth and VIIIth spinal nerve (Schulman and Weight, 1976; Jan *et al.*, 1979). There do not appear to be fibres capable of eliciting the ls-EPSP descending in the sympathetic chain from levels rostral to the VIIth ganglion. We have found that the ls-EPSP is abolished in a Ringer containing low Ca^{2+} and high Mg^{2+}, adding support to the designation of this long-lasting depolarization as a postsynaptic potential.

The ls-EPSP is generated in the presence of both nicotine and atropine indicating that it is a non-cholinergic response (Nishi and Koketsu, 1968a). Recent biochemical studies using the radioimmunoassay technique indicate that the transmitter mediating the ls-EPSP appears to be a peptide resembling luteinizing hormone-releasing factor (LH-RF) (Jan *et al.*, 1979) (for further discussion see chapter by Dun). Due to the very long duration of the ls-EPSP, its electrophysiological properties have not been investigated as extensively as those of the other PSPs in frog ganglia. Schulman and Weight (1976) reported that membrane resistance is usually increased during the ls-EPSP (Fig. 10A); that observation has been confirmed by Jan *et al.* (1980b). The electro-physiological properties of the slow depolarization elicited by the application of LH-RF appear to be identical to those of the ls-EPSP (Adams and Brown, 1980; Jan *et al.*, 1980b). In voltage-clamp experiments, the application of LH-RF has been found to reduce a voltage-dependent K^+ current, the 'M' current (Adams and Brown, 1980). Although this action appears to be identical to the effect of muscarinic receptor activation in B neurons (see above), it is not due to the release of ACh, because it persists in the presence of atropine. It thus appears that this peptide, acting on different receptors, has an action that is similar, if not identical, to that of muscarinic receptor activation. However, when the membrane is hyperpolarized to the K^+ equilibrium potential (E_K), most cells show a marked increase in the size of both the ls-EPSP and the LH-RF response (Jan *et al.*, 1980b). This suggests that, in addition to the decreased K^+ conductance, there may also be conductance increases involved in the ls-EPSP.

Although the ls-EPSP is generated in both B and C neurons, immuno-histochemical staining shows that the LH-RF-positive synaptic boutons are located mainly around the small (C) neurons, suggesting that ls-EPSP in B neurons results from diffusion of the peptide from terminals around C neurons (Jan *et al.*, 1980a). In addition, the cholinergic fibers that innervate C neurons have the same pattern of distribution as the LH-RF immunoreactive fibres, suggesting that ACh and the LH-RF-like peptide may exist in the same terminals, as has been observed in other tissues (see Hökfelt *et al.*, 1980).

MOLECULAR MECHANISMS AND POSTSYNAPTIC
POTENTIAL GENERATION

Cyclic nucleotides and postsynaptic potential generation

It has been proposed that the molecular mechanisms underlying the generation of both the s-IPSP and the s-EPSP involve cyclic nucleotides. Preganglionic stimulation increases the content of cyclic AMP in rabbit superior cervical ganglion (McAfee *et al.*, 1971). On the basis of that and the following electrophysiological observations in sucrose-gap experiments on the rabbit ganglion, McAfee and Greengard (1972) proposed that cyclic AMP acts as an intracellular second messenger mediating the generation of the s-IPSP: (1) cyclic AMP hyperpolarized postganglionic neurons; (2) the s-IPSP was blocked by prostaglandin E_1, a substance presumed to inhibit adenylate cyclase; (3) the s-IPSP was potentiated by theophylline, a drug that inhibits phosphodiesterase. In addition, they also reported that dibutyryl cyclic GMP depolarizes postganglionic neurons, and proposed that cyclic GMP mediates the generation of the s-EPSP (see also Bloom, 1975; Greengard, 1976; Nathanson, 1977). In frog sympathetic ganglia, preganglionic stimulation also increases the content of cyclic AMP, as well as cyclic GMP (Weight *et al.*, 1974). However, when the above electrophysiological experiments were repeated on frog ganglia using sucrose-gap recording, Busis *et al.* (1978) found: (1) the administration of cyclic AMP, cyclic GMP, or several of their derivatives produced little or no change in membrane potential; (2) prostaglandin E_1 did not block the s-PSPs; (3) theophylline produced membrane effects that were different from those associated with the s-PSPs, and, in addition, it reduced the s-EPSP and potentiated the slow IPSP. It appears likely that the potentiation of the s-IPSP by theophylline is not due to inhibition of phosphodiesterase on the basis of the following observations: (1) theophylline can potentiate other hyperpolarizing responses in frog ganglia by mechanisms independent of phosphodiesterase inhibition (Smith *et al.*, 1979); and (2) papaverine, a more potent phosphodiesterase inhibitor in frog ganglia (Smith *et al.*, 1979), does not potentiate but rather reduces the s-IPSP (Busis *et al.*, 1978). In addition, Weight *et al.* (1978) used intracellular recording techniques to study further the actions of cyclic nucleotides in bullfrog neurons. Despite a number of experimental procedures to optimize possible membrane actions, including the intracellular injection of cyclic nucleotides and several of their derivatives, they found that the majority of the neurons studied were neither hyperpolarized nor depolarized by cyclic GMP, cyclic AMP or several of their derivatives. Kuba and Nishi (1976) and Akasu and Koketsu (1977) have also reported that dibutyryl cyclic AMP does not hyperpolarize frog sympathetic neurons.

Two of the important criteria for establishing cyclic nucleotide mediation of a postsynaptic potential are: (1) demonstration that the effect of cyclic nucleotide application mimics the PSP; and (2) demonstration that agents that affect cyclic nucleotide metabolism appropriately affect the PSP (see Beam and Greengard, 1975; Greengard, 1976). The inability to satisfy convincingly these criteria does not provide support for the possibility that cyclic nucleotides mediate the generation of slow PSPs in frog sympathetic ganglia. It should be noted that a number of recent studies of rabbit and rat sympathetic ganglia have also reported data that do not support the cyclic nucleotide hypothesis for s-PSP generation (Dun *et al.*, 1977a, b; Dun and Karczmar, 1977; Gallagher and Shinnick-Gallagher, 1977; Kobayashi *et al.*, 1978; Brown *et al.*, 1979; Libet, 1979). For mammatian ganglia see Chapter by Kobayashi and Tosaka.

Calcium, protein phosphorylation, and membrane permeability

Although cyclic nucleotides do not appear to be involved in the molecular basis of membrane permeability changes in sympathetic ganglia, recent data suggest that calcium ions (Ca^{2+}) can function as an intracellular mediator of certain membrane permeability changes in sympathetic neurons. The intracellular injection of Ca^{2+} has been found to increase membrane K^+ permeability in several types of neurons (see Meech, 1978), including those in frog sympathetic ganglia (Kuba and Koketsu, 1978). In the sympathetic neurons of bullfrog, the after-hyperpolarization following a normal action potential consists of two components: (1) a short-duration voltage-sensitive K^+ conductance; and (2) a longer-duration calcium-sensitive K^+ conductance (Busis and Weight, 1976). The calcium-sensitive K^+ conductance is potentiated by theophylline, and that potentiation is independent of phosphodiesterase inhibition (Smith *et al.*, 1979).

In addition to prolonging the duration of the spike after-hyperpolarization, theophylline as well as caffeine induces the generation of spontaneous hyperpolarizations that occur rhythmically every 1–5 min (Kuba and Nishi, 1976; McCort and Weight, 1979; Kuba, 1980; Weight and McCort, 1981). These spontaneous hyperpolarizations are also generated by a calcium-sensitive K^+ conductance. The frequency of the rhythmic hyperpolarizations is increased by treatments that increase intracellular Ca^{2+} (A23187, increased extracellular Ca^{2+}, or increased extracellular K^+). On the other hand, the hyperpolarizations are decreased in frequency or abolished by dantrolene, a drug that decreases or blocks the intracellular release of Ca^{2+} from sarcoplasmic reticulum of muscle (Van Winkle, 1976; Desmedt and Hainaut, 1977). These observations suggest an involvement of intracellular Ca^{2+} release in the generation of the rhythmic hyperpolarizations. Recent experiments using the calcium-sensitive dye arsenazo III have revealed that an increase in intracellular Ca^{2+} is in fact associated with the generation of the spontaneous hyperpolarizations (Smith *et al.*, 1981).

Recent biochemical studies (Pant and Weight, 1980; Weight *et al.*, 1981), incubating intact frog ganglia in a Ringer containing ^{32}P, have shown that protein phosphorylation is decreased by treatments that increase intracellular Ca^{2+} (theophylline, A23187, increased extracellular Ca^{2+}, and increased extracellular K^+). On the other hand, protein phosphorylation is increased by dantrolene, which decreases intracellular Ca^{2+}. The largest change in ^{32}P incorporation is in protein bands at 12,000–14,000 and at 18,000–20,000 daltons. In homogenates of ganglia, protein phosphorylation is independent of cyclic nucleotides and dependent upon Ca^{2+}, with increased Ca^{2+} decreasing the phosphorylation. The data are consistent with the possibility that protein phosphorylation is involved in the membrane K^+ permeability activated by intracellular Ca^{2+}. However, further investigation is needed to establish whether the molecular basis of this membrane permeability change involves the phosphorylation of proteins.

POSTSYNAPTIC MODULATION OF MEMBRANE AND SYNAPTIC EXCITABILITY

Recent investigations indicate that the s-EPSP and the ls-EPSP increase both synaptic efficacy and neuronal excitability. Schulman and Weight (1976) studied the effect of muscarinic receptor activation on the f-EPSP in B neurons and found that both the amplitude and the duration of the f-EPSP are increased during the muscarinic response. The effect is not due to membrane depolarization, since it occurs when the membrane is held at the resting potential during the response and it does not occur with electrical depolarization of the membrane. Schulman and Weight (1976) also studied the effect of the ls-EPSP on the f-EPSP and found that both the amplitude and the duration of the f-EPSP are increased during the ls-EPSP (Fig. 10B). This observation has been confirmed by Jan *et al.* (1980b). The augmentation of the f-EPSP by either muscarinic receptor activation or the ls-EPSP often initiates the generation of postsynaptic action potentials. For example, in the experiment illustrated in Fig. 10C, following stimulation of the VIIIth nerve (S), the augmented f-EPSPs initiated the generation of action potentials for a period of more than 2 min. This indicates that stimulation of one synaptic pathway can result in a long-lasting increase in the efficacy of synaptic transmission in a second synaptic pathway by a postsynaptic mechanism. Furthermore, this enhancement of synaptic efficacy is long-lasting by virtue of the long duration of the postsynaptic response.

The excitability of the membrane is also increased by both the s-EPSP and the ls-EPSP (Schulman and Weight, 1976; Brown and Adams, 1980; Jan *et al.*, 1980b; Weight and MacDermott, 1981); viz. there is a marked facilitation of both the frequency and duration of repetitive spike firing during the response to either the synaptic or the pharmacological activation of

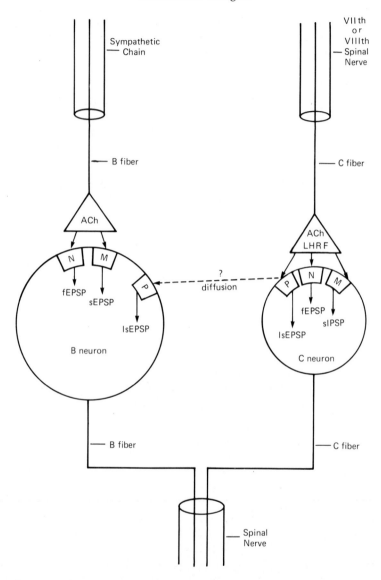

Figure 11 Schematic illustration of the suggested synaptic organization in the IXth and Xth paravertebral sympathetic ganglia of bullfrog. Left: B neuron innervated by cholinergic preganglionic axon with a B fibre conduction velocity that descends in the sympathetic chain. The neurotransmitter ACh is illustrated activating nicotinic postsynaptic receptors (N) to elicit the fast EPSP (fEPSP) and muscarinic postsynaptic receptors (M) to generate the slow EPSP (sEPSP). Right: C neuron innervated by a cholinergic preganglionic axon with a C fibre conduction velocity that enters the sympathetic chain from the VIIth or VIIIth spinal nerve. The neurotransmitter ACh is illustrated activating nicotinic postsynaptic receptors (N) to elicit the fast EPSP

muscarinic or LH-RF receptors. This increase of excitability is not due simply to depolarization since it cannot be elicited by depolarization of the membrane with current. In addition, a lowering of the threshold for action potential initiation and an activation of spike discharges at the termination of hyperpolarizing current pulses ('anodal break' response) are observed during both the s-EPSP and the ls-EPSP. The primary mechanism involved in these excitability changes is presumably the decreased K^+ conductance that is involved in the generation of these long-lasting PSPs, since membrane excitability of these neurons is also increased by Ba^{2+} as well as other pharmacological agents that decrease K^+ conductances (MacDermott and Weight, 1980; Nash and Weight, 1980; Weight and MacDermott, 1981).

The increase of both synaptic efficacy and membrane excitability during the s and the ls-EPSPs may prove to be the most functionally significant features of these long-lasting PSPs, since these membrane changes can alter the integrative functions of the neurons.

SUMMARY

This paper has reviewed our current understanding of the nature of synaptic mechanisms in amphibian sympathetic ganglia. During the 20 years since the first report of an intracellular investigation of frog ganglia, our knowledge has increased greatly with respect to both the synaptic organization and the mechanisms involved in the generation of several types of postsynaptic potentials in these ganglia. Our current understanding of the organization and synaptic mechanisms in the IXth and Xth sympathetic ganglia are summarized below and in Figs. 11 and 12.

In the IXth and Xth ganglia, B neurons receive synaptic connection from cholinergic preganglionic B fibres that enter the sympathetic chain from the IVth to VIth spinal nerves; C neurons are innervated primarily by cholinergic preganglionic C fibres that enter the chain via the VIIth and VIIIth spinal nerves (Fig. 11). Four types of postsynaptic potentials have been clearly delineated: (1) a fast EPSP (f-EPSP); (2) a slow EPSP (s-EPSP); (3) a slow IPSP (s-IPSP); and (4) a late-show EPSP (ls-EPSP). The *f-EPSP* is a nicotinic response with a duration of 30–50 msec. It generally mediates the transmission of preganglionic nerve impulses. The ionic mechanism underlying the

(fEPSP) and muscarinic postsynaptic receptors (M) to generate the slow IPSP (sIPSP) (see text for discussion). A neurotransmitter resembling luteinizing hormone-releasing factor (LHRF) is illustrated in the same preganglionic C fibre terminal as ACh (see text for details). The late-slow EPSP (lsEPSP) resulting from the activation of peptide receptors (P) is illustrated in the C neuron as due to the release of LHRF from the preganglionic C fibre, whereas in the B neuron it is illustrated as presumably resulting from diffusion of the peptide from the C fibre terminals on C neurons (see text for details). Modified from Weight and Smith (1980)

generation of the f-EPSP involves an increase in Na^+ and K^+ conductance that is similar in many respects to the end-plate potential at the neuromuscular junction (Fig. 12). The *s-EPSP* is a muscarinic response that lasts from 30 to 60 sec. It is elicited in B neurons by repetitive stimulation of preganglionic B fibres. The s-EPSP appears to be generated primarily by a decrease in K^+ conductance (Fig. 12), although in some cells a late increase in Na^+ and Ca^{2+} conductance may also be involved. The *s-IPSP* is generated in C neurons by stimulation of preganglionic C fibres in the VIIth and VIIIth spinal nerves. Its duration ranges from 4 to 20 sec. Although it had been proposed that the s-IPSP is mediated by a catecholamine released from an adrenergic interneuron, recent studies have failed to substantiate the observations on which that hypothesis was based. On the other hand, recent experiments have provided strong support for a proposal that the s-IPSP is mediated by a muscarinic postsynaptic action of ACh released from the cholinergic preganglionic fibres that innervate C neurons (Fig. 11). The ionic mechanism underlying the generation of the s-IPSP has been the subject of a number of experiments. One hypothesis proposed that the s-IPSP involves, in part, the synaptic activation of the electrogenic Na^+ pump. However, that hypothesis is not compatible with the observation that in curarized ganglia $1\,\mu M$ ouabain does not reduce the s-IPSP. On the other hand, recent evidence suggests that the s-IPSP might involve a decreased Na^+ conductance combined with an increased K^+ conductance (Fig. 12). The *ls-EPSP* is elicited in both B and C neurons by stimulation of preganglionic C fibres in the VIIth and VIIIth spinal nerves. Recent studies indicate that the transmitter mediating the ls-EPSP is an LH-RF-like peptide. Immunohistochemical techniques show that the LH-RF-staining boutons are located around C neurons, suggesting that the ls-EPSP in B neurons results from diffusion of the peptide from the terminals around C neurons (Fig. 11). The LH-RF-staining fibres have the same distribution pattern as the cholinergic fibres that innervate C neurons, suggesting that ACh and the LH-RF peptide may exist in the same terminals (Fig. 11). Although the ionic basis of the ls-EPSP has not been fully characterized, the investigations to date suggest that it involves primarily a decrease in K^+ conductance similar to that in the s-EPSP (Fig. 12), as well as possible increases in membrane conductance.

The molecular mechanisms that underlie the membrane permeability changes that generate the various PSPs are poorly understood. The hypothesis that cyclic GMP and cyclic AMP are intracellular second messengers mediating the generation of the s-EPSP and the s-IPSP, respectively, has not been supported by several recent investigations. On the other hand, recent data indicate that calcium ions can function as an intracellular mediator of a membrane permeability change—a calcium-sensitive K^+ conductance. In addition, the phosphorylation of certain proteins appears to be associated with intracellular Ca^{2+}. The observations are consistent with the possibility

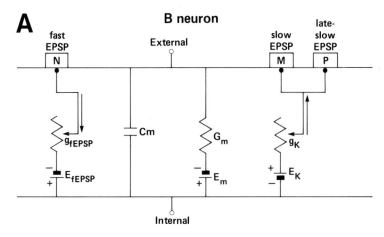

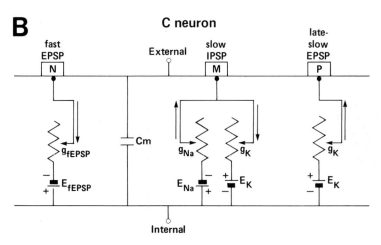

Figure 12 Electrical circuit diagrams which represent schematically the ionic mechanisms that are suggested to be involved in the generation of the postsynaptic potentials in B and C neurons in bullfrog sympathetic ganglia. (A) B neuron. f-EPSP: nicotinic receptor (N) activation increases Na^+ and K^+ conductances (g_{fEPSP}). s-EPSP: muscarinic receptor (M) activation primarily decreases a K^+ conductance (g_K). ls-EPSP: peptide receptor (P) activation by an LHRF-like peptide primarily decreases the same K^+ conductance (g_K) as muscarinic receptor activation. See text for details. Modified from Weight and Votava (1970). (B) C neuron: f-EPSP: nicotinic receptor (N) activation increases Na^+ and K^+ conductances (g_{fEPSP}). s-IPSP: muscarinic receptor (M) activation decreases Na^+ conductance (g_{Na}) and increases K^+ conductance (g_K). ls-EPSP: peptide receptor (P) activation by an LHRF-like peptide primarily decreases a K^+ conductance (g_K). See text for details. Modified from Weight and Padjen (1973a)

that the protein phosphorylation is involved in the membrane K^+ permeability activated by Ca^{2+}. However, further investigation is needed to establish whether protein phosphorylation is involved in this membrane permeability change.

Synaptic and membrane excitability are increased by both the s-EPSP and the ls-EPSP. Available data suggest that this facilitation of excitability is related to the decrease in K^+ conductance associated with both PSPs. It is possible that these excitability changes may prove to be the most functionally important feature of these long-lasting PSPs, since these membrane changes can increase the efficacy of synaptic transmission and alter the integrative functions of the neurons.

ACKNOWLEDGEMENTS

I thank Drs Amy B. MacDermott and Peter A. Smith for critically reviewing the manuscript, Ms Melpi K. Jeffries for technical assistance, and Ms Mary V. Kreysa and Ms Renee C. Nelson for typing and editing the manuscript.

REFERENCES

Adams, P. R., and Brown, D. A. (1980). Luteinizing hormone-releasing factor and muscarinic agonists act on the same voltage-sensitive K^+-current in bullfrog sympathetic neurones. *Br. J. Pharmacol.*, **68**, 353–355.

Akasu, T., and Koketsu, K. (1976). Ionic mechanisms of the slow inhibitory postsynaptic potential of sympathetic ganglion cells in bullfrogs. *Kurume Med. J.*, **23**, 183–188.

Akasu, T., and Koketsu, K. (1977). Effects of dibutyryl cyclic adenosine 3′,5′-monophosphate and theophylline on the bullfrog sympathetic ganglion cells. *Br. J. Pharmacol.*, **60**, 331–336.

Akasu, T., Omura, H., and Koketsu, K. (1978). Roles of electrogenic Na^+ pump and K^+ conductance in the slow inhibitory postsynaptic potential of bullfrog sympathetic ganglion cells. *Life Sci.*, **23**, 2405–2410.

Armet, C. I., and Ritchie, I. M. (1963). On the permeability of mammalian non-myelinated fibres to sodium and lithium ions. *J. Physiol. (London)*, **165**, 130–140.

Axelrod, J. (1966). Methylation reactions in the formation and metabolism of catecholamines and other biogenic amines: the enzymatic conversion of norepinephrine (NE) to epinephrine (E). *Pharmacol. Rev.*, **18**, 95–113.

Axelrod, J. (1973). The fate of noradrenaline in the sympathetic neurone. *Harvey Lect.*, **67**, 175–197.

Beam, K. G., and Greengard, P. (1975). Cyclic nucleotides, protein phosphorylation and synaptic function. *Cold Spring Harbor Symp. Quant. Biol.*, **40**, 157–168.

Beddoe, F., Nicholls, P. J., and Smith, H. J. (1971). Inhibition of muscarinic receptor by dibenamine. *Biochem. Pharmacol.*, **20**, 3367–3776.

Benfey, B. G., and Grillo, S. A. (1963). Antagonism of acetylcholine by adrenaline antagonists. *Br. J. Pharmacol.*, **20**, 528–533.

Blackman, J. G., Ginsborg, B. L., and Ray, C. (1963). Synaptic transmission in the sympathetic ganglion of the frog. *J. Physiol. (London)*, **167**, 355–373.

Bloom, F. E. (1975). The role of cyclic nucleotides in central synaptic function. *Rev. Physiol. Biochem. Pharmacol.*, **74**, 1–103.

Boyd, H., Burnstock, G., Campbell, G., Lowett, A., O'Shea, J., and Wood, M. (1963). The cholinergic blocking action of adrenergic blocking agents in the pharmacological analysis of autonomic innervation. *Br. J. Pharmacol.*, **20**, 418–435.

Brown, D. A., and Adams, P. R. (1980). Muscarinic suppression of a novel voltage-sensitive K^+ current in a vertebrate neurone. *Nature*, **283**, 673–676.

Brown, D. A., Caulfield, M. P., and Kirby, P. J. (1979). Relation between catecholamine-induced cyclic AMP changes and hyperpolarization in isolated rat sympathetic ganglia. *J. Physiol. (London)*, **290**, 441–451.

Brown, J. E., Muller, K. J., and Murray, G. (1971). Reversal potential for an electrophysiological event generated by conductance changes: mathematical analysis. *Science*, **174**, 318.

Busis, N. A., and Weight, F. F. (1976). Spike afterhyperpolarization of a sympathetic neurone is calcium sensitive and is potentiated by theophylline. *Nature*, **263**, 434–436.

Busis, N. A., Weight, F. F., and Smith, P. A. (1978). Synaptic potentials in sympathetic ganglia: are they mediated by cyclic nucleotides? *Science*, **200**, 1079–1081.

Cole, A. E., and Shinnick-Gallagher, P. (1980). Alpha-adrenoceptor and dopamine receptor antagonists do not block the slow inhibitory postsynaptic potential in sympathetic ganglia. *Brain Res.*, **187**, 226–230.

Cole, A. E., and Shinnick-Gallagher, P. (1981). Comparison of the receptors mediating the catecholamine hyperpolarization and slow inhibitory postsynaptic potential in sympathetic ganglia. *J. Pharmacol. Exp. Ther.*, **217**, 440–444.

Constanti, A., Adams, P. R., and Brown, D. A. (1981). Why do barium ions imitate acetylcholine? *Brain Res.*, **206**, 244–250.

Dennis, M. J., Harris, A. J., and Kuffler, S. W. (1971). Synaptic transmission and its duplication by focally applied acetylcholine in parasympathetic neurons of the heart of the frog. *Proc. Roy. S. London Ser. B.*, **177**, 509–539.

Desmedt, J. E., and Hainaut, K. (1977). Inhibition of the intracellular release of calcium by dantrolene in barnacle giant muscle fibres. *J. Physiol. (London)*, **265**, 565–585.

Dun, N. J., and Karczmar, A. G. (1977). A comparison of the effect of theophylline and cyclic adenosine 3′,5′-monophosphate on the superior cervical ganglion of the rabbit by means of the sucrose-gap method. *J. Pharmacol. Exp. Ther.*, **202**, 89–96.

Dun, N. J., and Karczmar, A. G. (1980). A comparative study of the pharmacological properties of the positive potential recorded from the superior cervical ganglia. *J. Pharmacol. Exp. Ther.*, **215**, 455–460.

Dun, N. J., Kaibara, K., and Karczmar, A. G. (1977a). Direct postsynaptic membrane effects of dibutyryl cyclic GMP on mammalian sympathetic neurons. *Neuropharmacology*, **16**, 715–717.

Dun, N. J., Kaibara, K., and Karczmar, A. G. (1977b). Dopamine and adenosine 3′, 5′-monophosphate responses of single mammalian sympathetic neurons. *Science*, **197**, 778–780.

Eccles, J. C. (1943). Synaptic potentials and transmission in sympathetic ganglion. *J. Physiol. (London)*, **101**, 465–483.

Eccles, J. C. (1964). *The Physiology of Synapses*, Springer-Verlag, Berlin, Gottingen, Heidelberg.

Eccles, R. M. (1952). Responses of isolated curarized sympathetic ganglia. *J. Physiol. (London)*, **117**, 196–217.

Eccles, R. M., and Libet, B. (1961). Origin and blockade of the synaptic responses of curarized sympathetic ganglia. *J. Physiol. (London)*, **157**, 484–503.

Freyburger, W. A., Graham, B. E., Rapport, M. M., Seay, P. H., Govier, W. M., Swoap, O. F., and Van der Brook, M. J. (1952). The pharmacology of 5-hydroxytryptamine (serotonin). *J. Pharmacol. Exp. Ther.*, **105**, 80–86.

Furchgott, R. F. (1954). Dibenamine blockade in strips of rabbit aorta and its use in differentiating receptors. *J. Pharmacol. Exp. Ther.*, **106**, 265–284.

Furchgott, R. F. (1955). The pharmacology of vascular smooth muscle. *Pharmacol. Rev.*, **7**, 183–265.

Furchgott, R. F. (1966). The use of beta-haloalkylamines in the differentiation of receptors and in the determination of dissociation constants of receptor–agonist complexes. *Adv. Drug Res.*, **3**, 21–55.

Gaddum, J. H., Hathaway, D. E., and Stephens, F. F. (1955). Quantitative studies of antagonists for 5-hydroxytryptamine. *Q. J. Exp. Physiol.*, **40**, 49–74.

Gallagher, J. P., and Shinnick-Gallagher, P. (1977). Cyclic nucleotides injected intracellularly into rat superior cervical ganglion cells. *Science*, **198**, 851–852.

Gallagher, J. P., Shinnick-Gallagher, P., Cole, A. E., Griffith, W. H., III, Williams, B. J. (1980). Current hypotheses for the slow inhibitory postsynaptic potential in sympathetic ganglia. *Fed. Proc.*, **39**, 3009–3015.

Gaupp, E. (1899). *Ecker's und Wiedersheim's Anatomie des Frosches*, Vol. 2, Veiweg, Braunschweig.

Ginsborg, B. L., and Guerrero, S. (1964). On the action of depolarizing drugs on sympathetic ganglion cells of the frog. *J. Physiol. (London)*, **172**, 189–206.

Graham, J. D. P., and Lewis, G. P. (1953). The antihistamine and antiadrenaline properties of a series of *N*-naphthylmethyl-2-haloethylamine derivatives. *Br. J. Pharmacol.*, **8**, 54–61.

Greengard, P. (1976). Possible role for cyclic nucleotides and phosphorylated membrane proteins in postsynaptic actions of neurotransmitters. *Nature*, **260**, 101–108.

Griffith, W. H., III, Gallagher, J. P., and Shinnick-Gallagher, P. (1980). Cholinergic slow potentials influence parasympathetic ganglionic transmission. *Neurosci. Abstr.*, **6**, 68.

Gyermek, L. (1966). Drugs which antagonize 5-hydroxytryptamine and related indolealkylamines. In *5-Hydroxytryptamine and Related Indolealkylamines, Handbook of Experimental Pharmacology* (Ed. V. Erspamer), Vol. 19, pp. 471–528, Springer-Verlag, Berlin.

Hartzell, H. C., Kuffler, S. W., Stickgold, R., and Yoshikami, D. (1977). Synaptic excitation and inhibition resulting from direct action of acetylcholine on two types of chemoreceptors on individual amphibian parasympathetic neurones. *J. Physiol. (London)*, **271**, 817–846.

Huber, G. C. (1900). A contribution on the minute anatomy of the sympathetic ganglion of the different classes of vertebrates. *J. Morphol.*, **16**, 27–86.

Hökfelt, T., Johansson, O., Ljungdahl, A., Lundberg, J. M., and Schultzberg, M. (1980). Peptidergic neurones. *Nature*, **284**, 515–521.

Iversen, L. L. (1975). Uptake process for biogenic amines. In *Handbook of Psychopharmacology* (Eds. L. L. Iversen, S. D. Iversen and S. Snyder), Vol. 3, pp. 381–442, Plenum Press, New York.

Jan, L. Y., Jan, Y. N., and Brownfield (1980a). Peptidergic transmitters in synaptic boutons of sympathetic ganglia. *Nature*, **288**, 380–382.

Jan, Y. N., Jan, L. Y., and Kuffler, S. W. (1979). A peptide as a possible transmitter in sympathetic ganglia of the frog. *Proc. Natl. Acad. Sci. U.S.A.*, **76**, 1501–1505.

Jan, Y. N., Jan, L. Y., and Kuffler, S. W. (1980b). Further evidence for peptidergic transmission in sympathetic ganglia. *Proc. Natl. Acad. Sci. U.S.A.*, **77**, 5008–5012.

Jenkinson, D. H. (1960). The antagonism between tubocurarine and substances which depolarize the motor end-plate. *J. Physiol. (London)*, **152**, 309–324.

Katz, B. (1966). *Nerve, Muscle and Synapse*, McGraw-Hill, New York.

Keynes, R. D., and Swan, R. C. (1959). The permeability of frog muscle fibres to lithium ions. *J. Physiol. (London)*, **147**, 626–638.

Kobayashi, H., and Libet, B. (1968). Generation of slow postsynaptic potentials without increases in ionic conductance. *Proc. Natl. Acad. Sci. U.S.A.*, **60**, 1304–1311.

Kobayashi, H., and Libet, B. (1970). Actions of noradrenaline and acetylcholine on sympathetic ganglion cells. *J. Physiol. (London)*, **208**, 353–372.

Kobayashi, H., and Libet, B. (1974). Is inactivation of potassium conductance involved in slow postsynaptic excitation of sympathetic ganglion cells? Effects of nicotine. *Life Sci.*, **14**, 1871–1883.

Kobayashi, H., Hashiguchi, T., and Ushiyama, N. (1978). Postsynaptic modulation of excitatory process in sympathetic ganglia by cyclic AMP. *Nature*, **271**, 268–270.

Koketsu, K. (1969). Cholinergic synaptic potentials and the underlying ionic mechanisms. *Fed. Proc.*, **28**, 101–131.

Koketsu, K., and Yamamoto, K. (1974). Effects of lithium ions on electrical activity in sympathetic ganglia of the bullfrog. *Br. J. Pharmacol.*, **50**, 69–77.

Koketsu, K., and Yamamoto, K. (1975). Unusual cholinergic response of bullfrog sympathetic ganglion cells. *Eur. J. Pharmacol.*, **31**, 281–286.

Koketsu, K., Nishi, S., and Soeda, H. (1968). Acetylcholine-potential of sympathetic ganglion cell membrane. *Life Sci.*, **7**, 741–749.

Kopin, I. J. (1972). Metabolic degradation of catecholamines. The relative importance of different pathways under physiological conditions and after the administration of drugs. In *Catecholamines* (Eds. H. Blaschko and E. Muscholl), *Handbuch der Experimentellen Pharmakologie*, Vol. 33, pp. 270–282, Springer-Verlag, Berlin.

Kuba, K. (1980). Release of calcium ions linked to the activation of potassium conductance in a caffeine-treated sympathetic neurone. *J. Physiol. (London)*, **298**, 251–269.

Kuba, K., and Koketsu, K. (1976). Analysis of the slow excitatory postsynaptic potential in bullfrog sympathetic ganglion cells. *Jpn. J. Physiol.*, **26**, 647–664.

Kuba, K., and Koketsu, K. (1978). Intracellular injection of calcium ions and chelating agents into the bullfrog sympathetic ganglion cells and effects of caffeine. In *Iontophoresis and Transmitter Mechanisms in the Mammalian Central Nervous System* (Eds. R. W. Ryall and J. S. Kelly), pp. 158–160, Elsevier, Amsterdam.

Kuba, K., and Nishi, S. (1976). Rhythmic hyperpolarizations and depolarization of sympathetic ganglion cells induced by caffeine. *J. Neurophysiol.*, **39**, 547–563.

Kuba, K., and Nishi, S. (1979). Characteristics of fast excitatory postsynaptic current in bullfrog sympathetic ganglion cells. *Pflügers Arch.*, **378**, 205–212.

Laporte, Y., and Lorente de Nó (1950). Potential changes evoked in a curarized sympathetic ganglion by presynaptic volleys of impulses. *J. Cell. Comp. Physiol.*, **35** (Suppl. 2), 61–106.

Libet, B. (1967). Long latent periods and further analysis of slow synaptic responses in sympathetic ganglia. *J. Neurophysiol.*, **30**, 494–514.

Libet, B. (1979). Which postsynaptic action of dopamine is mediated by cyclic AMP? *Life Sci.*, **24**, 1043–1058.

Libet, B. (1980). Functional roles of SIF cells in slow synaptic actions. In *Histochemistry and Cell Biology of Autonomic Neurons, SIF Cells and Paraneurons* (Eds. O. Eränkö, S. Soinila and H. Päivärinta), *Advances in Biochemical Psychopharmacology*, Vol. 25, pp. 111–118, Raven Press, New York.

Libet, B., and Kobayashi, H. (1974). Adrenergic mediation of slow inhibitory postsynaptic potential in sympathetic ganglia of the frog. *J. Neurophysiol.*, **37**, 805–814.

Libet, B., Chichibu, S., and Tosaka, T. (1968). Slow synaptic responses and excitability in sympathetic ganglia of the bullfrog. *J. Neurophysiol.*, **31**, 383–395.

Loew, E. R., and Micetich, A. (1948). Adrenergic blocking drugs: II. antagonism of histamine and epinephrine with N-(2-haloalkyl)-1-naphthalene-methylamine derivatives. *J. Pharmacol. Exp. Ther.*, **105**, 339–349.

MacDermott, A. B., and Weight, F. F. (1980). The pharmacological blockade of potassium conductances in voltage clamped bullfrog sympathetic neurons. *Fed. Proc.*, **39**, 2074.

MacDermott, A. B., Connors, E. A., Dionne, V. E., and Parsons, R. L. (1980). Voltage clamp study of fast excitatory synaptic currents in bullfrog sympathetic ganglion cells. *J. Gen. Physiol.*, **75**, 39–60.

Maizels, E. (1954). Active cation transport in erythrocytes. *Symp. Soc. Exp. Biol.*, **8**, 202–227.

McAfee, D. A., and Greengard, P. (1972). Adenosine 3',5'-monophosphate: electrophysiological evidence for a role in synaptic transmission. *Science*, **178**, 310–312.

McAfee, D. A., Schorderet, M., and Greengard, P. (1971). Adenosine 3',5'-monophosphate in nervous tissue: increase associated with synaptic transmission. *Science*, **171**, 1156–1158.

McCort, S. M., and Weight, F. F. (1979). Analysis of the role of calcium in rhythmic hyperpolarizations induced by theophylline in bullfrog sympathetic neurons. *Neurosci. Abstr.*, **5**, 47.

Meech, R. W. (1978). Calcium-dependent potassium activation in nervous tissue. *Annu. Rev. Biophys. Bioeng.*, **7**, 1–18.

Nakamura, J. (1978). The effects of neuroleptics on the dopaminergic and cholinergic systems in sympathetic ganglia. *Kurume Med. J.*, **25**, 241–253.

Nash, J. W., and Weight, F. F. (1980). Analysis of calcium and divalent cation activation of a potassium conductance. *Fed. Proc.*, **39**, 282.

Nathanson, J. A. (1977). Cyclic nucleotides and nervous system function. *Physiol. Rev.*, **57**, 157–256.

Nishi, S., and Koketsu, K. (1960). Electrical properties and activities of single sympathetic neurons in frog. *J. Cell. Comp. Physiol.*, **55**, 15–30.

Nishi, S., and Koketsu, K. (1967). Origin of ganglionic inhibitory postsynaptic potential. *Life Sci.*, **6**, 2049–2055.

Nishi, S., and Koketsu, K. (1968a). Early and late after-discharges of amphibian sympathetic ganglion cells. *J. Neurophysiol.*, **31**, 109–121.

Nishi, S., and Koketsu, K. (1968b). Analysis of slow inhibitory postsynaptic potential of bullfrog sympathetic ganglion. *J. Neurophysiol.*, **31**, 717–728.

Nishi, S., Soeda, H., and Koketsu, K. (1965). Studies on sympathetic B and C neurons and patterns of preganglionic innervation. *J. Cell. Comp. Physiol.*, **66**, 19–32.

Nishi, S., Soeda, H., and Koketsu, K. (1967). Release of acetylcholine from sympathetic preganglionic nerve terminals. *J. Neurophysiol.*, **30**, 114–134.

Nishi, S., Soeda, H., and Koketsu, K. (1969). Influence of membrane potential on the fast-acetylcholine potential of sympathetic ganglion cells. *Life Sci.*, **8**, 499–505.

Pant, H. C., and Weight, F. F. (1980). Effect of calcium and cyclic nucleotides on protein phosphorylation in bullfrog sympathetic ganglia. *Fed. Proc.*, **39**, 1626.

Schulman, J. A., and Weight, F. F. (1976). Synaptic transmission: long-lasting potentiation by a postsynaptic mechanism. *Science*, **194**, 1437–1439.

Skok, V. I. (1965). Conduction in tenth ganglion of the frog sympathetic trunk. *Fed. Proc.*, **24** (Transl. Suppl.), T363–T367.

Smith, P. A., and Weight, F. F. (1977). Role of electrogenic sodium pump in slow synaptic inhibition is re-evaluated. *Nature*, **267**, 68–70.

Smith, P. A., and Weight, F. F. (1981). Evidence for generation of the slow IPSP by the direct muscarinic hyperpolarizing action of acetylcholine in bullfrog sympathetic ganglia. *Neurosci. Abstr.*, **7**, 807.

Smith, P. A., Weight, F. F., and Lehne, R. A. (1979). Potentiation of calcium dependent potassium activation by theophylline is independent of cyclic nucleotide elevation in sympathetic neurons. *Nature*, **280**, 400–402.

Smith, S. J., MacDermott, A. B., and Weight, F. F. (1981). Intracellular calcium transients elicited by synaptic and electrical membrane activation and by theophylline measured in bullfrog neurons using arsenazo III. *Neurosci. Abstr.*, **7**, 15.

Steinbach, J. H., and Stevens, C. F. (1976). Neuromuscular transmission. In *Frog Neurobiology* (Eds. R. Llinas and W. Precht), pp. 33–92, Springer-Verlag, Berlin, Heidelberg, New York.

Stone, C. A., and Loew, E. R. (1952). Specificity and potency of aryl-haloalkylamine adrenergic blocking drugs as determined on isolated seminal vesicles of guinea pigs. *J. Pharmacol. Exp. Ther.*, **106**, 226–234.

Takeuchi, A. (1977). Junctional transmission I. Postsynaptic mechanisms. In *Handbook of Physiology. Sect. 1: The Nervous System. Vol. 1: Cellular Biology of Neurons, Part 1* (Vol. Ed. E. R. Kandel), pp. 295–327, American Physiological Society, Bethesda.

Taxi, J. (1976). Morphology of the autonomic nervous systems. In *Frog Neurobiology* (Ed. R. Llinas and W. Precht), pp. 93–150, Springer-Verlag, Berlin, Heidelberg, New York.

Thomas, R. C. (1972). Electrogenic sodium pump in nerve and muscle cells. *Physiol. Rev.*, **52**, 563–594.

Tosaka, T., Chichibu, S., and Libet, B. (1968). Intracellular analysis of slow inhibitory and excitatory postsynaptic potentials in sympathetic ganglia of the frog. *J. Neurophysiol.*, **31**, 396–409.

Van Winkle, W. B. (1976). Calcium release from skeletal muscle sarcoplasmic reticulum: site of action of dantrolene sodium? *Science*, **193**, 1130–1131.

Wang, C. M., and Narahashi, T. (1972). Mechanisms of dual action of nicotine on end-plate membranes. *J. Pharmacol. Exp. Ther.*, **182**, 427–441.

Watanabe, H. (1980). Ultrastructural study of the frog sympathetic ganglia. In *Histochemistry and Cell Biology of Autonomic Neurons, SIF Cells, and Paraneurons* (Eds. O. Eränkö, S. Soinila and H. Päivärinta), *Advances in Biochemical Psychopharmacology*, Vol. 25, pp. 153–171, Raven Press, New York.

Weight, F. F. (1973). Slow synaptic inhibition and adrenergic antagonism in sympathetic ganglion. *Soc. Neurosci., Third Annual Meeting Abstracts*, p. 312.

Weight, F. F. (1974). Physiological mechanisms of synaptic modulation. In *The Neurosciences: Third Study Program* (Eds. F. O. Schmitt and F. G. Worden), pp. 929–941, MIT Press, Cambridge, MA.

Weight, F. F., and MacDermott, A. B. (1981). Postsynaptic mechanisms in synaptic plasticity. *Adv. Physiol. Sci.*, **36**, 243–251.

Weight, F. F., and McCort, S. M. (1981). Intracellular calcium and the regulation of neuronal membrane permeability. In *Ion-selective Microelectrodes and Their Use in Excitable Tissues* (Eds. E. Syková, P. Hnik and L. Vyklicky), pp. 351–354, Plenum Press, New York, London.

Weight, F. F., and Padjen, A. (1973a). Slow synaptic inhibition: evidence for synaptic inactivation of sodium conductance in sympathetic ganglion cells. *Brain Res.*, **55**, 219–224.

Weight, F. F., and Padjen, A. (1973b). Acetylcholine and slow synaptic inhibition in frog sympathetic ganglion cells. *Brain Res.*, **55**, 225–228.

Weight, F. F., and Smith, P. A. (1980). Small intensely fluorescent (SIF) cells and the generation of slow postsynaptic inhibition in sympathetic ganglia. In *Histochemistry and Cell Biology of Autonomic Neurons, SIF Cells, and Paraneurons* (Eds. O. Eränkö, S. Soinila and H. Päivärinta), *Advances in Biochemical Psychopharmacology*, Vol. 25, pp. 159–171, Raven Press, New York.

Weight, F. F., and Smith, P. A. (1981). IPSP reversal: evidence for increased potassium conductance combined with decreased sodium conductance. *Adv. Physiol. Sci.*, **4**, 351–354.

Weight, F. F., and Votava, J. (1970). Slow synaptic excitation in sympathetic ganglion cells: evidence for synaptic inactivation of potassium conductance. *Science*, **170**, 755–757.

Weight, F. F., and Votava, J. (1971). Inactivation of potassium conductance in slow postsynaptic excitation. *Science*, **172**, 504.

Weight, F. F., and Weitsen, H. A. (1977). Identification of small intensely fluorescent (SIF) cells as chromaffin cells in bullfrog sympathetic ganglia. *Brain Res.*, **128**, 213–336.

Weight, F. F., Petzold, G., and Greengard, P. (1974). Guanosine 3′,5′-monophosphate in sympathetic ganglia: increase associated with synaptic transmission. *Science*, **186**, 942–944.

Weight, F. F., Smith, P. A., and Schulman, J. A. (1978). Postsynaptic potential generation appears independent of synaptic elevation of cyclic nucleotides in sympathetic neurons. *Brain Res.*, **158**, 197–202.

Weight, F. F., Schulman, J. A., Smith, P. A., and Busis, N. A. (1979). Long-lasting synaptic potentials and the modulation of synaptic transmission. *Fed. Proc.*, **38**, 2084–2094.

Weight, F. F., Pant, H. C., and McCort, S. M. (1981). Protein phosphorylation and membrane permeability change correlated with intracellular calcium in nervous tissue. *Proc. Eighth Int. Congr. Pharmacol.*, 317.

Weitsen, H. A., and Weight, F. F. (1977) Synaptic innervation of sympathetic ganglion cells in the bullfrog. *Brain Res.*, **128**, 197–211.

Yavari, P., and Weight, F. F. (1981). Effects of phentolamine on synaptic transmission in bullfrog sympathetic ganglia. *Neurosci. Abstr.*, **7**, 807.

Zerahn, K. (1955). Studies on the active transport of lithium in the isolated frog skin. *Acta Physiol. Scand.*, **33**, 347–358.

Note Added in Proof: Since completion of this review in 1981 the following relevant papers have been published: Adams, P. R. et al (1982), J. Physiol. (London) **330**, 537–572; *ibid*, **332**, 223–272; Dodd, J. and Horn, J. P. (1983), *J. Physiol. (London)* **334**, 255–291; Jan, L. Y. and Jan, Y. N. (1982) **327**, 219–246; Katayama, Y. and Nishi, S. (1982), *J. Physiol. (London)* **333**, 305–313; MacDermott, A. B. and Weight, F. F. (1982), *Nature*, **300**, 185–188; McCort, S. M., Nash, J. W. and Weight, F. F. (1982), *Neuroscience Abstr.* **8**, 501; Sejnowski, T. J. (1982) *Federation Proc.*, **41**, 2923–2928.

Autonomic Ganglia
Edited by Lars-Gösta Elfvin
© 1983 John Wiley & Sons Ltd

Peptide Hormones and Transmission in Sympathetic Ganglia

N. J. DUN

Department of Pharmacology, Loyola University,
Stritch School of Medicine, Maywood, Illinois 60153, USA

INTRODUCTION

Over the past 20 years investigations into the nature of chemical transmission in the vertebrate nervous system have implicated a wide variety of agents as proven or putative transmitters (see Krnjévic, 1974). In addition to the classical transmitters of small molecular weight, i.e. acetylcholine (ACh), monoamines, and γ-aminobutyric acid, a number of substances with large, complex structures such as polypeptides may be today considered as putative transmitters (see Bloom, 1972; Nicoll, 1976; Otsuka and Konishi, 1977; Hökfelt *et al.*, 1980). That peptides may be derived from neural elements was demonstrated as early as 1931 by von Euler and Gaddum as they isolated substance P from equine brain and peripheral tissues. The explosive increase in the past few years of the number of investigations of the effects of peptides on neuronal function was touched off by the intense progress made in peptide chemistry. As synthetic peptides became available, antibodies needed for carrying out sensitive radioimmunoassays and for immunohistochemical localization of endogenous peptides could be developed. In fact, it appears that the rate of adding to the number of identified endogenous peptides is limited only by the rate at which new antibodies can be obtained. Currently, more than 20 peptides have been detected in the vertebrate central and peripheral nervous system; a number of which have been shown to be present in sympathetic ganglia (Hökfelt *et al.*, 1978, 1980).

The aim of this review is to evaluate the present status of peptides in sympathetic ganglia. In this context, only those peptides demonstrated to be present in sympathetic ganglia (Table 1) will be discussed.

SUBSTANCE P

The presence of substance P, an undecapeptide (Chang *et al.*, 1971) or of a closely related peptide in various sympathetic ganglia was demonstrated

Table 1 Occurrence and localization of peptides in sympathetic ganglia

Peptide	Locali- zation	Sympathetic ganglia	Species	References
APP	PGN	SCG, stellate, CMG	Rat, cat	Lundberg *et al.* (1980a)
CCK	NF	IMG, CMG	Rat, guinea-pig	Larsson and Rehfeld (1979)
ENK	NF	IMG, CMG, SCG	Guinea-pig, rat	Schultzberg *et al.* (1979)
	PGN	SCG	Rat, guinea-pig	DiGiulio *et al.* (1978); Schultzberg *et al.* (1979)
	SIF	SCG, IMG, CMG	Guinea-pig, rat	Schultzberg *et al.* (1979)
	SIF	Paravertebral	Bullfrog	Kondo and Yui (1981)
LHRF	NF	Paravertebral	Bullfrog	Jan *et al.* (1979)
SOM	PGN	IMG, CMG, SCG	Guinea-pig, rat	Hökfelt *et al.* (1977a)
BOMB	SIF	Paravertebral	Bullfrog	Kondo (unpublished)
SP	NF	IMG, CMG, SCG	Guinea-pig, rat	Hökfelt *et al.* (1977c)
	Intrinsic	SCG	Rat	Robinson *et al.* (1980)
VIP	NF	IMG, CMG, SCG	Guinea-pig, rat	Hökfelt *et al.* (1977b)
	PGN	IMG, CMG	Guinea-pig	Hökfelt *et al.* (1977b)

Abbreviations: Inferior mesenteric ganglia (IMG); coeliac-superior mesenteric ganglia (CMG); superior cervical ganglia (SCG); small intensely fluorescent cells (SIF); nerve fibres (NF); principal postganglionic neurons (PGN); avian pancreatic polypeptide (APP); cholecystokinin (CCK); enkephalins (ENK); bombesin (BOMB); luteinizing hormone-releasing factor (LHRF); substance P (SP); somatostatin (SOM); vaosactive intestinal polypeptide (VIP).

by means of immunohistofluorescence (Hökfelt *et al.*, 1977c) and radio-immunoassay (Konishi *et al.*, 1979b; Robinson *et al.*, 1980; Gamse *et al.*, 1981) methods. In particular, inferior mesenteric and coeliac-superior mesenteric ganglia of the guinea-pig exhibited dense networks of substance P-positive fibres which appeared to come into close contact with the postganglionic neurons, while such fibres were not observed around small intensely fluorescent (SIF) cells; relatively few of these fibres were observed in the superior cervical ganglia of the same species (Hökfelt *et al.*, 1977c).

The origin of substance P-containing fibres in inferior mesenteric ganglia is not certain. As substance P is found to be concentrated in small primary sensory neurons of the spinal ganglia (Hökfelt *et al.*, 1975), substance P-containing fibres observed in the inferior mesenteric ganglia may represent axon collaterals of sensory neurons as they course to the gastrointestinal tract (Hökfelt *et al.*, 1977c, 1980). Following injection of horseradish peroxidase into the inferior mesenteric ganglia, peroxidase labellings could be traced to primary sensory neurons of the spinal ganglia; hence, there is a definite connection between some of the fibres in the inferior mesenteric ganglia and the primary sensory neurons (Elfvin and Dalsgaard, 1977). Most recently, Gamse *et al.* (1981) reported that injection of capsaicin caused a marked depletion of immunoreactive substance P in both the dorsal root ganglia and sympathetic ganglia; this finding is consistent with the notion that substance P-containing fibres may originate from primary sensory neurons (Elfvin and Dalsgaard, 1977; see also page 217 in chapter by Schultzberg *et al.*).

The situation appears to be different with regard to the superior cervical ganglia of the rat. In this case, substance P immunoreactivity was not appreciably altered by either decentralization of the ganglia or axotomy, suggesting that this peptide may be of intrinsic origin; the exact location, however, has not been established (Robinson *et al.*, 1980). Thus, the origin and localization of substance P in paravertebral ganglia appear to be different from that in prevertebral ganglia; the possibility that substance P may have different physiological roles in these two groups of ganglia should be explored.

The demonstration of substance P-containing fibres in sympathetic ganglia of the guinea-pig has led to a quantitative determination of substance P immunoreactivity at these sites. Among the ganglia studied, coeliac-superior mesenteric and inferior mesenteric ganglia contained the highest amount of substance P immunoreactivity, whereas less than 10% of that amount was found in superior cervical ganglia (Konishi *et al.*, 1979b; Gamse *et al.*, 1981). Moreover, the peptide content was markedly reduced after ligation or sectioning of fibres leading to the coeliac-superior mesenteric ganglia, and immersing the ganglia in a high K^+ solution caused a release of the peptide in a calcium-dependent manner (Konishi *et al.*, 1979b). These findings and the previous observation that substance P-containing fibres come into close contact with the postganglionic neurons (Hökfelt *et al.*, 1977c) raised the possibility that substance P may have a synaptic function in the inferior mesenteric ganglia.

Shortly after the demonstration of the presence of dense networks of substance P-containing fibres in the inferior mesenteric ganglia (Hökfelt *et al.*, 1977c), Neild (1978) reported that repetitive stimulation of preganglionic fibres elicited a slowly developing excitatory potential lasting for seconds to minutes in these ganglion cells; more importantly, this potential was not blocked by cholinergic antagonists. It must be stressed that a slow excitatory non-cholinergic potential can also be induced in the bullfrog sympathetic ganglion cells (Nishi and Koketsu, 1968) and myenteric neurons of the guinea-pig (Katayama and North, 1978). These findings led to a search in this laboratory for a possible link between substance P and the non-cholinergic excitatory potential.

First, we confirmed the report of Neild (1978) that repetitive stimulation of the hypogastric nerves elicits in inferior mesenteric ganglion cells of the guinea-pig a slow excitatory potential (Fig. 1A) which is not blocked by cholinergic antagonists, whereas it is abolished in a low Ca^{2+} solution (Dun and Karczmar, 1979). The amplitude and duration of the non-cholinergic

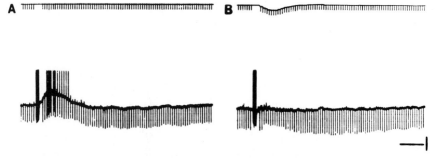

Figure 1 Non-cholinergic excitatory potential elicited in a guinea-pig inferior mesenteric ganglion cell. (A) Repetitive stimulation of both hypogastric nerves at a frequency of 30 Hz for 3 sec elicited spike discharges followed by a slow membrane depolarization lasting for about 40 sec. Hyperpolarizing electrotonic potentials (lower tracing) were induced by hyperpolarizing current pulses of 150 msec duration (upper tracing). The membrane resistance change was obscured by the occurrence of spike discharges during the generation of non-cholinergic excitatory potential. (B) Membrane depolarization was annulled by the passage of hyperpolarizing current through the recording electrode. Note that the membrane resistance showed an initial decrease followed by a more prolonged increase. Calibration: 10 mV, 1 nA and 20 sec

excitatory potential ranged from 2 mV to more than 10 mV and 20 sec to 3 min, respectively. In many instances, spontaneous discharges occurred during the generation of non-cholinergic potential (Fig. 1A); the spontaneous discharges were not blocked by cholinergic antagonists, but readily abolished by membrane hyperpolarization (Dun and Karczmar, 1979). In a portion of the neurons tested, the input resistance showed a biphasic change: an initial decrease was followed by a more prolonged increase (Fig. 1A). This biphasic membrane resistance change could also be demonstrated when the membrane potential was clamped manually at rest (Fig. 1B). In other neurons, the non-cholinergic potential was associated with either a monophasic increase of input resistance or no detectable change (Dun and Karczmar, 1979; Jiang and Dun, 1981).

Second, the effects of substance P on the membrane of inferior mesenteric ganglion cells were investigated. When applied to the neurons in the concentrations of less than 1 μM, substance P elicited a slow membrane depolarization that lasted for minutes (Fig. 2); the amplitude of depolarization varied from cell to cell (from 2 mV to more than 20 mV). A common feature of substance P depolarization was the occurrence of intense, repetitive spike discharges on the rising phase of the depolarization (Fig. 2). These spike discharges did not represent synaptic responses, as they were not abolished in a low Ca^{2+}–high Mg^{2+} solution which depressed transmitter release, or in a solution containing cholinergic antagonists (Dun and Karczmar, 1979; Dun and Minota, 1981). Substance P-induced depolarization was

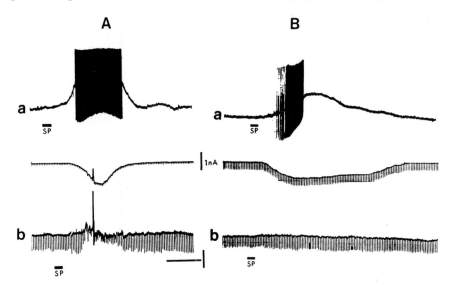

Figure 2 Membrane depolarization and membrane resistance change induced by substance P in two inferior mesenteric ganglion cells, A and B. Cell A: (a) membrane depolarization and intense neuronal discharge induced by substance P (0.5 μM). (b) membrane potential was clamped manually at the resting level (−58 mV), and hyperpolarizing electronic potentials (lower tracing) were elicited by hyperpolarizing current pulses (upper tracing) of 100 msec duration. Note that the membrane resistance was initially increased and then decreased to about 49% of its control value. Cell B: (a) membrane depolarization and spike discharge induced by substance P (0.5 μM). (b) membrane potential was clamped at the resting level of −53 mV. Note that substance P caused a prolonged increase of membrane resistance. Substance P was applied for 10 sec as indicated by the bars (SP). Calibration: 10 mV and 40 sec. From Minota *et al.* (1981); reproduced by permission of Elsevier/North-Holland Biomedical Press

associated with either a decrease or increase of membrane resistance (Dun and Karczmar, 1979; Dun and Minota, 1981; Minota *et al.*, 1981). The electrophysiological characteristics of substance P-induced depolarization thus appeared to be similar to those of the non-cholinergic potential elicited by preganglionic stimulation (Neild, 1978; Dun and Karczmar, 1979; Konishi *et al.*, 1979b; Jiang and Dun, 1981).

Pharmacological analysis showed that substance P probably depolarized the postganglionic neurons directly, and that this response was not due to peptide-induced release of another endogenous substance, as the response persisted in a low Ca^{2+}–high Mg^{2+} solution, or in a solution containing nicotinic and muscarinic antagonists (Dun and Karczmar, 1979; Dun and Minota, 1981). As specific pharmacological antagonists of substance P were not available, the procedure of desensitization was employed to evaluate the similarity between the receptors mediating substance P depolarization and the non-cholinergic depolarization elicited by nerve stimulation. The slow non-cholinergic potential evoked by nerve stimulation was markedly diminished following application of exogenous substance P to the ganglion cells suggesting that the transmitter mediating the slow non-cholinergic potential and substance P may be acting on the same receptors (Dun and Karczmar, 1979). On the basis of these electrophysiological and pharmacological findings, we suggested that substance P may be the putative transmitter responsible for the generation of the non-cholinergic potential in the inferior mesenteric ganglia of the guinea-pig (Dun and Karczmar, 1979). Konishi *et al.* (1979b) investigated independently the effects of substance P on the inferior mesenteric ganglion cells and arrived at a similar conclusion with respect to these cells.

Third, the ionic mechanism underlying substance P depolarization appears to be similar to that of the non-cholinergic potential (Dun and Minota, 1981; Jiang and Dun, 1981). When the membrane potential was manually clamped at rest between -50 and -60 mV, substance P caused two types of membrane resistance change. One pattern of change consisted of a brief, transient increase followed by a prolonged decrease of membrane resistance (Fig. 2A); in other neurons, a sustained increase of membrane resistance was observed (Fig. 2B). It should be pointed out that in the case of these two responses the change of membrane resistance, whether increase or decrease, was usually not marked (about 20%), and the two types of changes were observed in about an equal number of neurons (Dun and Minota, 1981). A third type of response was noticed in a few neurons in which substance P elicited a large depolarization accompanied by a several fold increase of membrane resistance. Further analysis revealed that this response occurred invariably in neurons exhibiting high (> -70 mV) resting membrane potential (Dun and Minota, 1981; Minota *et al.*, 1981). An example is illustrated in Fig. 3. A detailed investigation of membrane properties of the neurons in question revealed that the large increase in membrane resistance was due probably to anomalous rectification of the membrane, as the increase in membrane resistance became much smaller when the membrane potential was manually clamped (Fig. 3B). In this context, it is interesting to note that in myenteric neurons of the guinea-pig (Katayama and North, 1978; Katayama *et al.*, 1979) and cat cuneate neurons (Krnjévic, 1977), substance P depolarization was associated with a large increase in membrane resistance. The finding that substance P elicited both an increase and decrease of membrane resistance of the neurons of the inferior mesenteric ganglia is of significance as these effects are analogous to similar membrane resistance changes associated with the non-cholinergic potential elicited in these neurons by nerve stimulation (Neild, 1978; Dun and Karczmar, 1979; Konishi *et al.*, 1979b; Jiang and Dun, 1981).

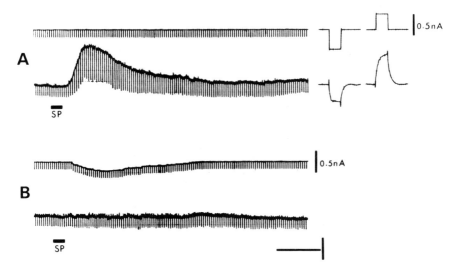

Figure 3 Substance P depolarization and membrane resistance change in a cell with high resting membrane potential (−72 mV). (A) Membrane depolarization and marked increase in neuronal input resistance. Hyperpolarizing electrotonic potentials (lower tracing) were induced by anodal current pulses of 100 msec duration (upper tracing). (B) Membrane potential was clamped at the resting level during depolarization. Note that the input resistance increase was small as compared with that obtained under A. Substance P (0.5 μM) was applied for 10 sec as indicated by the bars (SP). Recordings A and B were obtained from the same ganglion cell. Anomalous rectification revealed by means of small hyperpolarizing and large depolarizing electrotonic potentials induced by anodal and cathodal current pulses is shown in right hand corner inset. Calibration: 10 mV and 40 sec for records A and B, and 400 msec for the insert. From Minota *et al.* (1981); reproduced by permission of Elsevier/North-Holland Biomedical Press

In the case of cat cuneate (Krnjévic, 1977) and guinea-pig myenteric (Katayama *et al.*, 1979) neurons, the primary action of substance P appears to involve the inactivation of potassium conductance (G_K). In the case of inferior mesenteric neurons, the substance P depolarization was augmented upon conditioning hyperpolarization to the level of potassium equilibrium potential (E_K; Fig. 4); these findings are contrary to what could be expected if substance P caused an inactivation of G_K as suggested by Krnjévic (1977) and Katayama *et al.* (1979). However, as in a portion of inferior mesenteric ganglion cells substance P caused an increase of membrane resistance, the inactivation of G_K appears to be partially responsible for substance P-induced depolarization (Dun and Minota, 1981; Minota *et al.*, 1981). On the other hand, the observation that in some neurons substance P depolarization was associated with a decrease in membrane resistance indicates that the peptide may increase membrane permeability to certain ions (Dun and Minota, 1981;

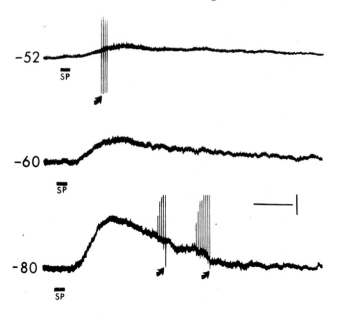

Figure 4 The effect of membrane hyperpolarization on substance P response. Substance P (0.5 µM) was applied for 10 sec as indicated by the bars. Arrows denote the peak of after-hyperpolarization of spike potential. Spontaneous spike potentials occurred at −52 mV. Cathodal current pulses were used to induce spike potentials at −80 mV. The peak of spike potentials was cut off. Note that the amplitude of substance P depolarization was increased upon membrane hyperpolarization. Calibration: 10 mV and 40 sec. From Minota *et al.* (1981); reproduced by permission of Elsevier/North-Holland Biomedical Press

Minota *et al.*, 1981). Moreover, as substance P depolarization was not appreciably altered in a low Cl⁻ or low Ca²⁺ solution, and as it was markedly reduced in a Na⁺-free medium, the peptide appeared to increase Na⁺ conductance (G_{Na}) Dun and Minota, 1981; Minota *et al.*, 1981). Taken together, these findings suggest that the electrogenic mechanism underlying substance P depolarization in inferior mesenteric ganglion cells includes both G_{Na} activation and G_K inactivation (Dun and Minota, 1981; Minota *et al.*, 1981). In this context, it is noteworthy that the electrogenic mechanism of muscarinic depolarization in bullfrog sympathetic neurons was suggested to be due to a combined mechanism of G_{Na} and G_{Ca} activation and G_K inactivation (Kuba and Koketsu, 1974, 1976, 1978). There appears then to be a close similarity between the mechanism of action of substance P and of muscarinic action of ACh on sympathetic neurons; it is plausible that a common cellular process leading to membrane depolarization is activated by these two pharmacologically distinct substances.

In summary, immunohistofluorescent, biochemical, electrophysiological and pharmacological evidence obtained thus far supports the contention that substance P may be the transmitter responsible for the generation of the non-cholinergic potential elicited in the inferior mesenteric ganglia of the guinea-pig (Hökfelt *et al.*, 1977c; Neild, 1978; Dun and Karczmar, 1979; Konishi *et al.*, 1979b; Dun and Minota, 1981; Jiang and Dun, 1981). In a similar context, it was suggested that substance P is the transmitter mediating the slow depolarization elicited in myenteric neurons of guinea-pig (Katayama and North, 1978; Morita *et al.*, 1980). Grafe *et al.* (1979) have obtained some evidence implicating serotonin rather than the peptide as the putative transmitter in this preparation.

Furthermore, substance P may exert modulatory effects on the sympathetic neurons. Indeed, it was noticed in the course of our study that when employed in concentrations that caused slight to negligible membrane depolarization substance P potentiated the amplitude of fast excitatory postsynaptic potential (f-EPSP); this effect resulted frequently in spike discharge (Dun and Karczmar, 1981). The mechanism of this action of substance P has not been investigated in detail.

The physiological role of substance P-containing fibres in sympathetic ganglia is intriguing. If indeed substance P-positive fibres are collaterals of primary sensory neurons (Elfvin and Dalsgaard, 1977), excitation of the primary sensory nerve endings would cause a release of substance P in the central nervous system as well as in the sympathetic ganglia. In a corollary, sensory activation may affect the activity of autonomic neurons via the release of substance P.

LUTEINIZING HORMONE-RELEASING FACTOR (LH-RF)

LH-RF is a decapeptide of hypothalamic origin; it stimulates the secretion of both luteinizing hormone and follicle-stimulating hormone from the anterior pituitary (Schally *et al.*, 1973). The occurrence and distribution of LH-RF in the peripheral autonomic nervous system has not been studied systematically. LH-RF or a closely related peptide has, however, been identified in bullfrog paravertebral ganglia, and implicated as the putative transmitter mediating the non-cholinergic late slow EPSP (ls-EPSP) in these ganglia (Nishi and Koketsu, 1968; Jan *et al.*, 1979, 1980a).

A long-lasting depolarization which was termed subsequently the ls-EPSP was first identified in bullfrog sympathetic ganglia following repetitive stimulation of preganglionic B and C fibres by Nishi and Koketsu (1968). As this potential was not blocked by nicotinic and muscarinic antagonists, but was eliminated in a low Ca^{2+} solution, it was proposed that it is generated by a non-cholinergic substance released presynaptically (Nishi and Koketsu, 1968). In the last few years the investigations carried out by Kuffler and his associates have led to the suggestion that LH-RF may be the putative transmitter responsible for the generation of ls-EPSP in bullfrog sympathetic ganglia (Jan *et al.*, 1979, 1980a). Their results may be summarized as follows.

First, the ganglionic contents of LH-RF or a closely related peptide were markedly reduced following sectioning of the preganglionic nerves. Second, it was shown that the LH-RF-like substance is released by isotonic KCl or nerve stimulation in a calcium-dependent manner (Jan *et al.*, 1979). Finally, immunohistochemical studies showed that LH-RF immunoreactivity is present in synaptic boutons terminating mainly on type C, but not on type B neurons (Jan *et al.*, 1980b). As a result, it was suggested that the ls-EPSP which can be recorded in B neurons is due to a diffusion of LH-RF released from nearby terminals impinging upon type C neurons (Jan *et al.*, 1980b). The question whether LH-RF is contained in cholinergic nerve fibres or present in a separate population of neurons remains to be answered.

The results obtained from electrophysiological and pharmacological study of the effects of LH-RF on bullfrog sympathetic neurons provide additional support that the peptide may be the mediator of the ls-EPSP. When applied by superfusion or pressure injection close to the ganglion cells, LH-RF produced a slow membrane depolarization associated with an increase in membrane resistance in the majority of neurons studied. In this connection, the ls-EPSP was also found to be associated with a rise in membrane resistance (Katayama and Nishi, 1977; Jan *et al.*, 1979, 1980a). The depolarizing effect of LH-RF persisted in a solution in which Ca^{2+} ions were removed, indicating that this peptide probably acted directly on the postganglionic neurons (Jan *et al.*, 1979). Furthermore, ls-EPSP was partially suppressed during depolarization elicited by LH-RF, and both the ls-EPSP and peptide-mediated depolarization were blocked by a LH-RF analogue, (D-pGlu[1], D-Phe[2], D-Trp[3,6])LH-RF, which was shown in an earlier study to antagonize the action of LH-RF in other tissues (Rivier and Vale, 1978). These results suggest that LH-RF and the transmitter generating the Is-EPSP probably act on the same receptors. It is also of interest to note that LH-RF as well as ls-EPSP may be involved in the modulation of membrane excitability, as during the course of the ls-EPSP as well as during LH-RF-induced depolarization, subthreshold f-EPSP was facilitated, and frequently generated action potentials (Jan *et al.*, 1980a).

The ionic mechanism underlying the LH-RF-induced depolarization as well as the ls-EPSP has not been fully elucidated. As the peptide-induced depolarization and the ls-EPSP were accompanied by an increase of membrane resistance in the majority of neurons, inactivation of G_K may be a plausible mechanism similar to that underlying the action of substance P on myenteric neurons (Katayama *et al.*, 1979). However, Jan *et al.* (1980a) emphasized that the action of LH-RF is probably not due to G_K inactivation alone, as both the response to LH-RF and ls-EPSP were enhanced in high K^+

solution upon conditioning hyperpolarization to the level of E_K. Furthermore, a decrease in membrane resistance has been noticed in some neurons treated with LH-RF (Jan *et al.*, 1980a). In this context, ls-EPSP that was associated with a decrease of membrane resistance has been reported for the bullfrog sympathetic neurons (Nishi and Koketsu, 1968). In this case, the ionic mechanism of ls-EPSP was suggested to result from an increase of G_{Na} and G_K (see Nishi, 1974). Ion-substitution studies will be needed to characterize fully the ionic mechanism of the effect of LH-RF on bullfrog sympathetic neurons, and for its identification as the transmitter generating the ls-EPSP. It is important to emphasize in this context that the ls-EPSP of the bullfrog sympathetic neurons, the mediator for which may be LH-RF, may be analogous to the slow non-cholinergic potential generated possibly by substance P in the inferior mesenteric ganglion cells of the guinea-pig (see above). As both increase and decrease of membrane resistance appear to occur in the case of the slow excitatory potential of both bullfrog and guinea-pig sympathetic neurons, a combined mechanism of G_{Na} activation and G_K inactivation may underlie the response in question (Dun and Minota, 1981).

The G_K inactivation phenomenon may be of particular interest in the case of the bullfrog ganglia, as using the voltage-clamp methods Adams and Brown (1980) demonstrated that LH-RF suppresses selectively a voltage-sensitive K^+ current (M current). The exact function of this voltage-sensitive K^+ current is not entirely clear; it may be associated with spike frequency regulation (Brown and Adams, 1980). Accordingly, the spike discharge associated with the application of LH-RF may be due to its ability to suppress selectively this outward K^+ current. Moreover, there is evidence that muscarine inactivated the voltage-sensitive K^+ current as well (Adams and Brown, 1980). The observation that the s-EPSP which is generated by a muscarinic action of ACh is greatly reduced during the ls-EPSP and during LH-RF-induced depolarization (Jan *et al.*, 1980a) may be explained if an ionic channel is commonly shared by these two substances.

In summary, there is substantial evidence indicating that the peptide LH-RF may be the putative transmitter responsible for the initiation of ls-EPSP in the bullfrog sympathetic ganglion cells (Jan *et al.*, 1979, 1980a). The physiological condition under which the ls-EPSP is initiated, as well as the role of LH-RF-containing fibres in bullfrog ganglia remains to be studied. The question whether or not LH-RF-positive fibres may represent sensory nerve fibres similar to that of substance P-containing fibres in mammalian sympathetic ganglia is also of interest.

ENKEPHALINS

Hughes *et al.* (1975) isolated from pig brain two short-chain pentapeptides with opioid activity which have been termed methionine- and leucine-

Autonomic Ganglia

enkephalin (Met- and Leu-enkephalin, respectively). Enkephalins have been found in varying amounts in effector tissues innervated by the peripheral autonomic nerves, sympathetic ganglia, peripheral nerves, and in chromaffin cells of the adrenal medulla (Hughes *et al.*, 1977; DiGiulio *et al.*, 1978; Schultzberg *et al.*, 1978, 1979). In sympathetic ganglia, the distribution and localization of enkephalin-like immunoreactivity appear to vary with species and, in a given species, from one ganglion to another. Thus, dense networks of enkephalin-positive fibres were observed in inferior mesenteric ganglia of the guinea-pig, while only a few positive fibres could be identified in superior cervical ganglia of the same species (Schultzberg *et al.*, 1979). Furthermore, a few immunoreactive SIF cells were observed in both mesenteric and superior cervical ganglia of the guinea-pig (Schultzberg *et al.*, 1979). Recently, enkephalin-immunoreactivity was observed in some SIF cells of the bullfrog sympathetic ganglia; enkephalins were not detected in principal neurons or in nerve fibres (Kondo and Yui, 1981). It is conceivable, however, that the level of enkephalin immunoreactivity in the latter two elements may have been too low to be detected.

At the present time, the origin of the enkephalin-positive fibres observed in the sympathetic ganglia has not been clearly identified. The finding that the enkephalin immunoreactivity disappeared from the sympathetic ganglia after decentralization (see Schultzberg *et al.*, 1979) suggests that the cell body of enkephalin-positive fibres may be of central origin (see also Dalsgaard and Elfvin, 1979 and page 217 in chapter by Schultzberg *et al.*). In the case of the superior cervical ganglia of the rat, the content of enkephalins was not affected by preganglionic denervation, whereas it was increased following transection of postganglionic fibres (DiGiulio *et al.*, 1978). On the basis of this finding, it was suggested that in the rat superior cervical ganglia enkephalins may be concentrated in the postganglionic neurons whose axons project outside the ganglia. Altogether, there is species difference with respect to the localization and density of enkephalin-like substance in sympathetic ganglia of the rat, guinea-pig and bullfrog. Whether or not this variation may represent a functional significance in the role of enkephalins in ganglionic transmission is not clear.

The effects of Met- and Leu-enkephalins on the guinea-pig coeliac-superior and inferior mesenteric ganglion cells (Konishi *et al.*, 1979a), rabbit and rat superior cervical ganglion cells (Dun and Karczmar, 1981) and guinea-pig myenteric neurons (North *et al.*, 1979) were investigated.

The most conspicuous effect of Met- or Leu-enkephalin when applied to the sympathetic neurons was a depression of the amplitude of fast EPSP (f-EPSP) (Konishi *et al.*, 1979a; Dun and Karczmar, 1981). In the concentrations of 0.05–5 μM, enkephalins reversibly depressed the amplitude of f-EPSP without causing much change of the membrane potential and input resistance in the majority of neurons studied. A slight depolarization or hyperpolarization was observed in a portion of the neurons (Dun and Karczmar, 1981). Met- and Leu-enkephalin were about equally effective in depressing the amplitude of f-EPSP and there was no apparent species difference between rat and rabbit sympathetic ganglia. It should be mentioned that about half of the neurons tested were sensitive to the depressant action of enkephalins (Dun and Karczmar, 1981).

While depressing the amplitude of f-EPSP, enkephalins did not affect appreciably the ACh potential induced by iontophoretic application of ACh onto the same ganglion cells from which the f-EPSP's were elicited (Fig. 5).

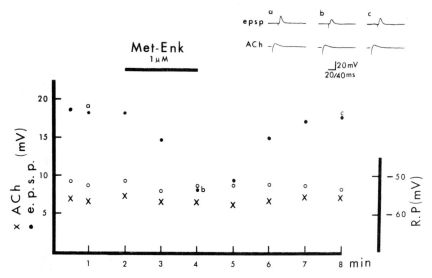

Figure 5 Effects of Met-enkephalin (1 µM) on the resting membrane potential, amplitude of f-EPSP and ACh potential of a single rabbit superior cervical ganglion cell. f-EPSPs were elicited by preganglionic nerve stimulation and ACh potentials were induced by iontophoresis of ACh onto the same ganglion cell. Met-enkephalin was applied to the ganglion cell for a period indicated by the solid bar. The solid and open circles represent the amplitude of f-EPSP and membrane potential, respectively, and X denotes the amplitude of ACh potential. Representative tracings taken from the graph can be seen in the upper right-hand column. Note that Met-enkephalin depressed the amplitude of f-EPSP while not affecting appreciably the membrane potential and ACh potential

The depressant effect of enkephalins was prevented by the opioid antagonists, naloxone and naltrexone (Konishi *et al.*, 1979a; Dun and Karczmar, 1981). The quantal content but not the quantal size of the f-EPSP evoked in a low Ca^{2+} solution was reduced by enkephalins (Konishi *et al.*, 1979a; Simmons *et al.*, 1981). These results taken together suggest that enkephalins may act on specific preganglionic opioid receptors, reducing the evoked release of ACh (Konishi *et al.*, 1979a; Dun and Karczmar, 1981).

In the case of the myenteric neurons of the guinea-pig ileum, Met- and Leu-enkephalin induced membrane hyperpolarization upon bath and iontophoretic application (North *et al.*, 1979). However, when iontophoretic methods were employed, hyperpolarization occurred only when enkephalins were applied away from the soma membrane, i.e. in the vicinity of the cell processes that release ACh (North *et al.*, 1979). As interpreted by North *et al.* (1979) these data suggest that enkephalins depressed ACh release, a finding comparable with the results obtained with the sympathetic neurons. It must be pointed out, however, that the inhibition of neuronal firing induced by enkephalins with respect to both central and peripheral neurons may result not only from presynaptic inhibitory effects of enkephalins, but also from postsynaptic effects that were also demonstrated with regard to myenteric neurons (North and Williams, 1976).

The precise mechanism by means of which enkephalins diminish the transmitter output is not clear. A change of the nerve terminal membrane potential and/or conductance induced by enkephalins would influence the amount of ACh liberated; this mechanism would be compatible with the observation of North *et al.* (1979) of presumably presynaptic hyperpolarizing effect of enkephalins. While the number of cells that exhibited such membrane hyperpolarization was limited (North *et al.*, 1979), a hyperpolarization of the preganglionic nerve terminals was, in fact, demonstrated by means of the sucrose-gap method in the case of the bullfrog sympathetic ganglia (Wouters and van den Bercken, 1980). However, it is difficult to ascertain whether the hyperpolarization recorded by this method occurs at the terminal membrane or somewhere along the distal portion of the axons. Alternatively, enkephalins may operate via a mechanism that does not involve membrane polarity change, namely by interfering with entry of Ca^{2+} ions into the nerve terminals; this possibility is suggested by the finding that the diminution of f-EPSP induced by enkephalins is partially antagonized in high Ca^{2+} (5–10 mM) solution (Simmons *et al.*, 1981). That Ca^{2+} ions may be involved in the action of opiates is indicated by several other studies; for example, the shortening by enkephalins of the plateau phase of the action potential of the cultured dorsal root ganglion cells was compatible with suppression of Ca^{2+} influx (Mudge *et al.*, 1979), and the inhibitory effect of relatively high concentrations of morphine on frog and rat sympathetic ganglionic transmission was partially reversed by elevation of extracellular Ca^{2+} concentrations (Minker *et al.*, 1980).

The results described so far do not demonstrate conclusively that endogenous enkephalins play a role in ganglionic transmission. However, slow ganglionic potentials, i.e. s-IPSP and s-EPSP, generated in the rabbit superior cervical ganglion cells via repetitive preganglionic stimulation, were markedly potentiated by naloxone and naltrexone (Dun and Karczmar, 1981). These results are compatible with the hypothesis that repetitive preganglionic stimulation causes a release of ganglionic enkephalins which, in turn, inhibit the liberation of transmitters responsible for the generation of slow ganglionic potentials; this would explain the facilitatory effect of opiate antagonists as resulting from a disinhibition of the depressant effect of enkephalins on transmitter output (Dun and Karczmar, 1981). On the other hand, the f-EPSP elicited by single preganglionic stimulation was not appreciably affected by opiate antagonists; this suggests that the amount of enkephalins released by a single impulse may be relatively small (Konishi *et al.*, 1979a; Dun and Karczmar, 1981).

Enkephalins appear to be at least 10–100 times more potent than catecholamines in depressing the release of ACh from preganglionic fibres of the sympathetic ganglia (Christ and Nishi, 1971; Dun and Nishi, 1974; Dun and Karczmar, 1977). It was suggested that the depressant effect of catecholamines on ganglionic transmission is primarily presynaptic in nature, and that it reflects the physiological role of these substances in the ganglia (Dun and Nishi, 1974; Dun and Karczmar, 1977; Martinez and Adler-Graschinsky, 1980). As enkephalins are present in sympathetic ganglia and as their action is similar to and more potent than the action of catecholamines, the physiological condition under which the peptides may be released in the autonomic ganglia is of particular interest.

SOMATOSTATIN

Somatostatin or growth hormone-release inhibiting hormone was identified as one of the hypothalamic-adenophypophyseal peptides; somatostatin was found subsequently to be a cyclic peptide consisting of 14 amino acids (Brazeau *et al.*, 1973).

The presence of somatostatin or a closely related peptide in peripheral sympathetic ganglia has been demonstrated (Hökfelt *et al.*, 1977a; Leranth *et al.*, 1980). The pattern of distribution of this peptide in sympathetic ganglia is distinctively different from that of substance P. In the case of somatostatin, the immunoreactivity was found to be localized mainly in the postganglionic neurons; a few SIF cells showed also somatostatin immunoreactivity (Hökfelt *et al.*, 1977a). It is interesting to emphasize that the coexistence of a neuropeptide with a bioamine neurotransmitter in a single neuron was first observed with respect to the presence of somatostatin in the noradrenergic postganglionic neurons of the guinea-pig sympathetic ganglia. Subsequently, this phenomenon was demonstrated with respect to a number of other autonomic and central neurons (see Hökfelt *et al.*, 1980).

The coexistence of somatostatin or like peptide in noradrenergic neurons of the sympathetic ganglia has been confirmed recently by means of the peroxidase–antiperoxidase technique which allows fine-structural visualization (Leranth *et al.*, 1980). It is noteworthy that in both studies somatostatin-positive neurons were found to be more numerous in coeliac-mesenteric ganglia complex than in superior cervical ganglia (Hökfelt *et al.*, 1977a; Leranth *et al.*, 1980). The functional implication of this observation is not clear.

Somatostatin has been shown to exert an inhibitory effect on central neurons (Renaud *et al.*, 1975); also, it inhibited the release of norepinephrine from central (Göthert, 1980) and peripheral (Cohen *et al.*, 1978) noradrenergic neurons, and of ACh from peripheral cholinergic nerve cells (Guillemin, 1976; Furness and Costa, 1979). However, the effect of somatostatin on sympathetic neurons and on the characteristics of ganglionic transmission has not been reported as yet. In this context, application of somatostatin to neurons of the myenteric plexus of the guinea-pig ileum caused no consistent membrane effect; neurons were either hyperpolarized, depolarized or not affected (Katayama and North, 1980). Thus, the physiological significance of the presence of somatostatin in sympathetic ganglia remains to be investigated. The possibility that this peptide may influence the activity of sympathetic neurons via its release from intraganglionic fibres as suggested by Leranth *et al.* (1980) is of particular interest.

OTHER PEPTIDES

The presence of vasoactive intestinal polypeptide (VIP; Hökfelt *et al.*, 1977b), cholecystokinin (CCK; Larsson and Rehfeld, 1979), avian pancreatic polypeptide (APP; Lundberg *et al.*, 1980a) and bombesin (Kondo, personal communication) in sympathetic ganglia has been demonstrated by immunohistochemical methods. Especially dense networks of VIP- and CCK-containing fibres were observed in inferior mesenteric ganglia of the guinea-pig; these fibres may originate in the gastrointestinal tract and may be involved in the reflex modulation of the activity of these ganglia arising upon the stimulation of the mechanoreceptors of the gastrointestinal tract (see Hökfelt *et al.*, 1980).

It is not known at this time whether or not VIP, CCK, APP and bombesin exert effects upon sympathetic neurons and on ganglionic transmission. However, it was shown that VIP and bombesin depolarize myenteric neurons of the guinea-pig (Williams and North, 1980) and spinal motoneurons of the frog (Nicoll, 1978), respectively.

CONCLUSIONS

The demonstration of the presence of a number of peptides in peripheral sympathetic ganglia aroused interest in the exploration of the ganglionic effects and the physiological function in the ganglia of these substances. Evidence is accumulating that peptides may serve as transmitters generating transmitter-specific synaptic potentials and/or as modulators in regulating the membrane excitability and transmitter release in sympathetic ganglia.

The evidence is particularly strong that substance P and LH-RF may mediate the non-cholinergic excitatory potential in guinea-pig inferior mesenteric and bullfrog sympathetic ganglia, respectively (Dun and Karczmar, 1979; Jan *et al.*, 1979; Konishi *et al.*, 1979b). It was also suggested that substance P may be the transmitter generating the slow depolarization in myenteric neurons of the guinea-pig (Katayama and North, 1978; Morita *et al.*, 1980; however, see Grafe *et al.*, 1979).

Peptides may exert a number of excitatory effects on sympathetic neurons and modulating action on ganglionic transmission. Substance P, LH-RF and angiotensin II may modulate ganglionic cell activity directly by enhancing spike discharge frequency (Dun *et al.*, 1978; Adams and Brown, 1980; Brown and Adams, 1980; Brown *et al.*, 1980). In addition, these peptides may facilitate synaptic transmission by converting subthreshold f-EPSP into spike potential (Brown *et al.*, 1980; Jan *et al.*, 1980a; Dun and Karczmar, 1981).

On the contrary, enkephalins exert an inhibitory effect on ganglionic transmission primarily by reducing the transmitter output from preganglionic fibres (Konishi *et al.*, 1979a; Dun and Karczmar, 1981). They seem to exert similar presynaptic effects in the myenteric plexus of the guinea-pig (North *et al.*, 1979). However, their involvement in the postsynaptic inhibition cannot be excluded. The finding that some SIF cells exhibit enkephalin immunoreactivity is of interest (Schultzberg *et al.*, 1979; Kondo and Yui, 1981). In this context it has been suggested that SIF cells are interneurons involved in the generation of the s-IPSP (Libet, 1970, 1979). However, the s-IPSP was not suppressed, rather it was augmented, by opiate antagonists (Dun and Karczmar, 1981). It appears unlikely that enkephalins are involved, via the SIF cells, in the generation of s-IPSP. The physiological function of enkephalins in SIF cells remains to be explored. Another candidate for the transmitter which is released from SIF cells in generating the s-IPSP is dopamine (Libet, 1970, 1979; see however, Dun, 1980). The presence of enkephalins, and possibly serotonin (Dun *et al.*, 1980; Verhofstad *et al.*, 1981), in SIF cells further complicates the issue of whether or not SIF cells are dopaminergic interneurons, and of the generation of s-IPSP (see for instance Dun, 1980; Dun and Karczmar, 1980).

Our present knowledge of the mode of action of peptides in sympathetic ganglia is by no means complete. The action of a number of peptides such as somatostatin, VIP, CCK, APP and bombesin has not been characterized or, indeed, studied, Information on the synthesis, storage, release and inactivation of peptides in sympathetic ganglia is at present not available. More searching questions concern the teleology of these substances. Indeed, what is the advantage in utilizing large, structurally complex molecules to transfer information as compared to utilization, for a similar purpose, of monoamines or other simple molecules? In a similar vein, why should a neuron release more than one transmitter? What additional coding value is contained in this mechanism? Is this value concerned with additional delivery of control and feedback processes?

It is noteworthy that the peptides which are present in the peripheral autonomic ganglia are identical with or closely related to the peptides found in the central nervous system and endocrine cells (see Hökfelt *et al.*, 1980); thus the same peptides are utilized in peripheral, central and endocrine systems and functions. As the anatomical arrangement of the peripheral ganglia is simple compared to that of the central nervous system, and as their physiology and pharmacology are relatively well defined, ganglia provide a unique model in the investigation of the physiological role of peptides in neuronal function and of the mechanisms involved.

Historically, the concept of neurohumoral transmission in vertebrate nervous system evolved from the classical studies of sympathetic ganglia by Langley and his associates (Langley, 1906). It is befitting in this respect that the study of the effect of peptides on sympathetic ganglia may lead to further insight into the complexity and the function of chemical transmission in vertebrate nervous system.

ACKNOWLEDGEMENTS

I thank Dr A. G. Karczmar for helpful comments in preparing the manuscript. Published and unpublished investigations were supported in part by USPHS Grant NS15848.

REFERENCES

Adams, P. R., and Brown, D. A. (1980). Luteinizing hormone-releasing factor and muscarinic agonists act on the same voltage-sensitive K^+-current in bullfrog sympathetic neurones. *Br. J. Pharmacol.*, **68**, 353–355.

Bloom, F. E. (1972). Amino acids and polypeptides in neuronal function. *Neurosci. Res. Prog. Bull.*, **10**, 121–251.

Brazeau, P., Vale, W. W., Burgus, R., Ling, N., Butcher, M., Rivier, J. E., and Guillemin, R. (1973). Hypothalamic polypeptide that inhibits secretion of immuno-reactive pituitary growth hormone. *Science*, **179**, 77–79.

Brown, D. A., and Adams, P. R. (1980). Muscarinic suppression of a novel voltage-sensitive K^+-current in a vertebrate neurone. *Nature*, **283**, 673–676.

Brown, D. A., Constanti, A., and Marsh, S. (1980). Angiotensin mimics the action of muscarinic agonists on rat sympathetic neurones. *Brain Res.*, **193**, 614–619.

Chang, M. M., Leeman, S. E., and Niall, H. D. (1971). Amino-acid sequence of substance P. *Nature*, **232**, 86–87.

Christ, D. D., and Nishi, S. (1971). Site of adrenaline blockade in the superior cervical ganglion of the rabbit. *J. Physiol. (London)*, **213**, 107–117.

Cohen, M. L., Rosing, F., Wiley, K. S., and Slater, I. H. (1978). Somatostatin inhibits adrenergic and cholinergic neurotransmission in smooth muscle. *Life Sci.*, **23**, 1659–1664.

Dalsgaard, C.-J., and Elfvin, L.-G. (1979). Spinal origin of preganglionic fibers projecting into the superior cervical ganglion and inferior mesenteric ganglion of the guinea pig, as demonstrated by the horseradish peroxidase technique. *Brain Res.*, **172**, 139–143.

DiGiulio, A. M., Yang, H. Y. T., Lutold, B., Fratta, W., Hong, J., and Costa, E. (1978). Characterization of enkephalin-like material extracted from sympathetic ganglia. *Neuropharmacology*, **17**, 989–992.

Dun, N. J. (1980). Ganglionic transmission: electrophysiology and pharmacology. *Fed. Proc.*, **39**, 2982–2989.

Dun, N., and Karczmar, A. G. (1977). The presynaptic site of action of norepinephrine in the superior cervical ganglion of guinea pig. *J. Pharmacol. Exp. Ther.*, **200**, 328–335.

Dun, N. J., and Karczmar, A. G. (1979). Actions of substance P on sympathetic neurons. *Neuropharmacology*, **18**, 215–218.

Dun, N. J., and Karczmar, A. G. (1980). A comparative study of the pharmacological properties of the positive potential recorded from the superior cervical ganglia of several species. *J. Pharmacol. Exp. Ther.*, **215**, 455–460.

Dun, N. J., and Karczmar, A. G. (1981). Multiple mechanisms in ganglionic transmission. In *Cholinergic Mechanisms: Phylogenetic Aspects, Central and Peripheral Synapses, and Clinical Significance* (Eds. G. Pepeu and H. Ladinsky), pp. 109–118, Plenum Press, New York.

Dun, N. J., and Minota, S. (1981). Effects of substance P on neurones of the inferior mesenteric ganglia of the guinea-pig. *J. Physiol. (London)*, **321**, 259–271.

Dun, N., and Nishi, S. (1974). Effects of dopamine on the superior cervical ganglion of the rabbit. *J. Physiol. (London)*, **239**, 155–164.

Dun, N. J., Nishi, S., and Karczmar, A. G. (1978). An analysis of the effect of angiotensin II on mammalian ganglion cells. *J. Pharmacol. Exp. Ther.*, **204**, 669–675.

Dun, N. J., Karczmar, A. G., and Ingerson, A. (1980). A neurochemical and neurophysiological study of serotonin in the superior cervical ganglia. *Soc. Neurosci. Abstr.*, **6**, 829.

Elfvin, L.-G., and Dalsgaard, C.-J. (1977). Retrograde axonal transport of horseradish peroxidase in afferent fibers of the inferior mesenteric ganglion of the guinea pig. Identification of the cells of origin in dorsal root ganglia. *Brain Res.*, **126**, 149–153.

Furness, J. B., and Costa, M. (1979). Actions of somatostatin on excitatory and inhibitory nerves in the intestine. *Eur. J. Pharmacol.*, **56**, 69–74.

Gamse, R., Wax, A., Zigmond, R. E., and Leeman, S. E. (1981). Immunoreactive substance P in sympathetic ganglia: distribution and sensitivity towards capsaicin. *Neuroscience*, **6**, 437–441.

Göthert, M. (1980). Somatostatin selectivity inhibits noradrenaline release from hypothalamic neurones. *Nature*, **288**, 86–88.

Grafe, P., Mayer, C. J., and Wood, J. D. (1979). Evidence that substance P does not mediate slow synaptic excitation within the myenteric plexus. *Nature*, **279**, 720–721.

Guillemin, R. (1976). Somatostatin inhibits the release of acetylcholine induced electrically in the myenteric plexus. *Endocrinology*, **99**, 1653–1654.

Hökfelt, T., Kellerth, J. O., Nilsson, G., and Pernow, B. (1975). Substance P: localization in the central nervous system and in some primary sensory neurones. *Science*, **190**, 889–890.

Hökfelt, T., Elfvin, L.-G., Elde, R., Schultzberg, M., Goldstein, M., and Luft, R. (1977a). Occurrence of somatostatin-like immunoreactivity in some peripheral sympathetic noradrenergic neurons. *Proc. Natl. Acad. Sci. U.S.A.*, **74**, 3587–3591.

Hökfelt, T., Elfvin, L.-G., Schultzberg, M., Fuxe, K., Said, S. I., Mutt, V., and Goldstein, M. (1977b). Immunohistochemical evidence of vasoactive intestinal polypeptide-containing neurons and nerve fibers in sympathetic ganglia. *Neuroscience*, **2**, 885–896.

Hökfelt, T., Elfvin, L.-G., Schultzberg, M., Goldstein, M., and Nilsson, G. (1977c). On the occurrence of substance P containing fibers in sympathetic ganglia: Immunohistochemical evidence. *Brain Res.*, **132**, 29–41.

Hökfelt, T., Elde, R., Johansson, O., Ljungdahl, A., Schultzberg, M., Fuxe, K., Goldstein, M., Nilsson, G., Pernow, B., Terenius, L., Ganten, D., Jeffcoate, S. L., Rehfeld, J., and Said, S. I. (1978). Distribution of peptide-containing neurons. In *Psychopharmacology: A Generation of Progress* (Eds. M. A. Lipton, A. DiMascio and K. F. Killam), pp. 39–66, Raven Press, New York.

Hökfelt, T., Johansson, O., Ljungdahl, A., Lundberg, J. M., and Schultzberg, M. (1980). Peptidergic neurones. *Nature*, **284**, 515–521.

Hughes, J., Smith, T. W., Kosterlitz, H. W., Forthergill, L. A., Morgan, B. A., and Morris, H. R. (1975). Identification of two related pentapeptides from the brain with potent opiate agonist activity. *Nature*, **258**, 577–579.

Hughes, J., Kosterlitz, H. W., and Smith, T. W. (1977). The distribution of methionine-enkephalin and leucine–enkephalin in the brain and peripheral tissue. *Br. J. Pharmacol.*, **61**, 639–647

Jan, Y. N., Jan, L. Y., and Kuffler, S. W. (1979). A peptide as a possible transmitter in sympathetic ganglia of the frog. *Proc. Natl. Acad. Sci. U.S.A.*, **76**, 1501–1504.

Jan, Y. N., Jan, L. Y., and Kuffler, S. W. (1980a). Further evidence for peptidergic transmission in sympathetic ganglia. *Proc. Natl. Acad. Sci. U.S.A.*, **77**, 5008–5012.

Jan, L. Y., Jan, Y. N., and Brownfield, M. A. (1980b). Peptidergic transmitters in synaptic boutons of sympathetic ganglia. *Nature*, **288**, 380–382.

Jiang, Z. G., and Dun, N. J. (1981). Multiple conductance change associated with the slow excitatory potential in mammalian sympathetic neurons. *Brain Res.*, **229**, 203–208.

Katayama, Y., and Nishi, S. (1977). The ionic mechanism of late slow epsp in amphibian sympathetic ganglion cells. *Proc. IUPS 27th*, **2**, 371.

Katayama, Y., and North, R. A. (1978). Does substance P mediate slow synaptic excitation within the myenteric plexus? *Nature*, **274**, 387–388.

Katayama, Y., and North, R. A. (1980). The action of somatostatin on neurones of the myenteric plexus of the guinea-pig ileum. *J. Physiol. (London)*, **303**, 315–323.

Katayama, Y., North, R. A., and Williams, J. T. (1979). The action of substance P on neurons of the myenteric plexus of the guinea-pig small intestine. *Proc. R. Soc. London Ser. B*, **206**, 191–208.

Kondo, H., and Yui, R. (1981). Enkephalin-like immunoreactivity in the SIF cells of sympathetic ganglia of frogs. *Biomed. Res.*, **2**, 338–340.

Konishi, S., Tsunoo, A., and Otsuka, M. (1979a). Enkephalins presynaptically inhibit cholinergic transmission in sympathetic ganglia. *Nature*, **282**, 515–516.

Konishi, S., Tsunoo, A., and Otsuka, M. (1979b). Substance P and non-cholinergic excitatory synaptic transmission in guinea pig sympathetic ganglia. *Proc. Jpn. Acad.*, **55**, 525–530.

Krnjević, K. (1974). Chemical nature of synaptic transmission in vertebrates. *Physiol. Rev.*, **54**, 418–540.

Krnjević, K. (1977). Effects of substance P on central neurons in cats. In *Substance P* (Eds. U. S. von Euler and B. Pernow), pp. 217–230, Raven Press, New York.

Kuba, K., and Koketsu, K. (1974). Ionic mechanism of the slow excitatory postsynaptic potentials in bullfrog sympathetic ganglion cells. *Brain Res.*, **81**, 338–342.

Kuba, K., and Koketsu, K. (1976). Analysis of the slow excitatory postsynaptic potential in bullfrog sympathetic ganglion cells. *Jpn. J. Physiol.*, **26**, 651–669.

Kuba, K., and Koketsu, K. (1978). Synaptic events in sympathetic ganglia. *Prog. Neurobiol. (Oxford)*, **11**, 77–169.

Langley, J. H. (1906). Croonian Lecture. On nerve endings and on special excitable substances in cells. *Proc. R. Soc. London Ser. B*, **78**, 170–194.

Larsson, L.-T., and Rehfeld, J. F. (1979). Localization and molecular heterogeneity of cholecystokinin in the central and peripheral nervous system. *Brain Res.*, **165**, 201–218.

Leranth, Cs., Williams, T. H., Jew, J. Y., and Arimura, A. (1980). Immunoelectron microscopic identification of somatostatin in cells and axons of sympathetic ganglia in the guinea pig. *Cell Tissue Res.*, **212**, 83–89.

Libet, B. (1970). Generation of slow inhibitory and excitatory postsynaptic potentials. *Fed. Proc.*, **29**, 1945–1956.

Libet, B. (1979). Slow postsynaptic actions in ganglionic functions. In *Integrative Functions of the Autonomic Nervous System* (Eds. C. McC. Brooks, K. Koizumi and A. Sato), pp. 197–222, University of Tokyo Press, Tokyo.

Lundberg, J. M., Hökfelt, T., Schultzberg, M., Uvnas-Wallensten, K., Kohler, C., and Said, S. I. (1979). Occurrence of vasoactive intestinal polypeptide (VIP)-like immunoreactivity in certain cholinergic neurons of the cat: evidence from combined immunohistochemistry and acetylcholinesterase staining. *Neuroscience*, **4**, 1539–1559

Lundberg, J. M., Hökfelt, T., Anggard, A., Kimmel, J., Goldstein, M., and Markey, K. (1980a). Coexistence of an avian pancreatic polypeptide (APP) immunoreactive substance and catecholamines in some peripheral and central neurons. *Acta Physiol. Scand.*, **110**, 107–109.

Lundberg, J. M., Hökfelt, T., Anggard, A., Uvnas-Wallensten, K., Brimijoin, S., Brodin, E., and Fahrnekrug, J. (1980b). Peripheral peptide neurons: distribution, axonal transport and some aspects on possible function. In *Neural Peptides and Neuronal Communication* (Eds. E. Costa and M. Trabucchi), pp. 25–36, Raven Press, New York.

Martinez, A. E., and Adler-Graschinsky, E. (1980). Release of norepinephrine induced by preganglionic stimulation of the isolated superior cervical ganglion of the cat. *J. Pharmacol. Exp. Ther.*, **212**, 527–532.

Minker, E., Vegh, A., and Osman-Taha, M. H. (1980). Inhibition of synaptic transmission by morphine and its antagonism by Ca^{++} in the isolated sympathetic ganglion of frog and rat. *Acta. Physiol. Acad. Sci. Hung.*, **55**, 379–384.

Minota, S., Dun, N. J., and Karczmar, A. G. (1981). Substance P-induced depolarization in sympathetic neurons: not simple K^+-inactivation. *Brain Res.*, **216**, 224–228.

Morita, K., North, R. A., and Katayama, Y. (1980). Evidence that substance P is a neurotransmitter in myenteric plexus. *Nature*, **287**, 151–152.

Mudge, A. W., Leeman, S. E., and Fischbach, G. D. (1979). Enkephalin inhibits release of substance P from sensory neurons in culture and decreases action potential duration. *Proc. Natl. Acad. Sci. U.S.A.*, **76**, 526–530.

Neild, T. O. (1978). Slowly-developing depolarization of neurones in the guinea-pig inferior mesenteric ganglion following repetitive stimulation of the preganglionic nerves. *Brain Res.*, **140**, 231–239.

Nicoll, R. A. (1976). Promising peptides. *Neurosci. Symp.*, **1**, 99–122.

Nicoll, R. A. (1978). The action of thyrotropin-releasing hormone, substance P and related peptides on frog spinal mononeurones. *J. Pharmacol. Exp. Ther.*, **207**, 817–824.

Nishi, S. (1974). Ganglionic transmission. In *The Peripheral Nervous System* (Ed. J. I. Hubbard), pp. 225–255, Plenum Press, New York.

Nishi, S., and Koketsu, K. (1968). Early and late afterdischarges of amphibian sympathetic ganglion cells. *J. Neurophysiol.*, **31**, 109–121.

North, R. A., and Williams, J. T. (1976). Enkephalin inhibits firing of myenteric neurones. *Nature*, **264**, 460–461.

North, R. A., Katayama, Y., and Williams, J. T. (1979). On the mechanism and site of action of enkephalin on single myenteric neurons. *Brain Res.*, **165**, 67–77.

Otsuka, M., and Konishi, S. (1977). Electrophysiological and neurochemical evidence for substance P as a transmitter of primary sensory neurones. In *Substance P* (Eds. U. S. von Euler and B. Pernow), pp. 207–214, Raven Press, New York.

Renaud, L. P., Martin, J. B., and Brazeau, P. (1975). Depressant action of TRH, LH–RH and somatostatin on activity of central neurones. *Nature*, **255**, 233–235.

Rivier, J. E., and Vale, W. W. (1978). (D-pGlu^1, D-Phe^2, D-Trp^{3,6})-LH-RH. A potent luteinizing hormone releasing factor antagonist *in vitro* and inhibitor of ovulation in the rat. *Life Sci.*, **23**, 869–876.

Robinson, S. E., Schwartz, J. P., and Costa, E. (1980). Substance P in the superior cervical ganglion and the submaxillary gland of the rat. *Brain Res.*, **182**, 11–17.

Schally, A. V., Arimura, A., and Kastin, A. J. (1973). Hypothalamic regulatory hormones. *Science*, **179**, 341–250.

Schultzberg, M., Lundberg, J. M., Hökfelt, T., Terenius, L., Brandt, J., Elde, R. P., and Goldstein, M. (1978). Enkephalin-like immunoreactivity in gland cells and nerve terminals of the adrenal medulla. *Neuroscience*, **3**, 1169–1186.

Schultzberg, M., Hökfelt, T., Terenius, L., Elfvin, L.-G., Lundberg, J. M., Brandt, J., Elde, R. P., and Goldstein, M. (1979). Enkephalin immunoreactive nerve fibres and cell bodies in sympathetic ganglia of the guinea-pig and rat. *Neuroscience*, **4**, 249–270.

Simmons, M. A., Jiang, Z. G., and Dun, N. J. (1981). Enkephalins and transmission in mammalian sympathetic ganglion cells. *Soc. Neurosci. Abstr.*, **7**, 185.11.

Verhofstad, A. A. J., Steinbusch, H. W. M., Penke, B., Varga, J., and Joosten, H. W. J. (1981). Serotonin-immunoreactive cells in the superior cervical ganglion of the rat. Evidence for the existence of separate serotonin- and catecholamine-containing small ganglionic cells. *Brain Res.*, **212**, 39–49.

von Euler, U. S., and Gaddum, J. H. (1931). An unidentified depressor substance in certain tissue extracts. *J. Physiol. (London)*, **72**, 74–87.

Williams, J. T., and North, R. A. (1979). Vasoactive intestinal polypeptide excites neurones of the myenteric plexus. *Brain Res.*, **175**, 174–177.

Wouters, W., and van den Bercken, J. (1980). Effects of met-enkephalin on slow synaptic inhibition in frog sympathetic ganglion. *Neuropharmacology*, **19**, 237–243.

Neurophysiology of Parasympathetic and Enteric Ganglia

J. D. WOOD

Department of Physiology, School of Medicine,
University of Nevada, Reno, Nevada 89557, USA

INTRODUCTION

This chapter's aim is to review the neurophysiology of parasympathetic and enteric ganglia. According to Langley's (1921) classic concept, the sympathetic, parasympathetic and enteric nervous systems comprise three divisions of the autonomic nervous system. Parasympathetic and enteric ganglia are situated in close proximity to their effector systems, both receive information from the central nervous system by way of cranial or pelvic neural pathways and information is transmitted by nicotinic-cholinergic synapses in both. Aside from these similarities, there are sufficient dissimilarities between enteric ganglia and parasympathetic ganglia to justify classification of enteric ganglia as a third subdivision of the autonomic nervous system. The major distinction is that parasympathetic ganglia of autonomic effector systems other than the gut function to relay and distribute commands from the central nervous system to the effector; whereas the enteric system is an integrative network that can control gastrointestinal effector systems independent of input from the brain and spinal cord. The enteric nervous system is a 'little brain' within the gastrointestinal tract and as such has many neurophysiological, neurochemical and structural properties that are commonly found in the central nervous system, but not in other autonomic ganglia. The parasympathetic and enteric ganglia, for this reason, will be compared as distinct subdivisions in the following account.

ENTERIC GANGLIA

Enteric ganglia are partitioned anatomically into the myenteric plexus and the submucosal plexus by the circular muscle coat of the gastrointestinal wall. Information is transferred over neural connections between the two plexuses, and although they are spatially separated, the ganglia of the two plexuses no doubt function together as a unit. Small ganglia that fit the classical description of parasympathetic ganglia are present on the serosal surface of the distal colon and rectum (Langley and Anderson, 1895). These ganglia function mainly as relay-distribution centres and do not show the variety of complex synaptic interactions that occur in the intramural ganglia of the gut (de Groat and Krier, 1976).

Similarities with central nervous systems

The neurobiological properties of enteric ganglia in many respects resemble central nervous system of both vertebrate and invertebrate animals. Enteric ganglia are similar to mammalian central nervous system in structural organization, neurochemistry, immunoreactivity of proteins, ontogeny, exchange of materials with blood-vascular system and integrative function of the neural circuits.

Enteric ganglia, unlike other autonomic ganglia, have compact organization of neural and glial elements, absence of collagen and paucity of extracellular space, all of which are common structural characteristics of the brain (Gabella, 1972). The enteric glial elements structurally resemble astroglia of the brain (Cook and Burnstock, 1976b; Gabella, 1971), and fibrillary acidic protein is immunologically specific for central nervous system astrocytes and enteric glial cells (Jessen and Mirsky 1980).

A dense synaptic neuropil exists within both enteric ganglia and central nervous systems. This is significant because in all integrative nervous systems, most of the information processing occurs in microcircuits within a synaptic neuropil. Axoaxonal and axodendritic synapses occur in the enteric neuropil and at least eight morphologically distinct types of axonal terminals can be seen in the neuropil (Cook and Burnstock, 1976a). Synapses occur also on enteric ganglion cell somas where three morphological types of axon endings can be distinguished ultrastructurally (Gabella, 1972).

Most putative neurotransmitters within the brain have been implicated as neurotransmitters in enteric ganglia. Furness and Costa (1979) reviewed the evidence for enteric transmitter function of acetylcholine, norepinephrine, dopamine, 5-hydroxytryptamine, purine nucleotides and an array of peptides that include substance P, somatostatin, vasoactive intestinal peptide, enkephalin and neurotensin. This suggests that the enteric nervous system uses as diverse an array of messenger molecules for transfer of information as the brain.

Enteric ganglion cells are derived from the neural plate of the embryonic ectoderm, and neurons with specific transmitter substances develop in a sequence that parallels development of some transmitter-specific neurons in the brain. Enteric cholinergic, serotonergic and intrinsic inhibitory neurons appear first during ontogeny and are followed by development of the adrenergic innervation. Peptidergic neurons are last to development (Gershon *et al.*, 1979).

Blood vessels do not enter enteric ganglia, and a blood–ganglion barrier analogous to the blood–brain barrier is interposed between the blood vasculature and the synaptic circuits of the ganglia (Gershon and Bursztajn, 1978). The blood–ganglion barrier has been demonstrated only for macromolecules and appears to be determined by properties of the capillary endothelium. It differs from the blood–brain barrier in this respect, but nevertheless represents another distinction of the enteric nervous system.

Many studies beginning with those of Trendelenburg (1917) have provided evidence that the neural circuitry of the enteric nervous system performs integrative function analogous to that of central nervous system. For example, the musculature of segments of intestine *in vitro* generates peristaltic patterns of intestinal motility (Brann and Wood, 1976; Frigo and Lecchini, 1970). Contractile activity continues, but the peristaltic propulsion is abolished both after blockade of enteric ganglion cells with tetrodotoxin (Frigo and Lecchini, 1970) and in segments of intestine from which enteric ganglia are congenitally absent (Brann and Wood, 1976). This indicates that neural control of the coordinated motor activity is dependent upon intact integrative circuitry within the enteric ganglia, and that this neural function is independent of input from the central nervous system. Relatively normal function of the gastrointestinal tract after vagotomy or sympathectomy is likewise indicative of the independence of enteric nervous function.

Enteric ganglia, unlike other autonomic ganglia, possess the full complement of constituents that characterize an integrative nervous system. They have sensory elements, interneurons and motor neurons. The sensory elements generate information on parameters such as the mechanical state of the gut wall or chemical composition of chyme. The internuncial integrative circuitry processes the sensory information and generates organized excitatory and inhibitory outflow in motor neurons to the musculature in much the same way that the internuncial circuitry of the central nervous system organizes motor outflow during somatomotor reflexes.

Spontaneous activity in enteric neurons

Enteric ganglion cells, unlike most autonomic neurons, are spontaneously active in isolated preparations without central nervous system input. Spontaneous activity is reflected by ongoing release of neurotransmitters (Paton *et al.*, 1971), by changes in contractile activity of the gastrointestinal musculature when the neural activity is blocked with drugs (Wood, 1972) and by ongoing spike discharge detected by extracellular and intracellular electrical recording (Wood, 1975, 1981). Spontaneous electrical activity consists of excitatory and inhibitory synaptic potentials (Wood and Mayer, 1978) and burst and single-spike patterns of action potential discharge.

Burst-type spike activity, as recorded with extracellular microelectrodes, occurs in two distinctive patterns that have been referred to as steady and erratic patterns (Wood, 1975). The steady bursters discharge bursts of spikes with relatively low statistical variance of the interburst interval; and when large variance of interburst interval does occur, it is as a distinct multiple of the shortest interburst interval (Wood and Mayer, 1973). The timing of the bursts seems to be determined by an oscillatory pacemaker mechanism analogous to the parabolic burster of the marine mollusc *Aplysia* (Strumwasser, 1967), rather than a synaptic mechanism, because blockade of synaptic transmission with elevated Mg^{2+} does not alter the discharge pattern (Wood, 1975; Kachalov, 1980).

The discharge patterns of erratic bursters are distinguished by irregular interburst intervals and periodic conversion to continuous spikes or spike doublets (Wood, 1973). The discharge of the erratic bursters appears to be dependent upon synaptic mechanisms because both the ongoing discharge and spike bursts evoked by electrical stimulation are blocked by elevated Mg^{2+} (Wood, 1975; Athey *et al.*, 1981). The discharge of the erratic bursters may be driven by synaptic input from the steady bursters. The identity of the transmitter substance that activates the erratic bursters is unknown. Several putative transmitter substances and synaptic blocking drugs have been tested and found not to affect stimulus-evoked spike bursts (Athey *et al.*, 1981). Nicotinic or muscarinic cholinergic receptor antagonists sometimes halt the ongoing discharge of the erratic bursters and acetylcholine and nicotine sometimes increase their discharge (Wood, 1970; Ohkawa and Prosser, 1972; Sato *et al.*, 1973; Kachalov *et al.*, 1978). These results suggest that cholinergic receptors may be present on the erratic bursters; however, the ongoing discharge seems to be driven by another uncommon transmitter substance.

The erratic burst-like discharge originates at sites distal to the cell soma and electrotonically invades the soma where it can be recorded intracellularly (Wood and Mayer, 1978). The bursts of electrotonic potentials that can be recorded in the cell body are probably dendritic spikes that are triggered by synaptic input within the ganglionic neuropil. Intracellular recording has not detected a counterpart of the extracellularly recorded steady burster; although it would be expected, if the steady bursters are indeed endogenous oscillators, that intracellular recording would detect neurons with rhythmic oscillations of membrane potential. Rhythmic oscillations sometimes occur in myenteric neurons (below), but the periods of those oscillations are much longer than the interburst intervals of the steady bursters. It could be that the intracellular method does not detect the steady bursters either because the somas are small and never impaled or because the oscillatory region of the neuron is remote from the cell soma.

Single-spike patterns of spontaneous activity can be recorded both extracellularly and intracellularly in enteric ganglia. This activity usually occurs at relatively low frequencies with no consistent pattern to the interspike intervals. The extracellularly recorded activity is sometimes altered but never blocked by elevated Mg^{2+}, indicating that it is independent of synaptic input. The noteworthy characteristic of these cells is that they are sensitive to nicotinic-cholinergic agonists; a property that is reminiscent of classic parasympathetic postganglionic neurons (Wood, 1975). Intracellular studies show that the single spikes are associated with ramp-like prepotentials or with nicotinic-cholinergic excitatory postsynaptic potentials (EPSPs). Intracellular recording also reveals low-frequency discharge of single spikes that reflects a tonic release of 5-hydroxytryptamine within myenteric ganglia. Continuous electrical stimulation of the interganglionic fibre tracts at low frequencies (0.5 Hz) elicits sustained discharge of single spikes in these cells (Wood and Mayer, 1978), and application of methysergide, which blocks postsynaptic receptors for serotonin (Wood and Mayer, 1979b), or norepinephrine, which prevents release of serotonin (Wood and Mayer, 1979c), stops the ongoing discharge. Intracellularly recorded single spikes occur also in neurons that do not receive serotonergic input. The intracellular observations indicate that the extracellularly recorded single-spike activity arises from a heterogeneous population of enteric neurons.

Another kind of spontaneous activity consists of slow sinusoidal-like oscillations of transmembrane voltage, which occur in less than 2% of the neurons impaled in the myenteric plexes of guinea-pig small intestine (Fig. 1).

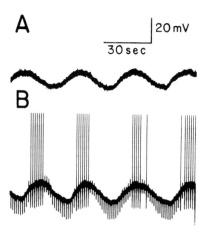

Figure 1 Electrical slow waves in a myenteric neuron of guinea-pig small intestine. (A) Intracellular recording of slow oscillatory potentials. (B) Intrasomatic injection of constant-current hyperpolarizing pulses reveals a progressive increase in the input resistance during the hyperpolarizing phase of the slow wave and progressive decrease in input resistance during the depolarizing phase of the slow wave. Action potentials at the offset of the hyperpolarizing pulse occur at the crest of the slow waves and reflect increased excitability at the crest of the wave

These waves have amplitudes of 10–15 mV and frequencies of about 2 per minute at 37 °C. The hyperpolarizing phase of the slow waves is associated with a progressive increase in input resistance and input resistance progressively decreases during the depolarizing phase. The excitability of the cell, as reflected by spike discharge evoked by intracellular current injection, is greatest at the crest of the slow wave. The slow waves occur between membrane potentials of −50 and −65 mV and disappear when the membrane is hyperpolarized beyond −65 mV.

Membrane properties of enteric neurons

Membrane potential, resistance and time constant   Membrane potentials of enteric ganglion cells range from −35 to −85 mV, input resistance is between 10 and 185 megaohms and membrane time constants range from 2 to 12 msec. Several factors influence these parameters and account for the wide variability in reported values. Use of high-resistance microelectrodes to study the cells and difficulties in balance of amplifier bridge circuits contribute to imprecise measurements. The different types of enteric neurons have different membrane properties and this increases the variability when expressed for enteric neurons as a single group. Another source of variability is change of the membrane properties with time. It is common during impalements of 6–8 hours to observe significant changes in membrane potential, input resistance and time constant. This seems to reflect periodic release of neuromodulator substances that change ionic conductance of the membrane because the changes are reversed by synapse-blocking drugs such as methysergide or by prevention of neurotransmitter release in the presence of elevated magnesium.

The ionic mechanism for the resting membrane potential of enteric ganglion cells is related to potassium conductance (G_K) as indicated by variations in the membrane potential that are predicted by the constant-field equation when the extracellular potassium concentration is altered (Grafe *et al.*, 1980). The membrane potential of enteric neurons is usually less than the potassium equilibrium potential (E_K). In the AH/type 2 neurons described below, a component of the resting G_K and consequently the resting potential seem to be dependent upon continuous influx of calcium and upon the level of free intracellular calcium (Grafe *et al.*, 1980). These membrane properties contribute to mechanisms for long-term modulation of neuronal excitability that involve action of neuromodulatory substances on calcium-dependent G_K. The significance of a membrane potential less than E_K is that it provides for modulation in either the hyperpolarizing or depolarizing direction depending upon whether the neuromodulator increases or decreases G_K.

Enteric neuronal classification

Four categories of enteric neurons are found in the guinea-pig small intestine. The neurons are classified as S/type 1, AH/type 2, type 3 or type 4 based on intracellularly recorded electrical behaviour of the cell body. This terminology is an arbitrary combination of terms used by the investigators who first reported on these neurons (Holman *et al.*, 1972; Nishi and North, 1973).

S/Type 1 neurons   These cells are distinguished by: (1) a low resting membrane potential relative to the other cell types; (2) high input resistance relative to the other cell types; (3) discharge of spikes during membrane depolarization that increases in frequency as a direct function of the amount of depolarization; (4) anodal-break excitation at the offset of intracellularly injected hyperpolarizing current pulses; (5) no hyperpolarizing after-potentials; and (6) tetrodotoxin-sensitive somal spikes.

AH/Type 2 neurons   Distinguishing characteristics of AH/type 2 cells are: (1) high resting membrane potential and low input resistance relative to S/type 1 neurons; (2) discharge of one or two spikes only at the onset of intracellular injection of prolonged depolarizing current pulses; (3) no anodal-break excitation; (4) long-duration postspike hyperpolarizing potentials; (5) tetrodotoxin-resistant action potentials; (6) membrane de-polarization and increased input resistance in the presence of calcium-channel blockers such as magnesium and manganese.

Type 3 neurons   These cells have high resting potentials and low input resistance similar to AH/type 2 neurons, but they do not discharge spikes to intracellularly injected depolarizing current pulses. They show prominent nicotinic-cholinergic EPSPs that never trigger spikes. Unlike AH/type 2 cells, elevated magnesium or manganese do not affect the cell.

Type 4 neurons   This cell type resembles AH/type 2 and type 3 neurons in having high resting membrane potentials ($> -65\,mV$) and low input resist-ance (<40 megaohms). Neither synaptic potentials nor somal action poten-tials can be evoked in these cells immediately after impalement. Earlier they were thought to be glial cells (Nishi and North, 1973); however, intracellular injection of dyes reveals these cells as neurons. These initially inexcitable cell bodies often begin to behave like AH/type 2 neurons 20–30 min after impalement (Hodgkiss and Lees, 1978) or after treatment with calcium antagonists (Grafe *et al.*, 1980).

When large numbers of preparations are tallied, all four neuronal types are impaled with about equal frequency in the cat and guinea-pig small intestinal myenteric plexus (Wood and Mayer, 1978; Wood, 1981); whereas S/type 1 neurons predominate in the guinea-pig submucosal plexus (Hirst and McKirdy, 1975). The situation differs for individual myenteric preparations where a preponderance of one or the other of the cell types is usually found.

Postspike hyperpolarizing potentials

Hyperpolarizing after-potentials (AH) are characteristic of AH/type 2 neurons. They begin from 45 to 80 msec after the spike and last for periods up to 20 sec (Wood and Mayer, 1978). The amplitude of the AH summates when more than one spike is discharged during the time course of the AH, and the input resistance of the cell is reduced during the AH. The AH reflects a postspike increase in calcium-dependent potassium conductance (Hirst and Spence, 1973; North, 1973). An inward calcium current during the rising phase of the somal action potential appears to increase intracellular calcium which leads to increased G_K. The functional significance of the AH relates to a decreased safety factor and decreased probability of repetitive spike discharge by the cell soma.

Topographic heterogeneity

Several lines of evidence suggest that the multipolar myenteric ganglion cells might be multifunctional integrative units with specialized kinds of integrative functions occurring at different topographic regions of the same neuron. This is like some of the complexly branched invertebrate ganglion cells where spikes with different characteristics can originate independently at multiple sites such as the cell body, the axon hillock, a neurite between axon hillock and axon branch point, or the dendrites. The mollusc, *Aplysia*, has sensorimotor neurons consisting of sensory and motor processes emanating from a single cell body (Coggeshall, 1971).

Topographic heterogeneity in myenteric neurons is suggested by distinct differences in the membrane properties of the cell soma and its attached processes. The processes of AH/type 2 neurons are readily excitable by electrical stimulation when the somal membrane of the cell is relatively inexcitable. Differences between the soma and its processes are reflected also by the presence of tetrodotoxin-insensitive, calcium spikes in the soma and classical tetrodotoxin-sensitive, sodium spikes in the processes (North, 1973). Another indication of multiple sites of spike initiation is the spontaneous occurrence of patterned bursts of electrotonic spike potentials in the cell soma which reflects spike activity originating at sites remote from the soma (Wood and Mayer, 1978). Topographical differences in excitability between the soma and initial segments of its processes can often be demonstrated by intrasomatic injection of depolarizing current that fires the initial segment, but not

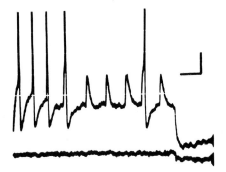

Figure 2 Differential excitability between the cell soma and one of its neurites in a myenteric neuron of guinea-pig small intestine. Intrasomatic injection of a depolarizing current pulse fired the soma and the neurite; however, the neurite fired more often (low-amplitude electrotonic potentials) than the soma, indicating that the neurite was more excitable than the soma. Vertical calibration 10 mV; horizontal calibration 25 msec

the soma (Fig. 2). The low safety factor for spike discharge in the soma functions to isolate the initial segments of each process so that action potential discharge by one initial segment does not influence spike activity of another at an opposite pole of the soma. If independent excitatory synaptic input occurred at the initial segments, as is indicated by ultrastructural and electrophysiological studies, this would permit independent spike initiation in each of the cell processes. Independence of the cell processes might be of functional significance in terms of neural economy in that one ganglion cell could function as several separate neurons depending on the number of processes. The isolation of the processes by low excitability of the soma represents one of two different functional states of the neuron; in a second functional state, increased excitability of the cell body allows synchronous discharge of all of the processes of the multipolar cell. Later discussion will show how slow synaptic excitation of the cell soma provides for synchronization of the processes by the soma.

Relationships between electrophysiology and morphology

Dogiel (1899) described three morphological types of enteric ganglion cells. Type I cells had short club-shaped processes and one long slender process that exited the ganglion in an interganglionic fibre tract. Type II cells had many long smooth processes several of which exited the ganglion in interganglionic connectives. Type III cells were multipolar with processes of intermediate length that terminated in the same ganglion or projected to adjacent ganglia. Two groups of workers have attempted to associate morphology of enteric neurons with electrophysiological characteristics by intracellular injection of dye from the recording electrode (Hodgkiss and Lees, 1980; Erde *et al.*, 1980). This method reveals characteristic Dogiel morphology; however, association between electrophysiological and morphological types has been impossible. Electrophysiological characteristics of S/type 1 neurons may occur in any of the Dogiel cell types; whereas, ganglion cells with AH/type 2, type 3 or type 4 electrophysiological behaviour are usually Dogiel type II or type III cells. These studies have not yielded useful information for improving the presently inadequate schemes of classification of enteric ganglion cells.

Enteric sensory receptors

Enteric ganglia, unlike other autonomic ganglia, contain sensory elements that generate information for processing by integrative circuitry within the synaptic network of the ganglia. This was first recognized when Trendelenburg (1917) demonstrated the peristaltic reflex in segments of intestine without central nervous input *in vitro*.

Extracellular recording from single units within the myenteric plexus reveals neural elements that respond with an increased rate of discharge to mechanical distortion of the ganglion, and behave like mechanoreceptors (Wood, 1970; Mayer and Wood, 1975; North and Williams, 1977; Yokoyama and Osaki, 1978). One kind of mechanosensitive unit behaves like a slowly adapting mechanoreceptor in that sustained spike discharge without signs of adaptation occurs during a constant intensity stimulus, and the frequency of discharge is directly related to the stimulus intensity. A second kind of unit with properties of a fast-adapting mechanoreceptor responds to mechanical stimulation with an intensity-dependent discharge at the onset of the stimulus and quickly stops firing during a sustained stimulus. The generator regions of these units appear to be within the periganglionic connective tissue.

The discharge patterns of the fast- and slowly adapting mechanosensitive neurons, when recorded at the ganglion, resemble patterns of discharge recorded in gastrointestinal afferent fibres in the vagus (Iggo, 1957; Davison, 1972) and splanchnic nerves (Ranieri *et al.*, 1973). The general assumption is that the sensory elements of the gut are processes of cell bodies in the dorsal root or vagal sensory ganglia; nevertheless, results obtained by Dr Erzsébet Fehér (personal communication) with horseradish peroxidase (HRP) tracing techniques indicate that some centrally directed afferent fibres in intestinal mesenteric nerves arise from cell bodies in the myenteric plexus. Horseradish peroxidase reaction product appears in cell somas of multipolar ganglion cells (Dogiel type II or III) in myenteric ganglia after HRP is applied to the mesenteric nerves and sufficient time allowed for retrograde transport of the HRP in the centrally directed fibres. This result is consistent with the view expressed above on topographical and functional heterogeneity of the processes of multipolar neurons in the myenteric plexus. The sensory elements in the intestine have not been identified morphologically, and it can be questioned whether the terminals of some of the processes that arise from the multipolar ganglion cells might be the sensory elements. With this kind of organization the same sensory receptor could provide information to both the enteric integrative circuitry and the central nervous system.

Synaptic transmission in enteric ganglia

Transfer of information within the enteric plexuses occurs at axosomatic, axoaxonal and axodendritic synapses. The latter two contribute to synaptic circuitry in a neuropil with microcircuitry for information processing and neural pattern generation that is unlike autonomic ganglia elsewhere in the body. Microcircuitry in the neuropil is derived in part from processes of enteric interneurons. The term interneuron is used with reservation here because neither interneurons, sensory neurons nor motor neurons have been unequivocally identified by electrophysiological techniques in the enteric nervous system, as they have been in the central nervous system. The possibility exists that the enteric ganglion cells are not functionally unique; it could be that somal isolation of functionally different nerve fibres nourished by the same cell body confers functional heterogenity to the multipolar neurons (refer to above section on topographic heterogeneity). Nevertheless, all existing information on enteric synaptic mechanisms obtained by intracellular recording methods is restricted to the cell soma. No electrophysiological information on synaptic mechanisms exists for the neuropil, although this aspect of ganglionic function probably exceeds axosomatic mechanisms in functional importance.

All of the electrophysiological information on neurochemical transmission that follows below was obtained from the guinea-pig and cat small intestine. Results from these two species show that both fast synaptic potentials with durations of less than 50 msec and slow synaptic potentials lasting several seconds can be recorded in cell bodies of enteric ganglion cells. These synaptic events may be excitatory postsynaptic potentials (EPSPs) or inhibitory postsynaptic potentials (IPSPs), and they can be evoked experimentally by electrical stimulation of presynaptic fibres or they may occur spontaneously. Presynaptic inhibitory mechanisms are operative at both the fast and slow synaptic junctions.

Neurotransmitter substances

Table 1 lists the substances that are putative neurotransmitters in enteric ganglia. The list has rapidly expanded from addition of a large number of peptide neurotransmitters in recent years. This reflects the rapid development and increased popularity of immunocytochemical techniques for

Table 1 Putative neurotransmitter or neuromodulatory substances in the enteric
nervous system

Acetylcholine	Neurotensin
Angiotension	Norepinephrine
Bombesin	Prostaglandins
Cholecystokinin	Purine nucleotides
Dopamine	Secretin
Enkephalins	Serotonin
γ-Aminobutyric acid	Somatostatin
Gastrin	Substance P
Glycine	Thyrotropin releasing hormone
Histamine	Vasoactive intestinal peptide
Motilin	

intracellular localization of peptides and an often unjustified tendency to ascribe messenger function to a substance solely on the basis of its presence in nerve cells. The advances in the immunocytochemistry of the enteric nervous system (see chapter by Llewellyn-Smith *et al.*) have surged far ahead of the electrophysiological studies that are required to establish firmly neurotransmitter function for these substances. In spite of this, it is clear that the electrophysiological studies do not show a sufficient variety of synaptic potentials to allow for a neurotransmitter role for all of the putative transmitter substances; unless of course, some of these substances function at synapses in the neuropil that have been inaccessible to electrical recording.

Some of the putative neurotransmitter substances evoke membrane potential changes in enteric neurons, but cannot be confirmed to function as transmitters because no synaptic input to the cell that mimics the action of the substance can be demonstrated. This is the case for γ-aminobutyric acid (GABA). GABA is present in enteric neurons (Jessen *et al.*, 1979), and it produces picrotoxin-sensitive depolarization of myenteric neurons (Grafe *et al.*, 1979a); however, no picrotoxin-sensitive synaptic potentials can be evoked in the cells that are affected by exogenous GABA. The functional significance of extrasynaptic receptors like these is unknown in this system.

Acetylcholine, norepinephrine and 5-hydroxytryptamine (5-HT) are the substances that meet most of the necessary criteria for neurotransmitter function at synapses in enteric ganglia. A transmitter function for most of the enteric peptides is not yet supported by firm electrophysiological evidence, and the temptation to exaggerate their roles as neurotransmitters at enteric synapses without adequate supporting evidence should be avoided.

The order of appearance of acetylcholine and 5-HT in the fetal development of the intestine is consistent with a key neurotransmitter role for these substances in the integrative circuitry of the enteric ganglia; whereas the development of some of the putative peptide transmitters is not consistent with a major role for these substances (reviewed by Gershon *et al.*, 1979).

Cholinergic and serotonerric neurons develop first, and this coincides with the earliest indication of neural control in intestinal motor activity. Noradrenergic sympathetic fibres appear next in the developing gut while the putative peptidergic transmitters do not appear until after birth—long after maturation of the cholinergic, serotonergic and noradrenergic synaptic mechanisms.

Serotonin-binding protein is an example of an immunoreactive substance that appears in enteric neurons, but does not function as a neurotransmitter. It is packaged in synaptic vesicles with 5-HT, and is released with 5-HT by a calcium-dependent and tetrodotoxin-sensitive process (Jonakait *et al.*, 1979). Serotonin-binding protein probably functions to reduce the number of osmotically active particles within the synaptic vesicles and permits 5-HT to be concentrated without osmotic swelling of the vesicle. It should be considered that this might be the functional significance of some of the other peptides that are detected by immunocytochemistry in enteric ganglion cells.

Fast EPSPs

Fast EPSPs (f-EPSPs) occur in both myenteric and submucosal ganglion cells (Nishi and North, 1973; Hirst *et al.*, 1974; Hirst and McKirdy, 1975; Wood, 1981). They occur in S/type 1, AH/type 2 and type 3 ganglion cells. f-EPSPs usually have smaller amplitudes in AH/type 2 neurons than in the other neuronal types (Grafe *et al.*, 1979b). This reflects synaptic input to a region of the cell distal to the recording site in the cell body and a short space constant associated with low membrane resistance of AH/type 2 neurons. The membrane resistance also determines the membrane time constant and time course of decay of the f-EPSP which is variable in some ganglion cells because of sporadic intraganglionic release of neuromodulatory substances that produce long-term changes in membrane resistance. Multiple fast synaptic inputs converge on the enteric ganglion cells and both spatial and temporal summation of the synaptic potentials occur.

All of the f-EPSPs in enteric ganglion cells of the small intestine appear to be mediated by nicotinic-cholinergic receptors. Iontophoretic application of acetylcholine mimics the EPSPs, acetylcholine esterase inhibitors prolong them and nicotinic-blocking drugs such as hexamethonium and *d*-tubocurarine reduce or abolish the EPSPs. The ionic mechanisms of the cholinergic f-EPSPs has not been investigated in enteric ganglia.

The amplitude of f-EPSPs is often progressively decreased when they are evoked repetitively by electrical stimulation applied to the ganglion surface. The rundown in amplitude occurs at stimulus frequencies as low as 0.1 Hz, and the rate of rundown is a direct function of stimulus frequency. This phenomenon is probably a reflection of presynaptic inhibition of acetylcholine release by additional transmitter substances released within the ganglion by the electrical stimulation. It cannot be explained by a postsynaptic mechanism because no rundown occurs during repetitive iontophoretic applications of acetylcholine. A presynaptic mechanism is suggested by observations that the rate of rundown is often directly related to the strength of stimulation, and sometimes rundown does not occur if the stimulus strength is reduced to the threshold for just evoking the EPSP.

Fast IPSPs

Relatively short-duration hyperpolarizing potentials occur spontaneously and can be evoked by electrical stimulation in myenteric neurons (Wood and Mayer, 1978). These putative IPSPs summate in amplitude during repetitive stimulation. They reverse polarity at membrane potentials greater than $-90\,mV$, and they are associated with a decrease in the cell's input resistance. The spontaneously occurring IPSPs are similar to the hyperpolarizing potentials that are induced by caffeine in hamster submandibular ganglia (Suzuki and Kusano, 1978). The identity of the neurotransmitter and the ionic mechanism for the f-IPSP are unknown.

Slow synaptic excitation

Electrical stimulation of the ganglion surface or of the interganglionic fibre tracts of the myenteric plexus evokes a slowly rising depolarization (slow EPSP) that lasts for a minute or more after termination of the stimulation (Fig. 3). The slow EPSP (s-EPSP) occurs in AH/type 2 neurons, and it is characterized by increased input resistance and augmented excitability of the somal membrane. The augmented excitability has the following characteristics: (1) the neuron sometimes discharges a prolonged train of action potentials which continues for several seconds after termination of the stimulus; (2) intrasomatic injection of a depolarizing current pulse elicits repetitive spike discharge throughout the current pulse in cells that discharge only a single spike to the same current pulse in the absence of the EPSP; (3) electrotonic spike potentials that invade the soma from its processes, trigger somal action potentials (Fig. 4); (4) the characteristic postspike hyperpolarizing potentials of AH/type 2 neurons are greatly reduced or abolished (Grafe *et al.*, 1980).

The transmitter for the s-EPSP appears to be 5-HT. The myenteric neurons contain 5-HT (Tafuri and Raick, 1964; Gershon *et al.*, 1977), and the enzymatic pathways for synthesis of 5-HT from the precursor tryptophan are present in the neurons (Dreyfus *et al.*, 1977a). Release of H^3-labeled 5-HT and its binding protein occurs during transmural electrical stimulation of intestinal segments *in vitro*, and this release is blocked by tetrodotoxin (Jonakait *et al.*, 1979). Tetrodotoxin-sensitive release of endogenous neuronal stores of 5-HT can also be evoked by electrical field stimulation (M. D. Gershon, personal communication). Microiontophoretic application of 5-HT to the AH/type 2 neurons mimics the stimulus-evoked s-EPSP (Wood and Mayer, 1979b). Both the transmitter substance and 5-HT produce membrane depolarization, both increase the input resistance of the neuron, both reduce or abolish the postpike hyperpolarizing potentials, and oth augment membrane excitability. During tachyphylaxis to excess 5-HT in the bathing solution or in the presence of methysergide, the stimulus-evoked s-EPSP is blocked. The blocking action of methysergide is at the postsynaptic receptors, rather than presynaptic prevention of transmitter release, because methysergide quickly aborts a s-EPSP that is in progress; whereas agents that act presynaptically to block the s-EPSP do not abort an ongoing EPSP but do prevent the stimulus-evoked response (Wood and Mayer, 1979c). Myenteric neurons have a high-affinity uptake mechanism for 5-HT that could accomplish termination of action of the transmitter at the postsynaptic membranes (Dreyfus *et al.*, 1977b). In short, 5-HT satisfies all criteria for establishing a substance as the transmitter for a synaptic event.

An important objection to 5-HT as the transmitter for the s-EPSP is that application of some other putative neurotransmitter substances also depolarizes and increases the input resistance of myenteric ganglion cells. Both substance P (Fig. 3) and histamine (C. J. Mayer, personal communication) act this way. Although substance P has been proposed as the transmitter for the s-EPSP (Katayama and North, 1978; Morita *et al.*, 1980), its action does not resemble the action of the endogenous transmitter as closely as does 5-HT. The following observations of the action of substance P are inconsistent with it being the transmitter for the s-EPSP: (1) substance P application does not always mimic the s-EPSP (Fig. 3); (2) substance P does not reduce the postspike hyperpolarizing potentials in AH/type 2 cells as does both the transmitter for the s-EPSP and 5-HT (Katayama *et al.*, 1979); (3) methysergide blocks both the s-EPSP and the action of 5-HT, but does not affect the action of substance P (Grafe *et al.*, 1979); (4) the s-EPSP can be evoked after desensitization to substance P; (5) substance P effects are not specific for AH/type 2 neurons.

The mechanism for slow synaptic excitation in the AH/type 2 neurons appears to be a synaptically mediated decrease in the resting membrane conductance for potassium ions that is reflected by depolarization of the membrane potential and increase in the input resistance of the cell. The reversal potential has been reported by Grafe *et al.* (1980) to be between -70 and $-75\,\text{mV}$ and by Johnson *et al.* (1980) to be greater than $-90\,\text{mV}$. These values are near the potassium equilibrium potential. Neither alteration of extracellular chloride nor intracellular injection of chloride ions alters the s-EPSP.

The high resting potassium conductance (G_K) in the AH/type 2 neurons is

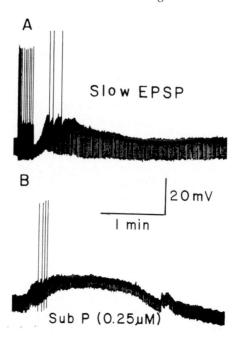

Figure 3 Comparison of the s-EPSP and the action of substance P on a myenteric neuron of guinea-pig intestine. (A) Intracellular recording of stimulus-evoked s-EPSP. Action potentials were evoked by the train of stimulus pulses that precedes the EPSP. (B) Action of substance P added to the superfusion solution of the same neuron. Constant-current hyperpolarizing pulses were injected continuously into the cell. Note that the electrotonic potentials evoked by the current pulses increase during the s-EPSP but decrease during the depolarization produced by substance P, indicating that the input resistance increased during the s-EPSP, and was decreased by substance P

calcium-dependent, and both the transmitter for the s-EPSP and 5-HT appear to decrease resting G_K by decreasing the level of free intracellular calcium. Accumulated evidence obtained mainly from invertebrate ganglion cells indicates that the resting permeability of some neuronal membranes for potassium is a direct function of the concentration of free calcium in the cytoplasm (Meech, 1974; Connor, 1979). Resting G_K in AH/type 2 neurons appears also to be calcium-dependent because application of di- and trivalent cations (e.g. manganese, magnesium and lanthanum) that impede transmembrane movement of calcium and block calcium-dependent neuronal processes mimicks the stimulus-evoked s-EPSP and the action of 5-HT (Grafte *et al.*, 1980). The characteristics common to both the s-EPSP and the effects of calcium-antagonistic ions are: (1) depolarization of the membrane potential; (2) increased input resistance; (3) augmented excitability; (4) reduction or blockade of postspike hyperpolarizing potentials; (5) reversal potential between -70 and $-75\,\mathrm{mV}$. The relationship between external potassium concentration and the membrane potential of these neurons is best described by the constant-field equation. Comparison of this relationship in the presence and absence of calcium antagonistic ions indicates that resting potassium permeability is decreased by about 50% in the presence of the calcium antagonists (Grafe *et al.*, 1980), and can account for the depolarization and increased input resistance of the cell when calcium influx is reduced.

The organic calcium antagonists verapamil and D-600, which reduce transmembrane calcium fluxes in cardiac and smooth muscle cells, do not affect the calcium-dependent potassium conductance in myenteric neurons.

The somas of AH/type 2 neurons function between extremes of low and high excitability. The low excitability state is related to high resting membrane conductance for potassium that is dependent on availability of cytoplasmic calcium. The probability of action potential occurrence in this state is low; if a spike does occur, additional calcium enters the cell during the rising phase of the spike and further activates G_K. This in turn produces hyperpolarizing after-spike potentials that restrict repetitive spike discharge. Conversion to high excitability occurs when the chemical transmitter for the s-EPSP reduces the level of free intracellular calcium with concomitant decrease in resting G_K and reduces postspike hyperpolarization by preventing calcium entry during the action potential.

The functional significance of the s-EPSP is three-fold. First, is an increased probability of spike discharge in the AH/type 2 neuron that is transformed into excitation or inhibition at either the next order neuron or at an effector. Intestinal peristalsis, for instance, requires sustained discharge by some type of enteric neuron in order to account for the delays of several seconds between stimulus and coordinated responses and to account for sustained neural influence at the effector. Behaviour of the neuron during the s-EPSP fits the requirements for a neuronal unit whose functional significance would be production of either prolonged excitation or inhibition at neuronal or neuroeffector junctions within the intestinal wall.

The second functional aspect of the s-EPSP is a neuromodulatory function by which other synaptic inputs to the cell are altered. The increased membrane resistance and augmented excitability of the cell body during the s-EPSP increases the probability that a f-EPSP will trigger an action potential in the neuron.

The third functional aspect of the s-EPSP and the combined behaviour of the cell soma of AH/type 2 neurons is that a mechanism is provided by which the soma of the multipolar neuron can control the spread of excitation between the processes that arise from opposite poles of the soma (Fig. 4). Intracellular recording from the soma shows that electrical stimulation of the cell's processes elicits spikes that electrotonically invade the somal mem-

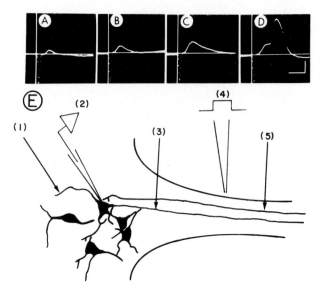

Figure 4 Functional significance of the s-EPSP in a multipolar myenteric neuron (A–D). Intracellular recordings of progressive changes in electrotonic potentials within the soma during repetitive stimulation of the fibre tract. Shocks were applied to the fibre tract at a frequency of 1 Hz, and A–D represent the 1st, 5th, 8th, and 10th stimuli, respectively. Note that the amplitude of the electrotonic potentials increased and the rate of decay increased as the s-EPSP developed with consecutive stimulus pulses. In D, spike threshold was reached and the soma fired a spike. (E) Diagram of the experiment. An intracellular electrode (2) recorded electrotonic changes within the soma. Fibre tract stimulation (4) activated both the cell's process (3) and presynaptic fibres to the soma (5). The somal membrane had low resistance due to high resting G_K, and spikes from the cell's process produced only small electronic potentials in the soma (A). During repetitive stimulation of the presynaptic fibre (5), the s-EPSP and associated increase in resistance and time constant of the somal membrane were reflected by increased amplitude and rate of decay of the electrotonic potentials (B, C). These observations suggest that the soma functions as a gate which permits transmission of spike information from processes at one pole of the soma (1) to processes at opposite poles (3) only during the s-EPSP. The presynaptic fibres for the s-EPSP projected from an adjacent ganglion, and the process of the AH/type 2 neuron projected to the adjacent ganglion, thereby establishing bidirectional flow of information between the two ganglia. Electrical records were plotted from computer memory. The initial downward deflection is the stimulus artifact. Vertical calibration 20 mV; horizontal calibration 2 msec

brane, and also that spontaneously occurring spike patterns in the processes spread electrotonically into the soma (Wood and Mayer, 1978; Wood and Mayer, 1979a). The probability that the passive current flow from these axonal or dendritic spikes will trigger a somal action potential is low in the absence of the s-EPSP and is increased during the augmented excitability of the s-EPSP.

Consequently, the spike activity associated with information processing in the synaptic neuropil is restricted to single processes of the cell in the absence of the s-EPSP; whereas, during the s-EPSP, the soma would relay spike information in one process to all other neurites arising from other poles of the soma. If the neurons were multiaxonal (this is unknown), discharge of all axons would be synchronized during the s-EPSP. The increased probability of passive current spread from axonal or dendritic spikes triggering a somal spike during the s-EPSP may be the mechanism that underlies transfer of information between adjacent ganglia within the neural plexus. The simultaneous occurrence of both the s-EPSP and an electrotonic or initial segment spike in the soma of the neurons during electrical stimulation of an interganglionic connective indicates that the neuron from which the recording is made sends one of its processes in the connective to the adjacent ganglion and in turn receives slow synaptic input from an axon projecting into the same connective from an adjacent ganglion (Fig. 4). This connectivity would enable a neuron (neuron A) in one ganglion to activate the soma of a second neuron (neuron B) in another ganglion to switch ongoing spike activity in the dendrites of neuron B to its axon which projects in the interganglionic connective to the ganglion containing neuron A. This suggests that the specialized properties of the AH/type 2 neurons and their synaptic input provide a mechanism whereby the integrative circuitry of one ganglion can control the information input it receives from an adjacent ganglion. This could be basic to the regulation of spread of neural information within the plexus.

Slow synaptic inhibition

Electrical field stimulation evokes s-IPSPs in about 30% of the submucosal ganglion cells of the small intestine (Hirst and McKirdy, 1975). These are slowly developing hyperpolarizing potentials that persist for 1–5 sec after termination of the stimulus. They occur in S/type 1 neurons, and are generated by a single synaptic input on the cell. Single input may not be an appropriate term for the slow modulatory potentials in enteric neurons because *en passant* release of transmitter from several synaptic varicosities of a single axon could be the case. The stimulus threshold for evoking the s-IPSP is higher than the threshold for eliciting f-EPSPs in the same neurons. A decrease in the input resistance of the cell occurs during the s-IPSP. The reversal potential for the s-IPSP is about $-86\,\text{mV}$, suggesting that the decrease in input resistance might be accounted for by a transmitter-induced increase in potassium conductance.

The putative neurotransmitter substance for the s-IPSP is a catecholamine (Hirst and Silinsky, 1975). Iontophoretic application of both norepinephrine and dopamine mimics the stimulus-evoked IPSP. Guanethidine blocks the IPSP, while propranolol does not affect the action of norepinephrine. Since methysergide does not block mammalian adrenergic receptors, Hirst and Silinsky (1975) suggested that the submucosal ganglion cells behave like molluscan neurons where methysergide blocks the inhibitory action of dopamine. The neurotransmitter for the s-IPSP must be released from neurons intrinsic to the enteric nervous system, because the s-IPSP still occurs after degeneration of sympathetic postganglionic fibres in the intestine. There is no evidence that the cell body of the neuron that releases the inhibitory transmitter is located in the submucous plexus; it could be in the myenteric plexus and have projections to the submucosal plexus. There is evidence that amine-accumulating neurons are located within myenteric ganglia (Gershon and Altman, 1971), but no intrinsic neurons contain tyrosine hydroxylase or dopamine β-hydroxylase (Furness *et al.*, 1979) suggesting that intrinsic enteric ganglion cells cannot synthesize the putative catecholaminergic transmitter for the submucosal s-IPSP.

Repetitive electrical simulation of the ganglionic surface also evokes a slowly developing hyperpolarization of the membrane of some AH/type 2 myenteric neurons (Johnson *et al.*, 1980). These potential changes are associated with a decrease in the input resistance, and they reverse polarity at membrane potentials more negative than -97 mV. The synaptic basis for these effects is uncertain. Opioid peptides, somatostatin, 5-HT, and norepinephrine are putative neurotransmitters that hyperpolarize and reduce the input resistance of some myenteric neurons. The stimulus-evoked hyperpolarizing responses are unaffected by naloxone and therefore probably are not mediated by opioid peptides. The hyperpolarizing action of norepinephrine probably reflects shut-off of the ongoing release of the neurotransmitter for the s-EPSP (Wood and Mayer, 1979c). Tonic release of the transmitter, which is probably 5-HT, maintains the AH/type 2 neurons of some preparations in a partially depolarized state with increased membrane resistance due to some degree of potassium inactivation, and norepinephrine reverses this by preventing the release of the transmitter (see section on presynaptic inhibition). An initial action of elevated magnesium or manganese also is a reduction in input resistance and hyperpolarization presumably produced by reduction of ongoing transmitter release (Hirst *et al.*, 1974); whereas methysergide reduces input resistance and hyperpolarizes the cell by blocking the receptors for the tonically released transmitter (Wood and Mayer, 1979b). The hyperpolarizing action of exogenous 5-HT (Johnson *et al.*, 1980) may reflect the desensitization phenomenon that occurs when these postsynaptic receptors are 'flooded' with artificially applied transmitter substances. Desensitization and blockade of the s-EPSPs by exogenous 5-HT occurs within 1–2 min at concentrations as low as 0.1 μM (Wood and Mayer, 1979b).

Presynaptic inhibition

Presynaptic inhibition within myenteric ganglia acts to prevent the release of acetylcholine and 5-HT from axonal terminals. These are axoaxonal synapses (Manber and Gershon, 1979) that function to inactivate the excitatory synaptic circuitry that mediates intestinal motor function. This is basic to the mechanism of sympathetic nervous shutdown of intestinal function.

Application of norepinephrine or electrical stimulation of sympathetic postganglionic neurons in the intestinal mesentery blocks the cholinergic f-EPSPs that are evoked by electrical stimulation, but does not affect the depolarizing response of the neuron to iontophoretically applied acetylcholine (Nishi and North, 1973; Hirst and McKirdy, 1974). Likewise, norepinephrine blocks the stimulus-evoked s-EPSP, but does not affect the action of exogenously applied 5-HT (Wood and Mayer, 1979c). Norepinephrine also prevents the release of 5-HT from isolated intestinal segments that is evoked by electrical field stimulation (Jonakait *et al.*, 1979). These findings indicate that norepinephrine acts at adrenergic receptors on the cholinergic and serotonergic nerve terminals to prevent release of the respective transmitter substances. The action of norepinephrine is prevented by α-adrenergic blocking drugs, suggesting that the presynaptic receptors are α-receptors.

Application of 5-HT to myenteric ganglia reduces the amplitude of stimulus-evoked f-EPSPs, but does not affect the depolarizing response of the neuron to iontophoretically applied acetylcholine (North *et al.*, 1980). This suggests a presynaptic action of 5-HT; however, the significance of the effect is uncertain, because it does not always occur and when it is observed it is much weaker than the effect of norepinephrine (Fig. 5). Methysergide reduces the f-EPSP amplitude by about the same amount as 5-HT. It might be that this effect of methysergide and 5-HT reflects a non-specific reduction in calcium influx at the axon terminal.

PARASYMPATHETIC GANGLIA

Introduction

Intracellular electrophysiological studies on mammalian parasympathetic ganglia have been reported for the ganglia associated with the urinary bladder (Booth and de Groat, 1979; Griffith *et al.*, 1980), submandibular ganglia that control salivary secretion (Suzuki and Sakada, 1972; Lichtman, 1977; Suzuki and Kusano, 1978; Suzuki and Volle, 1979) and the ciliary ganglion involved with pupillary miosis (Melnichenko and Skok, 1970). Most of these studies were done on ganglia *in vitro* because of technical difficulties of impaling the neurons with microelectrodes *in situ*. The work of Suzuki and Kusano (1978) is exceptional in that they compared the electrophysiological properties of

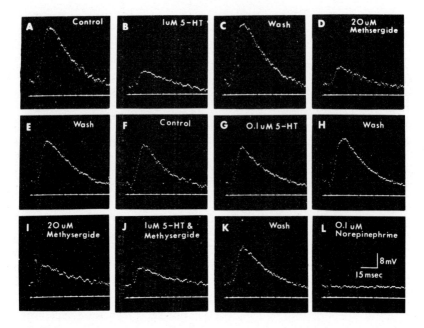

Figure 5 Comparison of action of 5-HT and norepinephrine on f-EPSPs in a myenteric neuron of guinea-pig small intestine. (A). Control EPSPs. (B) Reduction in amplitude of EPSPs by 1 μM 5-HT. (C) Recovery of amplitude after washout of 5-HT. (D) Reduction in amplitude of EPSPs by the 5-HT antagonist, methysergide. (E) After washout of methysergide. (F) Control for 0.1 μM 5-HT. (G) Small reduction of EPSP amplitude in 0.1 μM 5-HT. (H) After 5-HT washout. (I) Reduction of EPSP amplitude by methysergide. (J) Effect of 5-HT added in the presence of methysergide. (K) After washout of 5-HT and methysergide. (L) Abolition of the EPSPs by 0.1 μM norepinephrine. Records are computer averages of 10 or 12 EPSPs evoked at 2-sec intervals. Records were made in sequence from the same neuron. Drugs were added to the superfusion solution

hamster submandibular cells *in vitro* and *in vivo*. The results are encouraging for investigators who work with ganglion cells *in vitro*, because the properties of the cells do not seem to change in the *in vitro* situation.

Electrophysiological findings in parasympathetic ganglia indicate that the neurophysiology is more complex than simple nicotinic-cholinergic relay and divergence of preganglionic information to autonomic effector systems. The transfer function of these ganglia is no doubt specialized for compatibility with the effector system they control, and it is evident that this specialization is associated with heterogeneous synaptic interactions and with electrophysiological properties that are suggestive of integrative and modulatory functions within the ganglia. The emergent concept is that broad flexibility for the transfer of information from the central nervous system to autonomic effectors is incorporated within the neural circuits of both enteric and parasympathetic ganglia.

Spontaneous activity in parasympathetic ganglion cells

Of the three kinds of parasympathetic ganglia that have been studied with intracellular microelectrodes, only the urinary bladder neurons show persistent ongoing spike discharge (Griffith *et al.*, 1980; de Groat *et al.*, 1979). The spontaneous discharge occurs with various degrees of regularity at 0.5–14 Hz, and sometimes appears in bursts; although there is no patterned regularity to the bursts as in enteric neurons. Ramp-like prepotentials, suggestive of pacemaker potentials, precede the spikes. The discharge frequency is a direct function of the degree of depolarization produced by intrasomatic current injection and discharge stops when the cells are sufficiently hyperpolarized. Spontaneous discharge is an intrinsic property of the cell because it continues after synaptic blockade in elevated magnesium–zero calcium solutions. Only neurons that discharge spikes throughout prolonged depolarizing current pulses (see section on membrane properties below) show spontaneous spike discharge.

Spontaneously occurring hyperpolarizing potentials occur in submandibular ganglion cells (Suzuki and Kusano, 1978) and in the cardiac ganglion of *Necturus* (Hartzell *et al.*, 1977). These potentials reflect periodic increases in calcium-dependent G_K and are similar to the spontaneous IPSPs that occur in myenteric neurons (Wood and Mayer, 1978). However, they are not synaptic potentials in submandibular ganglion cells because they are unaffected by tetrodotoxin and can be induced with caffeine in calcium-free extracellular solutions. As in the case of AH/type 2 enteric neurons, a component of G_K appears to be a function of the free intracellular calcium in submandibular neurons, and the G_K-related fluctuations in membrane potential reflect alterations in intracellular calcium homeostasis.

Membrane properties of parasympathetic ganglion cells

The resting membrane potentials of submandibular ganglion cells and ganglion cells of the urinary bladder are similar in mean value and in the range of potentials encountered when large numbers of neurons are sampled. The mean resting potential and the range for bladder neurons are −51.7 mV and 40–73 mV (Griffith *et al.*, 1980), and for the salivary neurons the mean and range are −53 mV and 40–70 mV (Suzuki and Kusano, 1978). Mean input resistance in bladder neurons is 36 megaohms (range 9–85) and for salivary neurons mean input resistance is 40 megaohms (range 10–90). The low membrane potentials in some of those ganglion cells and in some enteric neurons appears to represent a functional state of the cell rather than being due to injury. Application of caffeine or calcium ionophores hyperpolarizes some of these neurons, suggesting that low membrane potentials and relatively high input resistances reflect some degree of inactivation of resting calcium-dependent G_K.

Three types of neurons can be distinguished on the basis of the nature of spike discharge evoked by intrasomatic injection of depolarizing current pulses in bladder ganglion cells (Griffith *et al.*, 1980). One type gives spike discharge throughout the depolarizing current pulses, and the discharge frequency is a direct function of the amount of depolarization. The second type fires a single spike only at the onset of depolarizing current pulses and comprises 6% of the sampled cells. Spike discharge cannot be evoked in the third type of cell, which has resting potentials greater than $-75\,mV$ and is either a neuron with an electrically inexcitable soma or a glial cell. Submandibular ganglion cells usually discharge a single spike only at the onset of depolarizing current pulses.

Hyperpolarizing after-potentials are associated with the spikes in all of these ganglion cells. The after-potentials summate and are prolonged when spikes are evoked repetitively; however, their durations are less than 1 sec, which is much shorter than the hyperpolarizing after-potentials in AH/type 2 enteric neurons. The ionic mechanism for the postspike hyperpolarization is an increase in calcium-dependent G_K that is triggered by influx of calcium during the rising phase of the action potential (Suzuki and Kusano, 1978), and is the same as the mechanism for postspike hyperpolarization in AH/type 2 enteric neurons. The functional significance of this mechanism in all of the neurons is to restrict the frequency of spike discharge.

Synaptic transmission in parasympathetic ganglia

Transfer of information within parasympathetic ganglia seems to be specialized for compatibility with the physiology of the effector system with which the ganglia are associated, and this is reflected in the specific characteristics of synaptic transmission in the ganglia that will be discussed below. Morphological studies indicate that axosomatic, axoaxonal and axodendritic synapses are present in the ganglia; although there is much variability between different ganglia and between the same ganglia in different species with respect to the length of dendrites, synaptic structure, etc. (see review by Gabella, 1976). This is an important consideration for understanding the synaptic circuitry of these ganglia because intracellular microelectrode studies of synaptic transmission have been limited to axosomatic synapses or axoaxonal synapses that are located on the axon hillock very near to the soma.

Intrasomatic recording from both urinary bladder ganglia and submandibular ganglia show fast and slow synaptic potentials. The fast potentials are excitatory. The slow potentials may be excitatory or inhibitory. Presynaptic inhibitory mechanisms appear to be present in bladder ganglia.

f-EPSPs in parasympathetic ganglia

Fast transmission between preganglionic and postganglionic parasympathetic neurons is mediated by nicotinic-cholinergic receptors in all ganglia; however, the behaviour of the nicotinic synapses is not the same in all of the ganglia. f-EPSPs with a high safety factor for evoking spikes occur in submandibular ganglia (Suzuki and Volle, 1979), ciliary ganglia (Melnichenko and Skok, 1970) and also in frog cardiac ganglia (Dennis *et al.*, 1971). Bladder ganglia, in contrast, show a low safety factor for spike initiation when the spike frequency in the preganglionic fibre is below 0.5 Hz and a high safety factor when the preganglionic spike frequency is sustained between 1 and 20 Hz (Booth and de Groat, 1979). This synaptic behaviour imparts a switching function to the ganglia that seems to be of adaptive significance in the normal physiology of the urinary bladder (de Groat, 1980). The 'high pass' property of the synapses prevents activation of the bladder muscle by random low-frequency activity in the preganglionic fibres during bladder filling, and it effectively 'opens the gate' for transmission of excitatory impulses to the bladder muscle when preganglionic firing is sustained at high frequency during the micturition reflex. This ganglionic gating property is accounted for by temporal facilitation of the amplitude of the f-EPSP that results from increased release of acetylcholine from the presynaptic terminals when they are activated repetitively.

s-EPSPs and s-IPSPs in parasympathetic ganglia

Stimulus-evoked s-EPSPs and s-IPSPs with durations as long as 20 sec can be recorded in bladder ganglion cells after nicotinic receptor blockade (Griffith *et al.*, 1981). These responses are mimicked by microiontophoretic application of muscarinic-cholinergic agonists, and are blocked by atropine. Although small intensely fluorescent (SIF) (catecholaminergic) neurons (Libet, 1970) are present in the ganglia, it is unlikely that the slow synaptic potentials are mediated by an interneuron because iontophoretic application of acetylcholine still mimics the s-EPSP and s-IPSP after synaptic blockade in elevated magnesium–low calcium solutions. Hartzell *et al.* (1977) reported s-IPSPs that were also mediated by muscarinic receptors in cardiac ganglion cells of *Necturus*. Suzuki and Kusano (1978) reported s-IPSPs in submandibular ganglion cells. The ionic mechanisms of the slow synaptic potentials in bladder ganglion cells have not been determined. The s-IPSP in amphibian cardiac ganglion cells is mediated by a conductance increase for potassium (Hartzell *et al.*, 1977). s-IPSPs in submandibular ganglia can be accounted for by a transmitter-induced increase in calcium-dependent G_K (Suzuki and Kusano, 1978). If the stimulus-evoked hyperpolarizing potentials in submandibular ganglia are indeed synaptic potentials, the nature of the postsynaptic receptors is uncertain. The muscarinic agonists, bethanechol and acetyl-β-methylcholine, either depolarize or hyperpolarize the submandibular ganglion cells and both of the potential changes are associated with an increase in input resistance (Suzuki and Volle, 1979). This argues against a muscarinic synaptic mechanism that increases G_K. Relatively large concentrations of the muscarinic agonists (25 μM to 1 mM) were required for these effects, which nevertheless were blocked by atropine.

Some responses evoked in parasympathetic ganglion cells by electrical stimulation of preganglionic fibres are biphasic, consisting of a depolarizing phase followed by hyperpolarization. Care in interpretation of such responses should be used because the hyperpolarizing phase is sometimes not due specifically to the action of the transmitter. These hyperpolarizing potentials are sometimes due to delayed rectification involving an increase in G_K that follows depolarizations produced by injection of a brief current pulse or short iontophoretic applications of acetylcholine (Dennis *et al.*, 1971).

The functional significance of the slow synaptic potentials in the parasympathetic ganglion cells, as in enteric ganglion cells, seems to be a neuromodulatory action that shifts the level of neuronal excitability both to alter the responsiveness to convergent inputs carried by other presynaptic channels and to modulate ongoing spike discharge that is intrinsic to the cell. This can be demonstrated in bladder ganglia where the frequency of spontaneous spike discharge is increased during the s-EISP and decreased during the s-IPSP (Griffith *et al.*, 1981).

Presynaptic inhibition

The only parasympathetic ganglia where there is evidence for presynaptic modulation of transmitter release is in the urinary bladder ganglia, and this evidence is equivocal. Ganglion cells containing catecholamines are present in these ganglia (Hamberger *et al.*, 1965), and either intra-arterial administration of catecholamines or electrical stimulation of the hypogastric nerves activates α-adrenoceptors that depress transmission through the vesical ganglia (de Groat and Saum, 1972). In addition, norepinephrine or dopamine depresses the amplitudes of f-EPSPs evoked by electrical stimulation of parasympathetic preganglionic inputs to the bladder ganglion cells (de Groat and Booth, 1980). On the other hand, large concentrations of catecholamines two or three orders greater than the concentrations required to depress the f-EPSP in enteric neurons are required to suppress the bladder EPSPs; and, unlike myenteric neurons, catecholamines have direct actions on the electrical activity of bladder neurons that are inconsistently reported by the two laboratories that have recorded intracellularly from these cells (cf. de Groat and Booth, 1980; Griffith *et al.*, 1979, 1981). Evidence that the response of the postsynaptic neurons to iontophoretic application of acetylcholine is unchanged when the stimulus-evoked f-EPSPs are suppressed by exogenous catecholamines or hypogastric nerve stimulation is lacking; however, this is needed to support the proposal of de Groat and Booth (1980) that presynaptic α-adrenoceptors have functional significance in modulation of transmission through the bladder ganglia.

CHALLENGES AND FRONTIERS

The neurobiology of enteric and parasympathetic ganglia is a relatively unexplored area of neuroscience. As such, it offers many investigative challenges and opportunities for advancement of basic knowledge of integrative function in neural networks of small ensembles of neurons outside the central nervous system, as well as improved understanding of nervous control of autonomic effector systems.

The enteric nervous system has many properties in common with the central nervous system. It is an independent integrative system with information-processing circuitry interposed between sensory receptors and motor neurons to gastrointestinal effector systems. Sparse knowledge of sensory mechanisms in the enteric system presents a major investigative challenge; not even the identity of the sensory elements is known. Precisely timed patterns of spike discharge of unknown functional significance are generated by poorly understood mechanisms within the enteric neural circuitry and represent another challenge for future research. Enteric ganglion cells and perhaps parasympathetic neurons are functionally heterogeneous with specialized kinds of integrative functions localized at topographically distinct regions of the same neuron. Developmental mechanisms of membrane heterogeneity in the individual neurons and the development of synaptic relationships within the ganglia is another fertile area for further study. Calcium-dependent potassium conductance in the membranes of both enteric and parasympathetic ganglion cells are basic to mechanisms involved in modulation of excitability of these neurons. Repetitive spike discharge in some of these neuronal somas is controlled by hyperpolarizing after-potentials that reflect an increase in potassium conductance that is activated by influx of calcium during the action potential. Neurotransmitter substances modulate neuronal excitability by preventing calcium influx during the action potential and also by decreasing calcium-dependent potassium conductance of the resting membrane. Although calcium-dependent changes in potassium conductance are the key to modulation of excitability of the ganglion cell membrane, little is known about mechanisms of intraneuronal calcium homeostasis or about the calcium channels and receptor mechanisms involved in synaptic modulation of calcium-dependent potassium conductance. Presynaptic receptors as well as fast and slow inhibitory and excitatory postsynaptic events that involve a diverse array of neurotransmitter substances occur within enteric ganglia. About two dozen putative neurotransmitters, over half of which are neuropeptides, are present within the enteric ganglion cells. Neurotransmitter function is not unequivocally established for any of these neuropeptides in enteric or parasympathetic ganglia. The functional significance of the great diversity of immunocytochemically demonstrable neuropeptides is enigmatic and another challenging research frontier.

REFERENCES

Athey, G. R., Cooke, A. R., and Wood, J. D. (1981). Synaptic activation of enteric burst-type myenteric neurons in cat small intestine. *Am. J. Physiol.*, **240**, G437–441.

Booth, A. M., and de Groat, W. C. (1979). A study of facilitation in vesical parasympathetic ganglia of the cat using intracellular recording techniques. *Brain Res.*, **169**, 388–392.

Brann, L., and Wood, J. D. (1976). Motility of the large intestine of piebald-lethal mice. *Am. J. Dig. Dis.*, **21**, 633–640.

Coggeshall, R. E. (1971). A possible sensory-motor neuron in *Aplysia californica*. *Tissue Cell*, **3**, 637–648.

Connor, J. A. (1979). Calcium current in molluscan neurones: measurement under conditions which maximize its visibility. *J. Physiol. (London)*, **286**, 41–60.

Cook, R. D., and Burnstock, G. (1976a). The ultrastructure of Auerbach's plexus in the guinea pig, I. Neuronal elements. *J. Neurocytol.*, **5**, 171–194.

Cook, R. D., and Burnstock, G. (1976b). The ultrastructure of Auerbach's plexus in the guinea pig. II. Non-neuronal elements. *J. Neurocytol.*, **5**, 195–206.

Davison, J. S. (1972). Response of single vagal afferent fibers to mechanical and chemical stimulation of the gastric and duodenal mucosa in cats. *Q. J. Exp. Physiol.*, **57**, 405–416.

de Groat, W. C., and Booth, A. M. (1980). Inhibition and facilitation in parasympathetic ganglia of the urinary bladder. *Fed. Proc.*, **39**, 2990–2996.

de Groat, W. C., and Krier, J. (1976). An electrophysiological study of the sacral parasympathetic pathway to the colon of the cat. *J. Physiol. (London)*, **260**, 425–445.

de Groat, W. C., and Saum, W. R. (1972). Sympathetic inhibition of the urinary bladder and of pelvic ganglionic transmission in the cat. *J. Physiol. (London)*, **220**, 297–314.

de Groat, W. C., Booth, A. M., and Krier, J. (1979). Interaction between sacral parasympathetic and lumbar sympathetic inputs to pelvic ganglia. In *Integrative Functions of the Autonomic Nervous System* (Eds. C. McC. Brooks, K. Koizuni and A. Sato), pp. 234–247, Elsevier/North-Holland Biomedical Press, Amsterdam.

Dennis, M. J., Harris, A. J., and Kuffler, S. W. (1971). Synaptic transmission and its duplication by focally applied acetylcholine in parasympathetic neurons in the heart of the frog. *Proc. R. Soc. London Ser. B*, **117**, 509–539.

Dogiel, A. S. (1899). Uber den Bau der Ganglien in den Geflachten des Darmes und der Gallenblase den Menschen und der Saugetiere. *Arch. Anat. Physiol. Leipzig Anat. Abt.*, 130–158.

Dreyfus, C. F., Bornstein, M. B., and Gershon, M. D. (1977a). Synthesis of serotonin by neurons of the myenteric plexus *in situ* and in organotypic tissue culture. *Brain Res.*, **128**, 125–139.

Dreyfus, C. F., Sherman, D., and Gershon, M. D. (1977b). Uptake of serotonin by intrinsic neurons of the myenteric plexus grown in organotypic tissue culture. *Brain Res.*, **128**, 102–123.

Erde, S. M., Gershon, M. D., and Wood, J. D. (1980). Morphology of electrophysiologically identified types of myenteric neurons: Intracellular recording and injection of Lucifer yellow in the guinea pig small bowel. *Neurosci. Abstr.*, **6**, 274.

Frigo, G. M., and Lecchini, S. (1970). An improved method for studying the peristaltic reflex in the isolated colon. *Br. J. Pharmacol.*, **39**, 346–356.

Furness, J. B., and Costa, M. (1980). Types of nerves in the enteric nervous system. *Neuroscience*, **5**, 1–20.

Furness, J. B., Costa, M., and Freeman, C. G. (1979). Absence of tyrosine hydroxylase activity and dopamine β-hydroxylase immunoreactivity in intrinsic nerves of guinea pig ileum. *Neuroscience*, **4**, 305–310.

Gabella, G. (1971). Glial cells in the myenteric plexus. *Z Naturforsch.*, **26B**, 244–245.

Gabella, G. (1972). Fine structure of the myenteric plexus in the guinea pig ileum. *J. Anat.*, **111**, 69–97.

Gabella, G. (1976). *Structure of the Autonomic Nervous System*, John Wiley and Sons, New York.

Gershon, M. D., and Altman, R. F. (1971). An analysis of the uptake of 5-hydroxytryptamine by the myenteric plexus of the small intestine of the guinea pig. *J. Pharmacol. Exp. Ther.*, **179**, 29–41.

Gershon, M. D., and Bursztajn, S. (1978). Properties of the enteric nervous system: Limitation of access of intravascular macromolecules to the myenteric plexus and muscularis externa. *J. Comp. Neurol.*, **180**, 467–488.

Gershon, M. D., Dreyfus, C. F., Pickel, V. M., John, T. H., and Reis, D. J. (1977). Serotonergic neurons in the peripheral nervous system: identification in gut by immunohistochemical localization of tryptophan hydroxylase. *Proc. Natl. Acad. Sci. U.S.A.*, **71**, 3086–3089

Gershon, M. D. Dreyfus, C. F., and Rothman, T. P. (1979). The mammalian enteric nervous system: a third autonomic division. In *Trends in Autonomic Pharmacology* (ed. S. Kalsner), Vol. I, pp. 59–102, Urban and Schwarzenberg, Baltimore.

Grafe, P., Galvin, M., and Mayer, C. J (1979a). Action of GABA on guinea pig myenteric neurons. *Pflügers Arch.*, **382**, R44.

Grafe, P., Wood, J. D., and Mayer, C. J. (1979b). Fast excitatory postsynaptic potentials in AH (type 2) neurons of guinea pig myenteric plexus. *Brain Res.*, **163** 349–352.

Grafe, P., Mayer, C. J., and Wood,. J. D. (1980). Synaptic modulation of calcium-dependent potassium conductance in myenteric neurons in the guinea pig. *J. Physiol. (London)*, **305**, 235–248.

Griffith, W. H., Gallagher, J. P., and Shinnick-Gallagher, P. (1979). Action of norepinephrine on neuronal activity recorded from cat parasympathetic ganglia. *Fed. Proc.*, **38**, 276.

Griffith, W. H., Gallagher, J. P., and Shinnick-Gallagher, P. (1980). An intracellular investigation of cat vesicle pelvic ganglia. *J. Neurophysiol.*, **143**, 343–354.

Griffith, W. H., Gallagher J. P., and Shinnick-Gallagher, P. (1981). Mammalian parasympathetic ganglia fire spontaneous action potentials and transmit slow synaptic potentials. In *Advances in Physiological Sciences, Proceedings of the 28th International Congress of Physiology Budapest: Vol. 4, Physiology of Excitable Membranes* (Ed. J. Salanki), Pergamon Press, New York.

Hamberger, B., Levi-Montalcini, R., Norberg, K. A., and Sjöqvist, F. (1965). Monoamines in immunosympathectomized rats. *Int. J. Neuropharmacol.*, **4,** 91–96.

Hartzell, H. C., Kuffler, S. W., Strickgold, R., and Yoshikami, D. (1977). Synaptic excitation and inhibition resulting from direct action of acetylcholine on two types of chemoreceptors on individual amphibian parasympathetic neurones. *J Physiol. (London),* **271,** 817–846.

Hirst, G. D. S., and McKirdy, H. C. (1974). Presynaptic inhibition at a mammalian peripheral synapse. *Nature,* **250,** 430–431.

Hirst, G. D. S., and McKirdy, H. C. (1975). Synaptic potentials recorded from neurones of the submucous plexus of guinea pig small intestine. *J. Physiol. (London),* **249,** 369–385.

Hirst, G. D. S., and Silinsky, E. M. (1975). Some effects of 5-hydroxytryptamine, dopamine and noradrenaline on neurones in the submucous plexus of guinea pig small intestine. *J. Physiol. (London),* **251,** 817–832.

Hirst, G. D. S. and Spence, I. (1973). Calcium action potentials in mammalian peripheral neurons. *Nature* (London), **243,** 54–56.

Hirst, G. D. S., Holman, M. E., and Spence, I. (1974). Two types of neurons in the myenteric plexus of duodenum in the guinea pig. *J Physiol. (London),* **236,** 303–326.

Hodgkiss, J. P., and Lees, G. M. (1978). Correlated electrophysiological and morphological characteristics of myenteric neurones. *J. Physiol. (London),* **285,** 19–20P.

Hodgkiss, J. P., and Lees, G. M. (1980). Morphological features of guinea pig myenteric plexus neurones. In *Gastrointestinal Motility* (Ed. J. Christensen), pp. 111–117, Raven Press, New York.

Holman, M. E., Hirst, G. D. S., and Spence, I. (1972). Preliminary studies of the neurones of Auerbach's plexus using intracellular microelectrodes. *Aust. J. Exp. Biol. Med.,* **50,** 795–801.

Iggo, A. (1957). Gastric mucosal chemoreceptors with vagal afferent fibers in the cat. *Q. J. Exp. Physiol.,* **42,** 398–409.

Jessen, K. R., and Mirsky, R. (1980). Glial cells in the enteric nervous system contain glial fibrillary acidic protein. *Nature,* **286,** 736–737.

Jessen, K. R., Mirsky, R., Dennison, M. E., and Burnstock, G. (1979). GABA may be a neurotransmitter in the vertebrate peripheral nervous system. *Nature,* **281,** 71–74.

Johnson, S. M., Katayama, Y., and North, R. A. (1980). Slow synaptic potentials in neurons of the myenteric plexus. *J. Physiol. (London),* **301,** 505–516.

Jonakait, G. M., Tamir, H., Gintzler, A. R., and Gershon, M. D. (1979). Release of [³H]serotonin and its binding protein from enteric neurons. *Brain Res.,* **174,** 55–69.

Kachalov, U. P. (1980). Activity of enteric ganglion cells with intact and disrupted interganglionic connections. *Fiziol. Zh. SSSR,* **66,** 962–970.

Kachalov, U. P., Nozdrachev, A. D., and Pogorelov, A. G. (1978). Effects of cholinergic substances on electrical processes in a ganglion of the enteric nervous system. *Fiziol. Zh. SSSR,* **64,** 1530–1539.

Katayama, Y., and North, R. A. (1978). Does substance P mediate slow synaptic excitation within the myenteric plexus? *Nature,* **274,** 387–388.

Katayama, Y., North, R. A., and Williams, J. T. (1979). The action of substance P on neurons of the myenteric plexus of the guinea pig small intestine. *Proc. R. Soc. London Ser. B,* **206,** 191–208.

Langley, J. N. (1921). *The Autonomic Nervous System,* Part I, W. Heffer and Sons, London.

Langley, J. N., and Anderson, H. K. (1895). On the innervation of the pelvic and adjoining viscera, Part I. The lower portion of the intestine. *J. Physiol. (London)*, **18**, 67–105.

Libet, B. (1970). Generation of slow inhibitory and excitatory postsynaptic potentials. *Fed. Proc.*, **29**, 1945–1956.

Lichtman, J. W. (1977). The reorganization of synaptic connections in the rat submandibular ganglion during postnatal development. J. Physiol. (London), **273**, 155–177.

Manber, L., and Gershon, M. D. (1979). A reciprocal adrenergic-cholinergic axo-axonic synapse in the mammalian gut. *Am. J. Physiol.*, **236**, E738–E745.

Mayer, C. J., and Wood, J. D. (1975). Properties of mechanosensitive neurons within Auerbach's plexus of the small intestine of the cat. *Pflügers Arch.*, **357**, 35–49.

Meech, R. W. (1974). The sensitivity of *Helix aspera* neurons to injected calcium ions. *J. Physiol. (London)*, **237**, 259–277.

Melnichenko, L. V., and Skok, V. I. (1970). Natural electrical activity in mammalian parasympathetic ganglion neurons. *Brain Res.*, **23**, 277–279.

Morita, K., North, R. A., and Katayama, Y. (1980). Evidence that substance P is a transmitter in the myenteric plexus. *Nature*, **287**, 151–152.

Nishi, S., and North, R. A. (1973). Intracellular recording from the myenteric plexus of the guinea pig ileum. *J. Physiol. (London)*, **231**, 471–491.

North, R. A. (1973). The calcium-dependent slow after-hyperpolarization in myenteric plexus neurons with tetrodotoxin-resistant action potentials, *Br. J. Pharmacol.*, **49**, 709–711.

North, R. A., and Williams, J. T. (1977). Extracellular recording from the guinea pig myenteric plexus and the action of morphine. *Eur. J. Pharmacol.*, **45**, 23–33.

North, R. A., Henderson, G., Katayama, Y., and Johnson, S. M. (1980). Electrophysiological evidence for presynaptic inhibition of acetylcholine release by 5-hydroxytryptamine in the enteric nervous system. *Neuroscience*, **5**, 581–586.

Ohkawa, H., and Prosser, C. L. (1972). Functions of enteric neurons in enteric plexuses of cat intestine. *Am. J. Physiol.*, **222**, 1420–1426.

Paton, W. D. M., Vizi, E. S., and Zar, M. A. (1971). The mechanism of acetylcholine release from parasympathetic nerves. *J. Physiol. (London)*, **215**, 819–848.

Ranieri, F., Mei, N., and Groussilat, J. (1973). Les afferences splanchniques provenant des mechano recepteurs gastrointestinaux et peritoneaux. *Exp. Brain Res.*, **16**, 276–290.

Sato, T., Tankayanagi, I., and Takagi, K. (1973). Pharmacological properties of electrical activities obtained from neurons in Auerbach's plexus. *Jpn. J. Pharmacol.*, **23**, 665–671.

Strumwasser, F. (1967). Types of information stored in single neurons. In *Invertebrate Nervous Systems* (Ed. C. A. G. Wiersma), pp. 291–320, University of Chicago Press, Chicago.

Suzuki, T., and Kusano, K. (1978). Hyperpolarizing potentials induced by Ca-mediated K-conductance increase in hamster submandibular ganglion cells. *J. Neurobiol.*, **9**, 367–392.

Suzuki, T., and Sakada, S. (1972). Synaptic transmission in the submandibular ganglion of the rat. *Bull Tokyo Dent. Coll.*, **13**, 145–164.

Suzuki, T., and Volle, R. L. (1979). Nicotinic, muscarinic and adrenergic receptors in a parasympathetic ganglion. *J. Pharmacol. Exp. Ther.*, **211**, 252–256.

Tafuri, W. L., and Raick, A. (1964). Presence of 5-hydroxytryptamine in the intramural nervous system of the guinea pig's intestines. *Z. Naturforsch.*, **19**, 1126–1128.

Trendelenburg, P. (1917). Physiologische und pharmakologische Versuche uber die Dundarmperistaltik. *Naunyn-Schmiedebergs Arch. Exp. Pathol. Pharmakol.*, **81**, 55–129.

Wood, J. D. (1970). Electrical activity from single neurons in Auerbach's plexus. *Am. J. Physiol.*, **219**, 159–169.

Wood, J. D. (1972). Excitation of intestinal muscle by atropine, tetrodotoxin and xylocaine. *Am. J. Physiol.*, **222**, 118–125.

Wood, J. D. (1973). Electrical discharge of single enteric neurons in guinea pig small intestine. *Am. J. Physiol.*, **225**, 1107–1113.

Wood, J. D. (1975a). Neurophysiology of Auerbach's plexus and control of intestinal motility. *Physiol. Rev.*, **55**, 307–324.

Wood, J. D. (1975b). Effects of elevated magnesium on discharge of myenteric neurons of cat small bowel. *Am. J. Physiol.*, **229**, 657–662.

Wood, J. D. (1980). Intracellular study of effects of morphine on electrical activity of myenteric neurons in cat small intestine. *Gastroenterology*, **79**, 1222–1230.

Wood, J. D. (1981). Intrinsic neural control of intestinal motility. *Annu. Rev. Physiol.*, **43**, 33–51.

Wood, J. D., and Mayer, C. J. (1973). Patterned discharge of six different neurons in a single enteric ganglion. *Pflügers Arch.*, **338**, 247–256.

Wood, J. D., and Mayer, C. J. (1978). Intracellular study of electrical activity of Auerbach's plexus in guinea pig small intestine. *Pflügers Arch.*, **374**, 265–275.

Wood, J. D., and Mayer, C. J. (1979a). Intracellular study of tonic-type enteric neurons in guinea pig small intestine. *J. Neurophysiol.*, **42**, 569–581.

Wood, J. D., and Mayer, C. J. (1979b). Serotonergic activation of tonic-type enteric neurons in guinea pig small intestine. *J. Neurophysiol.*, **42**, 582–593.

Wood, J. D., and Mayer, C. J. (1979c). Adrenergic inhibition of serotonin release from neurons in guinea pig Auerbach's plexus. *J. Neurophysiol.*, **42**, 594–693.

Yokoyama, S., and Osaki, T. (1978). Functions of Auerbach's plexus. *Jpn. J. Smooth Muscle Res.*, **14**, 173–187.

Development and Plasticity

Autonomic Ganglia
Edited by Lars-Gösta Elfvin
© 1983 John Wiley & Sons Ltd

The Effect of Nerve Growth Factor
on Autonomic Ganglion Cells

R. LEVI-MONTALCINI and L. ALOE

*Institute of Cell Biology, CNR Via Romagnosi 18/A,
00196 Rome, Italy*

INTRODUCTION

The discovery almost three decades ago, that mouse sarcomas 180 and 37 release a humoral factor which elicits a potent growth and differentiation effect on sympathetic immature nerve cells of chick embryos and promotes the excessive production and aberrant peripheral distribution of their axons (Levi-Montalcini and Hamburger, 1951), was the starting point of a long series of investigations which succeeded in identifying the protein molecule endowed with nerve growth promoting activity and uncovering its large spectrum of actions on sympathetic nerve cells from the time when they have still not acquired morphological and biochemical marks of their identity to their full maturity.

Here we shall at first briefly mention only the most relevant early findings and then report in more detail on recent developments of studies which illustrate the unique role of this protein molecule, known as the Nerve Growth Factor, in the life of the sympathetic nerve cells. Besides their contribution to our knowledge of the structural, biochemical and functional properties of sympathetic nerve cells, these studies offer a new approach to more general problems of neurogenesis which had defeated analysis prior to the discovery of this specific growth factor.

HISTORICAL SURVEY

Although the sympathetic nerve cells are considered as the specific target cells of the nerve growth factor (NGF) in view of the fact that they are highly receptive to its action from their early inception to full differentiation, the sensory rather than the sympathetic nerve cells provided the Ariadne thread which was to lead, through tortuous routes, to the discovery of this protein molecule.

The ingenious experiment performed in 1948 by Bueker to transplant a fragment of mouse sarcoma 180 into the body wall of a 3-day-old chick embryo (Bueker, 1948) was aimed at testing the capacity of neurons from the spinal cord and dorsal root ganglia to innervate fast-growing tissues such as malignant tumours. The finding that sensory fibres gained access and branched among the neoplastic cells, and that the ganglia of origin of these neurites, appeared a few days later, larger than the contralateral ganglia innervating the leg bud, seemed to agree with the prevailing view that the growth properties of nerve cells are under the control of other cells, with which they establish connections. The subsequent finding that sympathetic ganglia in embryos bearing transplants of mouse sarcoma 180 or 37 (the latter originates as the former from a mammary carcinoma and is practically indistinguishable from sarcoma 180 in its structure, growth properties and malignancy) undergo an even more pronounced volume increase than sensory ganglia, prompted a more detailed and systematic study of the effects produced by the transplanted tumours (Levi-Montalcini and Hamburger, 1951). The observation that nerve fibres produced in excess by the hypertrophic and hyperplastic sympathetic ganglia, entered in large number into most of the embryonic viscera, and even gained access to 'off-limit' territories such as the cavity of blood vessels of the host, called for a revision of the original hypothesis that attributed to the vigorous growth and histochemical properties of mouse sarcoma 180, the penetration of sensory fibres into the neoplastic tissue and the hypertrophy of neurons of origin of these axons. The suggestion that the effects elicited by these two like tumours were instead due to a humoral agent released by the neoplastic cells, found strong support from experiments of transplantation of fragments of one or the other of these tumours onto the chorioallantoic membrane of 4–6-day-old chick embryos, in such a position as to prevent the entrance of sensory or sympathetic nerve fibres into the mouse sarcomas. Under these conditions, the only connections between embryonic and neoplastic tissues were established through the common vascular system. Sympathetic and sensory ganglia of embryos bearing these chorioallantoic tumour transplants appeared a few days later markedly larger than control ganglia. The similarity between the effects elicited by intraembryonic and chorioallantoic transplants of these tumours was stressed by the finding that also in these latter experimental series were the viscera of the host embryo loaded with sympathetic nerve fibres (Levi-Montalcini, 1952; Levi-Montalcini and Hamburger, 1953). The puzzling finding of large ganglionic agglomerates in the abdominal cavity of embryos bearing intra- or extraembryonic transplants of sarcomas 180 or 37, morphologically indistinguishable from but topographically distinct from those of the coeliac and other abdominal plexuses, remained unexplained at that time (Levi-Montalcini and Hamburger, 1953). We shall return later to the origin of these ganglia (p. 417).

A tissue-culture technique developed one year later (Levi-Montalcini, 1953) offered a new and most favourable approach to the study of the chemical nature and properties of the still unknown humoral factor released by the two tumours. Sensory and sympathetic ganglia from 8-day chick embryos were explanted in a semi-solid medium consisting of rooster's plasma and embryonic chick extract, in close proximity to fragments of mouse sarcoma 180 or 37. In control cultures, fragments of other mouse tumours or of embryonic mouse or avian tissues were combined *in vitro* with the same ganglia. The sealed cultures were incubated at 38 °C and inspected at time intervals between 6 and 48 hours. At the end of the first day, all ganglia facing transplants of sarcoma 180 or 37, but none in control cultures, had developed a dense fibrillar halo which appeared particularly dense on the side facing the tumour (Levi-Montalcini *et al.*, 1954).

The subsequent finding that also the cell-free extract of these tumours added to the culture medium elicited the formation of a fibrillar nerve halo from sensory and sympathetic ganglia incubated in this medium, offered to Cohen the possibility of identifying the tumoural fraction endowed with nerve growth promoting activity. In 1954 it was reported that this activity resided in a nucleoprotein moiety isolated from both tumours, and the active particle was given the name nerve growth promoting factor, later to be shortened to Nerve Growth Factor (NGF) (Cohen *et al.*, 1954).

If the *in vitro* experiments afforded the possibility, unattainable in the developing embryos, to identify the nature of the tumoural nerve-growth promoting factor, their even more important contribution was to make available a fast and reliable assay to screen other normal and neoplastic tissues, as well as organic fluids, as potential sources of this factor. It was this technique which revealed, through fortuitous and most fortunate chance discoveries, the presence of two other much richer sources of NGF than mouse sarcomas, namely snake venom and the submaxillary salivary glands of adult male mice (Cohen and Levi-Montalcini, 1956; Levi-Montalcini and Cohen, 1956; Levi-Montalcini, 1958; Cohen, 1958). These discoveries not only invalidated the hypothesis that the nerve growth promoting activity of the two tumours could reside in some unique property of neoplastic cells (possibly the release of a virus particle), but made available much larger quantities of the NGF moiety which in turn afforded the possibility of studying its physicochemical properties and of exploring the characteristics of the growth response elicited in the living organism, in whole ganglia and in isolated nerve cells *in vitro*.

In 1956 Cohen identified the NGF isolated from snake venom as a protein molecule (Cohen and Levi-Montalcini, 1956), and in 1958 a molecule with similar if not identical properties to those of snake venom NGF was isolated and identified as the mouse salivary NGF (Cohen, 1958). At the biological level, the effects elicited by mouse sarcomas in the developing chick embryo and in sensory and sympathetic ganglia cultured *in vitro* were indistinguishable from the effects produced by injecting the embryos or adding to the culture medium minute amounts of the purified snake venom NGF or of the salivary NGF (Cohen, 1960; Levi-Montalcini and Booker, 1960a). However, while the exceedingly small amount of NGF that could be purified from mouse sarcomas, where it is present at very low concentration (Levi-Montalcini, 1958), have not permitted the assay of its biological activity in small mammals, the NGF isolated in milligram quantities from mouse salivary glands afforded the possibility of exploring its effects in neonatal and adult rodents as well as in other neonatal and young mammals. In view of their small size and breeding facilities, the mouse and later also the rat became the animals of choice for these studies.

The discovery in 1959 that injections of a specific antiserum to the salivary NGF produce the irreversible and almost total destruction of paravertebral sympathetic ganglia and of the coeliac and mesenteric ganglionic agglomerates in neonatal rodents and other neonatal mammals (Cohen, 1960; Levi-Montalcini and Booker, 1960b), gave evidence for the key role played by this molecule in the life of immature sympathetic nerve cells. Since the destruction of these ganglia by this procedure, which became known as 'immunosympathectomy' (Levi-Montalcini and Angeletti, 1966), does not interfere with the viability and normal somatic development of the rodents submitted in the first postnatal week to 3–5 injections of a specific antiserum to NGF, it became possible to produce colonies of mice and rats deprived since birth of the function of the paravertebral and prevertebral sympathetic ganglia (Steiner and Schönbaum, 1972). The unexpected finding that ganglia innervating the male and female internal genital tracts, positioned in close proximity to these structures, and other smaller ganglionic aggregates innervating the interscapular and the mediastinal brown adipose tissue and the heart atria (Sterner, 1972) are neither receptive to the growth stimulating properties of NGF, nor vulnerable to the action of antibodies to NGF, revealed hitherto unsuspected biological differences between sympathetic neurons lodged in the para- and prevertebral ganglia and those located close to the effector organs and structures mentioned above. The nerve cells of these latter ganglia were designated 'short adrenergic neurons' to distinguish them from those of para- and prevertebral ganglia which possess a long postganglionic axon and became known as 'long adrenergic neurons' (Owman and Sjöstrand, 1965). The hypothesis submitted by Owman *et al.* (1974), who explored in detailed studies the structural, biochemical and functional properties of the short adrenergic neurons, that they form a specific entity morphologically and functionally distinct from that of the long adrenergic neurons and that they serve a peripheral neuroendocrine function, puts into a new light these nerve cells which share with parasympathetic neurons the property of exerting effects restricted to the innervated structures. Their lack of response to NGF further stresses their difference from other adrenergic nerve cells even if they share many other morphological and functional properties in common with long adrenergic neurons.

In the present chapter we will consider the growth response of the long adrenergic neurons to NGF and the more recently discovered NGF effects on neoplastic chromaffin cells and on normal chromaffin cells at an early stage of their differentiation. The source of origin of NGF, its physicochemical properties, access and mechanism of action in its target cells which have been the object of recent extensive review articles (Levi-Montalcini, 1966; Levi-Montalcini *et al.*, 1972; Bradshaw, 1978; Server and Shooter, 1977; Greene and Shooter, 1980; Thoenen and Barde, 1980) will be only briefly mentioned here for space limitation and also in view of the fact that they are not directly pertinent to the main topic considered in this volume.

BIOLOGICAL SOURCES OF NGF

Ever since the discovery that NGF is present in the extract of the submaxillary salivary glands of adult male mice at a concentration about 10 000 times higher than in the mouse sarcomas 180 and 37 (Levi-Montalcini and Argeletti, 1968a), these glands became and remain to this day the richest available source of NGF. Investigations performed at the time of this discovery and extended in subsequent years (Caramia and Angeletti, 1962; Levi-Montalcini and Angeletti, 1964; Ishii and Shooter, 1975) showed that the NGF protein molecule is synthesized in the granular convoluted tubules of these glands, which are also endowed with the peculiar property of synthesizing a large number of other physiologically active polypeptides (Barka, 1980). The release in the mouse saliva of NGF, reported in early experiments (Levi-Montalcini and Angeletti, 1961), was subsequently the object of more detailed studies which, however, gave conflicting results. In 1976 Wallace and Partlow compared the NGF concentration in the mouse saliva stimulated by different secretagogues and came to the conclusion that the release of saliva rich in NGF, evaluated by *in vitro* bioassay and by radial immunodiffusion, is primarily regulated through α-adrenergic receptors (Wallace and Partlow, 1976). In 1978 Burton *et al.* confirmed these findings which had been refuted in 1977 by Murphy *et al.* These authors reported that an exceedingly high NGF concentration is normally found in the saliva of the male mouse even without resorting to α-adrenergic stimulation. The finding that sialoadenectomy does not lower the normally very low levels of circulating NGF, seemed to the same authors to disprove any possible endocrine role of the salivary glands with respect to the NGF. This conclusion has been challenged by the very recent finding that β-adrenergic stimulation in adult male mice results in a markedly increased level of NGF in the circulating blood (Levi-Montalcini and Aloe, 1980a). Furthermore, and of great interest in connection with a possible endocrine role of NGF released into the blood stream, is the observation that the enhanced NGF blood level, upon β-adrenergic stimulation, is accompanied by marked hypertrophy of intact long adrenergic neurons and by enhanced speed of regeneration of transected postganglionic roots of the superior cervical ganglion (Levi-Montalcini and Aloe, 1980a).

It remains to be assessed whether the same or different cells lining the granular convoluted tubules of the mouse salivary glands release the NGF into the saliva or into the blood, depending on the activation of α- or β-adrenergic secretagogues, and to elucidate the role of the salivary and circulating NGF in the differentiation and maintenance of sympathetic nerve cells. Studies in progress show that NGF administered orally to neonatal rodents produces marked hypertrophy of the long adrenergic neurons, thus suggesting that also the NGF released into the saliva may become available through reabsorption in the digestive tract to the differentiating long adrenergic nerve cells (Aloe *et al.*, unpublished observations).

Studies performed in the last two decades have shown that a large number of neoplastic and normal vertebrate cell lines are endowed with the property of synthesizing and releasing minute amounts of NGF (Levi-Montalcini and Angeletti, 1968a; Young *et al.*, 1975). The recent reports that NGF is normally present in measurable quantities in the human placenta (Goldstein *et al.*, 1978) and in larger amounts in the guinea-pig prostate and in the seminal vesicles of a large number of species, man included (Harper *et al.*, 1979; Harper and Thoenen, 1980), while giving evidence for the ubiquitousness of this molecule increase the difficulty of defining its source(s) as well as the biological role of the NGF released in large quantities from vastly different glands such as snake venom gland, mouse salivary glands, prostate and seminal vesicles, or in barely appreciable amounts from normal and neoplastic cell lines.

PHYSICOCHEMICAL PROPERTIES OF THE SALIVARY NGF

With the non-highly sophisticated techniques available in the late fifties, Cohen succeeded in identifying the mouse salivary NGF as a protein molecule with an estimated molecular weight of 44 000 (Cohen, 1960). With the advent of ion-exchange chromatography and gel filtration, it became possible to obtain NGF samples of sufficient purity to permit structural studies of the NGF molecule to be performed.

Using a modification of the procedure devised by Cohen, Bocchini and Angeletti (1969) purified a biologically active moiety with a sedimentation coefficient of 2.5 S and an apparent molecular weight of 30 000. Subsequent studies by Zanini *et al.* (1968) indicated that the NGF activity could be recovered from two fractions of molecular weight 28 000 and 14 000. Following a different procedure, other investigators reported that NGF activity in the mouse salivary glands is present in a protein moiety with a sedimentation coefficient of 7 S and a molecular weight of 130 000. This high molecular weight NGF consists of three different types of subunits; only one of these subunits, the β-subunit, is endowed with NGF activity. The other two subunits became known as the α- and γ-subunits (Varon *et al.*, 1968). The γ-subunit was identified as an arginine esteropeptidase of molecular weight 26 000; it is possibly involved in the processing of the β-NGF from a larger precursor (Berger and Shooter, 1977, 1978); the α-subunit consists of an acidic group of proteins of undetermined biological activity (Greene and Shooter, 1980). The 2.5 S NGF according to the studies performed by Zanini and Angeletti (1971), or the β-subunit according to the purification procedures of Varon and Shooter, are endowed with identical biological activity and differ from each other only in the absence from the 2.5 S NGF of an N-terminal octopeptide present in the β-subunit (Greene and Shooter, 1980). Using the purification procedure devised by Bocchini and Angeletti, Angeletti and Bradshaw (1971) determined the amino acid sequence of the 2.5 S NGF. They showed that it consists of two identical subunits with a molecular weight of 26 518; each of the two polypeptide chains contains 118 amino acids and has a molecular weight of 13 259, possessing amino-terminal serine and carboxyl-terminal arginine. Three disulphide bridges impart a rigid structure to the NGF molecule, as indicated by its striking resistance to enzymatic, chemical and heat denaturation (Angeletti and Bradshaw, 1971). A further step in the elucidation of the structural properties of NGF has been achieved by its crystallization (Wlodawer *et al.*, 1975). The NGF crystal is described as hexagonal bipyramids up to 0.7 mm long and 0.25 mm across. Since the biological identity and uniqueness of a protein molecule reside in its entire three-dimensional structure which comprises not only the amino acid sequence but also its folding and superfolding to form a globular entity, X-ray analysis of NGF crystals, a method that has provided invaluable information on the three-dimensional structure of proteins, should allow us to extend our knowledge of NGF structure.

STRUCTURAL, ULTRASTRUCTURAL AND METABOLIC EFFECTS OF NGF

The most outstanding feature of the growth response elicited by NGF, and in fact the first to have revealed the existence of this factor, was, as mentioned on p. 402, the precocious and exhuberant production of nerve fibres by sensory and sympathetic ganglionic cells in chick embryos bearing transplants of mouse sarcoma 180 to 37. The *in vitro* effect elicited by the purified salivary NGF protein is illustrated in Fig. 1, in which are reproduced two living sympathetic ganglia dissected out from 8-day chick embryos and cultured in the absence (Fig. 1a) or presence (Fig. 1b) of 10 ng of NGF per ml of culture

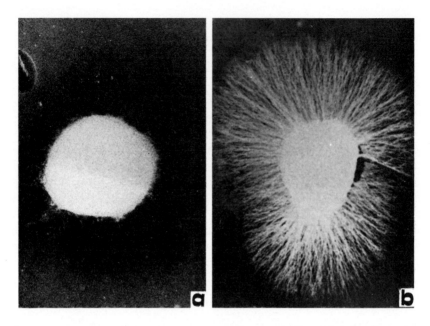

Figure 1   Dark-field microphotos of living sensory ganglia of 8-day chick embryos, cultured for 24 hours in a semisolid medium in the absence (a) or presence (b) of 1 BU of NGF. ×42

medium for a 24-hour period. The production of the dense and regular halo of nerve fibres in the NGF-rich medium became known as the growth response to 1 biological unit (BU) of NGF. The regularity and constancy of the effect elicited by 1 BU of NGF, whatever its source, became a most valuable index of the presence of the NGF protein in known and putative NGF-releasing tissues or organic fluids. A growth–response curve to the purified salivary NGF showed that the addition to the culture medium of 10 BU of NGF evokes the formation of a much shorter and denser fibrillar halo. Higher NGF concentrations (100 BU) produce what at first appeared to be an inhibitory effect of excess NGF, namely the total lack of the fibre outgrowth around the cultured ganglia. Subsequent studies showed that the failure of high NGF doses to evoke the effect produced by 1 BU NGF is due to an abrupt change from a radial to a circular pattern of nerve fibre outgrowth and to the formation of a progressively larger fibrillar capsule around the ganglionic explant (Levi-Montalcini and Angeletti, 1968b). A recent reinvestigation of this effect offered a very plausible explanation of this puzzling effect. In the presence of a high NGF concentration, an increasing larger number of nerve cells are stimulated and produce axons which aggregate in thick bundles. The elastic tension of these bundles resulting from fibre-to-fibre lateral adhesion not counteracted by a compensatory increase in their adherence to the substrate results in their detachment from it, and in their circular rather than radial outgrowth (Rutishauer and Edelman, 1980).

As soon as the highly purified salivary NGF became available in milligram quantities, its effects were assayed in neonatal rodents, other newborn mammals and in adult mice. Here only a condensed report of studies performed in neonatal rodents will be presented. The effects elicited by subcutaneous daily injections of the salivary NGF vary according to the purity of the preparation, the amount injected per dose and to the length of the treatment. This accounts for the marked discrepancies in the results reported from different laboratories.

In our earlier experiments performed with the still not highly purified salivary NGF, the volume increase of paravertebral sympathetic ganglia upon a 3-week treatment from the day of birth did not exceed six times the volume of control ganglia (Levi-Montalcini and Booker, 1960a). In more recent studies performed with a highly purified salivary NGF preparation, the sympathetic ganglia underwent in a 10-day treatment a volume increase 10–12 times that of controls (Levi-Montalcini *et al.*, 1972). Figure 2a–c illustrate the effect of a 5-day NGF treatment in neonatal rats.

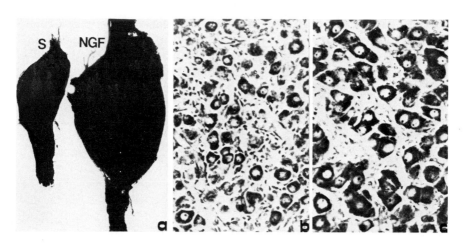

Figure 2 (a) Whole mounts of superior cervical ganglia of 5-day-old littermate rats injected since birth with saline solution (S) or with NGF. ×17. (b, c) Transverse sections of superior cervical ganglia reproduced in (a). ×380

This volume increase produced by daily injections of $5\,\mu l/g$ body weight of a NGF preparation containing $200\,\mu g$ of NGF per ml, results from a precocious differentiation of immature sympathetic nerve cells, neuronal hypertrophy (the cells attain a size much larger than that of fully differentiated neurons of untreated adult rodents), and marked increase in width of axons which find accommodation inside the ganglia before assembling in the postganglionic nerves. The numerical increase in nerve cells, which was at first attributed to a mitotic effect of NGF (Levi-Montalcini and Booker, 1960a), was subsequently shown to be due instead to a 'NGF rescue effect' of immature nerve cells doomed to death during the first postnatal week (Hendry, 1977). This process, which became known as 'neurothanasia' (Hollyday and Hamburger, 1976), occurs in a large number of developing nerve centres (Levi-Montalcini, 1950; Hamburger, 1975; Oppenheim and Chu-Wang, 1977; Pilar and Landmesser, 1976). Its occurrence is attributed to the now widely accepted competition hypothesis which postulates a competition of axons at the target areas and degeneration of the neurons that failed in the race for a limited number of synaptic sites and/or trophic substances released from peripheral tissues (Cowan, 1973; Pittman *et al.*, 1978; Borsellino, 1950). Injections of NGF in quantities largely exceeding those normally released by peripheral tissues, permit the survival of all nerve cells that underwent incipient differentiation, as long as the exogeneous NGF is made available to them. Discontinuation of the treatment results in the abrupt death of nerve cells produced in excess of peripheral synaptic sites (Levi-Montalcini and Angeletti, 1968; Levi-Montalcini *et al.*, 1972).

Ultrastructural studies performed in ganglia cultured *in vitro* in the presence or absence of NGF, and *in vivo* in sympathetic ganglia of control and NGF—injected neonatal rodents, showed that the most striking and precocious event elicited by NGF is the massive increase in cytoskeletal structures. Microtubules, microfilaments and intermediate filaments fill all available space in the cytoplasmic compartment (Levi-Montalcini *et al.*, 1968). Other features of the changes elicited by NGF in the fine structure of the target nerve cells are: rise in free and membrane-bound ribosomes, dilation and increase in the vesicles and membranes of the Golgi apparatus. The entire cellular synthetic machinery undergoes activation as indicated by metabolic studies which showed that NGF enhances all anabolic processes (Angeletti *et al.*, 1968). Inhibition of protein synthesis by puromycin and cyclohexamide causes a severe reduction in the growth of the fibrillar halo when these inhibitors are added at a concentration that practically blocks amino acid incorporation (Angeletti *et al.*, 1965). Early experiments by Cohen (1958), confirmed in subsequent studies, showed that the growth response is accompanied by marked enhancement of oxidative processes. The presence of a proper energy source is required for the outgrowth of nerve fibres; in its absence their growth starts but ceases almost immediately. Experiments with specifically labelled glucose indicate that this stimulation occurs mainly through a direct oxidative pathway (Angeletti *et al.*, 1964a). The NGF in fact significantly increases the release of CO_2 from glucose labelled in position 1, suggesting that the growth factor selectively enhances the synthesis of substances such as nucleotides and nucleic acids which contain pentoses. Lipid biosynthesis is also markedly stimulated, as shown by the marked enhanced incorporation of labelled acetate into lipids, already apparent after 4 hours of incubation in a NGF-rich medium (Angeletti *et al.*, 1964b). Differences in the rate of incorporation of labelled precursors into ganglia incubated in NGF-poor or -rich medium, however, may be due, at least in part, as suggested by Larrabee (1972), to the better maintenance of nerve cells in the presence of NGF, even if the incubation time was in all these *in vitro* experiments reduced to a minimum to avoid deterioration of control cells. The problem was recently the object of a reinvestigation which made use of more sophisticated techniques such as two-dimensional gel electrophoresis. A comparative analysis of more than 800 proteins in control and NGF-treated pheochromocytoma PC12 cells (a NGF target cell which will be considered on p. 417) showed that none of these proteins were qualitatively repressed after NGF treatment, and no new proteins appeared after NGF treatment, resulting in the transformation of the neoplastic chromaffin cells into a line exhibiting the typical phenotype of sympathetic nerve cells (Garrels and Schubert, 1979). These findings add further to the notion, gathered from earlier experiments with sensory and sympathetic nerve cells *in vitro*, that NGF causes quantitative modulation of protein synthesis rather than qualitative changes.

Of particular interest is the finding that NGF not only stimulates differentiative and metabolic processes but also enhances the specific function of sympathetic nerve cells. Treatment of newborn rats with NGF for a 10-day period results in the selective induction of the two rate-limiting enzymes in the synthesis of the adrenergic neurotransmitter noradrenaline: i.e. tyrosine hydroxylase (TH) and dopamine β-hydroxylase (DBH). Tyrosine hydroxylase underwent an 18-fold increase over the control and dopamine β-hydroxylase a 13-fold increase, whereas the activity of two other enzymes involved, respectively, in the biosynthesis and metabolic degradation of noradrenaline (namely, DOPA decarboxylase and monoamine oxidase) rose only in proportion to the increased protein content of the volume-increased NGF-treated sympathetic ganglia (Thoenen *et al.*, 1971; Yu *et al.*, 1977).

EVIDENCE FOR THE ESSENTIAL ROLE OF NGF IN GROWTH AND DIFFERENTIATION OF SYMPATHETIC NERVE CELLS

Early studies

The destruction of para- and prevertebral sympathetic ganglia by subcutaneous injections of a specific NGF antiserum (AS-NGF) in neonatal rodents and other mammals (Levi-Montalcini and Booker, 1960b) provided the first dramatic evidence for the unique role played by this molecule in the

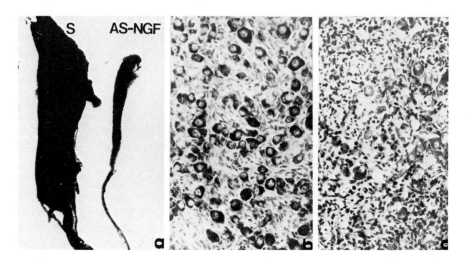

Figure 3 (a) Whole mounts of superior cervical ganglia of 10-day-old littermate rats injected for the first five postnatal days with saline solution (S) or with a specific antiserum to NGF (AS-NGF). ×21. (b, c) transverse sections of superior cervical ganglia reproduced in (a). Note disappearance of nerve cells following AS-NGF treatment. ×250

development of sympathetic adrenergic nerve cells (Fig. 3). Two hypotheses were submitted to account for these findings: nerve cell destruction could result from a cytotoxic complement-mediated effect, or alternatively, the cause of death could be due to the inactivation by circulating antibodies of the NGF released from endogenous sources and supplemented to nursing babies through the milk where it is present in measurable amounts (Levi-Montalcini and Angeletti, 1968a). While the former hypothesis was favoured at first, the latter gained progressively more support from the following experimental findings: (1) sensory and sympathetic embryonic nerve cells dissociated by trypsin and cultured in a minimum essential medium in the absence of NGF, undergo massive degeneration and death in the first 24 hours, while they survive for an indefinite time and build a dense fibrillar net which extends over the entire surface of the culture dish in the presence of one or more biological units of NGF (Levi-Montalcini and Angeletti, 1963); (2) recent experiments, to be considered in a following section, showed that delayed administration of NGF to infant rodents injected at birth with AS-NGF results in the survival of nerve cells otherwise doomed to death by AS-NGF administration, a result incompatible with the hypothesis of a cytotoxic effect of NGF.

Recent studies

The massive death of immature sympathetic nerve cells upon AS-NGF injections in neonatal rodents, which contrasts with the reversible lesions inflicted by the same treatment in adult animals (Levi-Montalcini and Angeletti, 1968a), suggested the exploration of the effects of pharmacological agents which, through different mechanisms, block the transmission of the nerve impulse from sympathetic nerve cells to their effectors. A summary report of these studies, described in detail in previous publications, is a necessary prerequisite for an understanding of the effects elicited by the simultaneous or delayed administration of NGF with each one of these pharmacological compounds.

The first agent assayed for its effects in immature sympathetic nerve cells of neonatal rodents was 6-hydroxydopamine (6-OHDA), a dopamine derivative which in adult animals blocks for a 6–8-week period the transmission of the adrenergic nerve impulse (Porter *et al.*, 1963). It was shown that this effect is due to an acute but reversible degeneration produced by the accumulation of 6-OHDA in the noradrenergic nerve endings (Thoenen, 1971; Tranzer and Richards, 1971; Sachs and Johnson, 1975).

Injections of 6-OHDA in neonatal rodents at the same doses as used in adult animals (100 µg/g body weight), result in the massive degeneration of sympathetic para- and prevertebral sympathetic ganglia. The effect is of the same magnitude as that produced by injections of AS-NGF and is likewise irreversible (Angeletti and Levi-Montalcini, 1970). Electron-microscopic studies showed that the lesions produced by 6-OHDA are restricted to the nerve end terminals while the cell perikarya appear normal (Aloe *et al.*, 1975).

The second compound investigated for its potential destructive effects in immature sympathetic nerve cells was guanethidine, an agent introduced in the medical treatment of arterial hypertension in 1959 (Page and Dustan, 1959) for its property of producing an acute but transient ganglion-blocking effect on sympathetic nerves. Electron-microscopic studies showed that guanethidine accumulates outside the noradrenaline storage granules and exerts a direct toxic effect on mitochondria, blocking oxidative phosphorylation (Juul and Sand, 1971).

Daily injections of guanethidine sulphate in neonatal rodents at doses of 50–100 µg/g body weight from the day of birth to the end of the second week, result in the massive destruction of sympathetic para- and prevertebral ganglia, to the same extent as treatment with AS-NGF or 6-OHDA (Eränkö and Eränkö, 1971; Angeletti *et al.*, 1972). Under the electron microscope the mitochondria appear enormously dilated and the cristae are disrupted or entirely destroyed; these alterations are followed by progressive cell deterioration and death (Angeletti *et al.*, 1972).

The third compound which upon injection in neonatal rodents produces the almost total destruction of sympathetic para- and prevertebral sympathetic ganglia is the *Vinca* alkaloid vinblastine. After one week of daily injections of 1 nmol of vinblastine per g body weight, the sympathetic ganglia are reduced to sclerotic nodules of diminutive size. Ultrastructural studies performed after a single does of vinblastine showed that the most precocious and prominent alterations consist of marked swelling of the axons, alterations of microtubules and the formation of large electron-dense intra-axonal inclusions which are then found also in the nuclear compartment (Calissano *et al.*, 1976; Menesini Chen *et al.*, 1977).

The massive destruction of sympathetic para- and prevertebral ganglia by these pharmacological compounds became known, ever since it was first described in rodents treated at birth with 6-OHDA, as chemical sympathectomy (Angeletti and Levi-Montalcini, 1970).

Surgical axotomy performed on postganglionic roots of the superior cervical ganglion in neonatal rodents (Hendry and Campbell, 1976) results likewise in the irreversible destruction of immature sympathetic neurons of this ganglion. Electron-microscopic studies showed a striking similarity between the effects produced by surgical axotomy and chemical axotomy by 6-OHDA. In both instances the earliest degenerative events consist of alterations localized in the adrenergic nerve endings, followed almost immediately by detachment and degeneration of preganglionic synaptic terminals from the apparently still intact perikarya of sympathetic nerve cells (Aloe and Levi-Montalcini, 1979a).

RESCUE EFFECTS OF NGF ON SYMPATHETIC NERVE CELLS LETHALLY INJURED BY IMMUNOLOGICAL, CHEMICAL OR SURGICAL PROCEDURES

The results to be summarized in this section provide strong evidence in favour of the hypothesis that the massive destruction of immature sympathetic nerve cells produced by administration to neonatal rodents of AS-NGF, 6-OHDA, or vinblastine, or by surgical transection of postganglionic roots of the superior cervical ganglion, results from the abrupt deprivation of NGF from these cells. This concept, elaborated in detail by Johnson and Aloe (1978), finds confirmation from the more recent studies of the effects of NGF in AS-NGF-treated neonatal rodents. In all instances the delayed or simultaneous supply of large doses of salivary NGF not only protects the cells from the otherwise destructive effects of these different treatments, but results in a volume enlargement of sympathetic ganglia which may be less pronounced than that elicited by treatment with NGF alone, equal to, or even, paradoxically, much more marked than the effect elicited by NGF alone.

Injections of NGF, even if delayed 24 or 48 hours after administration of one AS-NGF dose to neonatal rodents (Thoenen and Barde, 1980), bring to a halt the degenerative processes which, three days after the injection of antibodies to NGF, are already rather advanced, as indicated by the much smaller size of sympathetic ganglia in experimental than in control littermates. Morphological and electron-microscopic studies showed that, three days after the AS-NGF injection, the ganglia consist of nerve cells in an advanced state of degeneration and of closely packed still undifferentiated cells. These cells, which apparently did not suffer irreversible damage, undergo progressive hypertrophy, an effect which accounts for the rapid and progressive volume increase of the ganglia, which attain in a period of a week a size larger than that of controls (Aloe and Levi-Montalcini, unpublished observations).

Two different mechanisms would account for the property of NGF to counteract the destructive effects of 6-OHDA, surgical axotomy and vinblastine. Injections of the dopamine derivative or surgical axotomy prevent the uptake of NGF from peripheral tissues, while vinblastine interferes with its retrograde axonal transport through its disruptive action on microtubules. The paradoxical volume enlargement of ganglia submitted to dual 6-OHDA and NGF treatment, in which they may attain a size 30 times larger than controls in a 3-week period (Aloe *et al.*, 1975), results from the hypertrophy of sympathetic nerve cells but, to a much larger extent, from the production of collateral fibres from the proximal segment of the stem axon. These minute but exceedingly numerous collaterals find accommodation inside the ganglion and around it, where they form a dense fibrillar capsule. The volume increase and altered profile of ganglia submitted to dual NGF and 6-OHDA treatment are illustrated in Fig. 4. The mechanism underlying this paradoxical effect

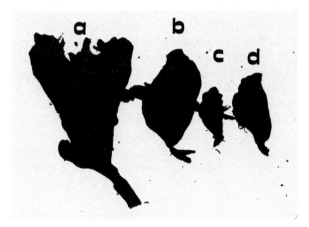

Figure 4 Whole mounts of superior cervical ganglia of 12-day littermate rats injected since birth with (a) NGF + 6-OHDA, (b) NGF, (c) 6-OHDA, (d) saline. Explanation in text. ×6. From Aloe *et al.* (1975); reproduced by permission of Prof. O. Pompeiano

which occurs also, even if to a lesser extent, in surgically axotomized and NGF-treated ganglia, is extensively considered in the original articles (Aloe *et al.*, 1975; Aloe and Levi-Montalcini, 1979a). NGF likewise counteracts the destructive effects of vinblastine. *In vitro* and *in vivo* studies showed that NGF exerts its protective action by favouring the assembly and organization of microtubules even in the presence of the *Vinca* alkaloid (Calissano *et al.*, 1976; Menesini Chen *et al.*, 1977). While in all the above instances the exogenous supply of NGF neutralizes and even overcompensates for the destruction, or prevented access of endogenous NGF to the target nerve cells, in the case of guanethidine treatment neither the primary cause of sympathetic nerve cell death nor the protective mechanisms of NGF have yet been elucidated, as already remarked by Johnson and Aloe (1978).

NEUROTROPIC EFFECTS OF NGF

A central issue in developmental neurobiology is the building of neuronal circuits in the cerebrospinal axis and the establishment of specific connections between nerve centres and the periphery. The problem of whether growing and regenerating nerve fibres are receptive to chemical signals issued from end-organs, as first put forward by Cajal, has remained unanswered until now, due to the extreme difficulty of isolating and identifying these putative neurotropic factors. The discovery of the nerve growth factor and its identification as a protein molecule synthesized and released in minute amounts by most normal and neoplastic vertebrate tissues, offered for the first time the possibility of approaching this problem. The experiments which gave the first unequivocable evidence for an *in vivo* neurotropic effect of NGF consisted of the intracerebral injection of NGF into neonatal rodents. The experiments were directed towards assessing a possible role for NGF in the growth and differentiation of monoaminergic intracerebral nerve cells. While the results of these experiments did not provide evidence for such an effect, they brought to light an unanticipated effect elicited by accumulation of NGF in the brain-stem and cerebrospinal axis. Sympathetic nerve fibres emerging from adjacent enlarged paravertebral ganglia in much larger number than from control ganglia, produced collaterals which stemmed out from axons directed to the periphery and entered in large fascicles inside the spinal cord and brain-stem in conjunction with the dorsal root fibres of spinal and cephalic ganglia. Once inside the central nervous system they took up a position in the dorsal funiculi of the spinal cord and ventrolateral column of the medulla oblongata, where they subsisted as a parasitic system, apparently devoid of function, as long as an exogenous supply of NGF was made available through daily intracerebral injections. They disappeared as soon as the treatment was discontinued (Menesini Chen *et al.*, 1978). Experiments indicative of an *in vitro* neurotropic effect of NGF had previously been reported by another group (Charlwood *et al.*, 1972). Much more compelling and indeed unequivocable evidence for an *in vitro* neutrotropic effect of NGF was recently presented in a series of most ingenious experiments performed in different laboratories (Campenot, 1977; Letourneau, 1979; Gundersen and Barrett, 1979).

PHENOTYPIC MODULATION OF NGF ON NEOPLASTIC CHROMAFFIN CELLS AND NORMAL CHROMAFFIN CELL PRECURSORS

In 1975 Tischler and Greene discovered that a clonal cell line, known as PC12 line, derived from a rat pheochromocytoma, responds to NGF by exhibiting morphological features of sympathetic nerve cells (Tischler and Greene, 1975). The property of neoplastic pheochromocytoma cells to acquire morphological biochemical and functional characteristics indistinguishable from those of genuine sympathetic nerve cells opened to a new and most fertile field of investigation on the mechanism of action of NGF and newly discovered property of diverting chromaffin neoplastic cells from glandular to a nervous phenotypic cell type. Limitations of space prevent even a cursory report on the extensive literature which in a few years has accumulated on this new and most promising approach to the study of the multiple properties and mechanism of action of NGF. We refer readers to recent original and review articles on this topic (Greene and Rein, 1977; Greene *et al.*, 1979; Greene and Shooter, 1980). Here we shall briefly consider the effects of NGF on normal rather than neoplastic chromaffin cells exposed to NGF when they have still not acquired the differentiative marks of adrenomedullary cells.

Two parallel sets of experiments performed in the last few years in the chick embryo and rat foetuses showed that injection of NGF in the chick embryo at day 4 of incubation and in the rat foetus between the fifteenth and sixteenth day of pregnancy, results in the massive transformation of chromaffin cells precursors and of immature chromaffin cells in sympathetic neurons. We refer readers to recent articles where these effects are described in detail (Aloe and Levi-Montalcini, 1979b; Levi-Montalcini and Aloe, 1980b). Here it suffices to mention that the NGF treated chromaffin cells give origin in the chick embryo to enormous ganglionic agglomerates which fill the abdominal cavity and innervate adjacent blood vessels. Their derivation from adrenal chromaffin cells which normally would have migrated inside the adrenal gland is demonstrated by the diminutive size of this gland which consists only of cordons of cortical cells surrounded by the large sympathetic nerve cell agglomerates. In rat foetuses, the whole medullary part of the adrenal gland is transformed into a large sympathetic cell aggregate (Fig. 5a, b). These cells when processed with formaldehyde-induced fluorescence exhibit a green

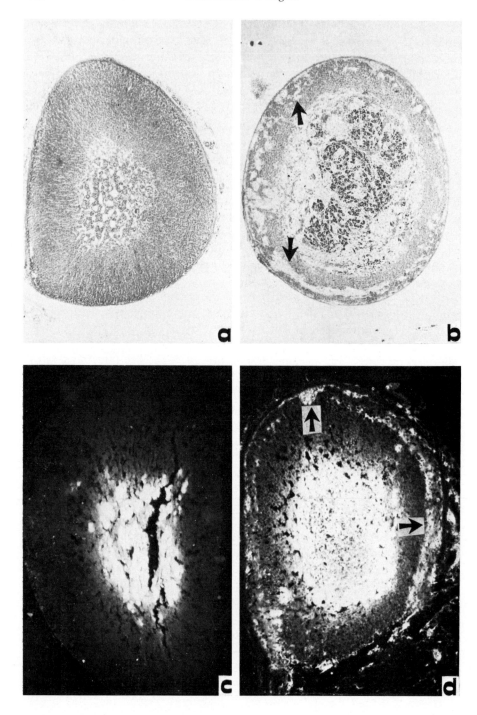

rather than yellow colour typical of sympathetic noradrenergic neurons. The fibres emerging from these cells branch in large fibre bundles among the external cortical layer of the gland (Fig. 5c, d). The transformation of chromaffin cells in sympathetic cells occurs also in abdominal ganglia and in the carotid body (Levi-Montalcini and Aloe, 1980b). Other authors in this volume will present evidence for the *in vitro* effects of NGF on fully differentiated glandular chromaffin cells.

ACCESS AND MECHANISM(S) OF ACTION OF NGF IN ITS TARGET CELLS

An important and still unsolved question is the extent to which immature and fully differentiated nerve cells are receptive to the action of trophic or toxic agents which may exert their action on the cell perikarya or after binding to nerve endings and retrograde axonal transport. The results of studies on NGF–sympathetic nerve cell interaction indicate the coexistence of both systems, although they do not permit an evaluation of their relative efficiency during developmental and postdevelopmental stages. The existence of a non-axonal-mediated transport system is indicated by three lines of evidence: (1) the NGF growth response occurs in embryonic nerve cells in the developing organism (chick embryos and rat foetuses) even before the formation of the axon, and in precursors of the glandular chromaffin cells; (2) the *in vitro* response materializes in embryonic nerve cells divested of their axon through mechanical or enzymatic dissociation; (3) specific high-affinity receptors for NGF were detected by different groups of investigators and different methodologies on the target-cell perikarya (Greene and Shooter, 1980; Thoenen and Barde, 1980).

A NGF–retrograde axonal transport system first demonstrated by Hendry *et al.* (1974) and its functional role have been firmly established through this and subsequent investigations.

The demonstration that NGF after binding to receptors distributed on the target-cell perikarya or localized on the nerve endings becomes internalized and gains access to the cell cytoplasm or, according to different groups (Yankner and Shooter, 1979; Andres *et al.*, 1977; Marchisio *et al.*, 1980), also to the nuclear compartment, afforded new approaches to the study of the mechanisms of action of this protein molecule. Since it is impossible to present even in a summary fashion the many hypotheses put forward in recent

Figure 5 Transverse sections of adrenal glands of 10-day-old rats treated pre- and postnatally with saline (a, c) or with NGF (b, d). (a, b) Toluidine stain, ×45 (c, d) Histofluorescence technique, ×64. Note in (b) and (d) the invasion of the external gland cortical layer by nerve fibres (arrows) emerging from the newly formed sympathetic nerve cell aggregates in the adrenal medulla

years, we shall list here only those now under intensive investigation in different laboratories.

The main, still unanswered, question is whether the multiple effects of NGF in its target cells involve multiple mechanisms of action or can be traced to a single action which in turn would promote a cascade of sequential processes leading to enhanced production of axonal material cell, hypertrophy and the other effects described in previous pages. In their recent review article Greene and Shooter (1980) favour the first alternative.

Another equally open question is whether the NGF molecule exerts a direct regulatory effect on the expression of genetic information at the nuclear transcription or ribosomal translational levels, or whether it acts through a second messenger. In discussing this problem and expressing a preference for the second-messenger hypothesis' which in turn could act on the genome expression or on cytoplasmic constituents, Thoenen and Barde (1980) consider it unlikely that cyclic AMP and cyclic GMP act as second messengers and they leave unanswered the question of the nature of this putative second messenger.

A different viewpoint is championed by Calissano and coworkers. These authors demonstrated a direct and selective *in vitro* binding of the NGF molecule to tubulin and actin, the two respective precursors of microtubules and microfilaments (Calissano and Cozzari, 1974). In subsequent studies they showed that NGF interacts in a highly specific fashion with cytoskeletal filamentous structures (Calissano *et al.*, 1978, 1980). These findings would favour the hypothesis that the primary and possibly main if not necessarily only mechanism of action of NGF consists in its selective binding to microtubule and microfilament precursors directly or through the agency of associated proteins.

CONCLUDING REMARKS

Almost three decades after the discovery of the release by some mouse sarcomas of a protein molecule endowed with a potent nerve growth promoting activity in sympathetic nerve cells of chick embryos, we believe that we have barely uncovered the most striking effects elicited by this molecule, whose (according to the authors) mechanism of action at the molecular level is still largely a matter of speculation and of future work. Even if much remains to be learned about the spectrum of action of NGF, the main contribution which we owe to the discovery of this remarkable stimulus–response system is to have focussed attention once again on the peripheral adrenergic neuron. It should be remembered that this cell has already many times in the past given invaluable contributions to our knowledge of fundamental properties of nerve cells, irrespective of their location in the central or peripheral nervous system and of their specific function. Without the sympathetic nerve cells, which hold a most favourable position for their inspection and experimental analysis, the humoral nature of the transmission of the nerve impulse, the metabolic pathways which lead to the biosynthesis of this and of other neurotransmitters, as well as their enzymatic degradation, release and reuptake mechanisms, would probably still be shrouded in mystery. Today this cell has come again to the forefront of research with the revelation of the all-powerful role played by NGF in its growth and differentiation and in the guidance of sympathetic nerve fibres. Apart from the significance of these findings for our understanding of the ontogenesis and functional organization of autonomic ganglia, perhaps the most significant contribution of these investigations is again, as it has been in the past, to have provided a unique model to uncover principles of general validity for the billions of nerve cells which form the central and peripheral nervous system.

ACKNOWLEDGEMENT
This investigation was supported in part by the 'Progetto Finalizzato Medicina Preventiva e Riabilitativa' of the Italian National Research Council (C.N.R.).

REFERENCES

Aloe, L., and Levi-Montalcini, R. (1979a). Nerve growth factor induced overgrowth of axotomized superior cervical ganglia in neonatal rats: similarities and differences with NGF effects in chemically axotomized sympathetic ganglia. *Arch. Ital. Biol.*, **117**, 287–307.

Aloe, L., and Levi-Montalcini, R. (1979b). Nerve Growth Factor *in-vivo* induced transformation of immature chromaffin cells in sympathetic neurons: effects of antiserum to the Nerve Growth Factor. *Proc. Natl. Acad. Sci. U.S.A.*, **76**, 1246–1250.

Aloe, L., Mugnaini, E., and Levi-Montalcini, R. (1975). Light and electron micro-scope studies on the excessive growth of sympathetic ganglia in rats injected daily from birth with 6-OHDA and NGF. *Arch. Ital. Biol.*, **113**, 326–353.

Andres, R. Y., Jeng, I., and Bradshaw, R. A. (1977). Nerve growth factor receptors: Identification of distinct classes in plasma membranes and nuclei of embryonic dorsal root neurons. *Proc. Natl. Acad. Sci. U.S.A.*, **74**, 2785–2789.

Angeletti, R. H., and Bradshaw, R. A. (1971). Nerve growth factor from mouse submaxillary gland: Amino acid sequence. *Proc. Natl. Acad. Sci. U.S.A.*, **68**, 2417–2420.

Angeletti, P. U., and Levi-Montalcini, R. (1970). Sympathetic nerve cell destruction in newborn mammals by 6-hydroxydopamine. *Proc. Natl. Acad. Sci. U.S.A.*, **65**, 114–121.

Angeletti, P. U., Liuzzi, A., Levi-Montalcini, R., and Gandini Attardi, D. (1964a). Effects of a nerve growth factor on glucose metabolism by sympathetic and sensory nerve cells. *Biochim. Biophys. Acta*, **90**, 445–450.

Angeletti, P. U., Liuzzi, A., and Levi-Montalcini, R. (1964b). Stimulation of lipid biosynthesis in sympathetic and sensory ganglia by a specific nerve growth factor. *Biochim. Biophys. Acta*, **84**, 778–781.

Angeletti, P. U., Gandini Attardi, D., Toschi, G., Salvi, M. L., and Levi-Montalcini, R. (1965). Metabolic aspects of the effect of nerve growth factor on sympathetic and sensory ganglia: protein and ribonucleic acid synthesis. *Biochim. Biophys. Acta*, **95**, 111–120.

Angeletti, P. U., Levi-Montalcini, R., and Calissano, P. (1968). The nerve growth factor: chemical properties and metabolic effects. *Adv. Enzymol.*, **31**, 51–75.

Angeletti, P. U., Levi-Montalcini, R., and Caramia, F. (1972). Structural and ultrastructural changes in developing sympathetic ganglia induced by guanethidine. *Brain Res.*, **43**, 515–525.

Barka, T. (1980). Biologically active polypeptides in submandibular glands. *J. Histochem. Cytochem.*, **28**, 836–859.

Berger, E., and Shooter, E. M. (1977). The biosynthesis and processing of pro β-NGF, a biosynthetic precursor to β-nerve growth factor. *Proc. Natl. Acad. Sci. U.S.A.*, **74**, 3647–3651.

Berger, E. A., and Shooter, E. M. (1978). The biosynthesis of β-nerve growth factor in mouse submaxillary gland. *J. Biol. Chem.*, **243**, 804–810.

Bocchini, V., and Angeletti, P. U. (1969). The nerve growth factor: purification as a 30 000 molecular weight protein. *Proc. Natl. Acad. Sci. U.S.A.*, **64**, 787–794.

Borsellino, A. (1980). Neuronal death in embryonic development: a model for selective cell competition and dominance. In *Multidisciplinary Approach to Brain Development* (Eds. C. Di Benedetta, R. Balazs, G. Gambos, and G. Porcellati), pp. 495–502, Elsevier/North-Holland Biomedical Press, Amsterdam.

Bradshaw, R. A. (1978). Nerve growth factor. *Annu. Rev. Biochem.*, **47**, 191–216.

Bueker, E. D. (1948). Implantation of tumors in the hind limb field of the embryonic chick and the developmental response of the lumbosacral nervous system. *Anat. Rec.*, **102**, 369–389.

Burton, L. E., Wilson, W. H., and Shooter, E. M. (1978). Nerve growth factor in mouse saliva. Rapid isolation procedures for and characterization of 7S nerve growth factor. *J. Biol. Chem.*, **253**, 7807–7812.

Calissano, P., and Cozzari, C. (1974). Interaction of nerve growth factor with the mouse brain neurotubule protein(s). *Proc. Natl. Acad. Sci. U.S.A.*, **71**, 2131–2135.

Calissano, P., Monaco, G., Levi, A., Menesini Chen, M. G., Chen, J. S., and Levi-Montalcini, R. (1976). New developments in the study of NGF-tubulin interaction. In *Contractile Systems in Non-muscle Tissues* (Eds. S. V. Perry, A. Margreth and R. S. Adelstein), pp. 201–211, Elsevier/North-Holland, Biomedical Press, Amsterdam.

Calissano, P., Monaco, G., Castellani, L., Mercanti, D., and Levi, A. (1978). Nerve growth factor potentiates actomyosin ATPase. *Proc. Natl. Acad. Sci. U.S.A.*, **75**, 2210–2215.

Calissano, P., Castellani, L., Monaco, G., Mercanti, D., and Levi, A. (1988). Studies on the mechanism of NGF-induced neurite growth. In *Nerve Cells, Transmitters and Behaviour* (Ed. R. Levi-Montalcini), pp. 65–86, Elsevier/North-Holland Biomedical Press, Amsterdam.

Campenot, R. B. (1977). Local control of neurite development by nerve growth factor. *Proc. Natl. Acad. Sci. U.S.A.*, **74**, 4516–4519.

Caramia, F., and Angeletti, P. U. (1962). Differentiation of serous and mucous components of salivary gland by alcian blue and a counterstain. *Stain Technol.*, **37**, 125–127.

Charlwood, K. A., Lamont, D. M., and Banks, B. E. C. (1972). Apparent orienting effects produced by nerve growth factor. In *Nerve Growth Factor and its Antiserum* (Eds. E. Zaimis and J. Knight), pp. 102–107, Athlone Press of the University of London.

Cohen, S. (1958a). A nerve growth-promoting protein. In *Chemical Basis of Development* (Eds. W. D. McElroy and B. Glass), pp. 665–667, Johns Hopkins Press, Baltimore.

Cohen, S. (1960). Purification of a nerve growth promoting protein from the mouse salivary gland and its neurocytotoxic antiserum. *Proc. Natl. Acad. Sci. U.S.A.*, **46**, 302–311.

Cohen, S., and Levi-Montalcini, R. (1956). A nerve growth factor stimulating factor isolated from snake venom. *Proc. Natl. Acad. Sci. U.S.A.*, **42**, 571–574.

Cohen, S., Levi-Montalcini, R., and Hamburger, V. (1954). A nerve growth stimulating factor isolated from sarcoma 37 and 180. *Proc. Natl. Acad. Sci. U.S.A.*, **40**, 1014–1018.

Cowan, M. V. (1973). Neuronal death as a regulative mechanism in the control of cell number in the nervous system. In *Development and Aging in the Nervous System* (Eds. M. Rockstein and L. M. Sussman), pp. 19–41, Academic Press, New York, London.

Eränkö, O., and Eränkö, L. (1971). Histochemical evidence of chemical sympathectomy of guanethidine in newborn rats. *Histochem. J.*, **3**, 451–456.

Garrels, I. J., and Schubert, D. (1979). Modulation of protein synthesis by nerve growth factor. *J. Biol. Chem.*, **254**, 7978–7985.

Goldstein, L. A., Reynolds, C. P., and Perez-Polo, J. R. (1978). Isolation of human nerve growth factor from placental tissue. *Neurochem. Res.*, **3**, 175–183.

Greene, L. A., and Rein, G. (1977). Release storage and uptake of catecholamines by a clonal cell line of nerve growth factor (NGF) responsive pheochromocytoma cells. *Brain Res.*, **129**, 247–263.

Greene, L. A., and Shooter, E. M. (1980). The nerve growth factor. Biochemistry synthesis and mechanism of action. *Annu. Rev. Neurosci.*, **3**, 353–402.

Greene, L. A., Burnstein, D. E., McGuire, J., and Black, C. (1979). Cell culture studies on mechanism of action of nerve growth factor. *Soc. Neurosci. Symp.*, **4**, 153–171.

Gundersen, R. W., and Barrett, J. N. (1979). Neurnal chemotaxis. Chick dorsal root axons turn toward high concentration of nerve growth factor. *Science*, **206**, 1079–1080.

Hamburger, V. (1975). Cell death in the development of the lateral motor column of the chick embryo. *J. Comp. Neurol.*, **160**, 535–546.

Harper, G. P., and Thoenen, H. (1980). The distribution of nerve growth factor in the male sex organs of mammals. *J. Neurochem.*, **77**, 391–402.

Harper, G. P., Barde, Y. A., Burnstock, G., Carstairs, J. R., Dennison, M. E., Suda, K., and Vernon, C. A. (1979). Guinea pig prostate is a rich source of nerve growth factor. *Nature*, **279**, 160–162.

Hendry, I. A. (1977). Cell division in the developing sympathetic nervous system. *J. Neurocytol.*, **6**, 299–309.

Hendry, J. A., and Campbell, J. (1976). Morphometric analysis of rat superior cervical ganglion after axotomy and nerve growth factor treatment. *J. Neurocytol.*, **5**, 351–360.

Hendry, I. A., Stockel, K., Thoenen, H., and Iversen, L. L. (1974). The retrograde axonal transport of nerve growth factor. *Brain Res.*, **68**, 103–121.

Hollyday, M., and Hamburger, V. (1976). Reduction of the naturally occurring motor neuron loss by enlargement of the periphery. *J. Comp. Neurol.*, **170**, 311–320.

Ishii, D. N., and Shooter, E. M. (1975). Regulation of nerve growth factor synthesis in mouse submaxillary glands by testosterone. *J. Neurochem.*, **25**, 843–851.

Johnson, E. M., and Aloe, L. (1978). Suppression of the *in-vitro* and *in-vivo* cytotoxic effects of guanethidine in sympathetic neurons by concomitant administration of nerve growth factor. *Brain Res.*, **141**, 105–118.

Juul, P., and Sand, O. (1971). Guanethidine determination in rat sympathetic ganglia following prolonged administration of guanethidine. *Acta Pharmacol. Toxicol.*, **29**, 25.

Larrabee, M. G. (1972). Metabolism during development in sympathetic ganglia of chickens: effects of age, Nerve Growth Factor and metabolic inhibitors. In *Nerve Growth Factor and its Antiserum* (Eds. E. Zaimis and J. Knight), pp. 71–88, The Athlone Press of the University of London.

Letourneau, P. C. (1979). Chemotactic response of nerve fibre elongation to Nerve Growth Factor. *Dev. Biol.*, **66**, 183–196.

Levi-Montalcini, R. (1950). The origin and development of the visceral system in the spinal cord of the chick embryo. *J. Morphol.*, **86**, 253–284.

Levi-Montalcini, R. (1952). Effect of mouse tumour transplantation on the nervous system. *Ann. N.Y. Acad. Sci.*, **55**, 330–343.

Levi-Montalcini, R. (1953). *In-vivo* and *in-vitro* experiments on the effect of mouse sarcoma 180 and 37 on the sensory and sympathetic system of the chick embryo. *Proc. XIV Int. Cong. Zool. Copenhagen*, 309.

Levi-Montalcini, R. (1958). Chemical stimulation of nerve growth. In *Chemical Basis of Development* (Eds. W. D. McElroy and B. Glass), pp. 646–664, Johns Hopkins Press, Baltimore.

Levi-Montalcini, R. (1966). The nerve growth factor: its mode of action on sensory and sympathetic nerve cells. *Harvey Lect.*, **60**, 217–259.

Levi-Montalcini, R., and Aloe, L. (1980a). Synthesis and release of the nerve growth factor from the mouse submaxillary salivary glands: Hormonal and neuronal regulatory mechanisms. In *Hormones and Cell Regulation* (Eds. J. A. Dumont and J. Nunez), Elsevier/North-Holland Biomedical Press, Amsterdam.

Levi-Montalcini, R., and Aloe, L. (1980b). Tropic, trophic and transforming effects of nerve growth factor. In *Histochemistry and Cell Biology of Autonomic Neurons, SIF Cells and Paraneurons* (Eds. O. Eränkö, S. Soinila and H. Päivärinta), *Advances in Biochemical Psychopharmacology*, Vol. 25, pp. 3–16, Raven Press, New York.

Levi-Montalcini, R., and Angeletti, P. U. (1961). Biological properties of a nerve growth promoting protein and its antiserum. In *Regional Neurochemistry, Proceedings 4th International Neurochemical Symposium* (Eds. S. S. Kety and J. Elkes), pp. 362–376, Pergamon Press, New York.

Levi-Montalcini, R., and Angeletti, P. U. (1963). Essential role of the nerve growth factor in the survival and maintenance of dissociated sensory and sympathetic nerve cells *in vitro*. *Dev. Biol.*, **7**, 655–659.

Levi-Montalcini, R., and Angeletti, P. U. (1964). Hormonal control of the NGF in the submaxillary glands of mice. In *Salivary Glands and Their Secretion* (Eds. L. M. Sreenby and J. Mayer), pp. 129–141, Pergamon Press, New York.

Levi-Montalcini, R., and Angeletti, P. U. (1966). *Immunosympathectomy*. Pharmacol. Rev., **18**, 619–628.

Levi-Montalcini, R., and Angeletti, P. U. (1968a). Nerve growth factor. *Physiol. Rev.*, **48**, 534–565.

Levi-Montalcini, R., and Angeletti, P. U. (1968b). Biological aspects of the nerve growth factor. In *Growth of the Nervous System, Ciba Foundation Symposium* (Eds. G. E. W. Wolstenholme and M. O'Connor), pp. 126–147, Churchill, London.

Levi-Montalcini, R., and Booker, B. (1960a). Excessive growth of the sympathetic ganglia evoked by a protein isolated from mouse salivary glands. *Proc. Natl. Acad. Sci. U.S.A.*, **46**, 373–384.

Levi-Montalcini, R., and Booker, B. (1960b). Destruction of the sympathetic ganglia in mammals dy an antiserum to the nerve growth protein. *Proc. Natl. Acad. Sci. U.S.A.*, **46**, 384–391.

Levi-Montalcini, R., and Cohen, S. (1956). *In vitro* and *in-vivo* effects of a nerve growth stimulating agent isolated from snake venom. *Proc. Natl. Acad. Sci. U.S.A.*, **42**, 695–699.

Levi-Montalcini, R., and Hamburger, V. (1951). Selective growth-stimulating effects of mouse sarcoma on the sensory and sympathetic nervous system of the chick embryo. *J. Exp. Zool.*, **116**, 321–362.

Levi-Montalcini, R., and Hamburger, V. (1953). A diffusible agent of mouse sarcoma producing hyperplasia of sympathetic ganglia and hyperneurotization of viscera in the chick embryo. *J. Exp. Zool.*, **123**, 233–278.

Levi-Montalcini, R., Meyer, H., and Hamburger, V. (1954). *In-vitro* experiments on the effects of mouse sarcoma 180 and 37 on the spinal and sympathetic ganglia of the chick embryo. *Cancer Res.*, **14**, 49–57.

Levi-Montalcini, R., Caramia, F., Luse, S. A., and Angeletti, P. U. (1968). *In-vitro* effects of the nerve growth factor on the fine structure of the sensory nerve cells. *Brain Res.*, **8**, 347–362.

Levi-Montalcini, R., Angeletti, R. H., and Angeletti, P. U. (1972). The nerve growth factor. In *The Structure and Function of Nervous Tissues* (Ed. H. G. Bourne), pp. 1–38, Academic Press, New York and London.

Marchisio, P. C., Naldini, L., and Calissano, P. (1980). Intracellular distribution of NGF in rat pheochromocytoma PC12 cells: evidence for a perinuclear and intra-nuclear location. *Proc. Natl. Acad. Sci. U.S.A.*, **77**, 1656–1660.

Menesini Chen, M. G., Chen, J. S., Calissano, P., and Levi-Montalcini, R. (1977). Nerve growth factor prevents vinblastine destructive effects on sympathetic ganglia in newborn mice. *Proc. Natl. Acad. Sci. U.S.A.*, **74**, 5559–5563.

Menesini Chen, M. G., Chen, J. S., and Levi-Montalcini, R. (1978). Sympathetic nerve fibers ingrowth in the central nervous system of neonatal rodents upon intracerebral NGF injection. *Arch. Ital. Biol.*, **116**, 53–84.

Murphy, R. A., Saide, J. D., Blanchard, M. H., and Young, M. (1977). Nerve growth factor in mouse serum and saliva: role of the submandibular gland. *Proc. Natl. Acad. Sci. U.S.A.*, **74**, 2330–2333.

Oppenheim, R. W., and Chu-Wang, I. Wu (1977). Spontaneous cell death of spinal motor neurons following peripheral innervation in the chick embryo. *Brain Res.*, **125**, 154–160.

Owman, C., and Sjöstrand, N. O. (1965). Short adrenergic neurons and catechola-mine-containing cells in vas deferens and accessory male genital glands of different mammals. *Z. Zellforch. Mikrosk. Anat.*, **66**, 300–320.

Owman, C., Sjöberg, N. O., and Sjöstrand, N. O. (1974). Short adrenergic neurons, peripheral neuroendocrine mechanisms. In *Amine Fluorescence Histochemistry* (Eds. M. Fujiwara and C. Tanaka), pp. 47–66, Igaku Shoin, Tokyo.

Page, I. H., and Dustan, H. P. (1959). A new potent antyhypertensive drug. Preliminary study of [2-(octahydro-1-azocinyl)-ethyl] guanethidine sulfate (guanethidine). *J. Am. Med. Assoc.*, **170**, 1265–1271.

Pilar, G., and Landmesser, L. (1976). Ultrastructural differences during embryonic cell death in normal and peripherally deprived ciliar ganglia. *J. Cell Biol.*, **68**, 339–359.

Pittman, R., Oppenheim, R. W., and Chu-Wang, I. Wu. (1978). Beta-bungarotoxin induced neuronal degeneration in the chick embryo spinal cord. *Brain Res.*, **153**, 199–204.

Porter, C. C., Totaro, J. S., and Stone, C. A. (1963). Effect of 6-hydroxydopamine and some other compounds on the concentration of norepinephrine in the hearts of mice. *J. Pharmacol.*, **140**, 308–316.

Rutishauer, U., and Edelman, G. M. (1980). Effects of fasciculation on the outgrowth of neurites from spinal ganglia in culture. *J. Cell Biol.*, **87**, 370–378.

Sachs, C., and Johnson, G. (1975). Mechanisms of action of 6-hydroxydopamine. *Biochem. Pharmacol.*, **24**, 1–8.

Server, A., and Shooter, E. M. (1977). Nerve growth factor. *Adv. Protein Chem.*, **31**, 339–409.

Steiner, G. (1972). Immunosympathectomy as a tool in metabolic studies. In *Immunosympathectomy* (Eds. G. Steiner and E. Schönbaum), pp. 159–175. Elsevier, Amsterdam.

Steiner, G., and Schönbaum, E. (Eds.) (1972). *Immunosympathectomy*, Elsevier, Amsterdam.

Thoenen, H. (1971). Biochemical alterations induced by 6-hydroxydopamine in peripheral adrenergic neurons. In *6-Hydroxydopamine and Catecholamine Neurons* (Eds. T. Malmfors and H. Theonen), pp. 75–86, North-Holland, Amsterdam.

Thoenen, H., and Barde, Y. A. (1980). Physiology of nerve growth factor. *Physiol. Rev.*, **60**, 1284–1335.

Thoenen, H., Angeletti, P. U., Levi-Montalcini, R., and Kettler, R. (1971). Selective induction by nerve growth factor of tyrosine hydroxylase and dopamine-β-hydroxylase in the rat superior cervical ganglia. *Proc. Natl. Acad. Sci. U.S.A.*, **68**, 1598–1602.

Tischler, A. S., and Greene, L. A. (1975). Nerve growth factor-induced process formation by cultured rat pheochromocytoma cell. *Nature*, **258**, 341–342.

Tranzer, J. P., and Richards, J. G. (1971). Fine structural aspects of the effect of 6-hydroxydopamine on peripheral adrenergic neurons. In *6-Hydroxydopamine and Catecholamine Neurons* (Eds. T. Malmfors and H. Thoenen), pp. 15–32, North-Holland, Amsterdam.

Varon, S., Nomura, J., and Shooter, E. M. (1968). Reversible dissociation of the mouse nerve growth factor protein into different subunits. *Biochemistry*, **7**, 1296–1303.

Wallace, L. J., and Partlow, L. M. (1976). α-Adrenergic regulation of secretion of mouse saliva rich in nerve growth factor. *Proc. Natl. Acad. Sci. U.S.A.*, **73**, 4210–4214.

Wlodawer, A., Hodgson, K. O., and Shooter, E. M. (1975). Crystallization of nerve growth factor from mouse submaxillary glands. *Proc. Natl. Acad. Sci. U.S.A.*, **72**, 777–779.

Yankner, B. A., and Shooter, E. M. (1979). Nerve growth factor in the nucleus: Interaction with receptors on the nuclear membrane. *Proc. Natl. Acad. Sci. U.S.A.*, **76**, 1269–1273.

Young, M., Oger, J., Blanchard, M. H., Asdourian, H., Amos, H., and Arnason, B. G. W. (1975). Secretion of a nerve growth factor by primary chick fibroblast cultures. *Science*, **187**, 361–362.

Yu, M. W., Nikoduevic, B., Laksmanan, J., Rowe, V., MacDonnem, P., and Guroff, G. (1977). Nerve Growth Factor and the activity of tyrosine hydroxylase in organ cultures of superior cervical ganglia. *J. Neurochem.*, **28**, 835–842.

Zanini, A., and Angeletti, P. U. (1971). Studies of the nerve growth factor by microcomplement fixation. Effects of physical, chemical and enzymatic treatments. *Biochim. Biophys. Acta*, **229**, 724–729.

Zanini, A., Angeletti, P. U., and Levi-Montalcini, R. (1968). Immunochemical properties of the nerve growth factor. *Proc. Natl. Acad. Sci. U.S.A.*, **61**, 835–842.

Differentiation of Avian Autonomic Ganglia

N. M. LE DOUARIN and J. SMITH

Institut d'Embryologie du CNRS et du Collège de France,
49 bis, Avenue de la Belle-Gabrielle,
94130 Nogent-sur-Marne, France

The embryonic origin of the autonomic nervous system from the neural crest has become a particularly well-documented subject during the last ten years. The introduction of appropriate methods to investigate the migration of cells during embryogenesis and the development of increasingly efficient cell-culture techniques have significantly increased our knowledge of the development of the ganglia and nerves which innervate the smooth muscles and glands of the body.

This chapter will be devoted first to the *in vivo* study of the development of the autonomic nervous system in the birds as carried out by means of the quail-chick chimaera system in the laboratories of the authors and others. Secondly, the *in vitro* analysis of the differentiation of the autonomic ganglion cells will be reviewed, once again with particular reference to the avian model.

The avian embryo, actually that of the chick (*Gallus gallus* L.), has long been the choice material on which the investigations on the development of the peripheral nervous system have been carried out. This was made possible by the availability of the embryo during the full span of development. Such an experimental model allowed free rein to the ingenuity of a number of experimenters who were able to disturb, in a controlled manner, the normal course of development in order to discover its rules. The various techniques used for this purpose have been reviewed several times: see, for example, Hörstadius (1950), Weston (1970), Le Douarin (1976, 1980, 1982).

EMBRYONIC ORIGIN OF THE AUTONOMIC GANGLIA AND PLEXUSES

Historical survey

Mesodermal origin of autonomic ganglia

The differentiation of local mesodermal cells into visceral neurons was, historically, the oldest theory put forward to account for the emergence of the autonomic system (Remak, 1847). This view was developed later by several authors (Fusari, 1893; Tello, 1924, 1925, 1945; Levi-Montalcini, 1947; Keuning, 1948). Tello (1945) described the formation of two cellular trunks close to the aorta in the chick embryo from 68 to 82 hours of incubation. He noticed that these cells aggregate about the segmental arteries and migrate along them to form the sympathetic trunk. The apparent similarity between the sympathoblasts and the endothelium of the aorta revealed with the techniques used in those days suggested to him that they might have a common origin.

Origin of autonomic ganglia from the neural primordium

These ganglia were first thought to be derived from the spinal ganglia, or from the neural crest via the spinal ganglia (Schenk and Birdsall, 1880; Onodi, 1886; His, 1897; Müller and Ingvar, 1923; Van Campenhout, 1931, 1947; Yntema and Hammond, 1945; Hammond and Yntema, 1947; Hammond, 1949; Wenger, 1950). The opinion also prevailed in certain quarters that autonomic ganglion cells originate primarily, if not entirely, from the neural tube (Kuntz, 1910, 1926; Abel, 1912; Jones, 1937, 1941, 1942; Brizzee, 1949; Brizzee and Kuntz, 1950).

An attractive idea developed by these workers was that the sympathetic and parasympathetic ganglion cells could arise from the same region of the neural primordium (i.e. the ependymal epithelium of the neural tube itself) as that from which the preganglionic cells are derived. The migration pathway of the ganglionic neuronal precursors would be, according to this view, the ventral nerve roots and the vagus nerve for sympathetic and enteric neurons, respectively.

The hypothesis of a mesodermal origin for the autonomic system was ruled out by experiments in which the neural primordium was partly removed or destroyed *in situ*. Large deficiencies of the peripheral nervous system always resulted from such interventions, indicating that its origin was closely linked to the development of the neural primordium (Van Campenhout, 1930a; Yntema and Hammond, 1947; Strudel, 1953). In view of the fact that the wide potentialities of migration and differentiation of neural crest cells were already a well-documented matter, it was accepted by most authors in the fifties that the peripheral nervous system arises mostly, if not entirely, from the neural crest itself rather than from the neural tube (see Hörstadius, 1950).

However, the purely neural crest origin of all the cell components of the peripheral nerves, ganglia and plexuses could only be definitively demonstrated by experiments in which fragments of labelled neural crest were implanted, for example, between the neural tube and the somitic axis (Le Lièvre et al., 1980) or in an orthotopic situation after removal of the host neural crest (Johnston, 1966; Noden, 1978a, b). The label, which was provided either by the quail-chick combination system (Le Douarin, 1969, 1971, 1973) or by the isotopic labelling of the nucleus (Weston, 1963), showed the peripheral host ganglia to be made up of elements belonging to the graft. Furthermore, selective removal of the neural crest in the embryo *in situ* has also been performed and has resulted in the lack of peripheral ganglia at the level of the operation.

Finally, heterospecific grafting of the neural crest (excluding the neural tube) between quail and chick embryos demonstrated an exclusively neural crest origin of the Schwann cells lining the peripheral nerves (Teillet, unpublished observations).

Level of origin and migration pathways of autonomic ganglion cell precursors

Sympathetic chains, plexuses, adrenal medulla, enteric ganglia

After the ganglia of the autonomic nervous system and the adrenal medulla had been recognized to arise from the neural primordium, the level of origin of their various components remained for a while a controversial matter. Some authors considered the vagal level of the neural primordium to be the only source of enteric ganglia (Yntema and Hammond, 1945, 1947, 1954, 1955), while others also attributed a role in the constitution of these structures to the trunk crest (Abel, 1909, 1912; Andrew, 1964, 1969, 1970, 1971; Van Campenhout, 1930b, 1931, 1932; Kuntz, 1953; Uchida, 1927).

In view of these discrepancies, it seemed worthwhile to apply to this problem the quail-chick chimaera system which, due to differences in the distribution of heterochromatin in the resting nucleus of quail and chick cells, provided a marking technique by which neural crest cell migration could be followed throughout ontogeny (Le Douarin, 1969, 1971, 1973). This study, carried out by Le Douarin and Teillet (1971, 1973), consisted in grafting fragments (corresponding to a length of 4 to 6 somites) of quail neural primordium into chick embryos (and vice versa) along the entire neural axis. The developmental stages of host and donor embryos were identical, but varied according to the level elected for the operation in order to ensure that crest cell migration had not started at the time of the intervention. The migrating neural crest cells were subsequently observed on serial sections of the trunk of the host (for the sympathetic chain and the adrenomedulla) and of its digestive tract (for the enteric and intravisceral ganglia). A correspondence was established between the level of the graft and the definitive location of the ganglion cells, as a result of the stability of the labelling provided by the quail-chick cell association. A fate-map of the autonomic structures could then be constructed in which the origin of the sympathetic and parasympathetic ganglia was traced back to the various levels of the neural axis (Fig. 1). The sympathetic chain derives from the entire length of the neural crest, from the

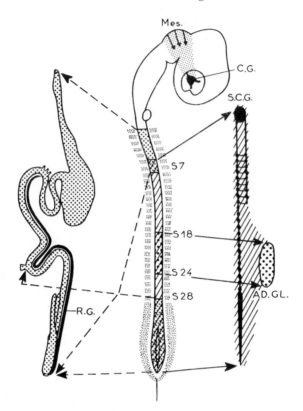

Figure 1 Levels of origin of adrenomedullary cells and autonomic ganglion cells. The spinal neural crest caudal to the level of the 5th somite gives rise to the ganglia of the orthosympathetic chain. The adrenomedullary cells originate from the spinal neural crest between the levels of somites 18 and 24. The vagal neural crest (somites 1–7) gives rise to the enteric ganglia of the preumbilical region, the ganglia of the postumbilical gut originating from both the vagal and lumbosacral neural crest. The ganglion of Remak (R.G.) is derived from the lumbosacral neural crest (posterior to the somite-28 level). The ciliary ganglion (C.G.) is derived from the mesencephalic crest (Mes.). AD. GL = adrenal gland; S.C.G. = superior cervical ganglion. Reproduced by permission of Ciba Foundation

level of the 6th somite caudad, with the chromaffin cells of the adrenal medulla originating specifically from the level of somites 18–24. The great majority of enteric ganglia arise from 'vagal' neural crest, opposite somites 1–7. Neural crest cells from this region start migrating (at around stage 8–10 somites) in a ventral direction and become localized in the area of the branchial arches (Le Lièvre and Le Douarin, 1975).

The precursors of the enteric ganglia become incorporated in the developing wall of the foregut, which is of mesodermal origin. Thereafter, they migrate caudally along the gut, colonizing it up to the cloacal end, and giving rise to Meissner's and Auerbach's plexuses. An additional, although minor, contribution to these structures in the postumbilical gut is made by the lumbosacral level of the crest, which gives rise essentially to the parasympathetic ganglion of Remak (Teillet, 1978). An interesting observation made during this study was that, in the area of the trunk between somites 7 and 28, neural crest cell migration was strictly confined to the dorsal mesenchymal region derived from the somites and the intermediate cell mass. Except for the Schwann cells that followed the nerve bundles to the periphery, neural crest derivatives were restricted to the sensory and sympathetic chain ganglia, the aortic and adrenal plexuses, and the adrenomedullary cords. No cells were ever found in the mesonephros or the gonads; more importantly, they never penetrated the dorsal mesentery.

In contrast, orthotopic grafts carried out at the vagal and lumbosacral levels of the neural primordium resulted in colonization both of the dorsal mesenchyme and, to a lesser extent, the splanchnopleure. In addition, the migration of the lumbosacral neural crest gives rise to the ganglion of Remak (See Fig. 5) and some of the intramural neurons of the gut, and also to the caudal part of the sympathetic chain and to the coeliac and pelvic plexuses.

That the largest contribution to the myenteric plexuses is made by the vagal neural crest was also found by Allan and Newgreen (1980) who transplanted fragments of the developing chick gut on the chorioallantoic membrane at different ages and could in this way follow the anteroposterior progression of the crest-derived neuroblasts in the gut wall mesenchyme. The timing of crest cell migration along the gut was deduced from grafting experiments in which the vagal quail neural primordium had been transplanted isotopically and isochronically into a chick. The stage at which the last cells leave the crest has been evaluated to be about the 14-somite stage. During their progression in the splanchnopleural wall of the gut, they appear dispersed in the loose mesenchyme of the gut wall. They reach the level of the pancreatic ducts at about stage 20 of Hamburger and Hamilton (1951) and the umbilicus at about 5 days of incubation. The colorectum is not fully colonized before 8 days. When the muscular and connective structures of the gut are organized, the neural crest cells become distributed into ganglia located on each side of the circular muscle layer.

The sympathetic system of birds develops through the formation of two ganglionated chains (His, 1897; Tello, 1925). The primary chain is the first to appear and is situated at the posterior aspect of the aorta, but it has only a transient existence and disappears nearly completely around the 5th day of incubation in the chick. Some remnants of the primary trunks persist in the upper thoracic and cervical regions as the irregular cervical sympathetic trunk including the superior cervical ganglia (Fig. 2). The definitive chain and plexuses, the adrenal medulla and other abdominal paraganglia begin to form

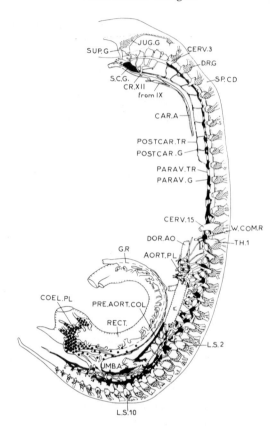

Figure 2 Diagram showing the general disposition of the sympathetic chains and plexuses of the 8-day-old chick embryo. AORT.PL = aortic plexus; CAR.A. = carotid artery; CERV.3 = cervical nerve 3; CERV.15 = cervical nerve 15; COEL.PL = coeliac plexus; CR.XII (from IX) = cranial nerve; DOR.AO = dorsal aorta; D.R.G. = dorsal root ganglion; G.R. ganglion of Remak; JUG.G. = jugular ganglion; L.S.2. = lumbosacral nerve 2; L.S.10 = lumbosacral nerve 10; PARAV.G = paravertebral ganglion; PARAV.TR = paravertebral trunk; POSTCAR.G = postcarotid ganglion; POSTCAR.TR = postcarotid trunk; PRE.AORT.COL = preaortic column; RECT. = rectum; S.C.G. = superior cervical ganglion; SP.CD = spinal cord; SUP.G = superior ganglion; TH.1 = thoracic nerve 1; UMB.A. = umbilical artery; W.COM.R = white communicating ramus. Modified from Yntema and Hammond (1945) and Hammond and Yntema (1947); reproduced by permission of Ciba Foundation

from day 5–6 in the chick. The superior cervical ganglion arises from the neural crest area corresponding to somites 5–10, as recently demonstrated by Teillet (unpublished). Behind the level of the 10th somite, sympathetic and dorsal root ganglia have a segmental distribution.

In our laboratory, the very early steps of gangliogenesis in the peripheral nervous system of the trunk have been the subject of investigations especially directed toward detailing the pathways followed by dorsal root and sympathetic precursor cells (Thiery *et al.*, 1982). It appeared that the first crest cells to migrate in a dorsoventral direction are those which penetrate the space located between two adjacent somites. The cells which leave the crest at the level of the bulk of the somitic block are stopped in their downward progression by the extreme narrowness of the extracellular space available at this stage between the somite and the neural tube. It is only later on (about 10 hours after the beginning of the migration) that this space widens. Although the precise mechanism of the sudden enlargement of the migration pathway is unknown, one possibility is that it is due to its high content of highly hydrophilic compounds such as hyaluronic acid and glycosaminoglycans (Pratt *et al.*, 1975; Derby, 1978), substances capable of increasing the extracellular space through a rapid hydration.

From about 10 hours following the onset of the migration, the stream of crest cells starts to slip down between somite and neural tube (Fig. 3a, b).

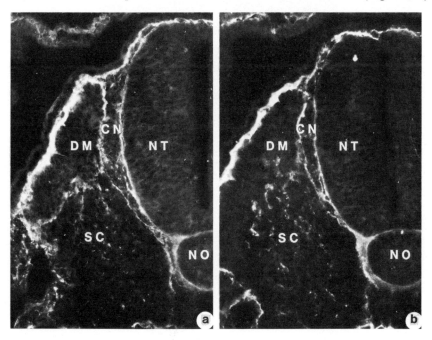

Figure 3 Transverse section of a 30-somite chick embryo at the level of the 15th somite. Immunocytochemical localization of fibronectin. (a) Section cut at the intersomitic level. Note the massive migration of crest cells (CN) in a fibronectin-rich space. (b) Section cut at the midsomite level. Crest-cell migration is relatively restricted. Note fibronectin-rich basement membrane of the dermomyotome (DM) and random deposits within the sclerotome (SC). NT = neural tube; NO = notochord. ×175

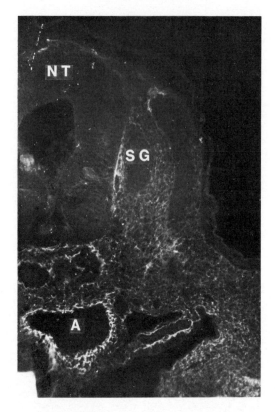

Figure 4 Transverse section of a 21-stage chick embryo at the level of the 15th somite. Fibronectin (revealed immunocytochemically) is abundant in the region of the aorta (A), but has completely disappeared within the developing sensory ganglion (SG). NT = neural tube. ×210

Simultaneously, the sclerotomal part of the somitic mesenchyme expands towards the mediodorsal line and the dorsoventral pathway then becomes obstructed. The crest cells are stopped and aggregate to form the primordium of the dorsal root ganglia at the transverse level of the somite (Fig. 4). Although it cannot be totally excluded that some of the neural cest cells which migrate at the transverse level of the somitic block reach more ventral areas (i.e. the level of the aorta and of the sympathetic chains), it seems very likely that two pathways of migration delineate the future sensory ganglion precursors from the autonomic cells from the beginning of the development of the neural crest.

According to the observations described above, the autonomic structures (sympathetic chains, plexuses, adrenal medulla and, posteriorly, the ganglion of Remak) arise from the cells which have migrated between two somites, whilst the sensory ganglia form from the cells migrating between somite and neural tube.

It was further observed that the migration phase of neural crest cells coincides with a period of time when the space in which the cells move is particularly rich both in hyaluronic acid and glycosaminoglycans (Toole and Trelstad, 1971; Toole, 1972; Meier and Hay, 1973; Trelstad *et al.*, 1974; Pratt *et al.*, 1975; Derby, 1978), and a large fibrillar molecule of the extracellular matrix, fibronectin (Duband and Thiery, 1982; Thiery *et al.*, 1982).

Ganglion of Remak

The main parasympathetic structure arising from the lumbosacral crest is the ganglion of Remak. The ontogeny of the Remak ganglion has been the subject of a detailed study by Teillet (1978). It is a complex structure, peculiar to birds, which develops in the dorsal mesentery (Fig. 1). The ganglioblasts arising from the neural crest posterior to the level of somite 28 accumulate first in the mesorectum at stage 24 of Hamburger and Hamilton in the chick, and at stage 18 of Zacchei (Zacchei, 1961) in the quail. They subsequently migrate cranially, along the ileum and jejunum, to reach the level of the hepatic and pancreatic ducts. In addition to masses of ganglion cells distributed throughout its length, the ganglion of Remak appears to be the route for descending and ascending nerve fibres. At the level of the cloaca, it is, as mentioned by Browne (1953), in close relationship with the pelvic plexus; the large nerve network that develops in the vicinity of the cloaca and the bursa of Fabricius contains mostly adrenergic cells which extend to the posterior end of the ganglion of Remak itself (Bennett and Malmfors, 1970; Teillet, 1978). The part of the ganglion corresponding to the anterior two-thirds of the rectum does not possess catecholamine(CA)-containing cells at any developmental stage, although numerous adrenergic fibres run along the whole length of the Remak ganglionated nerve.

The primordium of the ganglion of Remak was selectively labelled by means of a graft of quail neural primordium at the lumbosacral level of a chick embryo (Teillet, 1978). Subsequently, the complex consisting of colorectum plus mesorectum containing the labelled primordium of the Remak ganglion was taken from the chimaeric host at 5 days of incubation and grafted onto the chorioallantoic membrane of a chick host for 10 days. Passage of ganglioblasts from the ganglion of Remak to the gut was observed, showing that at least part of the lumbosacral ganglionic supply to the intramural innervation of the hind-gut migrated through the ganglion of Remak, in which the crest cells probably stop for a while before undertaking the last part of their ventral progression. Fig. 5 illustrates the different distribution of labelled cells arising in the autonomic trunk structures following isotopic grafts of the quail neural primordium at the vagal and lumbosacral regions of the neural axis of a chick embryo.

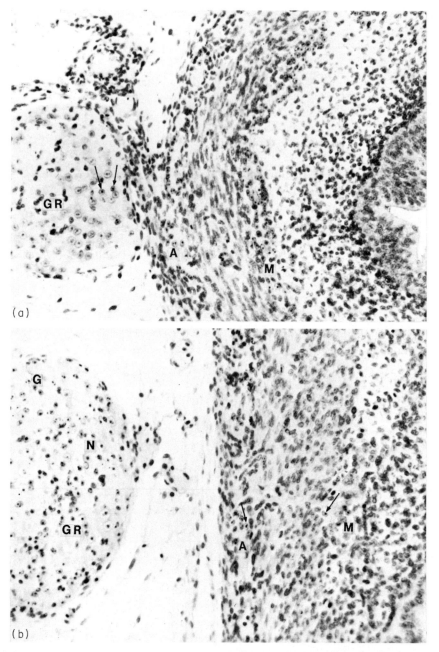

Figure 5 The embryological origin of the cells of the enteric nervous system of the
birds is evidenced on these sections of rectum by the quail-chick marking system. (a)
After an isotopic interspecific graft of the vagal neural primordium (somites 1–7)

The ciliary ganglion and other cephalic parasympathetic ganglia

The origin of the ciliary ganglion from the mesencephalic neural crest was first determined by Hammond and Yntema (1958) on the basis of extirpation experiments. This was later confirmed through the use of the quail-chick chimaera system by Narayanan and Narayanan (1978). Other parasympathetic ganglia besides the ciliary ganglion are present in the head, but there are relatively few studies on their ontogeny and on their structure and function. A neural crest origin has been mentioned by Noden (1978c) for lingual, submandibular, otic, sphenopalatine and ethnoid ganglia. This is supported by some of our observations on chimaeric embryos (Le Lièvre and Le Douarin, unpublished work).

PLASTICITY IN THE DEVELOPMENT OF AUTONOMIC GANGLION CELLS AS DEMONSTRATED BY *IN VIVO* TRANSPLANTATION EXPERIMENTS

Multipotentiality of the autonomic precursor population along the neural axis

The heterogeneity of neural crest with respect to its fate as cholinergic parasympathetic and adrenergic sympathetic autonomic derivatives (Fig. 1) suggested that the cells at each level of the crest were already determined before migration, i.e. that the crest was a mosaic-like structure made up of cells committed early to a given type of differentiation.

By changing the initial position of the crest cells along the neural axis before they started migrating, it could be shown that this interpretation was not correct. Both the cephalic and vagal neural crest, transplanted at the level of somites 18–24 ('adrenomedullary' level of the crest), provided adrenomedullary-like cells for the suprarenal paraganglia. Conversely, the cervicotruncal neural crest, grafted into the vagal region, colonized the gut and gave rise to cholinergic enteric ganglia (Le Douarin and Teillet, 1974; Le Douarin *et al.*, 1975).

intramural ganglia of the plexuses of Auerbach (A) and Meissner (M) are made up predominantly of quail cells. The ganglion of Remak (GR) is composed principally of host cells. A few quail cells (arrows) probably belong to descending vagal fibres. 10-day chick host. Feulgen staining, ×160. (b) After an isotopic interspecific graft of the lumbosacral neural primordium (somite 28 caudad), the ganglion of Remak is made up predominantly of quail neurons (N) and glial cells (G). Chick cells constitute the intraganglionic vascularity and some tentatively identified descending vagal fibres. Intramural ganglia of Auerbach's and Meissner's plexuses are made up principally of host cells. However, some quail cells (arrows) are found in these plexuses and probably represent a neural and glial participation of the lumbosacral neural primordium to the intramural innervation through the Remak ganglion. 14-day chick host. Feulgen staining, ×160

The latter finding was confirmed in a different experimental system. Culture of the hind-gut, taken from an embryo before it had received the ganglion precursor cells, on the chorioallantoic membrane for 7–10 days resulted in apparently normal muscular development but a total absence of ganglia (Smith *et al.*, 1977). When a fragment of a neural crest was associated with the aneural hind-gut before culture, enteric plexuses appeared, irrespective of whether the presumptive fate of crest cells was to give rise to enteric ganglia or to sympathoblasts and adrenomedullary cells. The cholinergic nature of the ganglia formed in the culture was attested to by the presence of choline acetyltransferase (CAT) activity and high levels of acetylcholinesterase, while neither tyrosine hydroxylase, the key enzyme for CA synthesis, nor formol-induced fluorescence (FIF) of CA was detected.

Lability of the differentiation in developing autonomic ganglia

The next series of experiments shows that the role of local environment on the differentiation of peripheral ganglion cells is not restricted to an early phase of development. Tissue environment obviously also plays a role during a long developmental period and seems to ensure the maintenance of the differentiated state as shown by Johnson *et al.* (1981) for the superior cervical ganglion of the adult rat.

In these experiments (Le Douarin *et al.*, 1978, 1979; Le Lièvre *et al.*, 1980), instead of exchanging neural primordia before the onset of migration and differentiation of neural crest cells, we back-transplanted, into a 2-day chick host crest derivatives that had terminated their normal migration and were in the process of differentiation, such as the ganglion of Remak, ciliary, sympathetic or spinal ganglia taken from 4- to 6-day quail embryos, i.e. at a stage when some of the ganglion cells have already expressed their typical phenotype (for instance presence of CA or ACh). The graft was inserted close to the host's own neural crest, between neural tube and somites, in the trunk region. Thus, differentiating crest-derived ganglia were subjected to the environment of the trunk of a younger embryo, at the stage of neural crest cell migration and differentiation. The evolution of these supernumerary grafts was observed subsequently, at various times after transplantation (Le Douarin *et al.*, 1978; Le Lièvre *et al.*, 1980). Three main results were obtained:

(1) During the first hours after implantation, cells from the periphery of the grafted ganglion detached from the implant and started to migrate along the side of the host's neural tube; after 24 to 48 hours, the cells of the graft were completely dispersed among the host's truncal tissues. If examined 4 to 6 days after grafting, the grafted quail cells were located exclusively in the normal sites of arrest of neural crest cells: ganglia of the peripheral nervous system, adrenal glands and plexuses and Schwann cells lining nerves. This means that,

although they had already undergone their migration at the time of transplantation, the ganglion cells behaved, when placed in the neural crest environment of the host, as premigratory, undifferentiated neural crest cells. They migrated anew and recognized the sites where neural crest cells normally stop.

(2) Not only did grafted ganglion cells locate at the normal sites of peripheral ganglion formation, but they also differentiated and expressed the phenotype corresponding to their environment; at least some of the quail ciliary ganglion cells originating from a cholinergic population, or sensory ganglion cells, when found in sympathetic ganglia or adrenal medulla of the host, responded positively to the FIF technique (Falck, 1962), which means that they contained CA and had become adrenergic.

(3) Spinal and autonomic grafted ganglia behaved differently in the host. Whereas the sensory ganglion-derived cells colonized not only the host's dorsal root ganglia but also the sympathetic chain and adrenal medulla, the autonomic ganglion cells were located only in the autonomic structures of the host. This result indicates that sensory and autonomic ganglion cells have different affinities for the sites of crest cell arrest.

Involvement of non-neural tissues in the chemical differentiation of autonomic neurons from neural crest precursors *in vivo*

The experiments already described highlight the importance of extrinsic signals in neural development; in particular, it is clear that the ultimate fate of neuron precursors, especially as concerns the choice of neurotransmitter to be produced, depends largely on the migratory pathways they follow during ontogeny. Stimuli could arise from tissues bordering these pathways and/or at the site of crest cell arrest. Knowledge of the routes followed by the presumptive neuroblasts is therefore an essential first step in any attempt to unravel the mechanism of their differentiation. As described in a previous section, a number of crest cell migration pathways have been worked out in the avian embryo. The results of such experiments, combined with those obtained by the application of neuron-specific biochemical or cytochemical techniques, provide a description of events occurring during the early phases of adrenergic and cholinergic ganglion formation and enable deductions to be made concerning the identity of the non-neural tissues involved.

Differentiation of adrenergic neurons

The appearance of adrenergic neuronal characteristics in developing neuroblasts of the sympathetic chain has been followed by a number of workers. In the chick embryo, FIF cannot be observed in neural crest cells either before or during their dorsoventral migration (Allan and Newgreen,

1977; our own results); the first CA-specific fluorescence is demonstrable at around 3.5 days, when the presumptive sympathoblasts of the primary sympathetic chains have already aggregated (Enemar *et al.*, 1965; Cohen, 1972; Allan and Newgreen, 1977), but while they are still dividing (Rothman *et al.*, 1978). The time-course of sympathoblast differentiation in the quail is essentially similar (unpublished results).

One may thus conclude that CA appears in crest-derived cells before they reach their definitive end-point, but only after they have undergone an initial period of migration. The neural tube and/or the somitic mesenchyme are possible candidates for a role in the initiation of the adrenergic phenotype. This eventuality was tested in a series of experiments involving tissue grafts on the chorioallantoic membrane *in vivo*. It was found that adrenergic (FIF-positive) cells developed from explanted neural crest only if the neural tube and somitic mesenchyme were present (Cohen, 1972). Later studies, in our laboratory, suggested that another embryonic tissue, the notochord, plays an important part in adrenergic differentiation. This transient axial structure is implicated in a number of embryonic induction processes. Furthermore, in the very early embryo, it is able to take up CA (Kirby and Gilmore, 1972; Lawrence and Burden, 1973; Allan and Newgreen, 1977; Rothman *et al.*, 1978). These facts, together with the observation that sympathoblasts develop in quite close proximity to the notochord, encouraged Teillet *et al.* (1978) to examine the influence of this structure on adrenergic differentiation in neural primordium (neural tube plus crest) explanted on the chorioallantoic membrane together with aneural colorectum taken from an embryo at 5 days of incubation. In the absence of notochord, it will be recalled (see previous section) that crest cells migrated into the gut, forming myenteric and submucous plexuses, but never expressed adrenergic properties; when notochord was associated, however, within 2 days groups of FIF-positive cells appeared along the developing circular muscle layer. If several fragments of notochord were added, about 80% of the experimental associations contained adrenergic cells (unpublished observations).

Notochord thus possesses the ability to promote adrenergic differentiation in crest cells placed in an otherwise unfavourable environment. Its participation in normal sympathoblast development awaits demonstration.

Formation of cholinergic ganglia

Analysis of early events in cholinergic neuron development are hampered by the lack of an adequately specific histo- or immunocytochemical technique for revealing the activity of CAT, the only really satisfactory marker of cholinergic differentiation (Hebb, 1956; Burt, 1968). Biochemical methods have, however, shown that CAT activity is present as soon as rudimentary parasympathetic or enteric ganglia have formed (Chiappinelli *et al.*, 1976;

Smith *et al.*, 1977; Le Douarin *et al.*, 1978). The extraintestinal migratory phase is not an essential prerequisite for cholinergic enteric neuron development, as was shown in experiments in which aneural colorectum was associated directly with neural crest on the chorioallantoic membrane (Smith *et al.*, 1977; Teillet *et al.*, 1978). It was concluded that the splanchnic mesenchyme itself (i.e. the end-point of migration) was responsible for the orientation of the neuroblasts towards the cholinergic pathway. However, more recent results, described below, have caused us to revise our opinion.

IN VITRO STUDIES ON THE DIFFERENTIATION OF NEURONS FROM NEURAL CREST CELLS

Developmental capacities of crest cells

In vitro culture techniques have been increasingly employed in attempts to define the conditions required for neuronal differentiation from neural crest. The earliest studies showed that CA-containing cells could develop *in vitro* from explants containing neural primordium (Bjerre, 1973) and confirmed that both neural tube and somitic mesenchyme were necessary for the appearance of FIF-positive cells (Norr, 1973). In later experiments, neural-tube-free cultures of crest were prepared by taking advantage of the fact that crest cells will migrate away from the tube if the total neural primordium is explanted on to a culture dish. After removal of the tube, crest-derived cells remain behind (Cohen and Konigsberg, 1975). Histiotypic cultures of trunk crest prepared in this way underwent extensive, 'spontaneous' adrenergic differentiation in the absence of other embryonic tissues (Cohen, 1977). Although the presence of contaminating non-crest cells in these cultures could not be excluded, subsequent studies in which crest cells were grown in secondary cultures at clonal density showed that direct cell-cell interactions during the entire culture period were not necessary for the development of FIF-positive cells *in vitro* (Sieber-Blum and Cohen, 1980). It is nonetheless possible that such interactions between neural crest cells and neural tube had already taken place during the first 24–48 hours of culture, when the tube was still present. CAT activity also appears in cultures both of mesencephalic and cervicothoracic crest (Greenberg and Schrier, 1977; Kahn *et al.*, 1980).

Recently we have published the results of a detailed study of the ability of quail neural crest to differentiate into autonomic neurons when cultured alone and in the presence of various young embryonic tissues (Fauquet *et al.*, 1981). This investigation was undertaken using neural crest excised from both the mesencephalic and truncal levels by a microsurgical technique, thus eliminating any possible stimulatory effect of the neural tube during the first few hours in culture. We examined systematically the ability of each culture to synthesize ACh and CA from radioactive precursors. This technique, which enables femtomole quantities of transmitter to be measured, allows convenient comparison of the relative importance of cholinergic and adrenergic activities under different culture conditions (Mains and Patterson, 1973).

In summary, our results confirmed the bipotentiality of the crest cell population with respect to the expression of cholinergic and adrenergic properties. In addition, they also revealed an important difference between the appearance of the two phenotypes: freshly excised mesencephalic crest was already capable of synthesizing ACh by a CAT-mediated reaction (Smith *et al.*, 1979) and a similar activity was also observed in crest taken from the trunk level (unpublished results). There is therefore no need to invoke exogenous stimuli during or after crest cell migration to account for the acquisition of cholinergic traits. ACh-synthesizing ability was equally present in all cultures and cocultures examined, irrespective of the axial level from which the crest had been taken. In contrast, CA was not produced by freshly removed crest, and even after culture its synthesis was only observed to any great extent when cells of non-crest origin were also present. Somites and notochord taken from 2-day quail embryos were quantitatively the most effective 'inducers' of adrenergic differentiation, but qualitatively their action was not specific: heart, and even hind-gut, were satisfactory substitutes. However, despite a certain level of biochemical differentiation, morphologically defined neuronal development was extremely limited under these conditions. Cultures of either mesencephalic or trunk crest, alone or in association with any of the above-mentioned tissues, contained very few cells resembling neurons in their phase-contrast appearance, and none that reacted positively to any of the cytological tests applied (in particular FIF).

The role of somites in sympathoblast differentiation

The relatively poor development of sympathetic neurons in cultures of excised trunk crest and 2-day somitic mesenchyme led us to examine the appearance of CA-containing cells in the presence of older somites. Such tissue, according to the experiments of Norr (1973), has received a stimulus from the neural tube and notochord that conditions it to stimulate sympathoblast differentiation. In the 3-day bird embryo, the somitic mesenchyme has already segregated into two distinct components, the dermomyotome and the sclerotome, which can be dissociated and cultured separately (Cheney and Lash, 1981). We were able to show (Fauquet *et al.*, 1981) that sclerotomes prepared in this way are intimately associated with migrating trunk crest cells, which, although lacking demonstrable neuronal characteristics at the time of explantation, undergo very rapid structural and biochemical maturation *in vitro*. ACh, but not CA, was synthesized by preparations of sclerotomes prior to culture (thus providing circumstantial evidence for the existence of cholinergic activity in the migrating trunk crest population). From 24 hours onward, however, both CA and ACh were produced by all cultures, with the molar ratio usually well in favour of the former transmitter. In addition, tyrosine hydroxylase was detected immunocytochemically in many of the cells. Cytological differentiation in general was excellent. Neurons were apparent within 24 hours of culture; after 7 days they were often grouped to form ganglion-like structures, joined by an extensive network of processes. CA fluorescence could be detected within 48 hours, and, several days later, large numbers of cells, fibres and varicosities were positive. Ultrastructural examination revealed the presence of many dense-core vesicles. Thus, in striking contrast to the 2-day somite, the 3-day sclerotome is a favourable environment, not only for the initiation of CA synthesis but also for an extensive structural neuronal maturation.

The nature of the factors involved in neuronal differentiation

One of the ultimate aims of the *in vitro* studies described above was, and remains, the identification and characterization of the agents responsible for neuronal differentiation. A similar approach has been successfully applied to neurons isolated from the central and peripheral nervous systems and has led to the compilation of a variety of 'factors' necessary for their development under these particular conditions. The term 'neuronal development' obviously covers a large number of phenomena, and different workers have concentrated on specific manifestations, such as neuronal survival, neurite outgrowth and the modulation of neurotransmitter-related properties. Nerve growth factor (NGF) is the classical and much-studied example of a molecule affecting all of these parameters in cultured sympathetic and sensory ganglia (see Vinores and Guroff (1980), Harper and Thoenen (1981), and also chapter by Levi-Montalcini and Aloe, for reviews). More recently, factors that can influence development of parasympathetic neurons in a similar way have been found in media conditioned by diverse types of non-neuronal cells.

Thus, the chick ciliary ganglion requires substances that are released into the medium by embryonic heart for survival, neurite elongation (Varon *et al.*, 1979; Nishi and Berg, 1979; Helfand *et al.*, 1976; Obata and Tanaka, 1980) and development of CAT (Varon *et al.*, 1979; Nishi and Berg, 1979). The trophic activity is present in many different regions of the chick embryo, and is particularly abundant in the part of the eye that contains the target tissues of ciliary ganglion neurons (Adler *et al.*, 1979; Landa *et al.*, 1980). The factors required for the development of parasympathetic nerve cells *in vitro* are different from NGF (Helfand *et al.*, 1978; Ebendal *et al.*, 1979), which itself is not unique as a sympathetic neurotrophic agent (Ebendal, 1979; Obata and Tanaka, 1980; Varon and Skaper, 1981). The nature and mechanism of action of these substances remain to be elucidated. Possibly they are examples of 'retrophins', a term that has been coined to designate substances synthesized and released by target tissues, taken up by nerve terminals and transported retrogradely to the perikaryon, where they exert their trophic effects (Hendry *et al.*, 1981).

What is the relationship of these findings to the development of neural crest cells? It must be borne in mind that all the neurotrophic factors so far described act on cells that already possess a neuronal imprint, even though certain structural features (e.g. neurites) may have been lost during establishment of the culture. It does not necessarily follow that the same factors also play a role in the earliest stages of neurogenesis, i.e. the initial acquisition of neuronal characters (including neurotransmitter choice) by crest cells or their derivatives.

As far as cholinergic differentiation of neuroblasts is concerned, the important point is that its initiation takes place early, i.e. at or before the formation of the neural crest (Smith *et al.*, 1979). However, the augmentation of the low initial activity in crest cells may involve interactions similar to those described above for maturing ciliary ganglion neurons, and ACh synthesis by cultured crest was indeed increased in the presence of various embryonic tissues (Fauquet *et al.*, 1981).

The appearance of the adrenergic phenotype in crest cells *in vitro* is a somewhat controversial point. In the experiments performed in the authors' laboratory (Fauqet *et al.*, 1981), catecholaminergic differentiation in cultures of neural crest alone was characterizable only by low levels of CA synthesis detected biochemically, and it was concluded that interactions between crest cells and the somitic mesenchymal derivatives were necessary for the full expression of the adrenergic phenotype. However in the *in vitro* studies of Sieber-Blum and Cohen (1980), continuous direct interactions with non-crest cells were not required for the development of adrenergic traits. This apparent contradiction can perhaps be resolved if it is conceded that somitic mesenchyme stimulates development via extracellular exudates deposited on the culture substrate and certain amounts of which may be present in normal serum and embryo extract. Addition to crest cultures of matrix derived from non-crest cells was indeed found to increase the number of FIF-positive cells (Sieber-Blum and Cohen, 1980) and a similar effect was observed with fibronectin (Sieber-Blum *et al.*, 1981), which, as emphasized by Thiery *et al.*, 1982 borders the neural tube, somites and notochord at the cervicothoracic level of the embryo.

Exogenous NGF is not needed for the earliest stages of adrenergic cell development *in vitro* (Norr, 1973; Fauquet *et al.*, 1981), although it cannot be excluded that an NGF-like factor is provided by the non-crest cells present in the culture or in the complex components of the medium.

Finally, one should not lose sight of the fact that the neural crest gives rise *in vivo* to several different kinds of CA-containing cells, which vary according to their size, presence and length of processes, nature of the CA produced and the diameter of their storage vesicles. The adrenergic cells developing in crest cultures appear to be predominantly of the small, intensely fluorescent (SIF) variety, and although many neuron-like cells did develop in sclerotome cultures (Fauquet *et al.*, 1981), numerous cells of the SIF type were also present. Evidence exists that small cells containing large, dense-core vesicles (intensely fluorescent) are the precursors of principal neurons (smaller vesicles, weakly fluorescent) of the avian sympathetic chain *in vivo* (Luckenbill-Edds and Van Horn, 1980; see Landis and Patterson, 1981, for discussion), but the situation is undoubtedly complex and continued efforts, employing a wide spectrum of experimental techniques *in vitro* and *in vivo*, will be required before it can be satisfactorily clarified.

CONCLUDING REMARKS

At the point reached in the experimental analysis of the development of the autonomic nervous system, a certain number of provisional conclusions can be drawn.

As so far investigated, it seems that the potentialities for giving rise to all cell types and all ganglionic and paraganglionic structures characterizing the various components of the autonomic nervous system exist in the whole population of neural crest cells, irrespective of their position (cephalic, cervicodorsal or lumbosacral) along the neural axis. However, the distribution and characteristics of the various ganglia and plexuses of the autonomic nervous system are highly specific in the various regions of the body. This variety is established during ontogeny through a complex interplay between the neural crest cells and the other tissues of the embryo. The latter first determine the migration pathways followed by the neural crest cells, which migrate preferentially within cell-free 'avenues' that contain an appropriate extracellular matrix, mainly produced by non-neuronal cells and the composition of which begins to be documented. It is rich in high-molecular-weight components such as hyaluronic acid, glycosaminoglycans and fibronectin. Crest cells also have the ability to penetrate certain tissues preferentially (e.g. the mesenchyme of the gut wall) in which they travel for long distances (see Le Douarin, 1980, 1982, for discussion). In contrast, they practically never migrate within somatopleure and in the limb-bud mesenchyme (except for the Schwann cells lining the nerve fibres and the melanoblasts). Nothing is known about the reasons why the penetrability of various tissues by migrating crest cells differs so much (see Le Douarin, 1982, for discussion). The sites where neural crest cells stop to form the ganglia and paraganglia of the peripheral nervous system also depend on the general morphogenesis of the embryo (i.e. on the non-neuronal tissues) since, under experimental conditions, gangliogenesis conforms to the target tissue of migration rather than to the specificity of the crest cells in terms of their origin (cephalic, cervicodorsal or lumbosacral) in the neural primordium.

Concerning the final differentiation of the autonomic nervous system precursors into the various kinds of autonomic nerve cells, the embryonic medium in which they develop governs the phenotype that they express. This could be restated as follows: 'When the neural crest cells stop at a certain point in the embryo they are "naive", i.e. undecided as to the type of ganglion they are going to construct'. Many latent potentialities exist in the young ganglia and changing the external conditions in which their development occurs (e.g. by transplanting them into a younger host embryo) will permit the expression of characters that would have been normally repressed (Le Douarin *et al.*, 1978; Le Douarin *et al.*, 1979; Le Lièvre *et al.*, 1980).

At what level is the selection of the environment exerted on the neural crest cells? Is it at the level of a single multipotential precursor or among a population of partly or totally committed cells? The answer to this crucial question cannot yet be provided, but as far as the biochemical differentiation of autonomic neurons into adrenergic or cholinergic cells is concerned, it seems reasonable to admit that a common bipotential precursor exists for these two kinds of nerve cells. The best arguments in favour of this view are (1) the unequivocal demonstration that both ACh and CA can be produced by a single neuron (Furshpan *et al.*, 1976; Landis, 1976), and (2) the possibility of instigating ACh synthesis in adrenergic sympathetic neurons of the adult rat (Johnson *et al.*, 1981).

The clear-cut conclusions that can be drawn concerning the role exerted by non-neuronal components of the body on the peripheral nerve cells do not allow us to grasp the molecular mechanisms through which these effects are regulated; hence the tendency of many workers interested in these problems to switch to cell-culture methods. The results so far obtained in culture of neural crest cells have revealed new aspects of this question, such as (1) the early appearance of ACh synthesis in migrating crest cells and the regular occurrence of ACh production in all types of crest cell cultures, (2) the ability of any crest cell population to produce simultaneously ACh and CA, (3) the possibility to modulate the production of one or the other of these two transmitters by modifying the cell culture substrate and medium.

In this review we have provided a number of examples of the way in which different experimental approaches can reveal fresh aspects of the problem of the ontogeny of the autonomic nervous system. There is undoubtedly a great deal more to learn, but if the rate of recent progress is any gauge, the next few years should see considerable advances in our understanding of the vexed question of the differentiation of the various types of autonomic ganglia.

REFERENCES

Abel, W. (1909). The development of the autonomic nerve mechanism in the alimentary canal of the chick. *Proc. R. Soc. Edinburgh*, **30**, 327–347.

Abel, W. (1912). Further observations on the development of the sympathetic nervous system of the chick. *J. Anat. Physiol.*, **47**, 35–72.

Adler, R., Landa, K. B., Manthorpe, M., and Varon, S. (1979). Cholinergic neuronotrophic factors: intraocular distribution of trophic activity for ciliary neurons. *Science*, **204**, 1434–1436.

Allan, I. J., and Newgreen, D. F. (1977). Catecholamine accumulation in neural crest cells and the primary sympathetic chain. *Am. J. Anat.*, **149**, 413–421.

Allan, I. J., and Newgreen, D. F. (1980). The origin and differentiation of enteric neurons of the intestine of the fowl embryo. *Am. J. Anat.*, **157**, 137–154.

Andrew, A. (1964). The origin of intramural ganglia. I. The early arrival of precursor cells in the presumptive gut of chick embryos. *J. Anat.*, **98**, 421–428.

Andrew, A. (1969). The origin of intramural ganglia. II. The trunk neural crest as a source of enteric ganglion cells. *J. Anat.*, **105**, 89–101.

Andrew, A. (1970). The origin of intramural ganglia. III. The 'vagal' source of enteric ganglion cells. *J. Anat.*, **107**, 327–336.

Andrew, A. (1971). The origin of intramural ganglia. IV. The origin of enteric ganglia: a critical review and discussion of the present state of the problem. *J. Anat.*, **108**, 169–184.

Bennett, T., and Malmfors, T. (1970). The adrenergic nervous system of the domestic fowl (*Gallus domesticus* L.). *Z. Zellforsch. Mikrosk. Anat.*, **106**, 22–50.

Bjerre, B. (1973). The production of catecholamine-containing cells *in vitro* by young chick embryos studied by the histochemical fluorescence method. *J. Anat.*, **115**, 119–131.

Brizzee, K. R. (1949). Studies on the origin of the sympathetic trunc ganglia in the chick. *Anat. Rec.*, **103**, 530.

Brizzee, K. R., and Kuntz, A. (1950). The histogenesis of sympathetic ganglion cells. *J. Neuropathol. Exp. Neurol.* **9**, 164–171.

Browne, M. J. (1953). A study of the sacral autonomic nerves in a chick and a human embryo. *Anat. Rec.*, **116**, 189–203.

Burt, A. M. (1968). Acetylcholinesterase and choline acetyltransferase activity in the developing chick spinal cord. *J. Exp. Zool.*, **169**, 107–112.

Cheney, C. M., and Lash, J. W. (1981). Diversification within embryonic chick somites: differential response to notochord. *Dev. Biol.*, **81**, 288–298.

Chiappinelli, V., Giacobini, E., Pilar, G., and Uchimura, H. (1976). Induction of cholinergic enzymes in chick ciliary ganglion and iris muscle cells during synapse formation. *J. Physiol. (London)*, **257**, 749–766.

Cohen, A. M. (1972). Factors directing the expression of sympathetic nerve traits in cells of neural crest origin. *J. Exp. Zool.*, **179**, 167–182.

Cohen, A. M. (1977). Independent expression of the adrenergic phenotype by neural crest cells *in vitro*. *Proc. Natl. Acad. Sci. U.S.A.*, **74**, 2899–2903.

Cohen, A. M., and Konigsberg, I. R. (1975). A clonal approach to the problem of neural crest determination. *Dev. Biol.*, **46**, 262–280.

Derby, M. A. (1978). Analysis of glycosaminoglycans within the extracellular environments encountered by migrating neural crest cells. *Dev. Biol.*, **66**, 321–336.

Duband, J. L., and Thiery, J. P. (1982). Distribution of fibronectin in the early phase of avian cephalic neural crest cell migration. *Dev. Biol.*, **93**, 308–323.

Ebendal, T. (1979). Stage-dependent stimulation of neurite outgrowth exerted by nerve growth factor and chick heart in cultured embryonic ganglia. *Dev. Biol.*, **72**, 276–290.

Ebendal, T., Belew, M., Jacobson, C. O., and Porath, J. (1979). Neurite outgrowth elicited by embryonic chick heart: partial purification of the active factor. *Neurosci. Lett.*, **14**, 91–95.

Enemar, A., Falck, B., and Hakanson, R. (1965). Observations on the appearance of norepinephrine in the sympathetic nervous system of the chick embryo. *Dev. Biol.*, **11**, 268–283.

Falck, B. (1962). Observations on the possibilities of the cellular localization of monoamines by a fluorescence method. *Acta. Physiol. Scand.*, **56** (Suppl. 197), 1–25.

Fauquet, M., Smith, J., Ziller, C., and Le Douarin, N. M. (1981). Differentiation of autonomic neuron precursors *in vitro*: cholinergic and adrenergic traits in cultured neural crest cells. *J. Neurosci.*, **1**, 478–492.

Furshpan, E. J., MacLeish, P. R., O'Lague, P. H., and Potter, D. D. (1976). Chemical transmission between rat sympathetic neurons and cardiac myocytes developing in microcultures: evidence for cholinergic, adrenergic, and dual-function neurons. *Proc. Natl. Acad. Sci. U.S.A.*, **73**, 4225–4229.

Fusari, R. (1893). Contribution à l'étude du développement des capsules surrénales et du sympathique chez le poulet et chez les Mammifères. *Arch. Ital. Biol.*, **18**, 161–182.

Greenberg, J. H., and Schrier, B. K. (1977). Development of choline acetyltransferase activity in chick cranial neural crest cells in culture. *Dev. Biol.*, **61**, 86–93.

Hamburger, V., and Hamilton, H. L. (1951). A series of normal stages in the development of the chick embryo. *J. Morphol.*, **88**, 49–92.

Hammond, W. S. (1949). Formation of the sympathetic nervous system in the trunk of the chick embryo following removal of the thoracic neural tube. *J. Comp. Neurol.*, **91**, 67–86.

Hammond, W. S., and Yntema, C. L. (1947). Depletions of the thoraco-lumbar sympathetic system following removal of neural crest in the chick. *J. Comp. Neurol.*, **86**, 237–266.

Hammond, W. S., and Yntema, C. L. (1958). Origin of ciliary ganglia in the chick. *J. Comp. Neurol.*, **110**, 367–389.

Harper, G. P., and Thoenen, H. (1981). Target cells, biological effects and mechanism of action of Nerve Growth Factor and its antibodies. *Annu. Rev. Pharmacol. Toxicol.*, **21**, 205–230.

Hebb, C. O. (1956). Choline acetylase in the developing nervous system of the rabbit and guinea-pig. *J. Physiol. (London)*, **133**, 566–570.

Helfand, S. L., Smith, G. A., and Wessels, N. K. (1976). Survival and development in culture of dissociated parasympathetic neurons from ciliary ganglia. *Dev. Biol.*, **50**, 541–547.

Helfand, S. L., Riopelle, R. J., and Wessells, N. K. (1978). Non-equivalence of conditioned medium and nerve growth factor for sympathetic, parasympathetic, and sensory neurons. *Exp. Cell Res.*, **113**, 39–45.

Hendry, I. A., Hill, C. E., and Bonyhady, R. H. (1981). Interaction between developing autonomic neurons and their target tissues. In *Development of the Autonomic Nervous System, Ciba Foundation Symposium*, **83**, pp. 194–212, Pitman Medical, London.

His, W. Jr. (1897). Ueber die Entwicklung des Bauch Sympathicus beim Hühnchen und Menschen. *Arch. Anat. Physiol. Anat. Abt.*, [1897] Suppl., 137–170.

Hörstadius, S. (1950). *The Neural Crest: Its Properties and Derivatives in the Light of Experimental Research*, Oxford University Press, London.

Johnson, M. I., Iacovitti, L., Higgins, D., Bunge, R. P., and Burton, H. (1981). Growth and development of sympathetic neurons in tissue culture. In *Development of the Autonomic Nervous System, Ciba Foundaion Symposium 83*, pp. 108–122, Pitman Medical, London.

Johnston, M. C. (1966). A radioautographic study of the migration and fate of cranial neural crest cells in the chick embryo. *Anat. Rec.*, **156**, 143–156.

Jones, D. S. (1937). The origin of the sympathetic trunk in the chick embryo. *Anat. Rec.*, **70**, 45–65.

Jones, D. S. (1941). Further studies on the origin of sympathetic ganglia in the chick embryo. *Anat. Rec.*, **79**, 7–15.

Jones, D. S. (1942). The origin of the vagi and the parasympathetic ganglion cells of the viscera of the chick. *Anat. Rec.*, **82**, 185–197.

Kahn, C. R., Coyle, J. T., and Cohen, A. M. (1980). Head and trunk neural crest *in vitro*: autonomic neuron differentiation. *Dev. Biol.*, **77**, 340–348.

Keuning, F. J. (1948). Histogenesis and origin of the autonomic nerve plexus in the upper digestive tube of the chick. *Acta Neerl. Morphol.*, **6**, 8–48.

Kirby, M. L., and Gilmore, S. A. (1972). A fluorescence study of the ability of the notochord to synthesize and store catecholamines in early chick embryos. *Anat. Rec.*, **173**, 469–477.

Kuntz, A. (1910). The development of the sympathetic nervous system in birds. *J. Comp. Neurol.*, **20**, 283–308.

Kuntz, A. (1926). The role of cells of medullary origin in the development of the sympathetic trunk. *J. Comp. Neurol.*, **40**, 389–408.

Kuntz, A. (1953). *The Autonomic Nervous System*, pp. 117–134, Baillière, Tindal and Cox, London.

Landa, K. B., Adler, R., Manthorpe, M., and Varon, S. (1980). Cholinergic neuronotrophic factors. III. Developmental increase of trophic activity for chick embryo ciliary ganglion neurons in their intraocular target tissues. *Dev. Biol.*, **74**, 401–408.

Landis, S. C. (1976). Rat sympathetic neurons and cardiac myocytes developing in microcultures: correlation of the fine structure of endings with neurotransmitter function in single neurons. *Proc. Natl. Acad. Sci. U.S.A.*, **73**, 4220–4224.

Landis, S. C., and Patterson, P. H. (1981). Neural crest cell lineages. *Trends Neurosci.*, **4**, 172–175.

Lawrence, I. E., and Burden, H. W. (1973). Catecholamines and morphogenesis of the chick neural tube and notochord. *Am. J. Anat.*, **137**, 199–208.

Le Douarin, N. M. (1969). Particularités du noyau interphasique chez la caille japonaise (*Coturnix coturnix japonica*). Utilisation de ces particularités comme 'marquage biologique' dans les recherches sur les interactions tissulaires et les migrations cellulaires au cours de l'ontogenèse. *Bull. Biol. Fr. Belg.*, **103**, 435–452.

Le Douarin, N. M. (1971). Caractéristiques ultrastructurales du noyau interphasique chez la caille et chez le poulet et utilisation de cellules de Caille comme 'marqueurs biologiques' en embryologie expérimentale. *Ann. Embryol. Morphog.*, **4**, 125–135.

Le Douarin, N. M. (1973). A biological cell labeling technique and its use in experimental embryology. *Dev. Biol.*, **30**, 217–222.

Le Douarin, N. M. (1976). Cell migration in early vertebrate development studied in interspecific chimaeras. In *Embryogenesis in Mammals, Ciba Foundation Symposium*, pp. 71–101, Excerpta Medica, Amsterdam.

Le Douarin, N. M. (1980). Migration and differentiation of neural crest cells. *Curr. Top. Dev. Biol.*, **16**, 31–85.

Le Douarin, N. M. (1982). *The Neural Crest*, Cambridge University Press.

Le Douarin, N. M., and Teillet, M. A. (1971). Localisation, par la méthode des greffes interspécifiques, du territoire neural dont dérivent les cellules adrénales surrénaliennes chez l'embryon d'oiseau. *C.R. Acad. Sci.*, **272**, 481–484.

Le Douarin, N. M., and Teillet, M. A. (1973). The migration of neural crest cells to the wall of the digestive tract in avian embryo. *J. Embryol. Exp. Morphol.*, **30**, 31–48.

Le Douarin, N. M., and Teillet, M. A. (1974). Experimental analysis of the migration and differentiation of neuroblasts of the autonomic nervous system and of neurecto-dermal mesenchymal derivatives, using a biological cell marking technique. *Dev. Biol.*, **41**, 162–184.

Le Douarin, N. M., Renaud, D., Teillet, M. A., and Le Douarin, G. H. (1975). Cholinergic differentiation of presumptive adrenergic neuroblasts in interspecific chimaeras after heterotopic transplantations. *Proc. Natl. Acad. Sci. U.S.A.*, **72**, 728–732.

Le Douarin, N. M., Teillet, M. A., Ziller, C., and Smith, J. (1978). Adrenergic differentiation of cells of the cholinergic ciliary and Remak ganglia in avian embryo after *in vivo* transplantation. *Proc. Natl. Acad. Sci. U.S.A.*, **75**, 2030–2034.

Le Douarin, N., Le Lièvre, C. S., Schweizer, G., and Ziller, C. M. (1979). An analysis of cell line segregation in the neural crest. In *Cell Lineage, Stem Cells and Cell Determination* (Ed. N. Le Douarin), pp. 353–365, Elsevier/North-Holland Biomedical Press, Amsterdam.

Le Lièvre, C. S., and Le Douarin, N. M. (1975). Mesenchymal derivatives of the neural crest: analysis of chimaeric quail and chick embryos. *J. Embryol. Exp. Morphol.*, **34**, 125–154.

Le Lièvre, C. S., Schweizer, G. G., Ziller, C. M., and Le Douarin, N. M. (1980). Restrictions of developmental capabilities in neural crest cell derivatives as tested by *in vivo* transplantation experiments. *Dev. Biol.*, **77**, 362–378.

Levi-Montalcini, R. (1947). Ricerche sperimentali sull'origine del simpatico toraco-lombare nell'embrione di pollo. *Atti Accad. Naz. Lincei Ser. 8a*, **3**, 140–144.

Luckenbill-Edds, L., and Van Horn, C. (1980). Development of chick paravertebral sympathetic ganglia. I. Fine structure and correlative histofluorescence of catechol-aminergic cells. *J. Compar. Neurol.*, **191**, 65–76.

Mains, R. E., and Patterson, P. H. (1973). Primary cultures of dissociated sympathetic neurons. I. Establishment of long-term growth in culture and studies of differenti-ated properties. *J. Cell Biol.*, **59**, 329–345.

Meier, S., and Hay, E. D. (1973). Synthesis of sulfated glycosaminoglycans by embryonic corneal epithelium. *Dev. Biol.*, **35**, 318–331.

Müller, E., and Ingvar, S. (1923). Über die Ursprung des Sympathicus beim Hühnchen. *Arch. Mikroskop. Anat. Entwicklungsmech.*, **99**, 650–671.

Narayanan, C. H., and Narayanan, Y. (1978). On the origin of the ciliary ganglion in birds studied by the method of interspecific transplantation of embryonic brain regions between quail and chick. *J. Embryol. Exp. Morphol.*, **47**, 137–148.

Nishi, R., and Berg, D. K. (1979). Survival and development of ciliary ganglion neurones grown alone in cell culture. *Nature*, **277**, 232–234.

Noden, D. M. (1978a). Interactions directing the migration and cytodifferentiation of avian neural crest cells. In *The Specificity of Embryological Interactions* (Ed. D. Garrod), Vol. 4, pp. 3–47, Chapman and Hall, London.

Noden, D. M. (1978b). The control of avian cephalic neural crest cytodifferentiation. I. Skeletal and connective tissues. *Dev. Biol.*, **67**, 296–312.

Noden, D. M. (1978c). The control of avian cephalic neural crest cytodifferentiation. II. Neural tissues. *Dev. Biol.*, **67**, 313–329.

Norr, S. C. (1973). *In vitro* analysis of sympathetic neuron differentiation from chick neural crest cells. *Dev. Biol.*, **34**, 16–38.

Obata, K., and Tanaka, H. (1980). Conditioned medium promotes neurite growth from both central and peripheral neurons. *Neurosci. Lett.*, **16**, 27–33.

Onodi, A. D. (1886). Ueber die Entwicklung des sympatischen Nervensystems. *Arch. Mikroskop. Anat. Entwicklungsmech.*, **26**, 553–580.

Pratt, R. M., Larsen, M. A., and Johnston, M. C. (1975). Migration of cranial neural crest cells in a cell-free hyaluronate-rich matrix. *Dev. Biol.*, **44**, 298–305.

Remak, R. (1847). *Ueber ein Selbständiges Darmnervensystem*, G. Reimer, Berlin.

Rothman, T. P., Gershon, M. D., and Holtzer, H. (1978). The relationship of cell division to the acquisition of adrenergic characteristics by developing sympathetic ganglion cell precursors. *Dev. Biol.*, **65**, 322–341.

Schenk, S. L., and Birdsall, W. R. (1880). Über die Lehre von der Entwicklung der Ganglien des Sympathicus. *Mitt. Embriol. Inst. Univ. Wien*, *5(N.S.)*, **1**, 213–228.

Sieber-Blum, M., and Cohen, A. M. (1980). Clonal analysis of quail neural crest cells: they are pluripotent and differentiate *in vitro* in the absence of non crest cells. *Dev. Biol.*, **80**, 96–106.

Sieber-Blum, M., Sieber, F., and Yamada, K. M. (1981). Cellular fibronectin promotes adrenergic differentiation of quail neural crest cells *in vitro*. *Exp. Cell Res.*, **133**, 285–295.

Smith, J., Cochard, P., and Le Douarin, N. M. (1977). Development of choline acetyltransferase and cholinesterase activities in enteric ganglia derived from presumptive adrenergic and cholinergic levels of the neural crest. *Cell Differ.*, **6**, 199–216.

Smith, J., Fauquet, M., Ziller, C., and Le Douarin, N. M. (1979). Acetylcholine synthesis by mesencephalic neural crest cells in the process of migration *in vivo*. *Nature*, **282**, 853–855.

Strudel, G. (1953). Conséquences de l'excision de tronçons du tube nerveux sur la morphogenèse de l'embryon de poulet et sur la différenciation de ses organes: Contribution à la genèse de l'orthosympathique. *Ann. Sci. Nat. Zool. 11e Sér.*, **15**, 251–329.

Teillet, M. A. (1978). Evolution of the lumbo-sacral neural crest in the avian embryo: origin and differentiation of the ganglionated nerve of Remak studied in interspecific quail-chick chimaerae. *W. Roux's Arch. Dev. Biol.*, **184**, 251–268.

Teillet, M. A., Cochard, P., and Le Douarin, N. M. (1978). Relative roles of the mesenchymal tissues and of the complex neural tube-notochord on the expression of adrenergic metabolism in neural crest cells. *Zoon*, **6**, 115–122.

Tello, J. F. (1924). La précocité embryonnaire du plexus d'Auerbach et ses différences dans les intestins antérieur et postérieur. *Trab. Lab. Invest. Biol. Univ. Madrid*, **22**, 317–328.

Tello, J. F. (1925). Sur la formation des chaînes primaires et secondaires du grand sympathique dans l'embryon de poulet. *Trab. Lab. Invest. Biol. Univ. Madrid*, **23**, 1–28.

Tello, J. F. (1945). Algunas observaciones mas sobre las primeras faces del desarollo del simpatico en el pollo. *Trab. Inst. Cajal Invest. Biol. (Madrid)*, **37**, 103–149.

Thiery, J. P., Duband, J. L., and Delouvée, A. (1982). Pathways and mechanisms of avian trunk neural crest cell migration and localization *Dev. Biol.*, **93**, 327–373.

Toole, B. P. (1972). Hyaluronate turnover during chondrogenesis in the developing chick limb bud and axial skeleton. *Dev. Biol.*, **29**, 321–329.

Toole, B. P., and Trelstad, R. L. (1971). Hyaluronate production and removal during corneal development in the chick. *Dev. Biol.*, **26**, 28–35.

Trelstad, R. L., Hayashi, K., and Toole, B. P. (1974). Epithelial collagens and glycosaminoglycans in the embryonic cornea. Macromolecular order and morphogenesis in the basement membrane. *J. Cell Biol.*, **62**, 815–830.

Uchida, S. (1927). Über die Entwicklung des sympatischen Nervensystems bei den Vögeln. *Acta Sch. Med. Univ. Kyoto*, **10**, 63–136.

Van Campenhout, E. (1930a). Historical survey of the development of the sympathetic nervous system. *Q. Rev. Biol.*, **5**, 23–50, 217–234.

Van Campenhout, E. (1930b). Expériences concernant l'origine et le développement du système nerveux viscéral. *C.R. Assoc. Anat.*, **25**, 78–79.

Van Campenhout, E. (1931). Le développement du système nerveux sympathique chez le poulet. *Arch. Biol.*, **42**, 479–507.

Van Campenhout, E. (1932). Further experiments on the origin of the enteric nervous system in the chick. *Physiol. Zool.*, **5**, 333–353.

Van Campenhout, E. (1947). Au sujet de l'origine et du développement de ganglions nerveux intraviscéraux du tube digestif chez l'embryon de poulet. *Arch. Biol.*, **58**, 1–14.

Varon, S., and Skaper, S. D. (1981). *In vitro* response of sympathetic neurons to nerve growth factor and other macromolecular agents. In *Development of the Autonomic Nervous System, Ciba Foundation Symposium 83*, pp. 151–176, Pitman Medical, London.

Varon, S., Manthorpe, M., and Adler, R. (1979). Cholinergic neuronotrophic factors: I. Survival, neurite outgrowth and choline acetyltransferase activity in monolayer cultures from chick embryo ciliary ganglia. *Brain Res.*, **173**, 29–45.

Vinores, S., and Guroff, G. (1980). Nerve Growth Factor: Mechanism of action. *Annu. Rev. Biophys. Bioeng.*, **9**, 223–258.

Wenger, E. L. (1950). An experimental analysis of relations between parts of the brachial spinal cord of the embryonic chick. *J. Exp. Zool.*, **114**, 51–85.

Weston, J. A. (1963). A radioautographic analysis of the migration and localization of trunk neural crest cells in the chick. *Dev. Biol.*, **6**, 279–310.

Weston, J. A. (1970). The migration and differentiation of neural crest cells. *Adv. Morphog.*, **8**, 41–114.

Yntema, C. L., and Hammond, W. S. (1945). Depletions and abnormalities in the cervical sympathetic system of the chick following extirpation of neural crest. *J. Exp. Zool.*, **100**, 237–263.

Yntema, C. L., and Hammond, W. S. (1947). The development of the automatic nervous system. *Biol. Rev.*, **22**, 344–357.

Yntema, C. L., and Hammond, W. S. (1954). The origin of intrinsic ganglia of trunk viscera from vagal neural crest in the chick embryo. *J. Comp. Neurol.*, **101**, 515–542.

Yntema, C. L., and Hammond, W. S. (1955). Experiments on the origin and development of the sacral autonomic nerves in the chick embryo. *J. Exp. Zool.*, **129**, 375–414.

Zacchei, A. M. (1961). Lo sviluppo embrionale della quaglia giapponese (*Coturnix coturnix japonica* T. e S.). *Arch. Ital. Anat. Embriol.*, **66**, 36–62.

Autonomic Ganglia
Edited by Lars-Gösta Elfvin
© 1983 John Wiley & Sons Ltd

Factors which Influence the Transmitter Functions of Sympathetic Ganglion Cells

STORY C. LANDIS

*Department of Neurobiology, Harvard Medical School,
Boston, Massachusetts 02115, USA*

The choice of neurotransmitter is an important one for developing neurons. Examination of two different experimental systems has made it clear that environmental influences can play an important role in determining this choice, at least for neurons derived from the neural crest. Studies of the embryonic development of peripheral ganglia in chick-quail chimeras have provided strong evidence that the environment through which neuroblasts migrate and/or the environment in which they settle to form ganglia can influence neurotransmitter choice (see chapter by Le Douarin). A second line of evidence for the role of environmental influences on neurotransmitter choice has come from studies of cultured neurons dissociated from sympathetic ganglia of newborn rats. *In vivo*, the majority of mature sympathetic principal neurons are noradrenergic and use norepinephrine (NE) as a neurotransmitter while a small minority are cholinergic and use acetylcholine (ACh). The correct selection of one of these neurotransmitters is critical since in many target tissues they have antagonistic actions. The studies summarized below demonstrate that postmitotic sympathetic neurons are plastic with regard to this neurotransmitter choice and that they can be influenced by their culture environment. In addition, recent studies are described which suggest that plasticity and environmental influences are also important during the development of cholinergic sympathetic neurons in the intact animal as well.

NEUROTRANSMITTER CHOICE *IN VITRO*

The neural crest cells that will give rise to sympathetic neurons receive an adrenergic signal from their environment early in development. The nature of this signal appears to involve interactions between migrating crest cells and tissues along their migration pathway, in particular somitic mesenchyme, ventral neural tube and notochord (Cohen, 1972; Norr, 1973; Teillet *et al.*, 1978). Despite this early signal, the crest cells do not express noradrenergic properties during their primary migration until after they reach the site of the future ganglia. In the chick, specific, formaldehyde-induced catecholamine fluorescence is evident in the primary sympathetic chain as it forms (Enemar *et al.*, 1965; Kirby and Gilmore, 1976) and these fluorescent cells are capable of further cell divisions (Cohen, 1974; Rothman *et al.*, 1978). Similarly, in the rat and mouse, catecholamine histofluorescence as well as tyrosine hydroxylase and dopamine β-hydroxylase activity and immunoreactivity are also detectable as soon as sympathetic neuroblasts coalesce into ganglia (De Champlain *et al.*, 1970; Coughlin *et al.*, 1978; Cochard *et al.*, 1978, 1979; Teitelman *et al.*, 1978, 1979). By birth in the rat, virtually all of the neurons exhibit catecholamine histofluorescence (Eränkö, 1972). When neurons are dissociated from the superior cervical ganglia (SCG) of newborn rats, all of them initially appear to synthesize and store catecholamines. Following permanganate fixation, which reveals vesicular stores of NE as small granular vesicles (SGV) (Richardson, 1966), the growth cones of these neurons contain numerous SGV (Landis, 1978) and all of the synapses and varicosities which form during the first four days after plating contain SGV (Fig. 1a) (Landis, 1980; see also Johnson *et al.*, 1976, 1980b). Finally, when young cultures are assayed for transmitter synthesis, only catecholamines are made in detectable amounts (Mains and Patterson, 1973; Patterson and Chun, 1977b).

Under certain culture conditions the dissociated sympathetic neurons continue to differentiate noradrenergically and develop many of the properties characteristic of sympathetic neurons *in vivo*. If the dissociated sympathetic neurons are maintained in the virtual absence of non-neuronal cells, the neurons synthesize and store the catecholamines, dopamine and NE (Mains and Patterson, 1973; Patterson and Chun, 1977a) and can take up and store exogenous catecholamines and then release them in a calcium-dependent manner (Burton and Bunge, 1975; Patterson *et al.*, 1975). *In vitro* as in *in vivo* these sympathetic neurons possess axonal varicosities which sometimes form morphologically specialized synapses on neuronal cell bodies and dendrites (Rees and Bunge, 1974; Buckley and Landis, unpublished data). Following permanganate fixation, the synaptic terminals and varicosities contain predominantly SGV (Fig. 1b) (Rees and Bunge, 1974; Landis, 1980) and appear similar to those which the neurons form in the SCG itself (Grillo, 1966; Matthews, 1974) and in target tissues such as the iris (Hökfelt, 1969). Synaptic interaction has not been detected between noradrenergic neurons in these cultures (O'Lague *et al.*, 1978a) as would be expected from the fact that the neurons are relatively insensitive to catecholamines (O'Lague *et al.*, 1978b; Wakshull *et al.*, 1979a).

If, however, the dissociated sympathetic neurons are grown in the presence of certain types of non-neuronal cells such as heart myocytes and fibroblasts (Fig. 1c), the cultures develop cholinergic properties as well as noradrenergic. Significant amounts of ACh as well as catecholamines are synthesized

(Patterson and Chun, 1974, 1977a), choline acetyltransferase (CAT) activity increases (Johnson *et al.*, 1976, 1980a; Patterson and Chun, 1977a) and the neurons form excitatory cholinergic synapses with each other (Fig. 1d) (O'Lague *et al.*, 1974, 1978a, b; Ko *et al.*, 1976; Wakshull *et al.*, 1979a) and with heart myocytes (Furshpan *et al.*, 1976) and skeletal myotubes (Nurse and O'Lague, 1975). The induction of cholinergic properties can occur through direct neuronal contact with the heart cell surfaces (Hawrot, 1980) or by growth in medium conditioned (CM) by the heart cells (Patterson *et al.*, 1975; Landis *et al.*, 1976; Patterson and Chun, 1977a). Growth in high concentrations of heart cell CM not only induces cholinergic properties but it causes a simultaneous decline in catecholamine synthesis (Patterson and Chun, 1977a; Reichardt and Patterson, 1977; Fukada, 1980). In addition to influencing neurotransmitter choice, CM affects the lectin- and toxin-binding properties of the neuronal surfaces (Schwab and Landis, 1981) and the expression of certain membrane proteins as well as secreted and substrate-attached proteins (Sweadner and Braun, 1979; Sweadner, 1981). Bunge and his colleagues have found that cholinergic function can be induced by growth in high concentrations of human placental serum and chick embryo extract in the absence of non-neuronal cells (Wakshull *et al.*, 1978). These agents do not, however, lead to a simultaneous fall in catecholamine synthetic enzymes as does a high concentration of CM (Higgins *et al.*, 1981; Iacovitti *et al.*, 1980).

Several of the properties of the diffusible cholinergic factor have been described and work is in progress to purify and characterize it. Production of CM factor is species-specific; primary cultures of a number of different rat tissues and several rat cell lines produce CM factor, but not chick or mouse cells. There is a rough correlation between the innervation that a particular tissue receives and the ability of the tissue to condition medium effectively; skeletal muscle which receives cholinergic innervation is very effective while liver which receives only an adrenergic innervation is relatively ineffective (Patterson and Chun, 1977a). The cholinergic factor has been partially purified from serum-containing CM and has an approximate molecular weight of 50 000. Although relatively stable to heat, urea, guanidine and mercaptoethanol, it is highly sensitive to periodate (Weber, 1981). Recent experiments have shown that heart cells can condition serum-free medium and demonstrated that the production or release of the cholinergic factor is influenced by certain hormones and growth factors; epidermal growth factor (EGF) increases its release while glucocorticoids decrease its release (Fukada, 1980) and therefore cholinergic induction (McLennan *et al.*, 1980). It is clear that the cholinergic factor is different from nerve growth factor (NGF) since NGF is required for survival and stimulates the growth and differentiation of both the noradrenergic and cholinergic neurons while CM has no effect on survival or growth but selectively increases cholinergic differentiation (Chun and Patterson, 1977a, b).

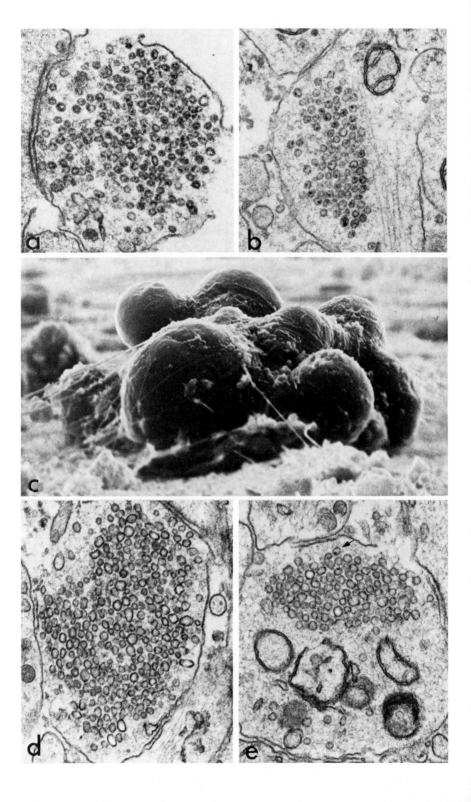

Several lines of evidence indicate that the cholinergic factor produced by non-neuronal cells induces neurons that have already begun to differentiate along a noradrenergic pathway to become cholinergic. As described above, shortly after plating, all the dissociated neurons exhibit noradrenergic properties and cholinergic ones appear only later (Johnson *et al.*, 1976, 1980b; Patterson and Chun, 1977b; Landis, 1980). Further, under the most cholinergic conditions, a reciprocity is evident between adrenergic and cholinerric functions (Patterson and Chun, 1977a; Reichardt and Patterson, 1977; Fukada, 1980), while neuronal number remains constant. Direct evidence for a transition has come from physiological and morphological studies of microcultures. These microcultures consist of one to several neurons growing on a small island of heart myocytes and fibroblasts; the myocytes are sensitive to both ACh and NE and serve as a bioassay for these two neurotransmitters in physiological studies. Many neurons have now been identified which are dual in function and release both ACh and NE and whose individual terminals appear intermediate in fine structure (Furshpan *et al.*, 1976; Landis, 1976; Potter *et al.*, 1980, 1981a, b). Amongst these single neurons, the relative balance of noradrenergic and cholinergic function, assayed both physiologically and morphologically, varies. This variation is consistent with a neurotransmitter shift. Further, repeated physiological assays of single neurons over time have disclosed transitions from noradrenergic to dual-function and dual-function to cholinergic and, most important, in one instance a complete transition from noradrenergic to dual-function to cholinergic has been demonstrated in a single neuron (Potter *et al.*, 1981b).

The effect of the cholinergic factor on neurotransmitter choice appears to be dose-dependent. In mass cultures containing several thousand neurons, the higher the proportion of CM in the growth medium, the more ACh is synthesized, the more cholinergic interactions are observed physiologically and the more apparently cholinergic synapses are identified morphologically (Landis *et al.*, 1976; Patterson and Chun, 1977a; Landis, 1980). Although at

Figure 1 (a) Four days after plating, all of the synapses and varicosities of neurons dissociated from the SCG of newborn rats contain numerous SGV after permanganate fixation. ×45 000. (b) Under noradrenergic growth conditions the synapses and varicosities present in mature cultures contain numerous SGV. Permanganate fixation. ×45 000. (c) Sympathetic neurons may be grown either alone or in the presence of non-neuronal cells as shown in this scanning electron micrograph. The neuronal cell bodies appear to sit on top of the monolayer of heart cells and axons rise from the monolayer and course over the cell bodies. ×1200. (d) When the neurons are grown in the presence of certain non-neuronal cells, or CM from them, many of the synapses and varicosities present in mature cultures lack SGV and endogenous catecholamines. Permanganate fixation, ×45 000. (e) A small percentage of the vesicles in such terminals can take up and store exogenous catecholamines in SGV (arrow). Permanganate fixation. ×45 000

low concentrations of CM catecholamine production is not decreased, at high concentrations it is significantly suppressed. Biochemical studies of single neurons indicate that the proportion of neurons which undergo transition is dependent upon the strength of the cholinergic stimulus (Reichardt and Patterson, 1977). In addition, physiological studies of the single neurons in microcultures make it clear that the rate of transition varies from neuron to neuron and suggest that the strength of the cholinergic stimulus is one of the factors that affect the rate (Potter *et al.*, 1980, 1981b). Thus, in general, transitions appear to occur more slowly in microcultures where relatively few heart cells are present than in mass cultures or single-neuron microcultures treated with high concentrations of CM (Patterson and Chun, 1977a, b; Reichardt and Patterson, 1977; Potter *et al.*, 1980, 1981a, b). In fact, neurons have been observed to remain in transition, secreting both NE and ACh, for several weeks (Potter *et al.*, 1980, 1981a, b). These observations indicate the induction of ACh synthesis need not result in the immediate turnoff of noradrenergic functions. Indeed, under culture conditions which apparently provide only a weak cholinergic stimulus, mass cultures show coordinate increases in both noradrenergic and cholinergic synthetic enzymes (Iacovitti *et al.*, 1980) and 90% of the neurons are immunoreactive for tyrosine hydroxylase in cultures where 85% of the cells interact cholinergically (Higgins *et al.*, 1981).

Not all noradrenergic properties are lost at the same rate. Biochemical (Reichardt and Patterson, 1977) and correlated physiological and morphological studies of single neurons (Furshpan *et al.*, 1976; Landis, 1976; Potter *et al.*, 1980, 1981b) have demonstrated that neurons which no longer synthesize or secrete detectable quantities of catecholamines can still take up and store exogenous catecholamines. Uptake and storage in SGV, however, is significantly decreased in older cultures grown under cholinergic conditions (Fig. 1e) (Johnson *et al.*, 1976, 1980b; Landis, 1980). These observations suggest that the ability to take up and store exogenous catecholamines in SGV is lost with time but that it disappears more slowly than the ability to synthesize catecholamines. This apparent difference in regulation could simply reflect a slower turnover rate for the membrane proteins responsible for uptake and storage than for the synthetic enzymes. In contrast, the high-affinity amine-uptake system of the plasma membrane may remain in neurons induced to become cholinergic and therefore be regulated independently of the catecholamine synthesis and vesicular storage systems (Wakshull *et al.*, 1978).

The ability of sympathetic neurons to respond to cholinergic factors appears to decrease with increasing age under some experimental conditions. When neurons are dissociated from the SCG of newborn rats they are more responsive to CM added during the first or second week than during the third or fourth (Patterson and Chun, 1977b). Cholinergic induction which is age-dependent has also been described in explant cultures. If explants of SCG are taken from neonatal rats, the neurons in these cultures will develop cholinergic properties; CAT activity and the number of apparently cholinergic endings increase with time in culture; coculture with heart muscle or growth in a cardiac extract causes greater cholinergic induction (Hill and Hendry, 1977; Ross *et al.*, 1977; Hill *et al.*, 1980; Johnson *et al.*, 1980a). However, as the explants are taken from increasingly older animals, the neurons become refractory to cholinergic influences (Hill and Hendry, 1977; Ross *et al.*, 1977; Johnson *et al.*, 1980a). If, instead of explant cultures, neurons from adult animals are dissociated and then grown in culture, at least some of these cells are able to form cholinergic synapses with each other and with skeletal myotubes (Johnson, 1978; Wakshull *et al.*, 1979a, b). It is unlikely that the dissociation procedure somehow selects for the small population of cholinergic sympathetic neurons thought to be present in the adult SCG, since preliminary examination of dissociated adult neurons in microcultures with cardiac myocytes has shown that many of these neurons initially release only NE and become dual-function with time, secreting both NE and ACh (Potter *et al.*, 1981b). Several explanations exist for the observed difference in plasticity between mature neurons in explants and after dissociation; for example, the organotypic environment of the explant may protect the neurons from cholinergic influences or the dissociation procedure may be more traumatic than explantation and cause the neurons to 'dedifferentiate' and become susceptible again to cholinergic influences.

In addition to the direct influence of the CM factor and the indirect effects of EGF and hydrocortisone, neuronal activity plays a role in influencing neurotransmitter choice in culture. The noradrenergic differentiation *in vitro* is stabilized and enhanced by growing the neurons under depolarizing conditions or by stimulating the neurons to fire electrophysiologically (Walicke *et al.*, 1977). Such conditions both increase catecholamine synthesis and prevent the neurons from responding to the cholinergic factor in CM. The effect of depolarization appears to be mediated by Ca^{2+} ions (Walicke and Patterson, 1981). However, evidence for the control of neurotransmitter choice by activity *in vivo* is lacking (Hill and Hendry, 1979).

NEUROTRANSMITTER CHOICE *IN VIVO*

In vivo, a small proportion of the principal sympathetic neurons are cholinergic. It is clearly of interest to ask whether these cholinergic sympathetic neurons *in vivo* possess the same developmental history as *in vitro*. Specifically, do they undergo a transition from noradrenergic to cholinergic function? If they do, do they retain any noradrenergic properties when they have acquired cholinergic ones? The cholinergic sympathetic neurons that have been most thoroughly characterized are those which innervate the eccrine sweat glands in the footpads of the cat. In the 1890's, Langley described a sympathetic outflow from the stellate and certain lumbar ganglia to the front and hind feet which caused secretion of sweat from the pads (Langley, 1891, 1894; see also Patton, 1948). A surprising finding was that the pharmacology of this sympathetic response was cholinergic rather than adrenergic: muscarinic agonists elicited sweating and adrenergic did not, while muscarinic antagonists blocked nerve-stimulation-induced sweating and adrenergic antagonists did not (Langley, 1922; Randall and Kimura, 1955; Foster and Weiner, 1970). Further evidence for the secretion of ACh from these sympathetic fibres was obtained by Dale and Feldberg (1934) who were able to demonstrate the presence of ACh in the venous effluent from footpads following nerve stimulation. The terminals around the sweat glands stain strongly for acetylcholinesterase (AChE) (Hellman, 1955; Sjöqvist, 1963a) and some neurons present in the stellate and 6th lumbar ganglia which provide innervation to the sweat glands in the front and hind feet are intensely AChE-positive (Sjöqvist, 1963a, b).

We have chosen to study the development of eccrine sweat glands in the rat (Landis and Keefe, 1980, 1981a, b) in part because the *in vitro* studies summarized above involved rat neurons. Rats, like cats, have sweat glands concentrated in the pads of their feet (Ring and Randall, 1947). Evidence for a cholinergic sympathetic innervation of the glands in the rat is not as complete as for the cat. It is known that sweating is induced by stimulation of peripheral nerves and that the effect of stimulation is produced by cholinergic agonists as in the cat (Ring and Randall, 1947; Sato and Sato, 1978). In the adult rat, each gland consists of a single, unbranched and tightly coiled tubule whose secretory portion lies in the subcutaneous tissue and is connected to the surface by a duct through the dermis leading to a tunnel through the epidermis (Ring and Randall, 1947; Sato and Sato, 1978). The secretory portion of the tubule is formed by secretory and myoepithelial cells (Weschler and Fisher, 1968) which abut onto thick basement membrane that is in turn surrounded by an incomplete sheath of fibrocytes. A plexus of fibres which stain heavily for AChE surround the tubule profiles in the gland. When such preparations are examined with the electron microscope, reaction product is found within and around all the bundles of axons in the glands. The pattern of innervation is characteristic of certain other autonomic junctions; the axons, even unsheathed varicosities, occur at a considerable distance from the target, are separated by fibrocyte processes as well as a basement membrane and exhibit no membrane specializations (Fig. 2a; see also Uno and Montagna, 1975). The varicosities contain small clear synaptic vesicles and larger, dense-core vesicles.

There is no evidence of adrenergic innervation of the sweat glands in adult rats, although in primates noradrenergic fibres have been observed in a small proportion of glands (Uno and Montagna, 1975). No fluorescent fibres are seen in the glands of the rat in Falck-Hillarp preparations and no small granular vesicles are present in the axon terminals after permanganate fixation (Fig. 2b). If, however, rats are injected with α-methylnorepinephrine (1–10 mg/kg i.p.) prior to sacrifice, then a catecholamine histofluorescent plexus is present in each of the sweat glands and its density and distribution matches that of the AChE-stained plexus. This uptake of exogenous catecholamine is blocked by prior injections with desmethylimipramine (30 mg/kg i.p.) as is uptake into adrenergic terminals (Iversen, 1967). Furthermore, the uptake is specific to cholinergic sympathetic fibres since cholinergic parasympathetic fibres in the irides and salivary glands of ganglionectomized rats do not show any catecholamine fluorescence after α-methylnorepinephrine injections. Similar loading of previously non-fluorescent terminals with exogenous catecholamines has been observed in primates but has been attributed to the sparse noradrenergic innervation rather than to the cholinergic innervation (Uno and Montagna, 1975). Ultrastructural examination after 5-hydroxydopamine loading (Tranzer and Thoenen, 1967) and permanganate fixation indicates that a few vesicles in all of the terminals in the sweat glands can take up and store some catecholamine (Fig. 2c).

The sweat glands and their innervation develop postnatally in the rat. Shortly after birth, the epidermis on the hind feet begins to invaginate at numerous points. Over the course of the next several days, these shallow invaginations form long straight tubules which begin to coil at about 10 days. At 14 days, the lumens of the glands are patent and differentiated myoepithelial and secretory cells are evident. A few faintly AChE-stained fibres are present in the forming glands at 7 days and the plexus increases in density and staining intensity as the glands mature. In contrast to the adult, numerous endogenously fluorescent catecholamine fibres are present around the glands at 7, 10 and 14 days. The fluorescent fibres are present as early as 4 days; thus the appearance of fluorescence in the plexus precedes that of the AChE staining. By 21 days, only an occasional and faintly fluorescent fibre is observed in the absence of exogenous catecholamine. Ultrastructural examination of developing terminals fixed with permanganate is in progress to determine whether all the innervating fibres initially appear noradrenergic and contain many SGV which are then gradually lost as one would expect if the fibres do indeed undergo a transition from noradrenergic to cholinergic.

These observations on the innervation of the sweat glands suggest that cholinergic sympathetic neurons *in vivo* share certain developmental properties with cholinergic sympathetic neurons *in vitro*: they are noradrenergic early in development and are able to take up catecholamines even when they no longer contain any endogenous catecholamines. These findings provide preliminary evidence for a transition from noradrenergic to cholinergic function in the normal development of these sympathetic neurons. Additional evidence for a transition comes from the observation that treatment of neonatal rats with 6-hydroxydopamine (6-OHDA) which specifically destroys

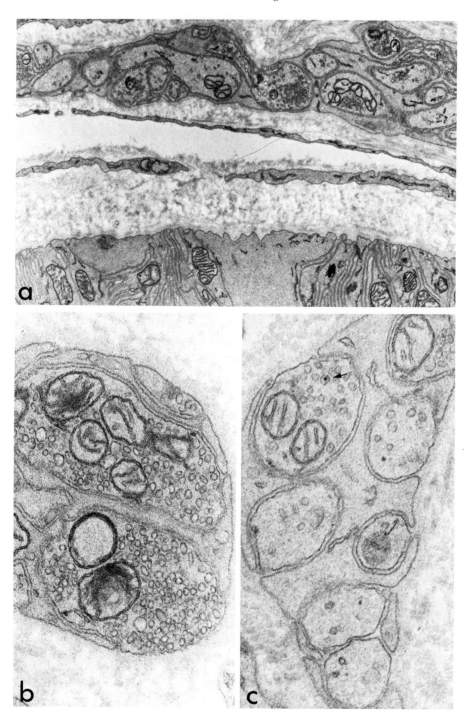

noradrenergic, but not other, neurons in newborn rats (Angeletti and Levi-Montalcini, 1970; Finch *et al.*, 1973) results in the virtual absence of an AChE-stained plexus around each gland when examined at four weeks. Further, no or very few terminals were seen in thin sections (Yodlowski and Landis, 1983). Treatment of adult animals with 6-OHDA had little effect on the mature innervation, probably because the catecholamine-uptake system which is required for 6-OHDA toxicity is reduced in adults (see Uno and Montagna, 1975). It is of interest that, in contrast to the apparent ineffectiveness of 6-OHDA treatment of adult rats, chronic treatment with guanethidine, another adrenergic neurotoxin, appears to cause the destruction of all sympathetic neuron cell bodies, cholinergic and noradrenergic (Heath and Burnstock, 1977).

A similar transmitter transition has been postulated for a population of neuron-like cells in the embryonic gut. At 11.5 days of gestation in the rat, noradrenergic cells appear in the developing gut; these neuroblasts stain immunocytochemically for tyrosine hydroxylase and dopamine β-hydroxylase and possess catecholamine histofluorescence. By 13.5 days, staining for the catecholamine synthetic enzymes and the catecholamine histofluorescence has disappeared (Cochard *et al.*, 1978, 1979; Teitelman *et al.*, 1978, 1979) although some cells present in the gut possess the ability to take up exogenous catecholamines until 17.5 days (Jonakait *et al.*, 1979). Treatment of fetuses with NGF (Kessler *et al.*, 1979) or elevation of maternal glucocorticoids (Jonakait *et al.*, 1980) postpones the normal disappearance of the noradrenergic properties for several days but does not apparently prevent their ultimate disappearance. One interpretation of these observations is that some enteric neuroblasts acquire the ability to synthesize catecholamines but then lose it as they acquire another transmitter, perhaps ACh, under the environmental influence of the gut. As in the sympathetic neuron cultures, the ability to store catecholamines is retained longer than synthetic abilities. It has not been possible, however, to determine the differentiated fate of these cells and exclude the possibility that they simply degenerate.

Figure 2 (a) The secretory tubule of the rat sweat gland, which contains secretory and myoepithelial cells, is surrounded by a thick basement membrane and fibrocyte processes. The innervating axons run in bundles of 10–12, and lie up to several micrometres away from the tubule. Permanganate fixation. ×15 000. (b) In adult rats there is no evidence of the presence of endogenous catecholamines in these terminals; for example, only clear synaptic vesicles are found after permanganate fixation. ×45 000. (c) A small percentage of the vesicles present in these terminals can take up and store exogenous catecholamines. One such vesicle is present in a single axon in this particular section (arrow). If, however, serial sections are examined, every varicosity contains a few loaded vesicles. ×45 000

SIF CELL PLASTICITY

In addition to principal neurons, many sympathetic ganglia contain small intensely fluorescent (SIF) cells. As described in the chapter by Taxi, these cells differ from principal neurons in several respects: they are small, 10 μm rather than 30–50 μm; they are brightly, rather than faintly, fluorescent; they store catecholamines predominantly in large dense-core vesicles (100–200 nm) rather than in small synaptic vesicles (50 nm); they extend relatively short processes, tens of micrometers rather than a centimeter or more; and they often occur in small clusters along blood vessels. Thus, in many of these properties, SIF cells appear intermediate between principal and chromaffin cells such as those in the adrenal medulla, which do not normally extend processes and contain very large storage granules (300 nm). All three populations of adrenergic cells—principal neurons, SIF cells and chromaffin cells—are derived from the neural crest and the question arises as to what influences determine the selection of phenotype.

Glucocorticoids represent one important developmental influence (Doupe and Patterson, 1981). One clue to the importance of glucocorticoids came from Lempinen's (1964) observation that the administration of hydrocortisone to neonatal rats not only prevents the normal developmental disappearance of extra-adrenal chromaffin tissue but results in an apparent hyperplasia of these tissues and the appearance of chromaffin-positive cells in sympathetic ganglia where they are never normally seen. Examination of the SCG of rat pups following hydrocortisone or dexamethasone treatment disclosed a marked increase in the number of SIF cells (Eränkö and Eränkö, 1972; Ciaranello *et al.*, 1973; Luizzi *et al.*, 1977). These SIF cells were often observed in atypical locations in the ganglion. A similar increase in the number of SIF cells has been observed when explants or whole ganglia from newborn rats have been cultured in the presence of high concentrations of glucocorticoids (Eränkö *et al.*, 1972a, b). Biochemical and immunocytochemical evidence indicates that the glucocorticoids not only cause an increase in the number of SIF cells but also the appearance of phenylethanolamine *N*-methyltransferase which converts NE into epinephrine (Ciaranello *et al.*, 1973; Koslow *et al.*, 1975; Gianutos and Moore, 1977; Luizzi *et al.*, 1977; Eränkö and Eränkö, 1979; Black *et al.*, 1980). The number of SIF cells appears to decrease after glucocorticoid treatment stops (Eränkö and Eränkö, 1980). Similar glucocorticoid treatment of adult animals does not cause an increase in the number of SIF cells (Eränkö and Eränkö, 1972; Ciaranello *et al.*, 1973). Thus there is a relatively narrow time span when cells are sensitive. The most common interpretation of these results has been that the glucocorticoids act on undifferentiated precursor cells and induce them to become SIF cells, some of which at least will produce epinephrine, but it has not been possible to exclude the possibility that some of these cells arise from division of already committed SIF cells or from conversion of neurons.

NGF represents a second developmental influence. Transplantation of adrenal medullary cells to the anterior chamber of adrenergically denervated eyes results in process outgrowth from the transplanted cells (Olson, 1970); these processes partially reinnervate the denervated host iris which has been shown to contain elevated levels of NGF (Ebendal *et al.*, 1980). The axons arise from groups of highly fluorescent cells. More direct evidence for the role of NGF comes from tissue-culture studies of rat adrenal medullary cells dissociated from week-old rats (Unsicker *et al.*, 1978). Treatment with NGF causes fibre outgrowth from the adrenal medullary cells. As in the transplantation studies, the cell bodies remain brightly fluorescent and thus resemble SIF cells more closely than principal neurons. This process outgrowth is blocked by glucocorticoids. Further, injections of NGF into 17- and 18-day rat fetuses followed by daily postnatal injections results in a striking transformation of the adrenal gland (Aloe and Levi-Montalcini, 1979). The entire adrenal medulla becomes filled with cells that resemble sympathetic neurons more than chromaffin cells and which extend processes that run in fascicles through the gland. It is of interest that most of the cell bodies still contain numerous large dense-core vesicles similar to those of chromaffin cells. Thus they also resemble SIF cells. In adult animals, NGF, like glucocorticoids, does not seem to affect phenotype of any of these adrenergic cells (Angeletti *et al.*, 1972; Aloe and Montalcini, 1979) although both NGF and glucocorticoids are able to modulate levels of enzyme activities (Harper and Thoenen, 1980; Doupe and Patterson, 1981).

The developmental influence of these hormones could be on the survival or mitosis of different populations of predetermined ganglionic cells or it could be on the phenotypic decision of individual cells. Further analysis of the actions of these hormones is being carried out in a dissociated cell culture system. If the cell suspension from dissociated sympathetic ganglia is plated into medium that contains dexamethasone, an antimitotic agent and no NGF, SIF cells develop in the virtual absence of neurons and non-neuronal cells (Doupe *et al.*, 1980) (cf. Fig. 3a, b). The cells are small, 10–15 μm, either round or flat and polygonal, and brightly fluorescent. They contain numerous large dense-core vesicles (100–250 nm) and lack processes. The glucocorticoids appear to affect the phenotype of undifferentiated cells since, initially after plating, no brightly fluorescent or granule-containing cells are present. Further, many of these cells are NGF-sensitive. Following exposure to NGF, they grow processes, and may lose their bright fluorescence and acquire a neuronal ultrastructure. These results suggest that there are cells in the SCG which have the potential to become either neurons or SIF cells, and that glucocorticoids and NGF influence this choice.

SUMMARY

In summary, it is clear from the work reviewed above and that detailed by Le Douarin (this volume) that environmental influences play an important

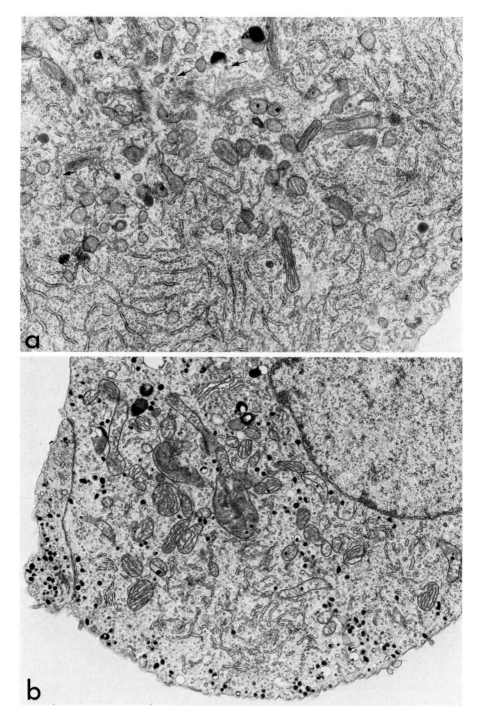

role in the phenotypic choices made by cells of the neural crest. In the case of the noradrenergic-cholinergic decision documented in cultures of rat sympathetic neurons, the culture environment can change the developmental fate of a postmitotic cell, even after it has begun to express one set of differentiated properties. Environmental influences can be mediated through specifying factors, such as the cholinergic factor, whose production and release is controlled in turn by growth factors and hormones. Alternatively, the growth factors and hormones may act directly on choice; thus, NGF and glucocorticoids appear to influence the decision of the adrenergic progeny of the crest to become either principal neurons, SIF cells or chromaffin cells. In both examples, transmitter choice and neuron-SIF-chromaffin cell choice, information has recently become available that suggests that developmental mechanisms explored in cell-culture systems will mirror those in the intact and developing animal.

ACKNOWLEDGEMENTS

I wish to thank Paul Patterson, David Potter and Ed Furshpan for their helpful discussions, and Dennis Keefe and Mary Hogan for their technical assistance. This research was supported by grants-in-aid from the Milton Fund and the American Heart Association (78–964) and US Public Health Service grants (NS 15549, NS 11576, NS 02253) from the National Institute of Neurological and Communicable Diseases and Stroke. S. L. is an Established Investigator of the American Heart Association.

REFERENCES

Aloe, L., and Levi-Montalcini, R. (1979). Nerve growth factor-induced transformation of immature chromaffin cells *in vivo* into sympathetic neurons: effect of antiserum to nerve growth factor. *Proc. Natl. Acad. Sci. U.S.A.*, **76**, 1246–1250.

Angeletti, P. U., and Levi-Montalcini, R. (1970). Sympathetic nerve cell destruction in newborn mammals by 6-hydroxydopamine. *Proc. Natl. Acad. Sci. U.S.A.*, **65**, 114–121.

Angeletti, P. U., Levi-Montalcini, R., Kettler, R., and Thoenen, H. (1972).

Figure 3 (a) When cells are dissociated from the SCG of newborn rats and grown in the presence of NGF and an antimitotic agent, they develop the ultrastructural characteristics of mature neurons; extensive stacks of rough endoplasmic reticulum, a well-organized Golgi apparatus and occasional large dense-core vesicles (80–100 nm, arrows) are present. Aldehyde-osmium fixation. ×18 000. (b) When cells are dissociated from the SCG of newborn rats and grown in the presence of dexamethasone and an antimitotic agent but without NGF, they develop the ultrastructural characteristics of SIF cells; numerous large dense vesicles (100–200 nm) and relatively scanty rough endoplasmic reticulum and Golgi apparatus are seen. Aldehyde-osmium fixation. ×18 000

Comparative studies on the effect of nerve growth factor on sympathetic ganglia and adrenal medulla in newborn rats. *Brain Res.*, **44**, 197–206.

Black, I. B., Bohn, M. C., Bloom, E. M., and Goldstein, M. (1980). Glucocorticoids induce expression of the adrenergic phenotype in a rat sympathetic ganglion. *Soc. Neurosci. Abstr.*, **6**, 408.

Burton, H., and Bunge, R. P. (1975). A comparison of the uptake and release of [3-H]-norepinephrine in rat autonomic and sensory ganglia in tissue culture. *Brain Res.*, **97**, 157–162.

Chun, L. L. Y., and Patterson, P. H. (1977a). Role of nerve growth factor in the development of rat sympathetic neurons *in vitro*. I. Survival, growth and differentiation of catecholamine production. *J. Cell Biol.*, **75**, 694–704.

Chun, L. L. Y., and Patterson, P. H. (1977b). Role of nerve growth factor in the development of rat sympathetic neurons *in vitro*. III. Effect on acetylcholine production. *J. Cell Biol.*, **75**, 712–718,

Ciaranello, R. D., Jacobowitz, D., and Axelrod, J. (1973). Effect of dexamethasone on phenylethanolamine *N*-methyltransferase in chromaffin tissue of the neonatal rat. *J. Neurochem.*, **20**, 799–805.

Cochard, P., Goldstein, M., and Black, I. B. (1978). Ontogenetic appearance and disappearance of tyrosine hydroxylase and catecholamines in the rat embryo. *Proc. Natl. Acad. Sci. U.S.A.*, **75**, 2986–2990.

Cochard, P., Goldstein, M., and Black, I. B. (1979). Initial development of the noradrenergic phenotype in autonomic neuroblasts of the rat embryo *in vivo*. *Dev. Biol.*, **71**, 100–114.

Cohen, A. M. (1972). Factors directing the expression of sympathetic nerve traits in cells of neural crest origin. *J. Exp. Zool.*, **917**, 167–182.

Cohen, A. M. (1974). DNA synthesis and cell division in differentiating avian adrenergic neuroblasts. In *Wenner-Gren Center International Symposium Series, Vol. 22, Dynamics of Degeneration and Growth in Neurons* (Eds. K. Fuxe, L. Olson and Y. Zotterman), pp. 359–370, Pergamon Press, Oxford.

Coughlin, M. D., Dibner, M. D., Boyer, D. M., and Black, I. B. (1978). Factors regulating development of an embryonic mouse sympathetic ganglion. *Dev. Biol.*, **66**, 513–528.

Dale, H. H., and Feldberg, W. (1934). The chemical transmission of secretory impulses to the sweat glands of the cat. *J. Physiol. (London)*, **82**, 121–128.

De Champlain, J., Malmfors, T., Olson, L., and Sachs, Ch. (1970). Ontogenesis of peripheral adrenergic neurons in the rat: pre- and postnatal observations. *Acta Physiol. Scand.*, **80**, 276–288.

Doupe, A. J., and Patterson, P. H. (1981). Glucocorticoids and the developing nervous system. *Curr. Top. Neuroendocrinol.*, in press.

Doupe, A. J., Patterson, P. H., and Landis, S. C. (1980). Dissociated cell culture of SIF cells: hormone-dependence and NGF action. *Soc. Neurosci. Abstr.*, **6**, 409.

Ebendal, T., Olson, L., Seiger, Å., and Hedlund, K.-O. (1980). Nerve growth factors in the rat iris. *Nature*, **286**, 25–28.

Enemar, A., Falck, B., and Håkanson, R. (1965). Observations on the appearance of norepinephrine in the sympathetic nervous system of the chick embryo. *Dev. Biol.*, **11**, 268–283.

Eränkö, L. (1972). Ultrastructure of the developing sympathetic nerve cell and the storage of catecholamines. *Brain Res.*, **46**, 159–172.

Eränkö, L., and Eränkö, O. (1972). Effect of hydrocortisone on histochemically demonstrable catecholamines in the sympathetic ganglia and extra-adrenal chromaffin tissue of the rat. *Acta Physiol. Scand.*, **84**, 125–133.

Eränkö, O., and Eränkö, L. (1979). Increase *in vivo* and *in vitro* of catecholamines and catecholamine-synthesizing enzymes in SIF cells of newborn rat superior cervical ganglia. In *Catecholamines: Basic and Clinical Frontiers* (Eds. E. Usdin, I. J. Kopin and J. Barchus), Vol. I, pp. 821–823, Pergamon Press, New York.

Eränkö, O., and Eränkö, L. (1980). Induction of SIF cells by hydrocortisone or human cord serum in sympathetic ganglia and their subsequent fate *in vivo* and *in vitro*. In *Histochemistry and Cell Biology of Autonomic Neurons, SIF Cells and Paraneurons* (Eds. O. Eränkö, S. Soinila and H. Päivärinta), *Advances in Biochemical Psychopharmacology*, Vol. 25, pp. 17–26, Raven Press, New York.

Eränkö, O., Eränkö, L., Hill, C. E., and Burnstock, G. (1972a). Hydrocortisone-induced increase in the number of small intensely fluorescent cells and their histochemically demonstrable catecholamine content in cultures of sympathetic ganglia of the newborn rat. *Histochem. J.*, **4**, 49–58.

Eränkö, O., Heath, J., and Eränkö, L. (1972b). Effect of hydrocortisone on the ultrastructure of the small, intensely fluorescent, granule-containing cells in cultures of sympathetic ganglia of newborn rats. *Z. Zellforsch. Mikrosk. Anat.*, **134**, 297–310.

Finch, L., Haeusler, G., and Thoenen, H. (1973). A comparison of the effects of chemical sympathectomy by 6-hydroxydopamine in newborn and adult rats. *Br. J. Pharmacol.*, **47**, 249–260.

Foster, K. G., and Weiner, J. S. (1970). Effects of cholinergic and adrenergic blocking agents on the activity of the eccrine sweat glands. *J. Physiol. (London)*, **210**, 883–895.

Fukada, K. (1980). Hormonal control of neurotransmitter choice in sympathetic neurone cultures. *Nature*, **287**, 553–555.

Furshpan, E. J., MacLeish, P. R., O'Lague, P. H., and Potter, D. D. (1976). Chemical transmission between rat sympathetic neurons and cardiac myocytes developing in microcultures: Evidence for cholinergic, adrenergic and dual-function neurons. *Proc. Natl. Acad. Sci. U.S.A.*, **73**, 4225–4229.

Gianutos, G., and Moore, K. E. (1977). Effects of pre- or postnatal dexamethasone, adrenocorticotrophic hormone and environmental stress on phenylethanolamine *N*-methyltransferase activity and catecholamines in sympathetic ganglia of neonatal rats. *J. Neurochem.*, **28**, 935–940.

Grillo, M. A. (1966). Electron microscopy of sympathetic tissues. *Pharmacol. Rev.*, **18**, 387–399.

Harper, G. P., and Thoenen, H. (1980). Nerve growth factor: biological significance, measurement and distribution. *J. Neurochem.*, **34**, 5–16.

Hawrot, E. (1980). Cultured sympathetic neurons: effects of cell-derived and synthetic substrata on survival and development. *Dev. Biol.*, **74**, 136–151.

Heath, J. W., and Burnstock, G. (1977). Selectivity of neuronal degeneration produced by chronic guanethidine treatment. *J. Neurocytol.*, **6**, 397–405.

Hellman, K. (1955). Cholinesterase and amine oxidase in the skin: a histochemical investigation. *J. Physiol. (London)*, **129**, 454–463.

Higgins, D., Iacovitti, L., Joh, T. H., and Burton, H. (1981). The immunocytochemical localization of tyrosine hydroxylase within rat sympathetic neurons that release acetylcholine in culture. *J. Neurosci.*, **1**, 126–131.

Hill, C. E., and Hendry, I. E. (1977). Development of neurons synthesizing noradrenaline and acetylcholine in the superior cervical ganglion of the rat *in vivo* and *in vitro*. *Neuroscience*, **2**, 741–749.

Hill, C. E., and Hendry, I. E. (1979). The influence of preganglionic nerves on the superior cervical ganglion of the rat. *Neurosci. Lett.*, **13**, 133–139.

Hill, C. E., Hendry, I. A., and McLennan, I. S. (1980). Factors influencing transmitter type in sympathetic ganglion cells. In *Histochemistry and Cell Biology of Autonomic Neurons, SIF Cells and Paraneurons* (Eds. O. Eränkö, S. Soinila and H. Päivärinta), *Advances in Biochemical Psychopharmacology*, Vol. 25, pp. 69–74, Raven Press, New York.

Hökfelt, T. (1969). Distribution of noradrenaline storing particles in peripheral adrenergic neurons as revealed by electron microscopy. *Acta Physiol. Scand.*, **76**, 427–440.

Iacovitti, L. I., Joh, T. H., Park, D. H., and Bunge, R. P. (1989). Dual expression of transmitter synthesis in cultured autonomic neurons. *Soc. Neurosci. Abstr.*, **6**, 329.

Iversen, L. L. (1967). *The Uptake and Storage of Noradrenaline in Sympathetic Nerves*, Cambridge University Press, Cambridge.

Johnson, M. (1978). Adult rat dissociated sympathetic neurons in culture: morphological and cytochemical studies. *Soc. Neurosci. Abstr.*, **4**, 116.

Johnson, M., Ross, D., Meyers, M., Rees, R., Bunge, R., Wakshull, E., and Burton, H. (1976). Synaptic vesicle cytochemistry changes when cultured sympathetic neurones develop cholinergic interactions. *Nature*, **262**, 308–310.

Johnson, M. I., Ross, C. D., and Bunge, R. P. (1980a). Morphological and biochemical studies on the development of cholinergic properties in cultured sympathetic neurons. II. Dependence on postnatal age. *J. Cell Biol.*, **84**, 692–704.

Johnson, M. I., Ross, C. D., Meyers, M., Spitznagel, E. L., and Bunge, R. P. (1980b). Morphological and biochemical studies of the development of cholinergic properties in cultured sympathetic neurons. I. Correlative changes in choline acetyltransferase and synaptic vesicle cytochemistry. *J. Cell Biol.*, **84**, 680–691.

Jonakait, G. M., Wolf, J., Cochard, P., Goldstein, M., and Black, I. B. (1979). Selective loss of noradrenergic phenotypic characters in neuroblasts of the rat embryo. *Proc. Natl. Acad. Sci. U.S.A.*, **76**, 4683–4686.

Jonakait, G. M., Bohn, M. C., and Black, I. B. (1980). Maternal glucocorticoid hormones influence neurotransmitter phenotypic expression in embryos. *Science*, **210**, 551–553.

Kessler, J. A., Cochard, P., and Black, I. B. (1979). Nerve growth factor alters the fate of embryonic neuroblasts. *Nature*, **280**, 141–142.

Kirby, M. I., and Gilmore, S. A. (1976). A correlative histofluorescence and light microscopic study of the formation of the sympathetic trunks in chick embryos. *Anat. Rec.*, **186**, 437–450.

Ko, C. P., Burton, H., Johnson, M. I., and Bunge, R. P. (1976). Synaptic transmission between rat superior cervical ganglion neurons in dissociated cell cultures. *Brain Res.*, **117**, 461–485.

Koslow, S. H., Bjegovic, M., and Costa, E. (1975). Catecholamines in sympathetic ganglia of rat: Effects of dexamethasone and reserpine. *J. Neurochem.*, **24**, 277–281.

Landis, S. C. (1976). Rat sympathetic neurons and cardiac myocytes developing in microcultures: Correlation of the fine structure of endings with neurotransmitter function in single neurons. *Proc. Natl. Acad. Sci. U.S.A.*, **73**, 4220–4224.

Landis, S. C. (1978). Growth cones of cultured sympathetic neurons contain adrenergic vesicles. *J. Cell Biol.*, **78**, R8–R14.

Landis, S. C. (1980). Developmental changes in the neurotransmitter properties of dissociated sympathetic neurons: a cytochemical study of the effects of medium. *Dev. Biol.*, **77**, 349–361.

Landis, S. C., and Keefe, D. (1980). Development of cholinergic sympathetic innervation of eccrine sweat glands in rat footpad. *Soc. Neurosci. Abstr.*, **6**, 379.

Landis, S. C., and Keefe, D. (1983a). Neurotransmitter plasticity *in vivo*. I. Properties of the cholinergic sympathetic fibers innervating the eccrine sweat glands in footpads of adult rats. In preparation.

Landis, S. C., and Keefe, D. (1981b). Neurotransmitter plasticity *in vivo*: II. Development of cholinergic sympathetic innervation of sweat glands in rat footpads. In preparation.

Landis, S. C., MacLeish, P. R., Potter, D. D., Furshpan, E. J., and Patterson, P. H. (1976). Synapses formed between dissociated sympathetic neurons: The influence of conditioned medium. *Soc. Neurosci. Abstr.*, **280**.

Langley, J. N. (1891). On the course and connections of the secretory fibres supplying the sweat glands of the feet of the cat. *J. Physiol. (London)*, **12**, 347–374.

Langley, J. N. (1894). Further observations on the secretory and vaso-motor fibres of the foot of the cat, with notes on other sympathetic fibres. *J. Physiol. (London)*, **17**, 296–314.

Langley, J. N. (1922). The secretion of sweat. Part. I. Supposed inhibitory nerve fibres on the posterior nerve roots. Secretion after denervation. *J. Physiol. (London)*, **56**, 110–119.

Lempinen, M. (1964). Extra-adrenal chromaffin tissue of the rat and the effect of cortical hormones on it. *Acta Physiol. Scand.*, **62** (Suppl. 231).

Luizzi, A., Foppen, F. H., Saavedra, J. M., Jacobowitz, D., and Kopin, I. J. (1977). Effect of NGF and dexamethasone on phenylethanolamine-*N*-methyl transferase (PNMT) activity in neonatal rat superior cervical ganglia. *J. Neurochem.*, **28**, 1215–1220.

Mains, R. E., and Patterson, P. H. (1973). Primary cultures of dissociated sympathetic neurons. I. Establishment of long-term growth in culture and studies of differentiated properties. *J. Cell Biol.*, **59**, 329–345.

Matthews, M. R. (1974). Ultrastructure of ganglionic junctions. In *The Peripheral Nervous System* (Ed. J. I. Hubbard), pp. 111–149, Plenum Press, New York.

McLennan, I. S., Hill, C. E., and Hendry, I. A. (1980). Glucocorticosteroids modulate transmitter choice in developing superior cervical ganglion. *Nature*, **283**, 206–207.

Norr, S. (1973). *In vitro* analysis of sympathetic neuron differentiation from chick neural crest cells. *Dev. Biol.*, **34**, 16–38.

Nurse, C. A., and O'Lague, P. H. (1975). Formation of cholinergic synapses between dissociated sympathetic neurons and skeletal myotubes of the rat in cell culture. *Proc. Natl. Acad. Sci. U.S.A.*, **72**, 1955–1959.

O'Lague, P. H., Obata, K., Claude, P., Furshpan, E. J., and Potter, D. D. (1974). Evidence for cholinergic synapses between dissociated rat sympathetic neurons in cell culture. *Proc. Natl. Acad. Sci. U.S.A.*, **71**, 3602–3606.

O'Lague, P. H., Furshpan, E. J., and Potter, D. D.(1978a). Studies on rat sympathetic neurons developing in cell culture. II. Synaptic mechanisms. *Dev. Biol.*, **67**, 404–423.

O'Lague, P. H., Potter, D. D., and Furshpan, E. J. (1978b). Studies on rat sympathetic neurons developing in cell culture. III. Cholinergic transmission. *Dev. Biol.*, **67**, 424–443.

Olson, L. (1970). Fluorescence histochemical evidence for axonal growth and secretion from transplanted adrenal medullary tissue. *Histochemie*, **22**, 1–7.

Patterson, P. H., and Chun, L. L. Y. (1974). The influence of non-neuronal cells on catecholamines and acetylcholine synthesis and accumulation in cultures of dissociated sympathetic neurons. *Proc. Natl. Acad. Sci. U.S.A.*, **71**, 3607–3610.

Patterson, P. H., and Chun, L. L. Y. (1977a). Induction of acetylcholine synthesis in primary cultures of dissociated rat sympathetic neurons. I. Effects of conditioned medium. *Dev. Biol.*, **56**, 263–280.

Patterson, P. H., and Chun, L. L. Y. (1977b). The induction of acetylcholine synthesis in primary cultures of dissociated sympathetic neurons. II. Developmental aspects. *Dev. Biol.*, **60**, 473–481.

Patterson, P. H., Reichardt, L. F., and Chun, L. L. Y. (1975). Biochemical studies on the development of primary sympathetic neurons in cell culture. *Cold Spring Harbor Symp. Quant. Biol.*, **40**, 389–397.

Patton, H. D. (1948). Secretory innervation of the cat's footpad. *J. Neurophysiol. (London)*, **11**, 217–227.

Potter, D. D., Landis, S. C., and Furshpan, E. J. (1980). Dual function during the development of rat sympathetic neurones in culture. In *Neurotransmission, Neurotransmitters and Neuromodulators* (Eds. E. A. Kravitz and J. E. Treherne), pp. 57–72, Cambridge University Press, Cambridge.

Potter, D. D., Landis, S. C., and Furshpan, E. J. (1981a). Chemical differentiation of sympathetic neurons. In *Neurosecretion and Brain Peptides: Implications for Brain Function and Neurological Disease* (Eds. J. Martin, S. Reichlin and K. L. Bick), pp. 275–285, Raven Press, New York.

Potter, D. D., Landis, S. C., and Furshpan, E. J. (1981b). Adrenergic-cholinergic dual function in cultured sympathetic neurones of the rat. In *The Development of the Autonomic Nervous System, Ciba Foundation Symposium 83*, Pitman Medical, London.

Randall, W. C., and Kimura, K. K. (1955). The pharmacology of sweating. *Pharmacol. Rev.*, **7**, 365–397.

Rees, R., and Bunge, R. P. (1974). Morphological and cytochemical studies of synapses formed in culture between isolated rat superior cervical ganglion neurons. *J. Comp. Neurol.*, **157**, 1–12.

Reichardt, L. F., and Patterson, P. H. (1977). Neurotransmitter synthesis and uptake by isolated sympathetic neurons in microcultures. *Nature*, **270**, 147–151.

Richardson, K. C. (1966). Electron microscopic identification of autonomic nerve endings. *Nature*, **210**, 756.

Ring, J. R., and Randall, W. C. (1947). The distribution and histological structure of sweat glands in the albino rat and their response to prolonged nervous stimulation. *Anat. Rec.*, **99**, 7–16.

Ross, D., Johnson, M., and Bunge, R. (1977). Development of cholinergic characteristics in adrenergic neurones is age dependent. *Nature*, **267**, 536–539.

Rothman, T. P., Gershon, M. D., and Holtzer, H. (1978). The relationship of cell division to the acquisition of adrenergic characteristics by developing sympathetic ganglion cell precursors. *Dev. Biol.*, **65**, 322–341.

Sato, F., and Sato, K. (1978). Secretion of a potassium-rich fluid by the secretory coil of the rat paw eccrine sweat gland. *J. Physiol. (London)*, **274**, 37–50.

Schwab, M., and Landis, S. (1981). Membrane properties of cultured rat sympathetic neurons: morphological studies of adrenergic and cholinergic differentiation. *Dev. Biol.*, **84**, 67–78.

Sjöqvist, F. (1963a). The correlation between the occurrence and localization of acetylcholinesterase-rich cell bodies in the stellate ganglion and the outflow of cholinergic sweat secretory fibres to the fore paw of the cat. *Acta Physiol. Scand.*, **57**, 339–351.

Sjöqvist, F. (1963b). Pharmacological analysis acetylcholinesterase-rich ganglion cells in the lumbo-sacral sympathetic system of the cat. *Acta Physiol. Scand.*, **57**, 352–362.

Sweadner, K. J. (1981). Environmentally regulated expression of soluble extracellular proteins of sympathetic neurons. *J. Biol. Chem.*, **256**, 4063–4070.

Sweadner, K. J., and Braun, S. J. (1979). Neurotransmitter-specific proteins of sympathetic neurons. *Soc. Neurosci. Abstr.*, **5**, 598.

Teillet M. A., Cochard, P., and Le Douarin, N. M. (1978). Relative roles of the mesenchymal tissues and of the complex neural tube–notochord on the expression of adrenergic metabolism in neural crest cells. *Zoon*, **6**, 115–122.

Teitelman, G., Joh, T. H., and Reis, D. J. (1978). Transient expression of a noradrenergic phenotype in cells of the rat embryonic gut. *Brain Res.*, **158**, 229–234.

Teitelman, G., Baker, Joh, T. H., and Reis, D. J. (1979). Appearance of catecholamine-synthesizing enzymes during development of rat sympathetic nervous system: possible role of tissue environment. *Proc. Natl. Acad. Sci. U.S.A.*, **76**, 509–513.

Tranzer, J. P., and Thoenen, H. (1967). Electron-microscopic localization of 5-hydroxydopamine (3,4,5-trihydroxy-phenylethylamine), a new 'false' sympathetic transmitter. *Experientia*, **23**, 743–745.

Uno, H., and Montagna, W. (1975). Catecholamine-containing nerve terminals of the eccrine sweat glands of macaques. *Cell Tissue Res*, **155**, 1–13.

Unsicker, K., Kirsch, B., Otten, U., and Thoenen, H. (1978). Nerve growth factor-induced fiber outgrowth from isolated rat adrenal chromaffin cells: impairment by glucocorticoids. *Proc. Natl Acad. Sci. U.S.A.*, **75**, 3498–3502.

Wakshull, E., Johnson, M. I., and Burton, H. (1978). Persistence of an amine uptake system in cultured rat sympathetic neurons which use acetylcholine as their transmitter. *J. Cell Biol.*, **79**, 121–131.

Wakshull, E., Johnson, M. I., and Burton, H. (1979a). Postnatal rat sympathetic neurons in culture. I. A comparison with embryonic neurons. *J. Neurophysiol.*, **42**, 1410–1425.

Wakshull, E., Johnson, M. I., and Burton, H. (1979b). Postnatal sympathetic neurons in culture. II. Synaptic transmission by postnatal neurons. *J. Neurophysiol.*, **42**, 1426–1436.

Walicke, P. A., and Patterson, P. H. (1981). On the role of Ca^{++} in the transmitter choice made by cultured sympathetic neurons. *J. Neurosci.*, **1**, 343–350.

Walicke, P. A., Campenot, R. B., and Patterson, P. H. (1977). Determination of transmitter function by neuronal activity. *Proc. Natl. Acad. Sci. U.S.A.*, **74**, 5767–5771.

Weber, M. (1981). A diffusible factor responsible for the determination of cholinergic functions in cultured sympathetic neurons: Partial purification and characterization. *J. Biol. Chem.*, **256**, 3447–3453.

Weschler, H. L., and Fisher, E. R. (1968). Eccrine glands of the rat. *Arch. Dermatol.*, **97**, 189–201.

Yodlowski, M., and Landis S. (1981). 6-Hydroxydopamine prevents the development of cholinergic sympathetic innervation: evidence for neurotransmitter plasticity *in vivo*. In preparation.

Autonomic Ganglia
Edited by Lars-Gösta Elfvin
© 1983 John Wiley & Sons Ltd

Cell and Tissue Culture Studies on the Sympathoadrenal System

K. UNSICKER

*University of Marburg, Department of Anatomy and Cell Biology,
Robert-Koch-Strasse 6, D-3550 Marburg, Federal Republic of Germany*

INTRODUCTION

Cell, tissue and organ cultures of sympathetic ganglia and adrenal medulla have become increasingly valuable tools during the past decade for investigating cell performances in defined environments. Differentiation, plasticity, regulation of transmitter synthesis, drug effects and interactions with various target tissues are specific issues that have been profitably studied with cultured sympathetic ganglia and adrenal medullae or with dissociated cells from these organs. The number of papers and the diversity of approaches have largely increased since the end of the 1960's. As with cultured nervous tissue from other sources, emphasis for *in vitro* studies of the sympathoadrenal system was initially on the preparation, maintenance and analysis of organotypic cultures and later proceeded to dissociated cells and cell lines (Bunge, 1975; Murray, 1977). Work on *in vitro* cultures of adrenal medulla and chromaffin cells started later than on sympathetic ganglia, presumably because of technical difficulties. Substantial reviews on culture work carried out with sympathetic ganglia and original papers reviewing the field are available (Burnstock and Costa, 1975; Burton and Bunge, 1981; Chamley *et al.*, 1972a, b; Crain, 1976; Fischbach and Nelson, 1977; Gabella, 1976; Murray, 1965, 1971; Nelson, 1975; Sato, 1973; Silberstein, 1973).

The aim of this chapter is to review morphological, physiological and biochemical data obtained with cultures from the sympathoadrenal system published mainly in the past decade. Two important aspects of sympathetic neurons *in vitro*, their dependence upon nerve growth factor (NGF) and their choice of transmitter, will be dealt with in separate chapters of this volume by Levi-Montalcini and Aloe and by Landis.

This review does not refer to *in vitro* work carried out with neuroblastoma and pheochromocytoma cells.

SYMPATHETIC GANGLIA AND DISSOCIATED SYMPATHETIC NEURONS IN CULTURE

Morphological studies

General organization of explant cultures

When sympathetic ganglia from mammals, chick and amphibia are explanted into culture, nerve fibres begin to grow out within 24 to 48 hours (Chamley *et al.*, 1972a; Hill and Burnstock, 1975; Hervonen, 1975a); addition of NGF may accelerate this process (Fig. 1a). At the electron-microscope

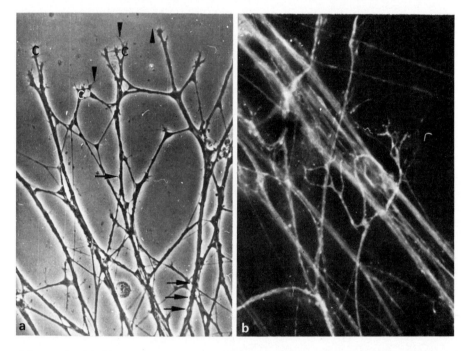

Figure 1 (a) Phase-contrast micrograph. (b) Catecholamine histofluorescence (glyoxylic acid). Neurite outgrowth from a sympathetic ganglion explant (perinatal rat, 72 hours in culture) grown in the presence of 50 ng/ml 2.5 S NGF. Neurites form mostly bundles with smooth and varicose (arrows) contours and end in typical growth cones (C) exhibiting thin filopodia (arrowheads). ×360

level one can observe that neurons together with satellite cells and fibroblasts are located centrally, whereas an abundance of nerve fibre bundles and fibroblasts occupy the surface and extend into the periphery. Distinct areas of neuropil are also found centrally (Olson and Bunge, 1973).

Types of neurons in explant cultures

Light- and electron-microscopic analysis of explanted ganglia from rat, guinea-pig and man provided evidence for the presence of two morphologically distinct types of neurons (Chamley *et al.*, 1972a,b; Murray and Stout, 1947; Olson and Bunge, 1973). The majority of neurons constituting approx. 90–95% of the total neuron population are large (from 24 × 16 μm to 45 × 32 μm (Chamley *et al.*, 1972a), contain prominent nuclei and nucleoli and have abundant cytoplasm and one or more processes (Chamley *et al.*, 1972a). These large neurons have a complete satellite cell encapsulation and rarely migrate outside of the explant. They exhibit weak catecholamine-specific histofluorescence (Chamley *et al.*, 1972a). Ultrastructural analysis of the large neurons reveals typical cytoplasmic organelles with prominent Golgi complexes and rough endoplasmic reticulum arranged in parallel sheaths (Olson and Bunge, 1973). There is consent that the large neurons observed in explant culture represent the principal ganglion cells (see Grillo, 1966, for review, and chapter by Dail and Barton).

A low percentage of neurons (5–10%) is characterized by smaller cell diameters (from 10 × 16 μm to 24 × 14 μm) and scant cytoplasm that gives an intense fluorescence reaction for catecholamines, which often extends into several long, branched processes. Cell bodies are often free of satellite cells and exhibit strong migratory ability (Chamley *et al.*, 1972a, b; Eränkö *et al.*, 1972b, c; Lever and Presley, 1971). Ultrastructurally the small neurons can be recognized by their large dense-core vesicles (110–280 nm in diameter) (Benitez *et al.*, 1974; Masurovsky *et al.*, 1972b; Olson and Bunge, 1973) and, hence, may be considered to be the small granule-containing cells or small intensely fluorescent (SIF) cells, respectively, of sympathetic ganglia (Eränkö and Eränkö, 1974; Matthews and Raisman, 1969; cf. Taxi *et al.*, this volume, and section on SIF cells of this chapter).

Chick sympathetic ganglia taken at various pre- and postnatal stages have been successfully maintained in long-term cultures and studied morphologically (Chamley *et al.*, 1972a; Hervonen, 1974, 1975a, b; Hervonen and Eränkö, 1975; Lever and Presley, 1971; Masurovsky *et al.*, 1972a; Mottram *et al.*, 1972; Murray and Benitez, 1967; Teichberg and Holtzman, 1973). With sympathetic ganglia of 5.5- or 6-day-old embryos the early development and differentiation of the primitive sympathoblast may be evaluated under *in vitro* conditions (Hervonen 1975a,b). The diameter of the sympathoblast perikarya doubles in two weeks, and after 3–4 weeks neurons dominate which display ultrastructural features such as catecholamine-storing vesicles and well-developed rough endoplasmic reticulum of *in vivo* matured principal neurons (Hervonen, 1975b).

No small granule-containing cells (SIF cells, 'interneurons') have been encountered in such cultures derived from immature ganglia (Benitez *et al.*,

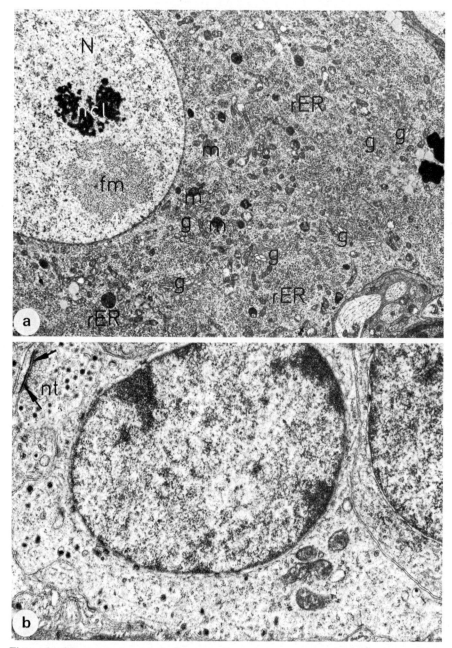

Figure 2   Electron micrographs of a principal neuron (a) and a small granule cell (b) in an organotypic culture of chick sympathetic ganglia after 3 weeks. The principal neuron has a large round nucleus (N) containing a prominent nucleolus (ncl) and a

1974; Hervonen, 1975b). Ganglia of 10- to 16-day-old embryos are already relatively mature (cf. Enemar *et al.*, 1965; Giacobini *et al.*, 1970; Ignarro and Shideman, 1968; Larrabee, 1970; Wechsler and Schmekel, 1966) and two types of neurons, perhaps less clearly separable by light-microscopic criteria than in mammalian ganglia (Chamley *et al.*, 1972a), have been distinguished. These are the principal neurons and SIF cells (Benitez *et al.*, 1974; Chamley *et al.*, 1972a, b; Hervonen, 1975a; Lever and Presley 1971). The large, principal neurons display vesicular nuclei with prominent nucleoli (Hervonen, 1975a), intranuclear rodlets (studied in detail by Masurovsky *et al.*, 1972a), rough surfaced endoplasmic reticulum in typical parallel arrangements (Hervonen, 1975a), smooth endoplasmic reticulum extending into the axon (Teichberg and Holtzman, 1973) and dense-core vesicles varying in size from 40 to 200 nm (Hervonen, 1975a, b; Teichberg and Holtzman, 1973) (cf. Fig. 2a). In contrast, SIF cells have larger granular vesicles (Fig. 2b) ranging from 100 nm to over 250 nm (Hervonen and Eränkö, 1975; for details see section on SIF cells, this chapter).

As in cultured mammalian and chick sympathetic ganglia, two types of neurons may be clearly distinguished in amphibian sympathetic ganglia *in vitro* (Hill and Burnstock, 1975), a large non-migrating and a smaller migrating neuron. The latter does not appear to be identical with chromaffin cells present in cultured amphibian sympathetic ganglia (Hill *et al.*, 1975; Hill and Burnstock, 1975).

Dissociated sympathetic neurons

The fine structure of the neurons which are generally taken from perinatal rat superior cervical ganglia is basically similar to that of superior cervical ganglia of the corresponding age (Bunge *et al.*, 1974; Claude, 1973; Eränkö, 1972; O'Lague *et al.*, 1976; Rees and Bunge, 1974). The isolated neurons adhere immediately to the collagen-coated coverslip and start to grow processes (Bray, 1970; Mains and Patterson, 1973a; Wakshull *et al.*, 1978, 1979a). With increasing age the cell bodies grow from 10–15 μm to 25–40 μm in diameter; the processes increase in length and form bundles up to 30 μm thick (Mains and Patterson, 1973a). The patterns of process ramification, which have been elucidated by injecting Procion yellow or horseradish

prominent assembly of probably filamentous material (fm). Cell organelles (m = mitochondria, g = Golgi complexes, p = pigment inclusions, rER = rough endoplasmic reticulum) are found in normal proportions and arrangements in the cytoplasm. ×7000. The small granule cell is characterized by a low cytoplasmic/nuclear ratio and large membrane-bound dense-core vesicles (diameter 70–120 nm). A nerve terminal (nt) containing small clear and slightly larger dense-core vesicles makes a synaptic contact (arrows) with a slender cytoplasmic process, whose identity in terms of belonging to a principle neuron or a small granule cell is not clear. ×16 200 peroxidase (HRP) into neurons (Ko *et al.*, 1976b; Liang and Perlman, 1979) range from simple to highly complex.

The yield of enzymatically dissociated neurons from perinatal rats is 40–60% and neuronal numbers remain constant after the first week *in vitro* (Wakshull *et al.*, 1979a), when NGF is added to the culture medium (Mains and Patterson, 1973a). A structural anomaly of completely dissociated sympathetic neurons *in vitro* is that they are not closely invested by non-neuronal cells (O'Lague *et al.*, 1976), even if culture conditions allow the presence of these cells. Antisera prepared against newborn rat sympathetic neurons may not only recognize these cells in immunofluorescence studies, but also cross-react with antigens from adrenal medullary, PC 12 pheochromocytoma and brain cells (Lee *et al.*, 1980).

SIF cells

SIF cells are present in varying numbers in almost all cultures of sympathetic ganglia (Benitez *et al.*, 1973, 1974; Chamley *et al.*, 1972b; Doupe *et al.*, 1980; Eränkö *et al.*, 1972b, c, 1976; Eränkö and Eränkö, 1980; Hervonen, 1975a; Hill and Burnstock, 1975; Jacobowitz and Greene, 1974; Jacobowitz *et al.*, 1976; Murray, 1976). Most of these studies, with few exceptions (Doupe *et al.*, 1980; Jacobowitz and Greene, 1974), were performed with explant cultures. SIF cells are readily identifiable by their intense green to yellow catecholamine histofluorescence, which, in contrast to principal neurons, is resistant to drugs such as α-methyl-*p*-tyrosine and reserpine (Benitez *et al.*, 1974; Murray, 1976). Processes of variable length may extend from the cell bodies (Benitez *et al.*, 1974; Chamley *et al.*, 1972b; Doupe *et al.*, 1980; Hervonen and Eränkö, 1975; Hervonen, 1975a; Jacobowitz and Greene, 1974; Jacobowitz *et al.*, 1976; Sano *et al.*, 1967). A prominent ultrastructural feature (Fig. 2b) of these cells are large dense-core vesicles averaging 140 nm in diameter (Benitez *et al.*, 1974). Two types of SIF cells have been described in dissociated rat superior cervical ganglia containing two different populations of dense-core vesicles (100 and 300 nm, respectively; Doupe *et al.*, 1980). SIF cells kept in organotypic cultures even establish the specific junctional relationships with each other and with principal neurons (Benitez *et al.*, 1974).

SIF cells in cultures of dissociated chick embryo sympathetic (Jacobowitz and Greene, 1974; Jacobowitz *et al.*, 1976) and rat superior cervical ganglia (Doupe *et al.*, 1980) may survive and extend long ramified processes in the absence of NGF. When treated with hydrocortisone (10 mg/l), cultures of both chick and rat sympathetic ganglia display a striking increase in the number of SIF cells (Eränkö *et al.*, 1972c, 1976; Eränkö and Eränkö, 1980; Hervonen and Eränkö, 1975). This increase is more likely to be due to an induction of potential precursors of SIF cells than to proliferation of already differentiated SIF cells, since it cannot be prevented by supplementing the cell culture medium with vinblastine sulphate (Eränkö and Eränkö, 1980). Induction of SIF cells by hydrocortisone *in vitro* is confined to ganglia taken during the first postnatal week. The increase in the number of SIF cells in cultured sympathetic ganglia by hydrocortisone is accompanied by an induction of the adrenaline-synthesizing enzyme phenylethanolamine *N*-methyltransferase (PNMT) (Eränkö and Eränkö, 1980). Adding human placental serum to the culture medium produces identical effects (Eränkö and Eränkö, 1980).

Carotid body cells in culture Cells resembling morphologically SIF cells of sympathetic ganglia are found in the carotid body (type I cells). They have been successfully maintained in culture (Pietruschka *et al.*, 1973), where they preserve their essential ultrastructural features (Pietruschka and Schäfer, 1976) and may be studied by electrophysiological methods (Acker and Pietruschka, 1977).

Nerve fibres, growth cones and synapses of cultured sympathetic neurons

The light-microscopic appearance, histochemistry (particularly with respect to transmitters; see section on histological studies), ultramorphology and dynamics of sympathetic neuronal processes in culture have been extensively studied. Both single fine fibres and bundles of axons often invested by Schwann cells grow out from rat, guinea-pig and chick sympathetic ganglia explants within 24 hours (Chamley *et al.*, 1972a). Varicosities that can easily be detected by catecholamine histochemistry are often found with single fibres, whereas bundles usually display smooth contours. Processes may branch extensively. Their growth rates may vary considerably; some neurons of dissociated ganglia may extend processes longer than 100 μm during their first 12 hours in culture (Bray, 1970; Mains and Patterson, 1973a); others do not elaborate processes within the first 14 hours (Mains and Patterson, 1973a).

By injecting HRP into dissociated neurons from rat superior cervical ganglia, Wakshull *et al.* (1979a) were able to demonstrate two basic types of processes: a large type that was smooth and rapidly tapering, and a thin, non-tapering one, which often exhibited varicosities. The authors suggested that the former corresponded to dendrites, whilst the latter acted as axons. No differences in the light-microscopic appearance of axons and dendrites were observed by Bray (1973). Differences in the pattern of fibre growth depending on the age of the animal at explantation have been described by Wakshull *et al.* (1979a) and Johnson *et al.* (1980a, b).

The ultrastructure of processes of isolated sympathetic neurons from chick, guinea-pig and rat in culture has been carefully analysed (Bunge, 1973;

Chamley *et al.*, 1972a; Teichberg and Holtzman, 1973). An integral structure of the fibres is an extensive network of sacs and tubules of agranular reticulum, which resembles the perikaryal endoplasmic reticulum both in terms of membrane thickness and histochemically demonstrable enzyme activities (Teichberg and Holtzman, 1973). The reticulum is sometimes filled with electron-dense material, and vesicles ranging in size from 40 to 100 nm in diameter appear to budd off the reticulum. Clear and granular vesicles measuring up to 150 nm are concentrated in the varicose regions (Chamley *et al.*, 1972a). Although polysomes may be seen, rough endoplasmic reticulum does not seem to occur in the fibres (Bunge, 1973).

Compositional biochemical analysis of axons from cultured sympathetic neurons has shown that there are no major differences in their polypeptide content as compared to the cell somata (Estridge and Bunge, 1978).

The leading tips of growing sympathetic nerve fibres form growth cones (Fig. 1a), which are highly mobile (Bray, 1970) and are equipped with numerous slender extensions, the filopodia. At an ultrastructural level, the filopodia have been shown to contain a distinctive network of (actin) microfilaments and membranous structures, but no other organelles. A full set of cell organelles, however, is present in the cone interior, although their concentration may vary greatly (Bunge, 1973). Growth cones of cultured sympathetic neurons store noradrenaline, as indicated by the presence of granular vesicles visualized after fixation with potassium permanganate (Landis, 1978). 'Mounds' protruding from the growth cone plasmalemma and containing 70–300 nm round vesicles have been interpreted to be sites of membrane addition (Pfenninger and Bunge, 1974; Pfenninger and Rees, 1976). This interpretation is derived from the observation that intra-membrane particles seen by freeze-fracture are less concentrated at mounds than over the rest of the growth cone plasmalemma (Pfenninger and Bunge, 1974). However, Rees and Reese (1981), by using freeze substitution on isolated sympathetic neurons to eliminate fixation artifacts, have provided evidence that mounds are a result of glutaraldehyde fixation. The plas-malemma of the growth cone differs from that of the rest of the neuronal membrane not only with respect to the density of intramembranous particles, but it also displays distinctive cytochemical properties, which allow its membrane to be distinguished from specialized synaptic membranes (Pfen-ninger and Rees, 1976). Growth cones from isolated sympathetic neurons may contact 'follower' neurons in cultures. In such instances pre- and postsynaptic membranes may develop increased densities (Claude, 1973; O'Lague *et al.*, 1974). During synaptogenesis there is an early increase in cell surface galactosyl and, probably, *N*-acetylgalactosaminyl residues at contact sites compared to non-synaptic areas, as indicated by lectin-binding studies (Simkowitz *et al.*, 1978).

The synaptic vesicle population is predominantly adrenergic in young cultures as seen by its capacity to take up 5-hydroxydopamine or by $KMnO_4$ fixation (Claude, 1973; Johnson *et al.*, 1980a, b; O'Lague *et al.*, 1974). In contrast, at 8 weeks, a majority of the boutons contain 80% clear non-adrenergic vesicles. This change in vesicle cytochemistry coincides with an increase in acetylcholine content and choline acetyltransferase activity in these cultures, indicating a progressive shift in transmitter production from noradrenaline to acetylcholine (see chapter by Landis, and section on developmental studies).

Glial and other accessory cells

Despite the important role glial cells are known to play for the trophic maintenance of neurons, and considerable progress that has been made in elucidating the functions of glial cells in the central nervous system by employing cell culture techniques, (cf. Hertz, 1977; Privat and Fulcrand, 1977; Sensenbrenner, 1977), relatively little work has been carried out with glial cells from sympathetic ganglia in culture. One central issue in studying accessory cells of sympathetic ganglia origin has been the decisive role they play for the determination of neurotransmitter function (see Patterson, 1978, and chapter by Landis, for reviews). A large number of accessory cells with differing morphological features have been described by Chamley *et al.* (1972b) in the outgrowth of explanted sympathetic ganglia from rat, guinea-pig and chick. Schwann cells are bi- or tripolar and either free or aligned along nerve fibres (see Murray and Stout, 1947; Ernyei and Young, 1966).

Satellite cells, which are closely associated with nerve cell bodies, are small and irregularly shaped (20–30 μm × 11–15 μm) and have 2–5 fine processes. In contrast to Schwann cells they do not show nuclear rockings and pulsations. Cells resembling oligodendrocytes and astrocytes were rarely observed. Their identity in terms of *in vivo* counterparts is unclear. Other accessory cells present in the outgrowth are peri- and epineural cells, macrophages, fibroblasts and endothelial cells. Similar types of non-neuronal cells have been observed in cultures of amphibian sympathetic ganglia (Hill and Burnstock, 1975).

A new potential for studying the morphology and function of accessory cells in culture has been introduced by McCarthy and Partlow (1976), who have developed a method for the preparation of 99% pure cultures of neurons and non-neuronal cells from chick sympathetic ganglia. They also noted a great diversity of morphological cell types among non-neuronal cells that ranged from spindle-shaped to fibroblast-like cells. The non-neuronal cultures lack detectable acetylcholinesterase. Their capacity to synthesize new DNA (shown by [3H]thymidine incorporation) is 300 to 600 times greater than that of pure neuronal cultures, indicating a considerable proliferative activity.

Histochemical, biochemical and pharmacological studies on sympathetic neurons in culture

There is general agreement that cultured sympathetic neurons store catecholamines as they do *in vivo* and do not lose this specific biochemical synthesis pathway. Histochemical studies have demonstrated catecholamine-specific histofluorescence in cultured neurons using the Falck-Hillarp or glyoxylic acid method for the visualization of catecholamines (Benitez *et al.*, 1973, 1974; Chamley *et al.*, 1972a, b; Hervonen, 1975a; Mains and Patterson, 1973a; Mottram *et al.*, 1972; Presley *et al.*, 1977; Sano *et al.*, 1967) (Fig. 1b). The fluorescence intensity is weak or moderate in the cell bodies of the principal neurons and bright in the varicosities of their axons, whilst SIF cells display an intense fluorescence throughout their cell bodies and processes. Treatment of cultures with the monoamine-oxidase inhibitor nialamide (Benitez *et al.*, 1974; Hervonen, 1974) or with biopterin, cofactor for tyrosine hydroxylase, increases neuronal fluorescence in principal neurons, whereas administration of reserpine causes fading (Benitez *et al.*, 1974). Measurements of noradrenaline fluorescence by microspectrophotometry have clearly documented the capacity of cultured sympathetic neurons axons to take up noradrenaline by a protríptyline- and phenoxybenzamine-sensitive uptake process (Presley *et al.*, 1977). Using cultured sympathetic ganglia, it has been shown that 6-hydroxydopamine and guanethidine, two drugs that cause a chemical sympathectomy *in vivo*, have a different mode and site of action upon the adrenergic neurons, 6-hydroxydopamine causing fibre fragmentation, while guanethidine causes nerve fibre retraction (Eränkö *et al.*, 1972a; Heath *et al.*, 1974; Hill *et al.*, 1973).

Biochemical analyses of catecholamine metabolism of cultured sympathetic neurons have further strengthened the view that sympathetic neurons may express many of their differentiated properties under culture conditions. Thus, it has been shown that not only do they take up catecholamines from the medium (Burdman, 1968; England and Goldstein, 1969; Goldstein, 1967; Patterson *et al.*, 1976; Reichardt and Patterson, 1977), but that they also synthesize and accumulate dopamine and noradrenaline from radioactive precursors (Mains and Patterson, 1973a; Reichardt and Patterson, 1977). The neurons also produce octopamine using tyramine as a precursor (Mains and Patterson, 1973a). The neurons' full capacity to synthesize noradrenaline depends on a sufficient supply of reduced ascorbic acid, the cosubstrate for dopamine β-hydroxylase (Mains and Patterson, 1973b), while biopterin only slightly enhances catecholamine biosynthesis (Côté *et al.*, 1975; Mains and Patterson, 1973b). The capacity of dissociated sympathetic neurons to synthesize catecholamines increases 50-fold during a 3-week period in culture, suggesting progressive maturation under culture conditions (Mains and Patterson, 1973c). Most of the intracellular noradrenaline synthesized from radioactive precursors is stored in vesicles and may be released by exocytosis (Patterson *et al.*, 1976). Release of [³H]noradrenaline from cultured chick embryo sympathetic neurons can be evoked by both nicotinic and muscarinic agonists (Greene and Rein, 1978). α-Bungarotoxin has been successfully used as a probe to label acetylcholine receptors in explants and dissociates of sympathetic ganglia (Gangitano, 1979; Greene *et al.*, 1973; Greene, 1976).

The catecholamine synthesizing enzymes tyrosine hydroxylase (TH), dopamine β-hydroxylase (DBH) and phenylethanolamine *N*-methyltransferase (PNMT) have been the objects of a large number of tissue culture studies using sympathetic ganglia. Both TH and DBH activities may be increased by potassium depolarization (Goodman *et al.*, 1974; MacKay and Iverson, 1972a, b; MacKay, 1974; Silberstein *et al.*, 1972a, b; Webb *et al.*, 1975; see, however, Otten and Thoenen, 1976a, b), nicotinic receptor agonists (Otten and Thoenen, 1976a), NGF and the synthetic glucocorticoid hormone dexamethasone (Nagaiah *et al.*, 1977). Dexamethasone has also been shown to augment PNMT activity and the adrenaline content in organ cultures of newborn rat superior cervical ganglia (Phillipson and Moore, 1975). For effects of NGF on cultured sympathetic ganglia see chapter by Levi-Montalcini and Aloe. In addition to catecholamines, cultured isolated sympathetic neurons and ganglia may produce acetylcholine in the presence of certain types of non-neuronal cells or in medium conditioned by these cells (Hill and Hendry, 1977; Hill *et al.*, 1980; Johnson *et al.*, 1980a, b; Patterson and Chun, 1974, 1977a, b; Patterson *et al.*, 1976; Reichardt and Patterson, 1977; for review see Patterson, 1978, and chapter by Landis).

Rat superior cervical ganglion neurons using acetylcholine as a transmitter can maintain their amine uptake system relatively unchanged (Wakshull *et al.*, 1978).

Developmental studies of sympathetic ganglia *in vitro*

Mechanisms regulating embryonic growth and development of sympathetic ganglia may be profitably studied in tissue cultures. Some of these studies describing mainly the morphological development of sympathetic ganglia *in vitro* have been reviewed in previous sections. However, more complete insight into the regulatory mechanisms of sympathetic neuron development comes from interdisciplinary studies that apply both morphological, histo- and immunocytochemical as well as biochemical techniques. Elegant examples for this type of approach have been provided by Black and his group, who have aimed at determining to what extent the *in vitro* development parallels that *in vivo*, and whether conditions favoring differentiation vary during the prenatal period (Black, 1978; Black and Coughlin, 1978; Coughlin *et al.*, 1977, 1978).

Explants of 13- to 15-day mice superior cervical ganglia display extensive spontaneous neurite outgrowth without added NGF and exhibit a marked increase in TH activity during the first 3 days in culture, which parallels that observed *in vivo*. Addition of NGF antiserum to the culture medium does not result in inhibition of neurite extension or increase in TH activity. Addition of NGF leads to an 8.6-fold increase in TH activity and a more pronounced fibre outgrowth, indicating that NGF is not required for the normal development in early fetal ganglia.

In contrast, ganglia from 18-day embryos fail to grow without added NGF: TH activity decreases by half and virtually no axon outgrowth occurs, suggesting an absolute requirement of sympathetic neurons for NGF at this later stage of development.

Studies on synapse formation and interactions of cultured sympathetic neurons with various target tissues

Cultured explants and dissociated neurons from sympathetic ganglia may be profitably used to study the specificity of synapse formation upon sympathetic neurons, the orientated growth of sympathetic nerves and their synaptic contacts in relation to various targets such as other neurons, smooth and striated muscle.

Superior cervical ganglia and isolated sympathetic neurons may become reinnervated in culture by spinal cord, but not cerebral cortex, neurons (Bunge *et al.*, 1974; Ko *et al.*, 1976a; Olson and Bunge, 1973; Rees *et al.*, 1976).

Two types of synapses can be observed, one containing adrenergic dense-core vesicles, the other type containing clear, presumably cholinergic vesicles. This latter type degenerates selectively after removal of the spinal cord explant. Intracellular recordings from dissociated neurons of the superior cervical ganglia established the occurrence of characteristic membrane resting and action potentials, spontaneous small depolarizations and excitatory postsynaptic potentials (EPSPs) in sympathetic neurons after spinal cord stimulation that are sensitive to Ca^{2+}, Mg^{2+}, D-tubocurare, hexamethonium and mecamylamine. These synaptic potentials can be mimicked by iontophoretic application of acetylcholine, but the synapses are not sensitive to α-bungarotoxin. These results suggest that spinal cord neurons form cholinergic nicotinic synapses on cultured sympathetic neurons, which are similar in function to the corresponding synapses *in vivo*.

Acetylcholine also produces depolarizations of isolated rat and chick sympathetic neurons cultured alone (Crain, 1976; Obata, 1974). Surprisingly, these sympathetic neurons are not only capable of forming adrenergic, but also excitatory cholinergic, synapses among each other after several weeks in culture (Ko *et al.*, 1976b; O'Lague *et al.*, 1974, 1976; Wakshull *et al.*, 1979b). These cholinergic synapses have been carefully characterized by electrophysiological and morphological means (cf. chapter by Landis). In addition, cholinergic synapses have been demonstrated between sympathetic neurons and both skeletal and cardiac muscle (Crain, 1976; Furshpan *et al.*, 1976; Nurse and O'Lague, 1975; Wakshull *et al.*, 1979b).

For a review of neurophysiologic studies on sympathetic neurons in culture, see also Crain (1976) and Burton and Bunge (1981). Cultures of sympathetic ganglia have been frequently utilized for studying mechanisms that regulate the reinnervation of various target organs. Noradrenergic nerve fibres grow abundantly into nearby iris tissue forming a dense plexus of fluorescent axons with patterns that resemble those observed *in vivo* (Hill *et al.*, 1976; Silberstein *et al.*, 1971). Using a photoelectrical recording technique Purves and associates (Hill *et al.*, 1976; Purves *et al.*, 1974) were able to demonstrate contractile activity of sphincter pupillae smooth muscle cells upon stimulation of the sympathetic ganglion, suggesting that sympathetic cholinergic fibres may substitute for the neuronal parasympathetic cholinergic fibres in the sphincter. A similar substitution may occur with sympathetic nerve fibres forming synaptic-like contacts upon isolated chromaffin cells (Unsicker *et al.*, 1978a). Effective junctions between sympathetic nerves and vas deferens smooth muscle or myocardial cells have also been reported (Purves *et al.*, 1974). Stimulation of sympathetic ganglia after 3–14 days *in vitro* evoked contractions of the vas deferens muscle and either excitatory and inhibitory responses in heart muscle. Functional interactions between dissociated (rat superior cervical) ganglion neurons and beating heart ventricular cells have been demonstrated in another type of experiment, where tyramine was used to release catecholamines from nerve terminals, which led to an increase in the contraction rate of the heart cells (King *et al.*, 1978).

Orientated growth of sympathetic nerve fibres occurs in culture towards targets, which normally receive a dense sympathetic nerve supply. When given an equal choice between explants of normally densely innervated tissues (vas deferens, atrium) and sparsely innervated tissues (kidney medulla, uterus, ureter and lung), sympathetic fibres grow preferentially towards the normally densely innervated tissues over distances of up to 2 mm (Burnstock, 1974; Chamley *et al.*, 1973a,b). Attraction of sympathetic nerve fibres towards explants of heart atrium has also been shown (Eränkö and Lahtinen, personal communication). These observations fit into the concept that target tissues regulate the ingrowth of neurites during development and regeneration, possibly by releasing trophic substances like NGF or other growth factors.

Analyses of interactions between sympathetic nerve fibres and isolated smooth muscle cells from various sources (Burnstock, 1974; Chamley *et al.*, 1973a; Chamley and Campbell, 1975, 1976; Mark *et al.*, 1973) or isolated adrenal cortical and medullary cells (Unsicker *et al.*, 1977, 1978a) using time-lapse microcinematography, have shown that long-lasting associations are preferentially made with cells, which normally receive a substantial sympathetic input. Thus, for example, sympathetic fibres form close, long-lasting contacts with smooth muscle cells from the ear artery, but only transitory relationships with cells from the aorta (Chamley and Campbell, 1976). Using cardiac muscle cells Campbell *et al.* (1978) have shown that neurotransmitter receptors are not involved in the mechanism of 'recognition' of the muscle cells by sympathetic nerves.

ADRENAL MEDULLARY AND EXTRA-ADRENAL CHROMAFFIN TISSUE AND DISSOCIATED CELLS IN CULTURE

Adrenal medullary and, to a lesser extent, extra-adrenal chromaffin cells, in culture have now become valuable tools not only for studying the development of endocrine neural crest-derived cells, but also for unravelling important neuronal functions such as transmitter synthesis, storage and release, enzyme induction, receptor regulation and phenotypic plasticity.

Morphological studies on chromaffin tissue and dissociated chromaffin cells in culture

Chromaffin cells, whether grown in explants or cultured as isolated cells, display ultrastructural features typical of this cell type. They store the large catecholamine-containing vesicles (Fenwick *et al.*, 1978; Hill *et al.*, 1975; Kilpatrick, 1980; *et al.*, Manuelidis, 1970; Manuelidis and Manuelidis, 1975; Tischler *et al.*, 1980; Unsicker and Chamley, 1977; Unsicker *et al.*, 1978b, 1980a), and the cell organelles appear normal even in long-term cultures (Unsicker *et al.*, 1980a). Morphological evidence has also been presented that cultured adrenal chromaffin cells release the contents of their granules by exocytosis (Unsicker and Chamley, 1977). Morphological phenomena associated with the secretory process and the movement of subcellular organelles within the cell, which is an important aspect of this process, have been analyzed by microcinematography and laser light scattering (Englert, 1980). Adrenal chromaffin cells store noradrenaline and adrenaline in separate cell entities, and granules storing the different amines may be distinguished by ultramorphological means. In culture there appears to occur a progressive loss of the capacity to produce adrenaline, which is more pronounced in rat (Unsicker *et al.*, 1978b) than in bovine (Kilpatrick *et al.*, 1980; Unsicker *et al.*, 1980a), human (Tischler *et al.*, 1980) and guinea-pig (Unsicker, to be published) chromaffin cells and which cannot be prevented by administration of dexamethasone (Unsicker *et al.*, 1978b). Although the morphology of cultured chromaffin cells parallels that of the cells *in vivo* to a great extent, the cultured cells also undergo changes, among which the extension of

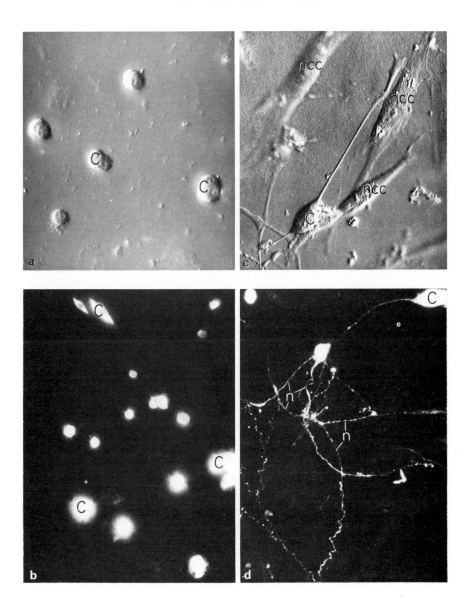

Figure 3 Phenotypic plasticity of rat adrenal chromaffin cells (C) in culture. (a, c) Nomarski micrographs; (b, d) catecholamine histofluorescence. Cells grown in the absence of NGF or non-chromaffin cells or in the presence of both NGF and dexamethasone (a, b) are round and phenotypically resemble their *in vivo* counterparts. In the presence of NGF and/or non-chromaffin cells (ncc) or a factor produced by these cells (c, d), chromaffin cells extend long neurite-like processes (n). ×340

neurite-like processes is the most prominent (Fig. 3). This 'neuronal transdifferentiation' not only occurs with chromaffin cells of embryonic origin (Hervonen *et al.*, 1971; Hervonen and Kanerva, 1973; Manuelidis and Manuelidis, 1975; Millar and Unsicker, 1980), but also with early postnatal (Unsicker and Chamley, 1976; Unsicker *et al.*, 1978b) and adult cells (Aunis *et al.*, 1980; Dean *et al.*, 1978; Livett *et al.*, 1978a; Trifaró and Lee, 1980; Unsicker *et al.*, 1980a).

Extension of processes goes along with a redistribution of catecholamine storage vesicles within the whole length of the processes including their growth cone-like terminations (Millar and Unsicker, 1981). Factors regulating process outgrowth have only partly been determined. NGF elicits process formation by cultured young rat (Unsicker *et al.*, 1978b, 1980b) (Fig. 3) and adult human (Tischler *et al.*, 1980) chromaffin cells, but not cultured chromaffin cells of newborn guinea-pigs (Unsicker, to be published) and adult cattle (Unsicker *et al.*, 1980a). NGF-induced neurite outgrowth from cultured rat chromaffin cells may be inhibited by dexamethasone (Unsicker *et al.*, 1978b), corticosterone and by adrenocorticotropin-stimulated adrenocortical cells present in the cultures (Goerke and Unsicker, to be published). Furthermore, dibutyryl cyclic AMP and cholera toxin, which elevates intracellular cyclic AMP levels by binding to its monosialoganglioside receptor, have also been shown to inhibit NGF-induced fibre outgrowth from rat chromaffin cells (Unsicker and Chamley, 1976; Ziegler and Unsicker, 1981). In addition to NGF, other factors evidently cause process formation of cultured chromaffin cells (Fig. 3). Thus, adrenal chromaffin cells from young rat and adult bovine glands extend processes when grown in the presence of adrenal non-chromaffin cells or cell-free extracts of these cells (Unsicker and Ziegler, 1981; Ziegler *et al.*, 1980). Organ extracts from bovine seminal vesicles, which contain NGF (Hofmann and Unsicker, 1981), but not the purified NGF from this source, elicit process formation by cultured bovine chromaffin cells (Unsicker and Hofmann, 1981). Finally, elevation of potassium levels in the culture medium has been shown to cause a dramatic increase in the number of process-extending bovine, but not rat, chromaffin cells (Unsicker and Hofmann, 1981). The pronounced ability of cultured chromaffin cells to acquire neuronal characteristics is consistent with the concept that both chromaffin cells and sympathetic neurons are closely related with respect to their neural crest origin. The close relationship of chromaffin cells and neurons is further strengthened by the observation that cultured chromaffin cells contain synaptic-like vesicles in addition to the large chromaffin storage granules (Manuelidis and Manuelidis, 1975; Tischler *et al.*, 1980; Unsicker and Chamley, 1977; Unsicker *et al.*, 1978b) and may become innervated by axons from cocultured para- and orthosympathetic ganglia (Unsicker *et al.*, 1977, 1978a).

Biochemical studies on adrenal medullae and dissociated chromaffin cells in culture

There is ample histo- and biochemical evidence that cultured chromaffin cells and adrenal medullae store and release catecholamines and possess the enzymes required for their synthesis. Formaldehyde- or glyoxylic acid-induced catecholamine histofluorescence reveals brightly fluorescent cell bodies and catecholamine stores in processes, including varicosities and growth cones (Brooks, 1977; Hill *et al.*, 1975; Livett *et al.*, 1978a; Millar and Unsicker, 1981; Tischler *et al.*, 1980; Unsicker *et al.*, 1978b, 1980a).

The intensity of the fluorescence reaction in cultured rat and human chromaffin cells decreases with age (Tischler *et al.*, 1980; Unsicker and Chamley, 1976). Microspectrofluorimetric studies on cultured rat chromaffin cells have shown that even in young cultures many cells store mixtures of noradrenaline and adrenaline (Hartwig and Unsicker, to be published). This observation would be in line with a suggestion based on ultramorphological analyses that have shown the simultaneous occurrence of noradrenaline- and adrenaline-typical storage granules within the same cell (Unsicker and Chamley, 1976).

Biochemical assays using mostly fluorimetry or high-performance liquid chromatography with electrochemical detection have provided further evidence that cultured chromaffin cells store catecholamines with both noradrenaline and adrenaline being present initially in proportions similar to those in the intact gland or in the primary cell suspension, respectively (Fenwick *et al.*, 1978; Hoch-Ligiti and Camp, 1959; Hochman and Perlman, 1976; Kilpatrick *et al.*, 1980; Müller and Unsicker, 1981) (Fig. 4).

In cultures of bovine chromaffin cells the absolute content of noradrenaline and adrenaline per cell remains constant up to day 10 (Müller and Unsicker, 1981) (Fig. 4b), and so does the noradrenaline/adrenaline ratio per culture (Kilpatrick *et al.*, 1980; Müller and Unsicker, 1981). In contrast, cultured chromaffin cells from 10-day-old rats rapidly lose the ability to store adrenaline and contain approximately 70% noradrenaline and 25% dopamine after 2 weeks (Müller and Unsicker, 1981) (Fig. 4a). Cultured bovine chromaffin cells also maintain their content of TH, DBH and PNMT during the first 2 weeks (Kilpatrick *et al.*, 1980; Waymire *et al.*, 1977). DBH is still demonstrable by immunocytochemistry in 3-week-old cultures (Unsicker, unpublished observation). Interestingly, the loss of PNMT activity, which occurs in older cultures of bovine chromaffin cells, cannot be prevented by administration of dexamethasone or cortisol (Hersey and DiStefano, 1979; Kilpatrick *et al.*, 1980), although in hypophysectomized animals glucocorticoid hormones may prevent the loss of adrenal PNMT (Wurtman *et al.*, 1972). This failure to induce PNMT activity by dexamethasone contrasts with an earlier report by Coupland and MacDougall (1966), who have found

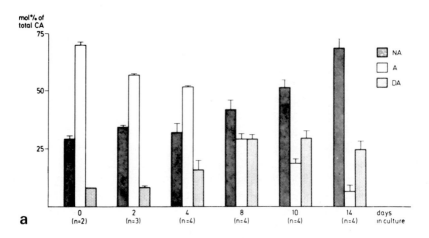

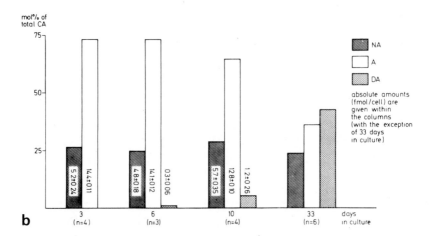

Figure 4   Determination of catecholamines in cultured rat (a) and bovine (b) chromaffin cells. For details see text

adrenaline formation in noradrenaline-storing cells *in vitro* to be induced by
corticosterone. In organ cultures of rat adrenal medullae, PNMT activity has
been shown to be regulated by the intracellular concentration of adrenaline
(Burke *et al.*, 1978).

Various compounds including acetylcholine, nicotine, veratridine, high
potassium and the Ca^{2+} ionophore ionimycin that stimulate the release of
catecholamines and DBH in perfused adrenal glands have similar effects
upon isolated adrenal chromaffin cells in culture (Aunis and Garcia, 1981;
Benitez *et al.*, 1973; Fenwick *et al.*, 1978; Kilpatrick *et al.*, 1980; Liang and
Perlman, 1979; Müller and Unsicker, 1981; Unsicker *et al.*, 1977).

The cholinergic receptor of cultured bovine chromaffin cells appears to be nicotinic, since catecholamine release is stimulated by nicotine and carbamyl-choline, but not by the muscarinic agonists pilocarpine and oxotremorine (Liang and Perlman, 1979; Unsicker *et al.*, 1977). Acetylcholine-induced catecholamine secretion is inhibited by hexamethonium, tubocurarine and atropine, but not by α-bungarotoxin (Hochman and Perlman, 1976; Liang and Perlman, 1979). Cultured chick adrenal chromaffin cells, however, seem to have muscarinic receptors only (Ledbetter and Kirshner, 1975). Both explants of adrenal medullary tissue and isolated chromaffin cells in culture have been widely used to study the induction of the catecholamine-synthesiz-ing enzymes. TH is induced in organ cultures of rat adrenal glands by high concentrations of potassium (Silberstein *et al.*, 1972a), which cause depolar-ization, release of catecholamines and consequently turn on synthesis of new TH molecules. Induction of both TH and DBH may be found in adrenal gland organ cultures and isolated cells after prior *in vivo* administration of reserpine (Gagnon *et al.*, 1976a, b; Goodman *et al.*, 1975; Wilson *et al.*, 1981. Another potent stimulator for TH activity in cultured adrenal chromaffin cells is cyclic AMP (Kumakura, 1979; Waymire *et al.*, 1977). The cyclic AMP-induced increase in enzyme activity is reflected at an ultrastructural level by a marked increase in the volume of the rough endoplasmic reticulum (Manu-eldis, 1976).

Adrenal chromaffin cells not only produce catecholamines, but have also been shown recently to be a rich source of opiate-like peptides including Met- and Leu-enkephalin (Schultzberg *et al.*, 1978; Stern *et al.*, 1979; Viveros *et al.*, 1979). This discovery has prompted a series of studies using cultured adrenal chromaffin cells in order to investigate the cellular distribution, synthesis, release, receptor binding and possible functions of these peptides. From an immunocytochemical study that demonstrated Leu- and Met-enkephalin to be present in both perikarya and processes of cultured bovine chromaffin cells, with a gradient increasing distally, it has been proposed that the peptides are axonally transported (Livett and Dean, 1980). The granular location of immunoreactivity is consistent with the concept of enkephalin storage in chromaffin granules (Stern *et al.*, 1979; Viveros *et al.*, 1979) and the corelease of enkephalin and catecholamines from cultured adrenal chromaf-fin cells in response to nicotine (Livett *et al.*, 1981). Catecholamine and opiate-like peptide biosynthesis appear to be coordinately regulated in cultured bovine chromaffin cells, since administration of reserpine causes an elevation of both TH activity and peptide content (Wilson *et al.*, 1981). Search for a physiological role of adrenal opioid peptides has led to investigations aimed at the characterization of specific opiate-binding sites in isolated bovine adrenal chromaffin cells. Kumakura *et al.* (1980) have reported that β-endorphin and other opiate compounds modulate the release of catecholamines in suspension cultures and postulated a relationship between the high-affinity opiate (naloxone) receptor and catecholamine release. More recently, however, Lemaire *et al.* (1980, 1981) have provided data suggesting that opiate modulation of catecholamine release from adrenal chromaffin cells is not related to the stimulation of the high-affinity stereo-specific opiate binding sites.

In addition to opioids, two other peptides, substance P and somatostatin, have been demonstrated to act as inhibitory modulators at the nicotinic receptor of cultured bovine chromaffin cells (Livett *et al.*, 1978b, 1979; Mizobe *et al.*, 1979a, b). Acetylcholine, which may act as a transmitter in cultured sympathetic neurons from newborn rats (see foregoing section on histochemical studies, and chapter by Landis) has not been demonstrated in cultured adrenal chromaffin cells so far, although acetylcholinesterase is present in cultured chromaffin cells (Millar, to be published) and may be released in response to acetylcholine stimulation (Mizobe and Livett, 1980). Cultured chromaffin cells have also been used as models to study the patterns of distribution of contractile proteins in neuronal cells (Aunis *et al.*, 1980). This study has provided evidence for the presence of α-actinin, actin and myosin immunoreactivity both in the perikarya and neurite-like expansions of cultured bovine chromaffin cells. Furthermore, actin- and α-actinin-like components were extracted from the chromaffin granule membrane.

Electrophysiological studies on cultured adrenal chromaffin cells

Recording of transmembrane potential with microelectrodes is a valuable tool for analyzing the function of various neuroeffector agents. However, because of technical difficulties, this method has only recently been applied to adrenal chromaffin cells. Douglas *et al.* (1966, 1976a, b) isolated adrenal medullary cells and impaled chromaffin cells, whose identity was later confirmed by a positive chromaffin reaction. They recorded resting potentials of 25–30 mV and discovered that acetylcholine in concentrations of 3×10^{-6} g/ml depolarizes the cells when applied to the culture medium or iontophoretically (Kanno and Douglas, 1967). Moreover, they found that the action potential in chromaffin cells has both sodium and calcium components. These results were later confirmed and extended by Biales *et al.* (1976) and Brandt *et al.* (1976). Both groups reported that chromaffin cells were capable of generating action potentials, similar to those generated by sympathetic neurons.

CONCLUSION

Cell and tissue culture studies on sympathetic neurons and adrenal chromaffin cells have become well-established and indispensable tools to evaluate the developmental potentials of these cells and to identify the environmental cues which influence their decisions in terms of phenotype, transmitter synthesis and contacts with various target cells. By making more extensive use of fully defined culture media and carefully separating and recombining the various cellular constituents of sympathetic ganglia and adrenal glands, it will become possible in the future to isolate and test hitherto undiscovered survival and maturation factors and to gain deeper insight into the mutual interactions of neurons and glial cells. Thus, cell and tissue culture of the sympathoadrenal system, which often has presented itself as an art in the past, will stand as a powerful analytical technique in the 1980's.

ACKNOWLEDGEMENTS

Work from our laboratory described in this article has been supported by grants from the Deutsche Forschungsgemeinschaft (Un 34/4–7, SFB 103). Thanks are due to Mr. Ch. Fiebiger and Mrs. I. Ganski for editorial help.

REFERENCES

Acker, H., and Pietruschka, F. (1977). Electrophysiologica characteristics of cultivated type I cells of carotid body. *Arzneim-Forsch.*, **27**, 452–453.

Aunis, D., and Garcia, A. G. (1981). Correlation between catecholamine secretion from bovine isolated chromaffin cells and ^3H-ouabain binding to plasma membranes. *Br. J. Pharmacol.*, **72**, 31–40.

Aunis, D., Guerold, B., Bader, M. F., and Cieselsi-Treska, J. (1980). Immunocytochemical and biochemical demonstration of contractile proteins in chromaffin cells in culture. *Neuroscience*, **5**, 2261–2277.

Benitez, H. H., Murray, M. R., and Côté, L. L. (1973). Response of sympathetic chain-ganglia isolated in organotypic culture to agents affecting adrenergic neurons: Fluorescence histochemistry. *Exp. Neurol.*, **39**, 424–448.

Benitez, H. H., Masurovsky, E. B., and Murray, M. R. (1974). Interneurons of the sympathetic ganglia, in organotypic culture. A suggestion as to their function, based on three types of study. *J. Neurocytol.*, **3**, 363–384.

Biales, B., Dichter, M., and Tischler, A. (1976). Electrical excitability of cultured adrenal chromaffin cells. *J. Physiol.*, **262**, 743–753.

Black, I. B.(1978). Regulation of autonomic development. *Annu. Rev. Neurosci.*, **1**, 183–214.

Black, I. B., and Coughlin, M. D. (1978). Ontogeny of an embryonic mouse sympathetic ganglion *in vivo* and *in vitro*. In *Maturation of Neurotransmission*. Satellite Symposium, 6th Meeting, International Society for Neurochemistry, Saint Vincent, 1977, pp. 65–75, Karger, Basel.

Brandt, B., Hagiwara, S., Kidokoro, Y., and Miyazaki, S. (1976). Action potentials in the rat chromaffin cell and effects of acetylcholine. *J. Physiol. (London)*, **263**, 417–439.

Bray, D. (1970). Surface movements during the growth of single explanted neurons. *Proc. Natl. Acad. Sci. U.S.A.*, **65**, 905–910.

Bray, D. (1973). Branching patterns of isolated sympathetic neurons. *J. Cell Biol.*, **56**, 702.

Brooks, J. C. (1977). The isolated bovine adrenomedullary chromaffin cell: A model of neuronal excitation–secretion. *Endocrinology*, **101**, 1369–1378.

Bunge, M. B. (1973). Fine structure of nerve fibres and growth cones of isolated sympathetic neurons in culture. *J. Cell Biol.*, **56**, 713–735.

Bunge, R. P. (1975). Changing uses of nerve tissue culture 1950–1975. In *The Nervous System* (Ed. D. B. Tower), Vol. 1, pp. 31–42, Raven Press, New York.

Bunge, R. P., Rees, R., Wood, P., Burton, H., and Ko, C. P. (1974). Anatomical and physiological observations on synapses formed on isolated autonomic neurons in tissue culture. *Brain Res.*, **66**, 401–412.

Burdman, J. A. (1968). Uptake of ^3H catecholamines by chick embryo sympathetic ganglia in tissue culture. *J. Neurochem.*, **15**, 1321–1323.

Burke, W. J., Davis, J. W., Joh, T. H., Reis, D. J., Horenstein, S., and Bhagat, B. D. (1978). The effect of epinephrine on phenylethanolamine *N*-methyltranferase in cultured explants of adrenal medulla. *Endocrinology*, **103**, 358–367.

Burnstock, G. (1974). Degeneration and oriented growth of autonomic nerves in relation to smooth muscle in joint tissue cultures and anterior eye chamber transplants. In *Dynamics of Degeneration and Growth in Neurons* (Eds. F. Fuxe, L. Olson, Y Zotterman), pp. 509–519, Pergamon Press, Oxford.

Burnstock, G., and Costa, M. (1975). *Adrenergic Neurons. Their Organization, Function and Development in the Peripheral System*, Chapman and Hall, London.

Burton, H., and Bunge, R. P. (1981). The expression of cholinergic and adrenergic properties by autonomic neurons in tissue culture. In *Excitable Cells in Tissue Culture* (Eds. P. G. Nelson and A. R. Lieberman), pp. 1–37, Academic Press, New York.

Campbell, G. R., Chamley, J. H., and Burnstock, G. (1978). Lack of effect of receptor blockers on the formation of long-lasting associations between sympathetic nerves and cardiac muscle cells *in vitro*. *Cell Tissue Res.*, **187**, 551–553.

Chamley, J. H., and Campbell, G. R. (1975). Isolated ureteral smooth muscle in culture. Including their interaction with intrinsic and extrinsic nerves. *Cytobiol.*, **11**, 358–365.

Chamley, J. H., and Campbell, G. R. (1976). Tissue culture. Interaction between sympathetic nerves and vascular smooth muscle. In *Vascular and Neuroeffector Mechanism*, 2nd International Symposium, Odense 1975 (Ed. J. A. Bevan), pp. 10–18, Karger, Basel.

Chamley, J. H., Mark, G. E., Campbell, G. R., and Burnstock, G. (1972a). Sympathetic ganglia in culture. I. Neurons. *Z. Zellforsch. Mikrosk. Anat.*, **135**, 287–314.

Chamley, J. H., Mark, G. E., and Burnstock, G. (1972b). Sympathetic ganglia in culture. II. Accessory cells. *Z. Zellforsch. Mikrosk. Anat.*, **135**, 315–327.

Chamley, J. H., Campbell, G. R., and Burnstock, G. (1973a). An analysis of the interactions between sympathetic nerve fibres and smooth muscle cells in tissue culture. *Dev. Biol.*, **33**, 334–361.

Chamley, J. H., Goller, I., and Burnstock, G. (1973b). Selective growth of sympathetic nerve fibres to explants of normally densely innervated autonomic effector organs in tissue culture. *Dev. Biol.*, **31**, 362–379.

Coupland, R. E., and MacDougall, J. D. B. (1966). Adrenaline formation in noradrenaline-storing chromaffin cells *in vitro* induced by corticosterone. *J. Endocrinol.*, **36**, 317–324.

Claude, P. (1973). Electron microscopy of dissociated rat sympathetic neurons *in vitro*. *J. Cell Biol.*, **59**, 57a.

Coughlin, M. D., Boyer, D. M., and Black, I. B. (1977). Embryonic development of a mouse sympathetic ganglion *in vivo* and *in vitro*. *Proc. Natl. Acad. Sci. U.S.A.*, **74**, 3438–3442.

Coughlin, M. D., Dibner, M. D., Boyer, D. M., and Black, I. B. (1978). Factors regulating development of an embryonic mouse sympathetic ganglion. *Dev. Biol.*, **66**, 513–528.

Côté, L. J., Benitez, H. H., and Murray, M. R. (1975). Biosynthesis of catecholamines in organotypic cultures of the peripheral autonomic nervous system: modification by biopterin and other agents. *J. Neurol.*, **6**, 233–243.

Crain, S. M. (1976). *Neurophysiologic Studies in Tissue Culture*, Raven Press, New York.

Dean, D. M., Bray, G. M., and Livett, B. G. (1978). Chromaffin cells in culture resemble adrenergic neurons. Can. Neurol. Sci. Meeting, Vancouver (abstract).

Douglas, W., Kanno, T., and Sampson, S. (1966). Intracellular recording from adrenal chromaffin cells: effects of acetylcholine, hexamethonium and potassium on membrane potentials. *J. Physiol. (London)*, **186**, 125–126.

Douglas, W. W., Kanno, T., and Sampson, S. R. (1967a). Effects of acetylcholine and other medullary secretagogues and antagonists on the membrane potential of adrenal chromaffin cells: an analysis employing techniques of tissue culture. *J. Physiol. (London)*, **188**, 107–120.

Douglas, W. W., Kanno, T., and Sampson, S. R. (1967b). Influence of the ionic environment on the membrane potential of adrenal chromaffin cells and on the depolarizing effects of acetylcholine. *J. Physiol. (London)*, **191**, 107–121.

Doupe, A. J., Patterson, P. H., and Landis, S. C. (1980). Dissociated cell culture of SIF cells: hormone dependence and NGF action. *Soc. Neurosci. Abstr.*, **6**, 409.

Enemar, A., Falck, B., and Håkanson, R. (1965). Observations on the appearance of norepinephrine in the sympathetic nervous system of the chick embryo. *Dev. Biol.*, **11**, 268–283.

Engand, J. M., and Goldstein, M. M. (1969). The uptake and localisation of catecholamines in chick embryo sympathetic neurons in tissue culture. *J. Cell. Sci.*, **4**, 677–691.

Englert, D. F. (1980). An optical study of isolated rat adrenal chromaffin cells. *Exp. Cell Res.*, **125**, 369–376.

Eränkö, L. (1972). Ultrastructure of the developing sympathetic nerve cell and the storage of catecholamines. *Brain Res.*, **46**, 159–175.

Eränkö, L., Hill, C., Eränkö, O., and Burnstock, G. (1972a). Lack of toxic effect of guanethidine on nerve cells and small intensely fluorescent cells in cultures of sympathetic ganglia of newborn rats. *Brain Res.*, **43**, 501–513.

Eränkö, O., and Eränkö, L. (1974). Small intensely fluorescent granule containing cells in the sympathetic ganglion of the rat. *Brain Res.*, **34**, 39–51.

Eränkö, O., and Eränkö, L. (1980). Induction of SIF cells by hydrocortisone or human cord serum in sympathetic ganglia and their subsequent fate *in vivo* and *in vitro*. *Histochemistry and Cell Biology of Autonomic Neurons, SIF Cells and Paraneurons* (Eds. O. Eränkö, S. Soinila and H. Päivärinta), *Advances in Biochemical Psychopharmacology*, Vol. 25, pp. 17–26, Raven Press, New York.

Eränkö, O., Eränkö, L., Hill, C., and Burnstock, G. (1972b). Hydrocortisone-induced increase in the number of small intensely fluorescent cells and their histochemically demonstrable catecholamine content in cultures of sympathetic ganglia of the newborn rat. *Histochem. J.*, **4**, 49–58.

Eränkö, O., Heath, J., and Eränkö, L. (1972c). Effect of hydrocortisone on the ultrastructure of small, intensely fluorescent, granule containing cells in cultures of sympathetic ganglia of newborn rats. *Z. Zellforsch. Mikrosk. Anat.*, **134**, 297–310.

Eränkö, O., Eränkö, L., and Hervonen, H. (1976). Cultures of sympathetic ganglia and the effect of glucocorticoides on SIF cells. *Fogarty Int. Cent. Proc.*, **30**, 196–214.

Ernyei, S., and Young, M. R. (1966). Pulsatile and myelin activities of Schwann cells *in vitro*. *J. Physiol. (London)*, **183**, 469–480.

Estridge, M. and Bunge, R. (1978). Compositional analysis of growing axons from rat sympathetic neuron. *J. Cell Biol.*, **79**, 138–155.

Fenwick, E. M., Fajdiga, P. B., Howe, N. B. S., and Livett, B. G. (1978). Functional and morphological characterization of isolated bovine adrenal medullary cells. *J. Cell Biol.*, **76**, 12–30.

Fischbach, G. D., and Nelson, P. G. (1977). Cell culture in neurobiology. In *Handbook of Physiology, Section I: The Nervous System*, Vol. I, Part 2, pp. 719–774, American Physiological Society, Washington, DC.

Furshpan, E. J., MacLeish, P. R., O'Laguè, P. H., and Potter, D. D. (1976). Chemical transmission between rat sympathetic neurons and cardiac myocytes developing in microcultures: evidence for cholinergic, adrenergic and dual-function neurons. *Proc. Natl. Acad. Sci. U.S.A.*, **73**, 4226–4229.

Gabella, G. (1976). *Structure of the Autonomic Nervous System*, Chapman and Hall, London.

Gagnon, C., Otten, U., and Thoenen, H. (1976a). Increased synthesis of dopamine β-hydroxylase in cultured rat adrenal medulla after *in vivo* administration of reserpine. *J. Neurochem.*, **27**, 259–265.

Gagnon, C., Schatz, R., Otten, U., and Thoenen, H. (1976b). Synthesis, subcellular distribution and turnover of dopamine β-hydroxylase in organ cultures of sympathetic ganglia and adrenal medullae. *J. Neurochem.*, **27**, 1083–1089.

Gangitano, C., Fumagalli, L., and Miani, N. (1979). Appearance of new α-bungaro-toxin–acetylcholine receptors in cultured sympathetic ganglia of chick embryos. *Brain Res.*, **161**, 131–141.

Giacobini, G., Marchiso, P. C., Giacobini, E., and Koslow, S. H. (1970). Develop-mental changes of cholinesterases and monoamine oxidase in chick embryo spinal and sympathetic ganglia. *J. Neurochem.*, **17**, 1177–1185.

Goldstein, M. N. (1967). Incorporation and release of H^3-catecholamines by cultured fetal human sympathetic nerve cells and neuroblastoma cells. *Proc. Soc. Exp. Biol.*, **125**, 993–996.

Goodman, R., Oesch, F., and Thoenen, H. (1974). Changes in enzyme patterns produced by high potassium concentration and dibutyryl cylic AMP in organ cultures of sympathetic ganglia. *J. Neurochem.*, **23**, 369–378.

Goodman, R., Otten, U., and Thoenen, H. (1975). Organ culture of the rat adrenal medulla: A model system for the study of trans-synaptic enzyme induction. *J. Neurochem.*, **25**, 423–427.

Greene, L. A. (1976). Binding of α-bungarotoxin to chick sympathetic ganglia: properties of the receptor and its rate of appearance during development. *Brain Res.*, **111**, 135–145.

Greene, L. A., and Rein, G. (1978). Release of norepinephrine from neurons in dissociated cell cultures of chick sympathetic ganglia via stimulation of nicotinic and muscarinic acetylcholine receptors. *J. Neurochem.*, **30**, 579–586.

Greene, L. A., Sytowski, A. J., Vogel, J., and Nirenberg, M. W. (1973). α-Bungaro-toxin used as a probe for acetylcholine receptors of cultured neurons. *Nature*, **243**, 163–166.

Grillo, M. A. (1966). Electron microscopy of sympathetic tissues. *Pharmacol. Rev.*, **18**, 387–399.

Heath, J. W., Hill, C. E., and Burnstock, G. (1974). Axon retraction following guanethidine treatment: studies of sympathetic neurons in tissue culture. *J. Neurocytol.*, **3**, 263–276.

Hersey, R. M., and DiStefano, V. (1979). Control of phenylethanolamine *N*-methyltransferase by glucocorticoids in cultured bovine adrenal medullary cells. *J. Pharmacol. Exp. Ther.*, **209**, 147–152.

Hertz, L. (1977). Biochemistry of glial cells. In *Cell, Tissue and Organ Culture in Neurobiology* (Eds. A. Federorff and L. Hertz), pp. 39–71, Academic Press, New York.

Hervonen, A., and Kanerva, L. (1973). Neuronal differentiation in human fetal adrenal medulla. *J. Neurosci.*, **5**, 43–46.

Hervonen, A., Hervonen, H., and Rechardt, L. (1971). Axonal growth from the primitive sympathetic elements of human fetal adrenal medulla. *Experientia*, **28**, 178–179.

Hervonen, H. (1974). Formaldehyde-induced fluorescence in sympathetic ganglia of chick embryo in maturing organotypic culture. *Med. Biol.*, **52**, 154–163.

Hervonen, H. (1975a). Histochemical and electron microscopical study on sympathetic ganglia of chick embryo in culture. *Acta Inst. Anat. Univ. Helsinki*, **8** (Thesis).

Hervonen, H. (1975b). Differentiation of sympathicoblasts in cultures of chick ganglia. *Anat. Embryol.*, **146**, 225–243.

Hervonen, H., and Eränkö, O. (1975). Fluorescence histochemical and electron microscopical observations on sympathetic ganglia of the chick embryo cultured with and without hydrocortisone. *Cell Tissue Res.*, **156**, 154–166.

Hill, C. E., and Burnstock, G. (1975). Amphibian sympathetic ganglia in tissue culture. *Cell Tissue Res.*, **162**, 209–233.

Hill, C. E., and Hendry, I. A. (1977). Development of neurons synthesizing noradrenaline and acetylcholine in the superior cervical ganglion of the rat *in vivo* and *in vitro*. *Neuroscience*, **2**, 741–749.

Hill, C. E., Mark, G. E., Eränkö, O., Eränkö, L., and Burnstock, G. (1973). Use of tissue culture to examine the actions of guanethidine and 6-hydroxydopamine. *Eur. J. Pharmacol.*, **23**, 162–174.

Hill, C. E., Hoult, M., and Burnstock, G. (1975). Extra-adrenal chromaffin cells grown in tissue culture. *Cell Tissue Res.*, **161**, 103–117.

Hill, C. E., Purves, R. D., Watanabe, H., and Burnstock, G. (1976). Specificity of innervation of iris musculature by sympathetic nerve fibres in tissue culture. *Pflügers Arch.*, **361**, 127–134.

Hill, C. E., Hendry, I. A., and McLennan, I. S. (1980). Development of cholinergic neurones in cultures of rat superior cervical ganglia. Role of calcium and macromolecules. *Neuroscience*, **5**, 1027–1032.

Hoch-Ligiti, C., and Camp, J. L., III. (1959). Catecholamine production in tissue cultures of human adrenal medullary tumors and of adrenal medulla. *Proc. Soc. Exp. Biol. Med.*, **102**, 692–693.

Hochman, J., and Perlman, R. L. (1976). Catecholamine secretion by isolated adrenal cells. *Biochim. Biophys. Acta*, **421**, 168–175.

Hofmann, H. D., and Unsicker, K. (1981). The seminal vesicle of the bull: A new source for nerve growth factor. *Neurosci. Lett. Suppl.*, **6**.

Ignarro, L. J., and Shideman, F. E. (1968). Appearance and concentrations of catecholamines and their biosynthesis in the embryonic and developing chick. *J. Pharmacol. Exp. Ther.*, **159**, 38–48.

Jacobowitz, D., and Greene, L. (1974). Histofluorescence study of chromaffin cells in dissociated cell cultures of chick embryo sympathetic ganglia. *J. Neurobiol.*, **5**, 65–83.

Jacobowitz, D. M., Greene, L. A., and Thoa, N. B. (1976). Chromaffin cells in culture. *Fogarty Int. Cent. Proc.*, **30**, 215–222.

Johnson, M. I., Ross, C. D., Meyers, M., Spitznagel, E. L., and Bunge, R. P. (1980a). Morphological and biochemical studies on the development of cholinergic properties in cultured sympathetic neurons. I. Correlative changes in choline acetyltransferase and synaptic vesicle cytochemistry. *J. Cell Biol.*, **84**, 680–691.

Johnson, M. I., Ross, C. D., and Bunge, R. P. (1980b). Morphological and biochemical studies on the development of cholinergic properties in cultured sympathetic neurons. II. Dependence on postnatal age. *J. Cell Biol.*, **84**, 692–704.

Kanno, T., and Douglas, W. W. (1967). Effect of rapid application of acetylcholine or depolarizing current on transmembrane potentials of adrenal chromaffin cells. *Proc. Can. Fed. Biol. Soc.*, **1**, 39.

Kilpatrick, D. L., Ledbetter, F. H., Carson, K. A., Kirshner, A. G., Slepetis, R., and Kirshner, N. (1980). Stability of bovine adrenal medulla cells in cultures. *J. Neurochem.*, **35**, 679–692.

King, K. L., Boder, G. B., Williams, D. C., and Harley, R. J. (1978). Chronotropic effect of tyramine on rat heart cells cultured with sympathetic neurons. *Eur. J. Pharmacol.*, **51**, 331–335.

Ko, C. H. P., Burton, H., and Bunge, R. P. (1976a). Synaptic transmission between rat spinal cord explants and dissociated superior cervical ganglion neurons in tissue culture. *Brain Res.*, **117**, 437–460.

Ko, C. H. P., Burton, H., Johnson, M. I., and Bunge, R. P. (1976b). Synaptic transmission between rat superior cervical ganglion neurons in dissociated cell cultures. *Brain Res.*, **117**, 461–485.

Kumakura, K., Guidotti, A., and Costa, E. (1979). Primary cultures of chromaffin cells: Molecular mechanisms for the induction of tyrosine hydroxylase mediated by 8-Br-cyclic AMP. *Molec. Pharmacol.*, **16**, 865–876.

Kumakura, K., Karoum, F., Guidotti, A., and Costa, E. (1980). Modulation of nicotinic receptors by opiate receptor agonists in cultured adrenal chromaffin cells. *Nature*, **283**, 489–490.

Landis, C. (1978). Growth cones of cultured sympathetic neurons contain adrenergic vesicles. *J. Cell Biol.*, **78**, 8–14.

Larrabee, M. G. (1970). Metabolism of adult and embryonic sympathetic ganglia. *Fed. Proc.*, **29**, 1919–1928.

Lee, V. M., Shelanski, M. L., and Greene, L. A. (1980). Characterization of antisera raised against cultured sympathetic neurons. *Neuroscience*, **5**, 2239–2245.

Ledbetter, F. H., and Kirshner, N. (1975). Studies of chick adrenal medulla in organ culture. *Biochem. Pharmacol.*, **24**, 967–974.

Lemaire, S., Lemaire, I., Dean, D. M., and Livett, B. G. (1980). Opiate receptors and adrenal medullary function. *Nature*, **288**, 303–304.

Lemaire, S., Livett, B., Tseng, R., Mercier, P., and Lemaire, I. (1981). Studies on the inhibitory action of opiate compounds in isolated bovine adrenal chromaffin cells: Noninvolvement of stereospecific opiate binding sites. *J. Neurochem.*, **36**, 886–892.

Lever, J. D., and Presley, R. (1971). Studies on the sympathetic neurone *in vitro*. *Prog. Brain Res.*, **34**, 499–512.

Livett, B. G., and Dean, D. M. (1980). Distribution of immunoreactive enkephalins in adrenal paraneurons: Preferential localization in varicose processes and terminals. *Neuropeptides*, **1**, 3–13.

Livett, B. G., Dean, D. M., and Bray, G. M. (1978a). Growth characteristics of isolated adrenal medullary cells in culture. *Soc. Neurosci. Abstr.*, **4**, 592.

Livett, B. G., Mizobe, F., Kozousek, V., and Dean, D. M. (1978b). Substance-P inhibits the nicotinic activation of adrenal paraneurons. *Clin. Res.*, **26**, 873A.

Livett, B. G., Kozousek, V., Mizobe, F., and Dean, D. M. (1979). Substance P inhibits nicotinic activation of chromaffin cells. *Nature*, **278**, 256–27.

Livett, B. G., Dean, D. M., Whelan, L. G., Udenfriend, S., and Rossier, J. (1981). Co-release of enkephalin and catecholamines from cultured adrenal chromaffin cells. *Nature*, **289**, 317–319.

MacKay, A. V. P., and Iversen, L. L. (1972a). Trans-synaptic regulation of tyrosine hydroxylase activity in adrenergic neurons: Effect of potassium concentration on cultured sympathetic ganglia. *Arch. Pharmacol.*, **272**, 225–229.

MacKay, A. V. P., and Iversen, L. L. (1972b). Increased tyrosine hydroxylase activity of sympathetic ganglia cultured in the presence of dibutyryl cyclic AMP. *Brain Res.*, **48**, 424–426.

MacKay, A. V. P. (1974). The long-term regulation of tyrosine hydroxylase activity in cultured sympathetic ganglia: Role of ganglionic noradrenaline content. *J. Pharmacol.*, **51**, 509–520.

Mains, R. E., and Patterson, P. H. (1973a). Primary cultures of dissociated sympathetic neurons. I. Establishment of long-term growth in culture and studies of differentiated properties. *J. Cell Biol.*, **59**, 329–345.

Mains, R. E., and Patterson, P. H. (1973b). Primary cultures of dissociated sympathetic neurons. II. Initial studies on catecholamine metabolism. *J. Cell Biol.*, **59**, 346–360.

Mains, R. E., and Patterson, P. H. (1973c). Primary cultures of dissociated sympathetic neurons. III. Changes in metabolism with age in culture. *J. Cell Biol.*, **59**, 361–366.

Manuelidis, L. (1970). Adrenal gland in tissue culture. *Nature*, **227**, 619–620.

Manuelidis, L. (1976). The effects of dbcAMP on adrenal chromaffin cells in organotypic culture. *J. Neurocytol.*, **5**, 1–10.

Manuelidis, L., and Manuelidis, E. E. (1975). Synaptic boutons and neuron-like cells in isolated adrenal gland cultures. *Brain Res.*, **96**, 181–186.

Mark, G. E., Chamley, J. H., and Burnstock, G. (1973). Interactions between autonomic nerves and smooth and cardiac muscle cells in tissue culture. *Dev. Biol.*, **32**, 194–200.

Masurovsky, E. B., Benitez, H. H., Kim, S. U., and Murray, M. R. (1972a). Origin, development and nature of intranuclear rodlets and associated bodies in chicken sympathetic neurons. *J. Cell Biol.*, **44**, 172–191.

Masurovsky, E. B., Benitez, H. H., and Murray, M. R. (1972b). Development of interneurons in long-arm organotypic cultures of rat cervical and stellate ganglia. *J. Cell Biol.*, **55**, 166A.

Matthews, M. R., and Raisman, G. (1969). The ultrastructure and somatic efferent synapses of small granule containing cells in the superior cervical ganglion. *J. Anat.*, **105**, 255–282.

McCarthy, K. D., and Partlow, L. M. (1976). Preparation of pure neuronal and non-neuronal cultures from embryonic chick sympathetic ganglia: A new method based on both differential cell adhesiveness and the formation of homotypic neuronal aggregates. *Brain Res.*, **114**, 391–414.

Millar, T. J., and Unsicker, K. (1981). *In vitro* development of rat adrenal medulla. *Vers. Anat. Ges. Würzburg, Anat. Anz.*, Jena, **149**, 95 (abstract)

Millar, T. J., and Unsicker, K. (1982). Ultramorphological analysis of growth cones formed by cultured rat chromaffin cells treated with nerve growth factor. *Dev. Brain Res.*, **2**, 577–582.

Mizobe, F., and Livett, B. G. (1980). Production and release of acetylcholinesterase by a primary cell culture of bovine adrenal medullary chromaffin cells. *J. Neurochem.*, **35**, 1469–1472.

Mizobe, F., Dean, D. M., Rorstad, O., Whelan, L. G., and Livett, B. G. (1979a). Substance P and somatostatin inhibit the nicotinic activation of adrenal paraneurons. *XIth International Congress of Biochemistry, Toronto*, Abstract.

Mizobe, F., Kozousek, V., Dean, D. M., and Livett, B. G. (1979b). Pharmacological characterization of adrenal paraneurons: Substance P and somatostatin as inhibitory modulators of the nicotinic response. *Brain Res.*, **178**, 555–556.

Mottram, D. R., Presley, R., Lever, J. D., and Ivens, C. (1972). Some characteristics of chick embryo sympathetic ganglion fragments in a simple culture system with and without nerve growth factor. *Z. Anat. Entwicklungsgesch.*, **138**, 127–133.

Müller, T. H., and Unsicker, K. (1981). High-performance liquid chromatography with electrochemical detection as a highly efficient tool for studying catecholaminergic systems. I. Quantification of noradrenaline, adrenaline and dopamine in cultured adrenal medullary cells. *J. Neurosci. Methods*, **4**, 39–52.

Murray, M. R. (1965). Nervous tissue *in vitro*. In *The Biology of Cells and Tissues in Culture* (Ed. E. N. Willmer), Vol. II, pp. 373–455, Academic Press, New York.

Murray, M. R. (1971). Nervous tissue isolated in culture. In *Handbook of Neurochemistry* (Ed. A. Lajtha), Vol. 5/A, pp. 373–438, Plenum Press, New York.

Murray, M. R. (1976). Sympathetic ganglia in organotypic culture: relationship between interneurons and principal cells. *Fogarty Int. Cent. Proc.*, 180–195.

Murray, M. R. (1977). Introduction. In *Cell, Tissue and Organ Cultures in Neurobiology* (Eds. S. Feoroff and L. Hertz), Academic Press, New York.

Murray, M. R., and Benitez, H. H. (1967). Deuterium oxide: direct action on sympathetic ganglia in culture. *Science*, **155**, 1021–1024.

Murray, M. R. and Stout, A. P. (1947). Adult human ganglion cells cultivated *in vitro*. *Am. J. Anat.*, **80**, 225–273.

Nagaiah, K., MacDonnell, P., and Guroff, G. (1977). Induction of tyrosine hydroxylase synthesis in rat superior cervical ganglia *in vitro* by nerve growth factor and dexamethasone. *Biochem. Biophys. Res. Commun.*, **75**, 832–837.

Nelson, P. G. (1975). Nerve and muscle in culture. *Physiol. Rev.*, **55**, 1–61.

Nurse, C. A., and O'Lague, P. H. (1975). Formation of cholinergic synapses between dissociated sympathetic neurons and skeletal myotubes of the rat in cell culture. *Proc. Natl. Acad. Sci. U.S.A.*, **72**, 1955–1959.

Obata, K. (1974). Transmitter sensitivities of some nerve and muscle cells in culture. *Brain Res.*, **73**, 71–88.

O'Lague, P. H., Obata, K., Claude, P., Furshpan, E. G., and Potter, D. D. (1974). Evidence for cholinergic synapses between dissociated rat sympathetic neurons in cell culture. *Proc. Natl. Acad. Sci. U.S.A.*, **71**, 3602–3606.

O'Lague, P. H., MacLeish, P. R., Nurse, C. A., Claude, P., Furshpan, E. J., and Potter, D. D. (1976). Physiological and morphological studies on developing sympathetic neurons in dissociated cell culture. *Cold Spring Harbor Symp. Quant. Biol.*, **40**, 399–407.

Olson, M. I., and Bunge, R. P. (1973). Anatomical observations on the specificity of synapse formation in tissue culture. *Brain Res.*, **59**, 19–33.

Otten, U., and Thoenen, H. (1976a), Mechanisms of tyrosine hydroxylase and dopamine β-hydroxylase induction in organ cultures of rat sympathetic ganglia by potassium depolarization and cholinomimetics. *Naunyn-Schmiedebergs Arch. Pharmacol.*, **292**, 153–159.

Otten, U., and Thoenen, H. (1976b). Role of membrane depolarization in transsynaptic induction of tyrosine hydroxylase in organ cultures of sympathetic ganglia. *Neurosci. Lett.*, **2**, 93–96.

Patterson, H. (1978). Environmental determination of autonomic neurotransmitter functions. *Annu. Rev. Neurosci.*, **1**, 1–17.

Patterson, P. H., and Chun, L. L. Y. (1974). The influence of non-neuronal cells on catecholamine and acetylcholine synthesis and accumulation in cultures of dissociated sympathetic neurons. *Proc. Natl. Acad. Sci. U.S.A.*, **71**, 3607–3610.

Patterson, P. H., and Chun, L. L. Y. (1977a). The induction of acetylcholine synthesis in primary cultures of dissociated rat sympathetic neurons. I. Effects of conditioned medium. *Dev. Biol.*, **56**, 263–280.

Patterson, P. H., and Chun, L. L. Y. (1977b). The induction of acetylcholine synthesis in primary cultures of dissociated rat sympathetic neurons. II. Developmental aspects. *Dev. Biol.*, **60**, 473–481.

Patterson, P. H., Reichardt, L. F., and Chun, L. L. Y. (1976). Biochemical studies on the development of primary sympathetic neurons in cell culture. *Cold Spring Harbor Symp. Quant. Biol.*, **40**, 389–397.

Pfenninger, K. H., and Bunge, R. P. (1974). Freeze-fracturing of nerve growth cones and young nerve fibres. A study of developing plasma membranes. *J. Cell Biol.*, **63**, 180–196.

Pfenninger, K. H., and Rees, R. P. (1976). From the growth cone to the synapse. Properties of membranes involved in synapse formation. In *Neuronal Recognition* (Ed. S. H. Barndes), pp. 131–178, Chapman and Hall, London.

Phillipson, C. T., and Moore, K. (1975). Effects of dexamethasone and nerve growth factor on phenylethanolamine *N*-methyltransferase and adrenaline in organ cultures of newborn rat superior cervical ganglion. *J. Neurochem.*, **25**, 295–298.

Pietruschka, F., and Schäfer, D. (1976). Fine structure of chemosensitive cells (glomus caroticum) in tissue culture. *Cell Tissue Res.*, **168**, 55–63.

Pietruschka, F., Acker, H., Gattermann, S., Seidl, E., and Lübbers, D. W. (1973). Cell of the carotid body in primary tissue cultures. *Arzneim-Forsch.*, **23**, 1607–1614.

Presley, R., Santer, R. M., Lu, K. S., and Lever, J. D. (1977). Measurements of noradrenaline fluorescence in axons of chick embryo sympathetic ganglia grown in three day culture. *Cell Tissue Res.*, **178**, 49–60.

Privat, A., and Fulcrand, J. (1977). Neuroglia—from the subventricular precursor to the mature cell. In *Cell, Tissue and Organ Cultures in Neurobiology* (Eds. S. Fedoroff and L. Hertz), pp. 11–37, Academic Press, New York.

Purves, R. D., Hill, C. E., Chamley, J. H., Mark, G. E., Fry, D. M., and Burnstock, G. (1974). Functional autonomic neuromuscular junctions in tissue culture. *Pflügers Arch.*, **350**, 1–7.

Rees, R., and Bunge, R. P. (1974). Morphological and cytochemical studies of synapses formed in culture between isolated rat superior cervical ganglion neurons. *J. Comp. Neurol.*, **157**, 1–2.

Rees, R. P., and Reese, T. S. (1981). New structural features of freeze-substituted neuritic growth cones. *Neuroscience*, **6**, 247–254.

Rees, R. P., Bunge, M. B., and Bunge, R. P. (1976). Morphological changes in the neuritic growth cone and target neuron during synaptic junction development in culture. *J. Cell Biol.*, **68**, 240–263.

Reichardt, L. F., and Patterson, P. H. (1977). Neurotransmitter synthesis and uptake by isolated sympathetic neurones in microcultures. *Nature*, **270**, 147–151.

Sano, Y., Odake, G., and Yonezawa, T. (1967). Fluorescence microscopic observations of catecholamines in cultures of the sympathetic chain. *Z. Zellforsch. Mikrosk. Anat.*, **80**, 345–352.

Sato, G. (1973). *Tissue Culture of the Nervous System*, Plenum Press, New York.

Schultzberg, M. Lundberg, J. M., Hökfelt, T., Terenius, L., Brandt, J., Elde, R. P., and Goldstein, M. (1978). Enkephalin-like immunoreactivity in gland cells and nerve terminals of the adrenal medulla. *Neuroscience*, **3,** 1169–1186.

Sensenbrenner, M. (1977). Dissociated brain cells in primary cultures. In *Cell, Tissue and Organ Cultures in Neurobiology* (Eds. S. Fedoroff and L. Hertz), pp. 191–213, Academic Press, New York.

Silberstein, S. D. (1973). *Sympathetic Ganglia in Organ Culture*, Academic Press, New York.

Silberstein, S. D., Johnson, D. G., Jacobowitz, D. M., and Kopin, I. J. (1971). Sympathetic reinnervation of the rat iris in organ culture. *Proc. Natl. Acad. Sci. U.S.A.*, **68,** 1121–1124.

Silberstein, S. D., Lemberger, L., Klein, D. C., Axelrod, J., and Kopin, I. J. (1972a). Induction of adrenal tyrosine hydroxylase in organ culture. *Neuropharmacology*, **11,** 721–726.

Silberstein, S. D., Brimijoin, S., Molinoff, P. B., and Lemberger, L. (1972b). Induction of dopamine β-hydroxylase in rat superior cervical ganglia in organ culture. *J. Neurochem.*, **19,** 919–921.

Simkowitz, P., Maylié-Pfenninger, M. F., and Pfenninger, K. H. (1978). Early changes in cell surface glycoconjugates during synaptogenesis. *J. Cell Biol.*, **79,** 60a.

Stern, A. S., Lewis, R. V., Kimura, S., Rossier, J., Gerber, L. D., Brink, L. Stein, S., and Udenfriend, S. (1979). Isolation of the opioid heptapeptide Met-enkephalin (Arg[6], Phe[7]) from bovine adrenal medullary granules and striatum. *Proc. Natl. Acad. Sci. U.S.A.*, **76,** 6680–6683.

Teichberg, S., and Holtzman, E. (1973). Axonal agranular reticulum and synaptic vesicles in cultured embryonic chick sympathetic neurons. *J. Cell Biol.*, **57,** 88–108.

Tischler, A. S., DeLellis, R. A., Biales, B., Nunnemacher, G., Carabba, V., and Wolfe, H. J. (1980). Nerve growth factor-induced neurite outgrowth from normal human chromaffin cells. *Lab. Invest.*, **43,** 399–409.

Trifaró, J. M., and Lee, R. W. H. (1980). Morphological characteristics and stimulus-secretion coupling in bovine adrenal chromaffin cell cultures. *Neuroscience*, **5,** 1533–1546.

Unsicker, K., and Chamley, J. H. (1976). Effects of dbcAMP and theophylline on rat adrenal medulla grown in tissue culture. *Histochemie.*, **46,** 97–201.

Unsicker, K., and Chamley, J. H. (1977). Growth characteristics of postnatal rat adrenal medulla in culture. *Cell Tissue Res.*, **177,** 247–268.

Unsicker, K. and Hofmann, H. D. (1981). Bovine chromaffin cells in culture: Changes in phenotype induced by organ extracts, elevated potassium and serum withdrawal, but not by nerve growth factor. *Soc. Neurosci. Abstr.*, **7,** 211.

Unsicker, K., and Ziegler, W. (1981). Spontaneous and nerve growth factor induced axon outgrowth from rat and bovine adrenal chromaffin cells in culture. *Soc. Neurosci, Abstr.*, **6,** 336.

Unsicker, K., Chamley, J. H., and Burnstock, G. (1977). Studies on the interactions between nerve fibres from para- and orthosympathetic ganglia and adreno-cortical and -medullary cells in joint culture. *Cell Tissue Res.*, **178,** 533–549.

Unsicker, K., Habura-Flueh, O., Zwarg, U., Tschechne, B., and Tschechne, D. (1978a). *Interactions Between Autonomic Nerves and Adrenal Chromaffin Cells in Culture and in Two In Vivo Transplant Systems*, In: Peripheral Neuroendocrine Interaction (R. E. Coupland and W. G. Forsmann, eds) pp. 60–69, Springer, Berlin.

Unsicker, K., Krisch, B., Otten, U., and Thoenen, H. (1978b). Nerve growth factor-induced fiber outgrowth from isolated rat adrenal chromaffin cells: Impairment by glucocorticoids. *Proc. Natl. Acad. Sci. U.S.A.*, **75,** 3498–3502.

Unsicker, K., Griesser, G. H., Lindmar, R., Löffelholz, K., and Wolf, U. (1980a). Establishment, characterization and fibre outgrowth of isolated bovine adrenal medullary cells in long-term cultures. *Neuroscience*, **5**, 1445–1460.

Unsicker, K., Rieffert, B., and Ziegler, W. (1980b). Effects of cell culture conditions. nerve growth factor, dexamethasone, and cyclic AMP on adrenal chromaffin cells *in vitro*. In: Histochemistry and Cell Biology of Autonomic Neurons, SIF Cells and Paraneurons (O. Tränkö, S. Soinila, H. Päivärinta, eds) pp. 51–59, Raven Press, New York.

Viveros, O. H., Diliberto, E. J., Jr., Hazum, E., and Chang, K. J. (1979). Opiate-like materials in the adrenal medulla: Evidence for storage and secretion with catecholamines. *Mol. Pharmacol.*, **16**, 1101–1108.

Wakshull, E., Johnson, M. I., and Burton, H. (1978). Persistence of an amine uptake system in cultured rat sympathetic neurons which use acetylcholine as their transmitter. *J. Cell Biol.*, **79**, 121–131.

Wakshull, E., Johnson, M. I., and Burton, H. (1979a). Postnatal rat sympathetic neurons in culture. I. A comparison with embryonic neurons. *J. Neurophysiol.*, **42**, 1410–1425.

Wakshull, E., Johnson, M. I., and Burton, H. (1979b). Postnatal rat sympathetic neurons in culture. II. Synaptic transmission by postnatal neurons. *J. Neurophysiol.*, **42**, 1426–1436.

Waymire, J. C., Waymire, K. G., Boehme, R., Noritake, D., and Wardell, J. (1977). Regulation of tyrosine hydroxylase by cyclic $3':5'$-adenosine monophosphate in cultured neuroblastoma and cultured dissociated bovine adrenal chromaffin cells. In *Structure and Function of Monoamine Enzymes*, pp. 327–363, Marcel Dekker, New York.

Webb, J. G., Berv, K. R., and Kopin, I. J. (1975). Induction of dopamine β-hydroxylase in superior cervical ganglia in organ culture. *Neuropharmacology*, **14**, 643–648.

Wechsler, W., and Schmekel, L. (1966). Elektronenmikroskopischer Nachweis spezifischer Grana in den Sympathicoblasten der Grenzstrangganglien von Hühnerembryonen. *Experientia*, **22**, 296–297.

Wilson, S. P., Abou-Donia, M. M., Chang, K. J., and Viveros, O. H. (1981). Reserpine increases opiate-like peptide content and tyrosine hydroxylase activity in adrenal medullary chromaffin cells in culture. *Neuroscience*, **6**, 71–79.

Wurtman, R. J., Pohorecky, L. A., and Baliga, B. S. (1972). Adrenocortical control of the biosynthesis of epinephrine and proteins in the adrenal medulla. *Pharmacol. Rev.*, **24**, 411–426.

Ziegler, W., and Unsicker, K. (1981). Differential effects of cyclic AMP and cholera toxin on nerve growth factor-induced neurite outgrowth from adrenal medullary chromaffin and pheochromocytoma cells. *Dev. Brain Res.*, **1**, 1–6.

Ziegler, W., Otten, U., and Unsicker, K. (1980). Possible involvement of non-adrenal cells in spontaneous axon outgrowth of chromaffin cells. *Eur. J. Cell Biol.*, **22**, 408.

NOTE

The final version of this article was submitted in July 1981. It is impossible to incorporate at this stage (January 1983) the vast literature which has contributed to this dramatically expanding field since then.

Autonomic Ganglia
Edited by Lars-Gösta Elfvin
© 1983 John Wiley & Sons Ltd

Adrenergic Nerve Growth Regulation: Nerve Fibre Formation by the Superior Cervical Ganglion, the Adrenal Medulla, and Locus Coeruleus—Similarities and Differences as Revealed by Grafting

LARS OLSON and ÅKE SEIGER

Department of Histology, Karolinska Institutet,
Box 60 400, S-104 01 Stockholm, Sweden

INTRODUCTION

The superior cervical ganglion (SCG), the adrenal medulla (AM) and locus coeruleus (LC) may be taken as typical representatives of the three principal classes of catecholamine-synthesizing cell systems in the body, namely peripheral postganglionic sympathetic neurons, chromaffin cells, and central adrenergic neurons, respectively. Although different in many respects they have certain common features. All three are dense aggregations of cells, permitting them to receive coherent afferent innervation. All three have remarkably widespread and diffuse target areas: SCG the entire head region except the brain, AM all catecholamine-sensitive tissues outside the blood–brain barrier, LC almost the entire brain and spinal cord. Thus, the functional responses mediated by these systems show a high degree of divergence. The fact that chromaffin cells form nervous processes under certain experimental conditions (Olson, 1970) makes it possible to add to the list of common features of the three cell groups also the ability to form nerve fibres.

In the following we will review factors that influence nerve fibre formation by SCG, LC and AM (cf. also Olson *et al.*, 1980a 1981a). In particular, we will evaluate the importance of the local environment for the differences in appearance by reviewing transplantation experiments in which the three cell groups have been placed in the same environment and systematically exposed to the same peripheral and central target tissues. In addition, the role of nerve growth factor (NGF) will be discussed.

INTRAOCULAR GRAFTING OF SUPERIOR CERVICAL GANGLION, LOCUS COERULEUS AND ADRENAL MEDULLA

Intraocular grafting in rodents is a useful tool in studies of nerve growth (see Olson *et al.*, 1983). It is rapid and simple and causes minimal harm to the host animal. It provides the investigator with a graft that can be visually inspected postoperatively and, at least in the case of monoamine neurons, a two-dimensional network of nerve fibres in the host iris that can be quantitatively studied in whole-mount preparations (Fig. 1). This is of particular value in studies of SCG and LC nerve fibre production, because it is virtually impossible to quantitate total nerve fibre production by these nerve cell groups *in situ*. The results are summarized in Fig. 2.

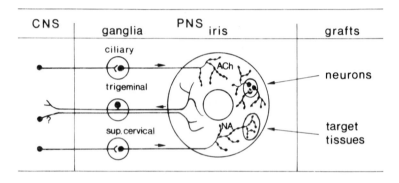

Figure 1   Schematic illustration of the iris innervation and the intraocular grafting experiments. The iris is innervated by three sets of nerves, each of which can be removed by lesioning of the corresponding input. Two types of grafts can be used: if tissues containing nerve cell bodies are grafted, outgrowth from these neurons may occur as a two-dimensional plexus on the host iris, in which case interaction between such fibres and iris innervation can be studied. When tissues that do not contain nerve cell bodies are grafted, they might become innervated by nerves formed by collateralization from the existing networks of the host iris. It is also possible to graft both neurons and target tissues, to study local interaction between grafts. CNS = central nervous system; PNS = peripheral nervous system; sup. = superior. From Olson *et al.* (1981); reproduced by permission of Pitman Books Limited

SCG grafts

When an adult SCG (decapsulated and divided) is grafted to a sympathetically denervated rat eye, it will effectively reinnervate the entire host iris in an organotypical fashion within a month (Fig. 3; Olson and Malmfors, 1970). If the sympathetic innervation of the host iris is left intact the same ganglion will survive and form a limited number of non-terminal axon bundles, but almost no varicose nerve terminals (i.e. no adrenergic ground plexus) will form.

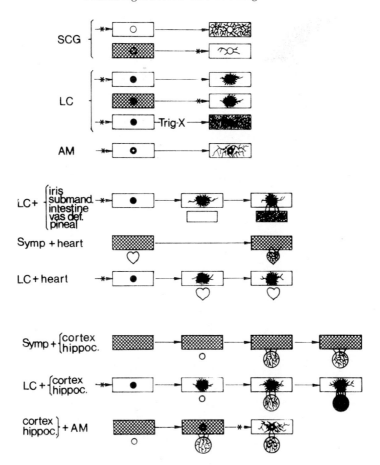

Figure 2 Summary of the main results. In all diagrams, host irides are depicted as large rectangles, and the presence of a normal sympathetic nerve plexus on the host irides indicated by a raster. Time flows from left to right as indicated by arrows. Removal of the sympathetic nerve plexus in the host iris is performed at various stages of the experiments and is indicated by an asterisk. Open circles on host irides: grafts of SCG. Filled circles: grafts of the developing LC. Filled circles with white centre grafts of AM. All drawings demonstrate the amount and distribution of catecholamine-containing nerve fibres as seen in whole mounts of irides and in freeze-dried sections of other types of grafts with Falck-Hillarp fluorescence histochemistry. From Olson *et al.* (1980a); reproduced from *Advances in Biochemical Psychopharmacology*, Vol. 25, by permission of Raven Press, New York

There seems to be little or no specificity between different sympathetic ganglia toward different target areas, since several other sympathetic ganglia than the SCG itself, when grafted to the eye chamber are also able to reinnervate a sympathetically denervated host iris (Olson and Malmfors,

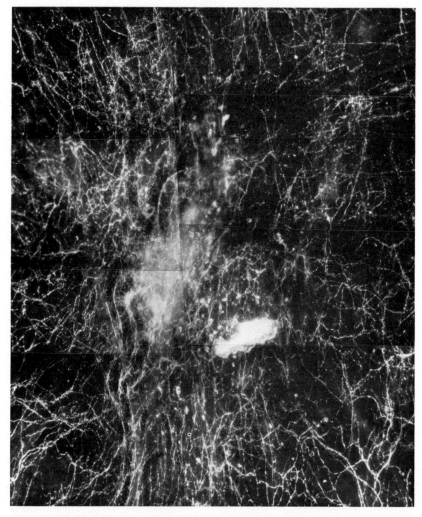

Figure 3 Outgrowth of sympathetic adrenergic nerves from SCG graft into a sympathetically denervated host iris. The site of attachment of the graft (which has been removed) is in the centre. Fluorescence microscopy photomontage of iris whole mount 6 weeks after grafting. ×90

1970). Even heterologous grafts (e.g. human SCG to rat eye) are able to form nerve fibres in the host iris although eventually rejection will take place (Olson and Malmfors, 1970). Interestingly, when fetal SCG are grafted, only a few adrenergic nerve cells, enough for complete innervation of the host iris, will survive. A considerably larger proportion of the grafted nerve cells will remain viable after grafting an adult SCG, suggesting that the immature ganglion is able to down-regulate the number of surviving nerve cells in response to the limited peripheral field provided by the iris. There is no evidence at present that nerve fibres from an intraocular SCG transplant are able to innervate structures outside the eye ball.

Recent studies have shown that fibre production from SCG grafted to eyes carrying a graft of the trigeminal ganglion is inhibited, particularly in areas innervated by the trigeminal ganglion graft (Seiger *et al.*, 1982). Perhaps this is an example of competition for available growth-stimulating factors such as NGF.

LC grafts

While SCG and AM grafts contain relatively homogeneous cell populations, LC grafts prepared from fetal brain tissue always contain also non-adrenergic neurons surrounding nucleus locus coeruleus. Using Falck-Hillarp histochemistry one is able to study selectively outgrowth of adrenergic nerve fibres from such grafts. It is possible, however, that the fibre growth responses of the locus coeruleus neurons to be described below are not only a result of interaction between these neurons and the various target tissues but that they are also influenced by other neuronal or glial components of the brain tissue graft. In marked contrast to SCG grafts, an LC graft, which in order to survive well must be taken from a fetus or a young postnatal animal, will only form a restricted halo of nerve fibres centred around the graft and covering no more than a third of the iris (Olson and Seiger, 1972; Seiger and Olson, 1977c). The formation of this halo also takes approximately a month (Fig. 4). Interestingly, this outgrowth of central adrenergic nerve fibres into a

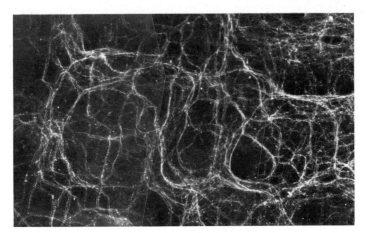

Figure 4   Outgrowth of adrenergic nerve fibres from a LC graft into a sympathetically denervated host iris. A network of varicose nerve fibres is seen in this field from the outer zone of innervation from the graft. Fluorescence microphotograph. ×90

peripheral environment is completely unaffected by the presence or absence of peripheral adrenergic nerves in the target tissue (Seiger and Olson, 1977a). Thus, although able partially to invade a peripheral environment, the growing LC-derived neurites do not seem to respond to sympathetic denervation. Parasympathetic cholinergic denervation of the host iris, by removal of the ciliary ganglion, is likewise without effect on amount or distribution of adrenergic fibre growth from an LC graft (Seiger and Olson, 1977a). Upon invading the iris tissue, the nerve fibres from the LC graft appear to change their morphology to become similar to the normally present SCG-derived sympathetic fibres. These changes include larger, more ovoid varicosities and clearly visible intervaricose parts. Bundles of axons from an LC graft seem to follow pre-existing circularly running axon bundles in the host iris. The important constituent of such axon bundles providing axon guidance (Weiss, 1941) for the growing LC fibres may be the sensory nerves. This is suggested by the marked directional influence that axon bundles formed from intraocular grafts of the trigeminal ganglion exert on growing axons from a subsequently grafted LC. In this case, LC fibres, reaching the area of outgrowth from the trigeminal ganglion, strictly follow the course of fibre bundles radiating out into the iris from neurons in the ganglion graft. In addition to axon guidance, this phenomenon seems to involve attraction of LC fibres by trigeminal fibre bundles (Seiger, 1980).

LC is not unique among central monoamine neurons in its ability to survive intraocular grafting and partially innervate the host iris. Principally the same result is observed with dopamine neurons in substantia nigra grafts and with 5-hydroxytryptamine neurons in grafts of the raphé nuclei (Olson and Seiger, 1972).

AM grafts

When pieces of the adult rat adrenal medulla are grafted to a sympathetically denervated host eye, nerve fibres will grow out from the grafts to innervate the iris (Fig. 5). The most interesting feature of this nerve fibre formation is the transformation of chromaffin cells into fibre-forming elements (Olson, 1970, see also Olson *et al.*, 1981b). The ability of chromaffin cells to form nerve fibres has been demonstrated for several species including man using grafting and tissue culture techniques (Olson *et al.*, 1981b; Unsicker *et al.*, 1980b; Tischler and Greene, 1980). In the following, the basic features of this phenomenon, as seen after intraocular grafting in rats, will be described.

Chromaffin cells will become elongated or polygonal, and some of them will migrate out into the host iris. The cell bodies and the most proximal parts of their newly formed processes show a typical chromaffin appearance in Falck-Hillarp fluorescence microscopy, with an extremely intense or rela-

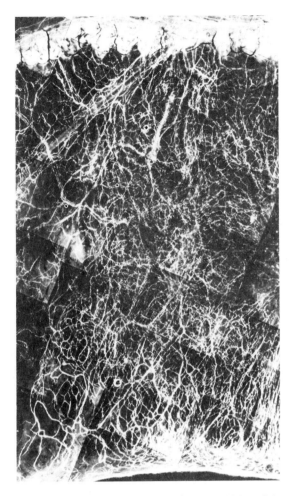

Figure 5 Outgrowth of adrenergic nerve fibres from an AM graft into a sympatheti-cally denervated host iris. From the area of attachment of the graft (right margin) a plexus of nerve terminals has formed that is very similar to the normally present sympathetic ground plexus. Corpus ciliare at top, sphincter margin at bottom. Fluorescence microphotomontage. ×40

tively intense fluorescence typical of noradrenaline and adrenaline cells, respectively. The proximal parts of the cellular processes are thick and irregularly bulgy. At longer distances from the cell bodies, however, many processes become indistinguishable from normal sympathetic nerve fibres. There is a marked tendency for AM-derived fibres to grow radially to the ciliary body and circularly within the ciliary body. From there, fibres re-enter the dilator plate at several points to reinnervate the iris proper. In optimal cases the end-result is complete adrenergic reinnervation of the host iris. There is, however, often a peculiar sparing of the sphincter region.

One problem in interpreting the results of AM grafting is the ganglion cells in the rat AM. Apparently, at least two cell types give rise to nerve fibres in AM grafts. Using multiple very small grafts to the iris it was found that only some grafts were surrounded by large plexuses of completely sympathetic-like fibres. These plexuses seemed to originate from large, polygonal, weakly fluorescent neuron-like cells. Other grafts contained only chromaffin-type cells. Of these grafts some had processes, others had not.

It is possible that a majority of the sympathetic-like fibres may originate from a minority of ganglion-like cells, while some of the sympathetic-like fibres and most of the coarse strongly fluorescent fibres originate from partly transformed chromaffin cells and that some chromaffin cells do not form fibres. It should be noted, however, that cells intermediate in character between chromaffin cells and ganglion cells (e.g. having a ganglion cell-like soma and chromaffin-like processes) are sometimes found. Thus, the relationship of the ganglion cells normally found in AM to the formation of fibres by AM grafts is at present somewhat unclear (Olson et al., 1981b).

The chromaffin granules can also be studied in iris whole-mounts prepared for Falck-Hillarp fluorescence histochemistry. Granules released to the vascular bed of the host iris, as well as granules in cell bodies and coarse processes, have been demonstrated.

The amount of nerve fibres formed by AM grafts is reduced if adrenal cortical tissue is included with the graft (Table 1; Olson *et al.*, 1980b). This is in line with the notion that chromaffin cells are driven towards an endocrine phenotype (adrenaline, no nerve fibres) by glucocorticoids. Conversely, NGF and absence of glucocorticoids drive the cells towards a neuronal phenotype (noradrenaline, nerve fibres). Thus, early NGF treatment *in vivo* converts chromaffin cells completely into sympathetic neurons (Levi-Montalcini and Aloe, 1980). Nerve fibre formation by neoplastic and normal chromaffin cells and the effects of glucocorticoids and NGF have also been demonstrated in tissue culture (Greene and Tischler, 1976; Unsicker and Chamley, 1977; Unsicker *et al.*, 1980a, b; Tischler and Greene, 1980).

ADDITION OF PERIPHERAL TISSUE GRAFTS TO SUPERIOR CERVICAL GANGLION, LOCUS COERULEUS OR ADRENAL MEDULLA *IN OCULO*

Double sequential grafting provides an opportunity to challenge the different grafted neuronal populations with potential target areas in a controlled manner. In all cases of double grafting to be described below, the first graft is an LC or AM graft. The second 'test' graft is introduced a month later and brought into contact with the first graft to study any possible

Table 1 Correlations between the medulla/cortex proportions in adrenal grafts and degree of innervation of central nervous system target region and host iris[a]

Case	Tissue components in adrenal graft		Amount of nerves formed by an adrenal graft in:	
	Medulla	Cortex	Cerebral cortex graft	Host iris
1	No graft		−	−
2	No graft		−	−
3	−	+++	−	−
4	−	+++	−	−
5	(+)	+++	−	−
6	(+)	+++	−	−
7	++	−	+++	−
8	++	(+)	+++	+++
9	++	++	+++	+++
		(Isolated)[b]		

[a] Amounts of medullary and cortical tissue in the adrenal grafts as well as the amounts of fluorescent nerves found in the cerebral cortex grafts and host irides in each case were estimated in the microscope using a scale from 0 (−) to 3 (+++). In cases 1 and 2, no adrenal tissue was grafted.

[b] In case 9, the adrenal cortical tissue was present as an isolated graft on the host iris several millimetres from the adrenal medullary graft. The isolated adrenal cortical graft was caused by fragmentation at grafting. The adrenal medullary tissue was fused with the central nervous system graft. From Olson *et al.* (1980b) by permission of Academic Press.

ingrowth of nerve fibres from the first graft. Obviously, since SCG-derived nerve fibres are normally present in the iris, ingrowth of such fibres into target tissues can be studied directly in single-graft experiments.

SCG + peripheral target

A wide range of muscular and glandular tissues, including irides and pieces from almost all organs in the digestive, urogenital, circulatory and endocrine systems grafted to the eye chamber, permit the following general conclusions: Sympathetic nerves of the host iris will branch to innervate all peripheral tissue grafts in an organotypical manner. Normally non-innervated tissues will remain non-innervated. In all cases where it has been tested (intestinal smooth muscle, portal vein, vas deferens: Olson and Malmfors, 1970; pineal gland: Bäckström *et al.*, 1976; heart: Olson and Seiger, 1976) the innervation leads to normally functioning noradrenergic neurotransmission between host nerves and grafted target tissue. A particularly illustrative example is provided by intraocular heart grafts. Such miniature hearts develop *in oculo* from grafts of the early embryonic heart anlage and become innervated by sympathetic and parasympathetic nerves from the host iris. They will exhibit rhythmic contractions with a frequency that becomes dependent upon the light influx to the host eye, since the heart grafts are now innervated by the same set of nerves that mediates the pupillary reflex (Fig. 6; Olson and Seiger, 1976).

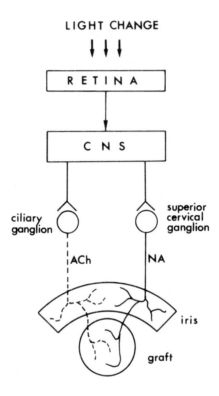

Figure 6 Schematic illustration of the use of the light reflex to activate specifically adrenergic and cholinergic pathways to intraocular grafts.

LC + peripheral targets

Adding an iris graft to an LC-carrying eye proved to be a key experiment in delineating differences in growth responses between SCG and LC (Seiger and Olson, 1977b). An iris graft promptly reinitiates fibre growth in LC neurons that have come to a rest intraocularly after having formed a halo of nerve fibres in the host iris. The iris graft will rapidly become completely innervated by LC fibres while the host iris remains only partially innervated. An iris graft becomes completely denervated by the grafting procedure. Since presence or absence of autonomic nerves, as discussed above, makes no difference for the outgrowth of LC nerves on an host iris, the sensory innervation provided by the trigeminal ganglion was next removed by stereotaxically lesioning the ophthalmomaxillary branch of the trigeminal nerve. Interestingly enough, this caused a rapid spreading of LC nerve fibres on the entire host iris (Olson *et al.*, 1978). The somewhat unexpected strong interaction between LC and fibres from the trigeminal ganglion can thus be summarized as both a guidance of LC fibre bundles by trigeminal ganglion-derived fibre bundles and an inhibition of terminal proliferation by LC in the presence of an intact trigeminal ganglion-derived innervation.

LC grafts have also been challenged with a series of other muscular, glandular and endocrine target tissue grafts (Seiger and Olson, 1978). In most cases, LC nerves are able to innervate these peripheral target tissues in a manner similar to the normal peripheral sympathetic innervation of the target grafts. A notable exception is heart tissue, which will not become innervated by LC. Hence, LC and SCG differ in this respect.

AM + peripheral targets

So far, only iris grafts have been added to AM-carrying eyes. Such iris grafts become effectively innervated by nerve fibres from the AM grafts.

ADDITION OF CENTRAL NERVOUS SYSTEM TISSUE GRAFTS TO SUPERIOR CERVICAL GANGLION, LOCUS COERULEUS OR ADRENAL MEDULLA *IN OCULO*

As described above, central LC-derived nerves are able to innervate peripheral tissues. The following experiments were designed to test if the reverse would also be true. In other words, can peripheral adrenergic nerves innervate brain tissue?

SCG + central targets

In most of these experiments ingrowth of sympathetic nerves from host iris into central nervous system targets was tested. Such ingrowth of peripheral sympathetic nerves can be demonstrated in brain cortices such as cerebellar cortex and parietal cerebral cortex, as well as into hippocampal and dentate gyri respectively (Hoffer *et al.*, 1975; Seiger and Olson, 1975; Freedman *et al.*, 1979; Goldowitz *et al.*, 1982). Ingrowing sympathetic nerves become morphologically similar to the normally present but now absent LC-derived fibres in these areas. In the two instances where it has been tested electrophysiologically (cerebellar grafts: Hoffer *et al.*, 1975; hippocampal grafts: Freedman *et al.*, 1979), the peripheral sympathetic nerves establish normal functional connections with the brain targets. In addition to sympathetic nerves, ingrowth of parasympathetic nerves into grafts of the hippocampal formation has been demonstrated (Freedman *et al.*, 1979). The ability of SCG to innervate cortex has also been demonstrated in double-graft design where adult or immature SCG and cortex were placed in contact in sympathecto-mized host eyes. Some SCG cells in this case became fully incorporated within the brain tissue graft (Seiger and Olson, 1975).

SCG does not, however, seem to be able to substitute for LC in all areas of the central nervous system. Thus, spinal cord grafts and grafts of the caudate nucleus do not become innervated to any appreciable degree by adrenergic nerves from the host iris (Olson *et al.*, 1979b, and unpublished observations).

LC + central targets

There is a rapid and initially organotypical innervation by LC of most central target areas placed in contact with a LC graft in the eye chamber. Thus, for example, coeruleocortical and coeruleohippocampal pathways can be made (Olson *et al.*, 1979b). In contrast to SCG, however, LC fibres will continue to invade the cortical target grafts until sometimes an extreme degree of hyperinnervation is reached (Olson *et al.*, 1980c). It has been shown that such hyperinnervation also results in adrenergic hyperfunction (Taylor *et al.*, 1980). It is possible that central adrenergic nerves growing into a central target area respond by fibre proliferation to the presumably large number of vacant synaptic sites present in a cortex graft, while peripheral adrenergic nerves in the same situation only recognize a limited proportion of such sites, perhaps only the adrenergic ones. Whatever the explanation may be, the above is yet another example of different responses by SCG and LC.

For reasons unknown, LC fibres are only capable of a very limited ingrowth into spinal cord grafts although spinal cord is a normal target for LC (Olson *et al.*, 1982).

AM + central targets

Grafts of the adrenal medulla are able to innervate later added grafts of parietal cerebral cortex (Fig. 7) as well as grafts of the hippocampal formation. The innervation will become similar to the innervation of those areas provided by peripheral adrenergic nerves although possibly somewhat more extensive. In addition, a subpopulation of thicker more chromaffin-like nerve fibres will be found throughout such cortical target grafts, particularly in relation to blood vessels (Olson *et al.*, 1980b). It was also shown that chromaffin tissue grafts are able to innervate grafts of cortex or hippocampus after intraocular maturation of the cortical targets by doing the double-grafting experiments in reverse order.

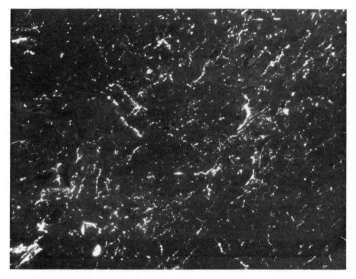

Figure 7 Section through an intraocular graft of cortex cerebri which has been innervated by an adjacent graft of AM. Fine (central nervous system-type), and coarse varicose nerve terminals are seen throughout the central nervous system graft. Fluorescence microphotograph. ×90

CONCLUDING REMARKS ON NERVE GROWTH REGULATION

The above experiments illustrate how the iris, its innervation apparatus, and intraocular grafting can be used to study nerve growth. We have discussed fibre growth responses by the superior cervical ganglion, the ciliary ganglion, and the trigeminal ganglion, as well as by grafts of adrenal medullary tissue, and central adrenergic neurons. A key issue in these experiments is under which conditions NGF and/or other chemical factors that influence nerve growth are present in the intraocular system and which of the above neuron types that are sensitive to such factors. One important difference between central and peripheral adrenergic neurons seems to be that central adrenergic neurons are not sensitive to NGF. Tissue culture experiments reveal that LC neurons are not stimulated by the presence of NGF, do not need NGF for fibre production, are not inhibited by antiserum against NGF and do not make NGF. Similarly, explants of immature cerebral cortex are unresponsive to NGF and its antiserum (Olson *et al.*, 1979a). The lack of NGF sensitivity may explain why LC is unable to innervate the host iris completely. Using an *in vitro* bioassay for NGFs employing chick sympathetic, ciliary and spinal ganglia, it was shown that the rat iris produces NGF in response to a sensory and/or sympathetic denervation (Ebendal *et al.*,

1980). As an iris graft becomes reinnervated from the host iris, the levels of NGF drop. The experiments also revealed the presence of a growth factor for cholinergic nerves that was released from freeze-killed iris tissue (Ebendal *et al.*, 1980). The appearance of NGF in a denervated host iris explains the extensive innervation of such irides by grafts of NGF-sensitive neurons such as SCG or by grafts of AM, and further explains the limited fibre growth by these structures on sympathetically innervated host irides. The lack of, or low levels of, NGF in central nervous system tissue may explain why AM tissue grafted to the brain produces far fewer nerve fibres (Freed *et al.*, 1981) than AM tissue combined with brain tissue in the eye chamber (Olson *et al.*, 1980b).

We conclude that SCG, LC and AM are highly plastic catecholamine-producing cell systems, all able to respond to a changing environment by nerve fibre production also in adulthood. Although able to substitute for each other in several situations, LC fibre growth is regulated by factors that differ from factors regulating NGF-sensitive tissues such as SCG and AM.

ACKNOWLEDGEMENTS

Work described in the chapter was supported by the Swedish Medical Research Council (14P-5867, 14X-03185, 25P-6326, 1YX-06555), the Magnus Bergvall Foundation, and funds from the Karolinska Institutet.

REFERENCES

Bäckström, M., Olson, L., and Seiger, Å. (1976). *N*-Acetyltransferase and hydroxyin-dole-*O*-methyltransferase activity in intraocular pineal transplants: Diurnal rhythm as evidence for a functional sympathetic adrenergic innervation. *Acta Physiol. Scand.*, **96**, 64–71.

Ebendal, T., Olson, L., Seiger, Å., and Hedlund, K.-O. (1980). Nerve growth factors in the rat iris. *Nature*, **286**, 25–28.

Freed, W. J., Morihisa, J. M., Spoor, E., Hoffer, B. J., Olson, L., Seiger, Å., and Wyatt, R. J. (1981). Transplanted adrenal chromaffin cells in rat brain reduce lesion-induced rotational behavior. *Nature*, **292**, 351–352.

Freedman, R., Taylor, D., Seiger, Å., Olson, L., and Hoffer, B. (1979). Seizures and related epileptiform activity in hippocampus transplanted to the anterior chamber of the eye. Modulation by cholinergic and adrenergic input. *Ann. Neurol.*, **6**, 281–295.

Goldowitz, D., Seiger, Å., and Olson, L. (1982). Anatomy of the isolated area dentata grown in the rat anterior eye chamber. *J. Comp. Neurol.*, **208**, 382–400.

Greene, L. A., and Tischler, A. S. (1976). Establishment of a noradrenergic clonal line of rat adrenal pheochromocytoma cells which respond to nerve growth factor. *Proc. Natl. Acad. Sci. U.S.A.*, **73**, 2424–2428.

Hoffer, B., Olson, L., Seiger, Å., and Bloom, F. (1975). Formation of a functional adrenergic input to intraocular cerebellar grafts: Ingrowth of inhibitory sympathetic fibres. *J. Neurobiol.*, **6**, 565–585.

Levi-Montalcini, R., and Aloe, L. (1980). Tropic, trophic, and transforming effects of nerve growth factor. In *Advances in Biochemical Psychopharmacology*, Vol. 25, *Histochemistry and Cell Biology of Autonomic Neurons, SIF Cells, and Paraneurons* (Eds. O. Eränkö, S. Soinila and H. Päivärinta) *Advances in Biochemical Psychopharmacology*, Vol. 25, pp. 3–13, Raven Press, New York.

Olson, L. (1970). Fluorescence histochemical evidence for axonal growth and secretion from transplanted adrenal medullary tissue. *Histochemie*, **22**, 1–7.

Olson, L., and Malmfors, T. (1970). Growth characteristics of adrenergic nerves in the adult rat. Fluorescence histochemical and ^{3}H-noradrenaline uptake studies using tissue transplantations to the anterior chamber of the eye. *Acta Physiol. Scand. Suppl.*, **348**, 1–112.

Olson, L., and Seiger, Å. (1972). Brain tissue transplanted to the anterior chamber of the eye: I. Fluorescence histochemistry of immature catecholamine and 5-hydroxytryptamine neurons reinnervating the rat iris. *Z. Zellforsch. Mikrosk. Anat.*, **135**, 175–194.

Olson, L., and Seiger, Å. (1976). Beating intraocular hearts: Light-controlled rate by autonomic innervation from host iris. *J. Neurobiol.*, **7**, 193–203.

Olson, L., Seiger, Å., and Ålund, M. (1978). Locus coeruleus fiber growth *in oculo* induced by trigeminotomy. *Med. Biol.*, **56**, 23–27.

Olson, L., Ebendal, T., and Seiger, Å. (1979a). NGF and anti-NGF: Evidence against effects on fiber growth in locus coeruleus from cultures of perinatal CNS tissues. *Dev. Neurosci.*, **2**, 160–176.

Olson, L., Seiger, Å., Hoffer, B., and Taylor, D. (1979b). Isolated catecholaminergic projections from substantia nigra and locus coeruleus to caudate, hippocampus and cerebral cortex formed by intraocular sequential double brain grafts. *Exp. Brain Res.*, **35**, 47–67.

Olson, L., Seiger, Å., Ebendal, T., and Hoffer, B. (1980a). Comparisons of nerve fiber growth from three major catecholamine producing cell systems; Adrenal medulla, superior cervical ganglion and locus coeruleus. In *Histochemistry and Cell Biology of Autonomic Neurons, SIF Cells and Paraneurons* (Eds. O. Eränkö, S. Soinila and H. Päivärinta), *Advances in Biochemical Psychopharmacology*, Vol. 25, pp. 27–34, Raven Press, New York.

Olson, L., Seiger, Å., Freedman, R., and Hoffer, B. (1980b). Chromaffin cells can innervate brain tissue: Evidence from intraocular double grafts. *Exp. Neurol.*, **70**, 414–426.

Olson, L., Seiger, Å., Taylor, D., and Hoffer, B. (1980c). Conditions for adrenergic hyperinnervation in hippocampus. I. Histochemical evidence from intraocular double grafts. *Exp. Brain Res.*, **39**, 277–288.

Olson, L., Björklund, H., Ebendal, T., Hedlund, K-O., and Hoffer, B. (1981a). Factors regulating growth of catecholamine-containing nerves, as revealed by transplantation and explantation studies. In *Development of the Autonomic Nervous System* (Eds. K. Elliott and G. Lawrenson), *Ciba Foundation Symposium 83*, pp. 213–226, Pitman Books Ltd., London.

Olson, L., Björklund, H., Hoffer, B. J., Palmer, M. R., and Seiger, Å. (1982). Spinal cord grafts: an intraocular approach to enigmas of nerve growth regulation. *Brain Res. Bull.*, **9**, 519–537.

Olson, L., Hamberger, B., Hoffer, B., Miller, R., and Seiger, Å. (1981b). Nerve fiber formation by grafted adult adrenal medullary cells. In *Chemical Neurotransmission 75 Years* (Eds. L. Stjärne, H. Lagercrantz, Å. Wennmalm and P. Hedqvist), Academic Press, London, pp. 35–48.

Olson, L., Seiger, Å., and Strömberg, I. (1983). Intraocular transplantation in rodents. A detailed account of the procedure and examples of its use in neurobiology with special reference to brain tissue grafting. In *Advances in Cellular Neurobiology*, (Ed. S. Fedoroff) **4**, pp. 407–442, Academic Press.

Seiger, Å. (1980). Growth interaction between locus coeruleus and trigeminal ganglion after intraocular double grafting. *Med. Biol.*, **58**, 149–157.

Seiger, Å., Johansen, L. E., and Ayer-Le Lievre, C. (1982). Influence of trigeminal sensory nerves on fibre growth from monoamine neurons grafted to the eye. Acta Physiol. Scand., Suppl. 508 p. 56.

Seiger, Å., and Olson, L. (1975). Brain tissue transplanted to the anterior chamber of the eye: 3. Substitution of lacking central noradrenaline input by host iris sympathetic fibers in the isolated cerebral cortex developed *in oculo. Cell Tissue Res.*, **159**, 325–338.

Seiger, Å., and Olson, L. (1977a). Growth of locus coeruleus neurons *in oculo* independent of simultaneously present adrenergic and cholinergic nerves in the iris. *Med. Biol.*, **55**, 209–223.

Seiger, Å., and Olson, L. (1977b). Reinitiation of directed nerve fiber growth in central monoamine neurons after intraocular maturation. *Exp. Brain Res.*, **29**, 15–44.

Seiger, Å., and Olson, L. (1977c). Quantitation of fiber growth in transplanted central monoamine neurons. *Cell Tissue Res.*, **179**, 285–316.

Seiger, Å., and Olson, L. (1978). Innervation of peripheral tissue grafts by locus coeruleus *in oculo*: Only partial correspondence with degree of sympathetic innervation. *Brain Res.*, **139**, 233–247.

Taylor, D., Freedman, R., Seiger, Å., Olson, L., and Hoffer, B. (1980). Conditions for adrenergic hyperinnervation in hippocampus. II. Electrophysiological evidence from intraocular double grafts. *Exp. Brain Res.*, **39**, 289–299.

Tischler, A. S., and Greene, L. A. (1980). Phenotypic plasticity of pheochromocytoma and normal adrenal medullary cells. In *Histochemistry and Cell Biology of Autonomic Neurons, SIF Cells, and Paraneurons* (Eds. O. Eränkö, S. Soinila and H. Päivärinta), *Advances in Biochemical Psychopharmacology*, Vol. 25, pp. 61–68, Raven Press, New York.

Unsicker, K., and Chamley, J. H. (1977). Growth characteristics of postnatal rat adrenal medulla in culture. A study correlating phase contrast, microcinematographic, histochemical and electron microscopical observations. *Cell Tissue Res.*, **177**, 249–268.

Unsicker, K., Griesser, G.-M., Lindmar, R., Löffelholz, K., and Wolf, U. (1980a). Establishment, characterization and fibre outgrowth of isolated bovine adrenal medullary cells in long-term cultures. *Neuroscience*, **5**, 1445–1460.

Unsicker, K., Rieffert, B., and Ziegler, W. (1980b). Effects of cell culture conditions, nerve growth factor, dexamethazone, and cyclic AMP on adrenal chromaffin cells *in vitro*. In *Histochemistry and Cell Biology of Autonomic Neurons, SIF Cells, and Paraneurons* (Eds. O. Eränkö, S. Soinila and H. Päivärinta), *Advances in Biochemical Psychopharmacology*, Vol. 25, pp. 51–59, Raven Press, New York.

Weiss, P. (1941). Nerve patterns: The mechanisms of nerve growth. *Growth Suppl.*, **5**, 163–203.

Index

Accessory cells in cultured sympathetic ganglia, 483
Acetylcholine (ACh), 102, 129, 190, 269, 281, 312, 453, 483
Acetylcholine, binding to nicotinic cholinergic receptors, 270
  muscarinically acting, 281
  nicotinically acting, 281
  receptor-α-BTX-binding site, 271
  release of, 269
Acetylcholinesterase (AChE), 43, 102, 133, 154, 161, 186, 190, 220, 222, 320, 443
Adenosine triphosphatase, 103
Adie's syndrome, 107
Adrenal medulla (AM), 429, 439, 475, 507
Adrenaline (A) Epinephrine (E), 79, 127, 186, 196, 235, 513
Adrenergic fibres in ciliary ganglion, 103
β-Adrenergic receptor adenylate cyclase complex, 240, 253
Agonist β-adrenergic, 253
Alkaline phosphatase, 103
AMP (3′, 5′-adenosine monophosphate), cyclic, 239, 286, 331
Amine-handling neurons in enteric ganglia, 153
Ampullary gland, 128
Angiotensin, 154
APUD (amine precursor uptake and decarboxylation) cells, 67
Atropine, 129, 282, 315
Attachment plaque, 47
Axon hillock, 186, 190

Bethanecol (BCh), 283
Bladder neck, 137
Blood-ganglion barrier, 369
Blood vessels in sympathetic ganglia, 7
Bombesin, 154, 207, 209, 346, 360
Brain cortices, intraocular grafts, 517

Bullfrog, sympathetic ganglia, 186, 309
α-Bungarotoxin (α-BTX), 104, 271, 485

Calcium ions (Ca^{2+}), 332
Cardiac ganglion of Necturus, 389
Carotid body, 13, 481
Catecholamine (histo)fluorescence, 9, 12, 67, 186, 477
Catecholamine(s) (CA), 13, 43, 435, 439, 441, 443, 445, 477, 507
Catechol O-methyltransferase (COMT), 285, 320
Cervix uteri, 132
Chimaera, 429, 437
Cholecystokinin (CCK), 154, 159, 207, 211, 346, 360
Choline acetyltransferase (CAT), 102, 134, 441, 443, 483
Cholinergic motor innervation in vas deferens, 129
Cholinergic nerves in uterus, 134
Cholinesterases, non-specific, 102
Chromaffin cells, 67, 235, 319, 464, 475, 507
Chromaffin granules, 490, 514
Chromaffin reaction, 67, 187
Chromaffin-like cells, 68, 126
Choroidal cells, 99
Ciliary body, 513
Ciliary cells, 99
Clonidine, 289
Coagulating gland, 127
Coexistence, 218, 222
Colchicine, 112
Conditioned medium, 455
Conduction velocities, 266
Convergence, 268
Corticosterone, 490
Crest cells, 433
Cyclic nucleotides, 281, 331
Cytochrome oxidase, 103